D1067850

WILLIAM F. MAAG LIBRARY
YOUNGSTOWN STATE UNIVERSITY

Perspectives in Exercise Science and Sports Medicine
Volume 3: Fluid Homeostasis During Exercise

Edited by

Carl V. Gisolfi, Ph.D.
University of Iowa

David R. Lamb, Ph.D.
The Ohio State University

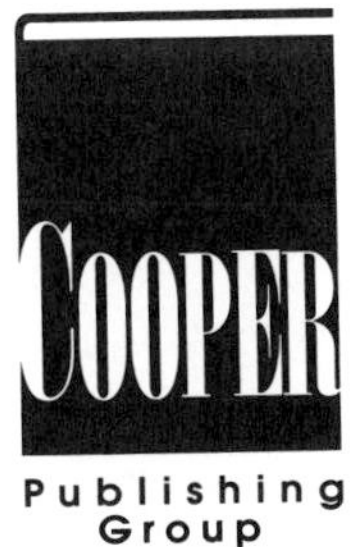

Publishing
Group

Copyright © 1990, by Cooper Publishing Group, LLC

ALL RIGHTS RESERVED.

Reproduction or translation of any part of this work beyond that permitted by Sections 107 and 108 of the 1976 United States Copyright Act without the permission of the copyright owner is unlawful. Requests for permission should be addressed to Publisher, Cooper Publishing Group, LLC., P.O. Box 562, Carmel, IN 46032.

Library of Congress Cataloging in Publication Data:

LAMB, DAVID R., 1939 -

GISOLFI, CARL V., 1942 -

Perspectives In Exercise Science and Sports Medicine
Volume 3: Fluid Homeostasis During Exercise

Library of Congress Catalog Card number: 88-70343

ISBN: 1-884125-07-7

Printed in the United States of America

10 9 8 7 6 5 4 3

The Publisher and Author disclaim responsibility for any adverse effects or consequences from the misapplication or injudicious use of the information contained within this text.

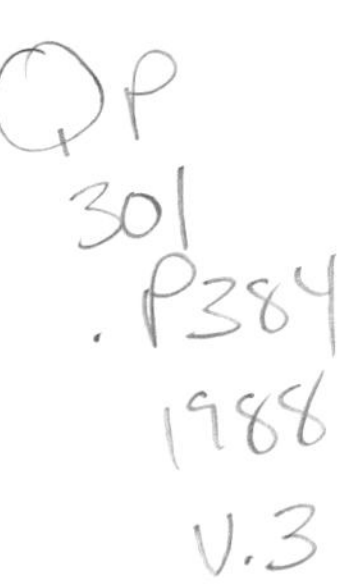
QP 301 .P384 1988 V.3

Contributors

Michael J. Brody, Ph.D.
Department of Pharmacology
2210 Bowen Sciences Building
University of Iowa
Iowa City, IA 52242
(319) 335-7943

Elsworth R. Buskirk, Ph.D.
Human Performance Lab
The Pennsylvania State University
119 Noll Laboratory
University Park, PA 16801
(814) 865-3453

Victor A. Convertino, Ph.D.
Human Performance Lab
Bionetics Corporation
Mail Code BIO-1
Kennedy Space Center, FL
(305) 867-4237

David L. Costill, Ph.D.
Ball State University
Human Performance Laboratory
Muncie, IN 47306
(317) 285-1156

Edward F. Coyle, Ph.D.
Exercise Physiology Laboratory
University of Texas at Austin
Bellmont 222
Austin, TX 78712
(512) 471-8596

J. Mark Davis, Ph.D.
Exercise Biochemistry Laboratory
Blatt Physical Education Center
University of South Carolina
Columbia, SC 29208
(803) 777-6881

Gerald F. DiBona, M.D.
Department of Internal Medicine
University of Iowa College of Medicine
Iowa City, IA 52242
(319) 338-0581

Carl V. Gisolfi, Ph.D.
Department of Exercise Science
The University of Iowa
Field House
Iowa City, IA 52242
(319) 335-9494

John E. Greenleaf, Ph.D.
NASA
Ames Research Center
Moffett Field, CA 94035
(415) 694-6604

Jack Harvey, M.D.
Ft. Collins Orthopaedic Associates P.A.
1227 Riverside
Ft. Collins, CO 80524
(303) 493-0161

Roger W. Hubbard, Ph.D.
Heat Research Division
USARIEM
Kansas Street
Natick, MA 01760
(617) 651-4873

Alan K. Johnson, Ph.D.
Department of Psychology
University of Iowa
E22 Sea Shore Hall
Iowa City, IA 52242
(319) 335-2423

William A. Kachadorian, Ph.D.
USPHS
National Institute of Aging
Bldg. 31, Rm. 5C27
Bethesda, MD 20205
(301) 550-1751

James P. Knockel, M.D.
Department of Internal Medicine
Veterans Administration Hospital
Dallas, TX 75216
(214) 372-7082

WILLIAM F. MAAG LIBRARY
YOUNGSTOWN STATE UNIVERSITY

David R. Lamb
Laboratory of Work Physiology
Ohio State University
337 W. 17th Avenue
Columbus, OH 43210
(614) 292-6887

James H. Meyer, M.D.
Veterans Administration Medical Center
16111 Plummer Street
Bldg. Code 1-11 G
B257 - Bldg. 3
Sepulvda, CA 91343
(818) 891-2496

Ethan R. Nadel, Ph.D.
John B. Pierce Foundation Laboratory
Yale University School of Medicine
290 Congress Avenue
New Haven, CT 06519
(203) 562-9901

M. Ian Phillips, Ph.D.
Department of Physiology
University of Florida
Gainesville, FL 32610
(904) 392-3791

Michael N. Sawka, Ph.D.
Military Ergonomics Division
Kansas Street
USARIEM
Natick, MA 01760
(617) 651-4831

Harold P. Shedl, M.D., Ph.D.
Department of Internal Medicine
University of Iowa College of Medicine
Rm C31G General Hospital
Iowa City, IA 52242
(319) 356-2742

W. Michael Sherman, Ph.D.
Ohio State University
School of HPER, 127 Larkins Hall
337 West 17th Avenue
Columbus, OH 43210
(614) 292-6887

Robert M. Summers, M.D.
Department of Internal Medicine
4426A John Colloton Pavilion
University of Iowa
Iowa City, IA 52242
(319) 356-2130

John R. Sutton, M.D.
Cumberland College of Health Sciences
East Street
P.O. Box 170
Lidcombe, New South Wales
AUSTRALIA, 2141
(02) 646-6444

Charles M. Tipton, Ph.D.
University of Arizona
Department of Exercise & Sport Sciences
108 Gittings Building
Tucson, AZ 85721
(602) 621-6990

Charles E. Wade, Ph.D.
Division of Military Trauma
SGRD-UL-MTR
Letterman Army Institute of Research
Presidio of San Francisco, CA 94129-6800
(415) 561-3385

Mohamed K. Yousef, Ph.D.
Department of Biological Sciences
University of Nevada
Las Vegas, NV 89154
(702) 739-3390

Edward J. Zambraski, Ph.D.
Department of Physiology
Thompson Hall, Rm. 130
Cook College
Rutgers University
New Brunswick, NJ 08903
(201) 932-9428

# *Acknowledgment*

The Quaker Oats Company and The Gatorade Sports Science Institute are proud to have facilitated the publication of this third volume in the series "*Perspectives in Exercise Science and Sports Medicine.*" The symposium on "Fluid Homeostasis During Exercise" and this publication represent the collective deliberations and contributions of many eminent scientists.

We at The Quaker Oats Company and Gatorade Sports Science Institute will continue our support of research and education in exercise science and sports medicine. By working with the scientific community, we hope to make a significant contribution to the science and medicine of exercise and sports.

Michael J. Callahan
Executive Vice President
The Quaker Oats Company

George A. Halaby, Ph.D.
Vice President
Research and Development

Foreword

I am pleased to introduce this third volume of the Quaker Series on sports medicine and exercise science to the scientific community on behalf of the American College of Sports Medicine.

Fluid homeostasis during exercise has been a topic of heated debate by both the exercise science community and medical clinicians in recent years. This subject has important implications for all segments of our society who exercise for performance or health, from elite athletes to octogenarians. Under the aegis of the Quaker Oats Company, a colloquium of international experts on this subject has been convened, and the results of the presentations, and debate, incorporated into the present volume by Drs. Gisolfi and Lamb.

The cooperation between the American College of Sports Medicine and the Quaker Oats Company which has resulted in this series *Perspectives in Exercise Science and Sports Medicine* could well serve as a model for support of our scientific community by American industry as a whole. Always supportive, never intrusive, Quaker Oats has demonstrated a concern for the long-term health issues of Americans which is truly worthy of respect.

Lyle J. Micheli, M.D.
President
American College of Sports Medicine

Preface

The impetus for developing this book was the lack of a synthesized body of knowledge on body fluid homeostasis during exercise and environmental stress. This important area of physiology is either superficially treated or simply not addressed in major textbooks dealing with the physiology of exercise and the environment. Several excellent reviews of limited aspects of this topic are available, but no attempt has been made to consolidate in one volume the physiology of fluid consumption, balance, and control. All of the authors, who are internationally recognized as leaders in their fields, not only provide a state-of-the-art review, but also present an historical perspective that culminates in recommendations for future research.

The volume begins with the physiological consequences of dehydration. This topic has been addressed by others, but Dr. Sawka brings us up to date and includes the effects of hypohydration on exercise performance. Dr. Hubbard explores the reasons for the fact that thirst is an inadequate stimulus to fully restore body water after dehydration. He includes a series of very instructive calculations for both experts and novices in the field.

Although we all recognize the symptoms of dehydration and the need to drink fluids, we rarely consider the crucial role of the gastrointestinal track in fluid homeostasis. Drs. Costill and Gisolfi discuss the important roles of gastric emptying and intestinal absorption, respectively, in achieving rehydration. Next, Dr. Nadel focuses on the recovery process following exercise and emphasizes the importance of sodium concentration in fluid replacement beverages.

The following two chapters deal with the important topic of controlling extracellular fluid volume and composition. Hormonal control is an extremely complex subject, and Dr. Wade does an excellent job of dealing with hormonal interactions in regulating body fluids. We often think of the kidney as an exocrine organ that contributes to the exercise response by tolerating a reduced blood flow; but what about the role of the kidney as an endocrine organ and as an endocrine target organ? Does the kidney actually respond inappropriately to exercise and the stress of fluid imbalance? Dr. Zambraski deals with these important questions.

Fluid homeostasis plays an important role in adapting to environmental stress. In his chapter, Dr. Greenleaf focuses on weightlessness and the importance of fluid balance to the physiological adjustments induced by microgravity. Next, Dr. Johnson discusses what we have learned about afferent signals, central integration, and the generation of efferent responses that govern fluid homeostasis. He synthesizes this vast literature into a logical, cogent, and exciting chapter that addresses the specific areas of the brain and putative neurotransmitters that participate in signal transduction in afferent and efferent pathways. Finally, Dr. Sutton addresses the important clinical implications of fluid imbalance, including the management of exertional heat stroke and the problems associated with overhydration.

The production of this volume is the third in the series PERSPECTIVES IN EXERCISE SCIENCE AND SPORTS MEDICINE. It represents only one of the many contributions that The Quaker Oats Company and Gatorade Thirst Quencher have made to foster exercise science and sports medicine. There are numerous people in the Quaker Oats Company that participated in this endeavor, but George Halaby, Ph.D., and Robert Murray, Ph.D., deserve special recognition. Without their support, ideas, and encouragement this scientific contribution would not have been possible.

We also acknowledge the crucial contribution of Leslie Walcyak and her colleagues at McCord Travel. The conference in Kauai, which served to improve the manuscripts for this book, was such a pleasant experience because Leslie worked behind the scenes to prevent and resolve problems before they became major issues. We also appreciate the efforts of Butch Cooper and Kendal Gladish of Benchmark Press for producing such a high-quality finished product.

Carl V. Gisolfi
David R. Lamb

Contents

1

Effects of Body Water Loss on Physiological Function and Exercise Performance

MICHAEL N. SAWKA, PH.D.

KENT B. PANDOLF, PH.D.

INTRODUCTION

Water is essential for human life, and the depletion of body water will not only adversely influence exercise performance, but more importantly the possible health and safety of the athlete/worker. Water provides the medium for biochemical reactions within cell tissues and is essential for maintaining an adequate blood volume and thereby the integrity of the cardiovascular system. Water is the largest component of the human body, representing about 60% of body weight and about 72% of lean body mass. Because water can be redistributed within the body's fluid-containing spaces, there is a reservoir to minimize the effects of a water deficit.

This chapter addresses the question of the magnitude of body water deficit that adversely affects exercise performance, and the physiological mechanism(s) responsible for the performance decrements. It becomes evident, upon reading this chapter, that the magnitude of performance decrement is related to how the water is lost, the magnitude of water deficit, the fluid-containing space that predominantly sustains the loss, the type of exercise, and the thermal environment to which the individual is exposed. For each combination of exercise and environment, there is a critical water deficit at which the exercise performance will be adversely affected.

Individuals in athletic, occupational, and military settings may have to perform physical exercise while incurring a body water deficit. Generally, the individual dehydrates during exercise because of fluid nonavailability or a mismatch between thirst and body water requirements. In these instances, the individual starts the exercise task as euhydrated but incurs an exercise-heat mediated dehydration over a prolonged period of time. This scenario is common for many athletic and occupational settings; however, in the military setting, particularly combat, the individual will often start the exercise task while already hypohydrated (Draper & Lombardi, 1986). There are also several sports (e.g., boxing, power lifting, wrestling) where the athlete may purposely achieve hypohydration prior to competition (Tipton & Tcheng, 1970; Zambraski, et al., 1976). These athletes desire to compete in a lower weight class to gain a size advantage over their competitors. In these instances, hypohydration might be achieved by a combination of restricted water and food intake, exercise-heat dehydration, and/or the use of diuretics (Caldwell et al., 1984; Strauss et al., 1983). Figure 1-1 provides an illustration of the magnitude and frequency of rapid weight loss in wrestlers during a typical season (Zambraski et al., 1976). Note that a wrestler will often lose 3–4 kg of body weight over a period of several days. Finally, the press have reported that some athletes are using diuretics to help conceal their use of anabolic steroids. If this is true, it is possible that those athletes might also be competing with a body water deficit.

Military personnel were the first to recognize the importance of water on man's ability to perform exercise; major battles have been decided by the availability of water to combatant troops. For example,

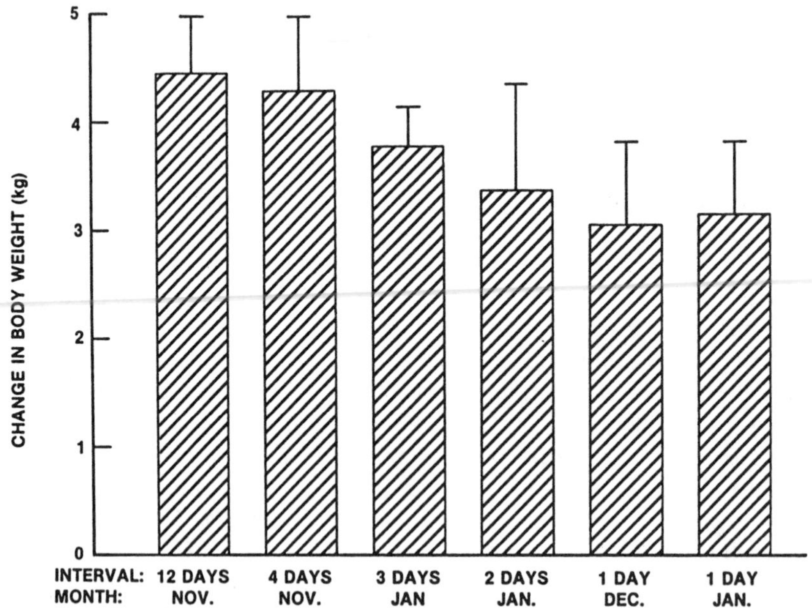

FIGURE 1-1. *Magnitude (+SE) and frequency of rapid weight loss in wrestlers throughout the competitive season (redrawn from Zambraski et al., 1976).*

dehydration-induced heat stroke was believed to be responsible for 20,000 deaths among Egyptian troops during the 1967 Six-Day War with Israel (Hubbard et al., 1982). Recognizing the importance of adequate hydration has resulted in military funding of comprehensive research programs concerning this topic, first at the Harvard Fatigue Laboratory (Horvath & Horvath, 1973), then at the Armored Medical Research Laboratory (Adolph & associates, 1947) and the Quartermaster Research Command, and now at the U.S. Army Research Institute of Environmental Medicine. Research from those institutions has led the military to change its interpretation of the term "water doctrine" from "withholding water for the toughening of troops" to the current "forced drinking."

The genesis of this current viewpoint required the dispelling of several myths concerning the benefits of water deprivation (Knochel, 1975). Unfortunately, myths may persist for some individuals responsible for supervising physical training. For example, during the summer of 1988, Massachusetts State Police recruits were limited access to water during training sessions, and 11 of them (from a class of 50) received serious heat injuries and were hospitalized; two underwent kidney dialysis, and one recruit required a liver transplant and later died (Commonwealth of Massachusetts, 1988).

Throughout this chapter, the term "euhydration" refers to "normal" body water content; whereas, "hypohydration" refers to body water deficit. The more common term "dehydration" denotes the dynamic loss of body water or the transition from euhydration to hypohydration. The term "hypovolemia" defines a steady-state blood volume that is less than normal.

BODY WATER LOSS

Physical exercise can increase total body metabolism by 5–20 times the resting rate to provide energy for skeletal muscle contraction. Depending upon the exercise task, between 70% and 100% of the metabolic rate results in heat and must be dissipated to restore body heat balance. Depending on environmental temperature, the relative contributions of evaporative and dry (radiative and conductive) heat exchange to the total heat loss vary. The hotter the environment the greater the dependence on evaporative heat loss, and thus on sweating (Nielsen, 1938). Therefore, in hot environments, a considerable amount of body water can be lost through eccrine sweat gland secretion to enable the evaporative cooling of the body (Wenger, 1972).

For a given person, sweating rate is dependent on environmental conditions (ambient temperature, dew point temperature, radiant load and air velocity), clothing (insulation and moisture permeability), and physical activity level (Adolph & associates, 1947; Molnar et al., 1946;

Shapiro et al., 1982; Strydom et al., 1966). Adolph and associates (1947) reported that for 91 men studied during diverse military activities in the desert, average sweating rate was 4.1 L every 24 h, but values ranged from 1–11 L every 24 h. During more intense physical exercise, much higher sweating rates can occur. Figure 1-2 provides an approximation of hourly sweating rates and therefore water requirements for runners based upon metabolic rate data from several laboratories and the prediction equation for sweating rates developed by Shapiro et al. (1982). Note that the amount of body fluid loss from sweat can vary greatly, and that sweating rates of $L \cdot h^{-1}$ are very common. The highest sweating rate reported in the literature is 3.7 $L \cdot h^{-1}$, which was measured for Alberto Salazar during the 1984 Olympic Marathon (Armstrong et al., 1986).

During physical exercise in the heat, the principal problem is to closely match the volume of fluid intake to the volume of sweat output. This is a difficult problem to solve because thirst does not provide a good index of body water requirements (Adolph & associates, 1947; Engell et al., 1987). Numerous investigators (Adolph & associates, 1947; Bar-Or et al., 1980; Phillips et al., 1984) report that *ad libitum* water intake results in incomplete water replacement or "voluntary" dehydration during exercise and/or heat exposure (see Chapter 2 for a detailed review). It is not

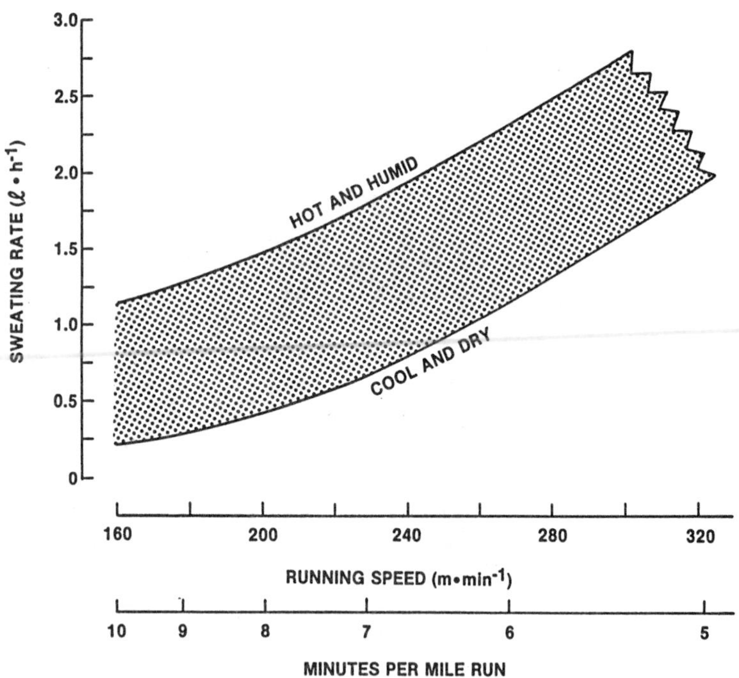

FIGURE 1-2. *An approximation of the hourly sweating rates for runners.*

uncommon for individuals to "voluntarily" dehydrate by 2-8% of their body weight during exercise-heat stress, despite the availability of adequate amounts of fluid to rehydrate (Adolph & associates, 1947; Armstrong et al., 1985b, 1986; Buskirk & Beetham, 1960; Hubbard et al., 1984; Pugh et al., 1967). The flavoring (Hubbard et al., 1984; Morimoto et al., 1981) and cooling (Armstrong, et al. 1985b) of ingested fluid increases its palatability and can help to minimize voluntary dehydration. Heat acclimation status may also influence the voluntary dehydration incurred during exercise in the heat. Although heat acclimation improves the relationship between thirst and body water needs (Eichna et al., 1945; Greenleaf et al., 1983), voluntary dehydration still occurs (Kristal-Boneh et al., 1988).

Thirst is probably not perceived until an individual has incurred a water deficit of ~2% of body weight (Adolph & associates, 1947). As a result, it is likely that unless forced hydration is stressed, some voluntary dehydration will occur during exercise in the heat. Neufer et al. (1989a) recently reported that hypohydration reduces gastric emptying rate of ingested fluids during exercise in the heat. They found an approximate 20-25% reduction in gastric emptying rate when their subjects were hypohydrated (5% body weight); the reduction was related to the increased thermal strain. Therefore, forced hydration during the early stages of exercise-heat stress is important, not only to avoid voluntary dehydration, but to maximize the bioavailability of the ingested fluids.

Sweat loss results in a reduction of total body water if an adequate amount of fluid is not consumed. Total body water constitutes approximately 60% (range 45–70%) of an average adult's body weight. Thus a 75 kg person has a total body water mass of about 45 kg. Therefore, a fluid loss equal to 5% of body weight could constitute 8% of total body water for this person. The question arises as to how water loss is partitioned between the body fluid spaces. As a consequence of free fluid exchange, hypohydration should affect each fluid space.

Figure 1-3 illustrates the findings of two studies on the redistribution of water between fluid spaces when hypohydrated (Sawka, 1988a). Costill et al., (1976) dehydrated subjects by using a combination of cycle ergometer exercise and heat exposure. Shortly after completing cycle ergometer exercise, blood and skeletal muscle samples were obtained from their subjects. Their data may be biased by the cessation of cycle ergometer exercise immediately prior to estimation of water distribution between fluid compartments. Durkot et al., (1986) dehydrated rats by using a passive heat exposure for several (5–11) hours and indicated that their data were slightly biased by the animals' appetite loss. The intent of Figure 1-3 is to present data trends, and not to imply that a given percent decrease of total body water is similar between man and rat. At low volumes of body water loss, the water deficit primarily comes from the

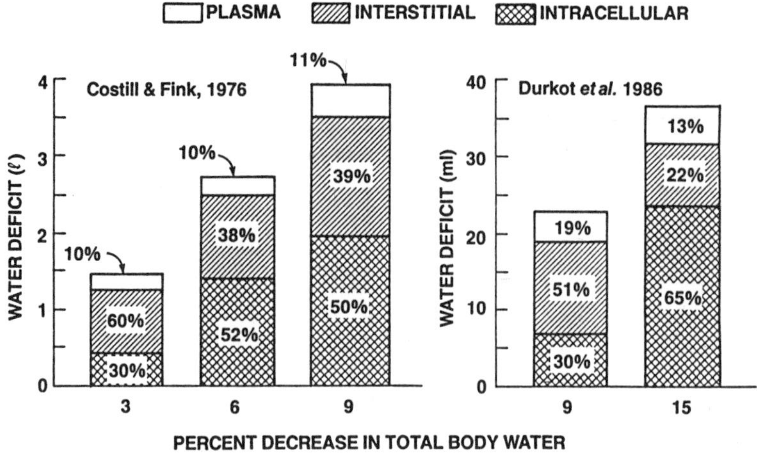

FIGURE 1-3. *The findings of two studies (Costill & Fink, 1976; Durkot et al., 1986) concerning the partitioning of water loss between fluid spaces during resting conditions (Sawka, 1988a).*

extracellular space. As the body water loss increases, a proportionately greater percentage of the water deficit comes from the intracellular space.

Nose and colleagues (1983) attempted to determine the distribution of body water loss not only among the fluid spaces, but also among different body organs. These investigators thermally dehydrated rats by 10% of body weight, and after the animals regained their normal core temperature, body water measurements were obtained. Figure 1-4 presents a summary of their findings. The water deficit was apportioned between the intracellular (41%), and extracellular (59%) spaces. Among the organs, 40% came from muscle, 30% from skin, 14% from viscera, and 14% from bone. Neither the brain nor liver lost significant water content. It was concluded that hypohydration results in water redistribution largely from the intracellular and extracellular spaces of muscle and skin to maintain blood volume. Homeostatic mechanisms seem to be present which defend the water content of organs (e.g., brain, liver) that are necessary to maintain life.

The method used to induce hypohydration may affect the partitioning of the remaining water between the body fluid spaces (Kozlowski and Saltin, 1964). For example, it has been estimated that 3–4 g of water is bound with each gram of glycogen (Olsson & Saltin, 1970), although this exact relationship can be variable (Sherman et al., 1982). Regardless, several papers (Costill et al., 1976, 1981; Costill & Saltin, 1975) have reported a substantial decrease of intracellular water content in skeletal muscle following 1.5–2.5 h of exercise dehydration. These investigators suggest that the loss of intracellular water may be the result of water

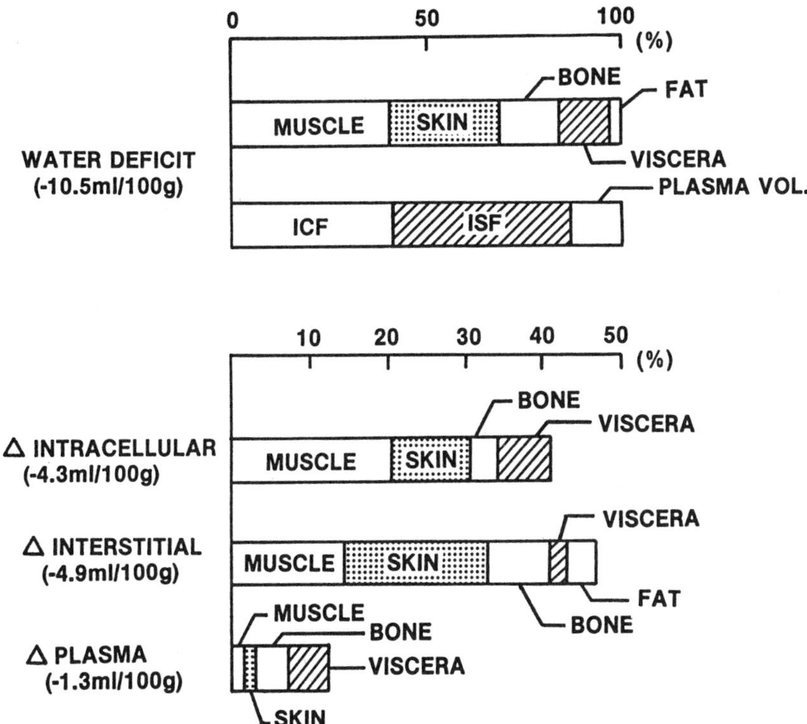

FIGURE 1-4. *Partitioning of water loss between the body fluid spaces and different body organs (redrawn from Nose et al., 1983).*

released with the breakdown of muscle glycogen. As a result, it could be hypothesized that exercise-induced hypohydration would result in a greater intracellular water loss than thermally induced hypohydration. Kozlowski and Saltin (1964) reported that exercise dehydration resulted in greater intracellular water loss than a comparable level of thermal dehydration. Costill and Saltin (1975), however, found no difference between exercise and thermal dehydration for the partitioning of water between the fluid spaces. Therefore, there is no clear evidence that exercise and thermally induced hypohydration caused a difference in the redistribution of water between fluid spaces.

The redistribution of water between the intracellular and extracellular space is dependent upon the osmotic gradient between these spaces. Cell membranes are freely permeable to water but only selectively permeable to various solutes. As a result, transient alterations in solute concentration cause water redistribution across the cell membrane until the two fluid spaces are again of equal osmolality. Therefore, if the methods used to induce hypohydration lead to differences in the intracellular

WILLIAM F. MAAG LIBRARY
YOUNGSTOWN STATE UNIVERSITY

and/or extracellular solute losses, the partitioning of water loss between the fluid spaces will vary accordingly.

It is well known that exercise or heat-induced hypohydration increases plasma osmotic pressure (Senay & Christensen, 1965). Eccrine sweat is hypotonic relative to plasma (Kirby and Convertino, 1986); therefore, the plasma becomes hyperosmotic when hypohydration is induced by sweat output (Sawka, 1988a; Senay, 1979). For resting subjects, plasma osmolality can increase from about 283 mosmol·kg^{-1} when euhydrated to values exceeding 300 mosmol·kg^{-1} when hypohydrated (Figure 1-5). Sodium, potassium, and their principal anion (chloride), are primarily responsible for the elevated plasma osmolality during hypohydration (Kubica et al., 1983; Senay, 1968). As re-emphasized by Nose et al., (1988), it is the plasma hyperosmolality which mobilizes fluid from the intracellular to the extracellular space to enable the defense of the blood (plasma) volume in hypohydrated subjects.

Sodium and chloride are the electrolytes that are principally lost in sweat, and both are primarily found in the extracellular fluid (Sawka, 1988a). The amount of electrolytes that are lost in sweat can be modified by an individual's state of heat acclimation (Allan & Wilson, 1971; Kirby & Convertino, 1986). For example, Kirby and Convertino (1986) reported that over the course of heat acclimation the sweat sodium concentration decreased, so that despite a 12% increase of sweating rate the sweat sodium losses decreased by 59%. Therefore, at a given sweating rate the heat-acclimated individual loses less solute from the plasma. It would seem logical that for a given amount of body fluid loss via sweat, in a heat-acclimated individual, a greater osmotic gradiant (because of lesser electrolyte loss in sweat) would move fluid from the intracellular to the extracellular space. The greater osmotic gradiant should enhance water redistribution and perhaps enable a better defense of blood (plasma) volume in hypohydrated subjects after heat acclimation.

In the early 1930s, investigators from the Harvard Fatigue Laboratory found that for a given loss of body water, via sweating, the blood volume decreased more in winter than in summer (Horvath & Horvath, 1973). This observation was made on one subject who voluntarily dehydrated over an extended period by performing physical exercise in the desert. Figure 1-6 presents recent data (Sawka, 1988a) showing the magnitude of hypovolemia associated with hypohydration of 5% of body weight both before and after a 10-day heat acclimation program. These data represent resting values; hypohydration was achieved by voluntary food and fluid denial combined with exercise in a hot environment. Subjects spent a period of ~15 h resting in a comfortable environment (while hypohydrated) prior to the measurements (Sawka et al., 1983). An identical program of exercise-heat stress, but with full fluid replacement, was completed on the day prior to the euhydration measurements (dotted

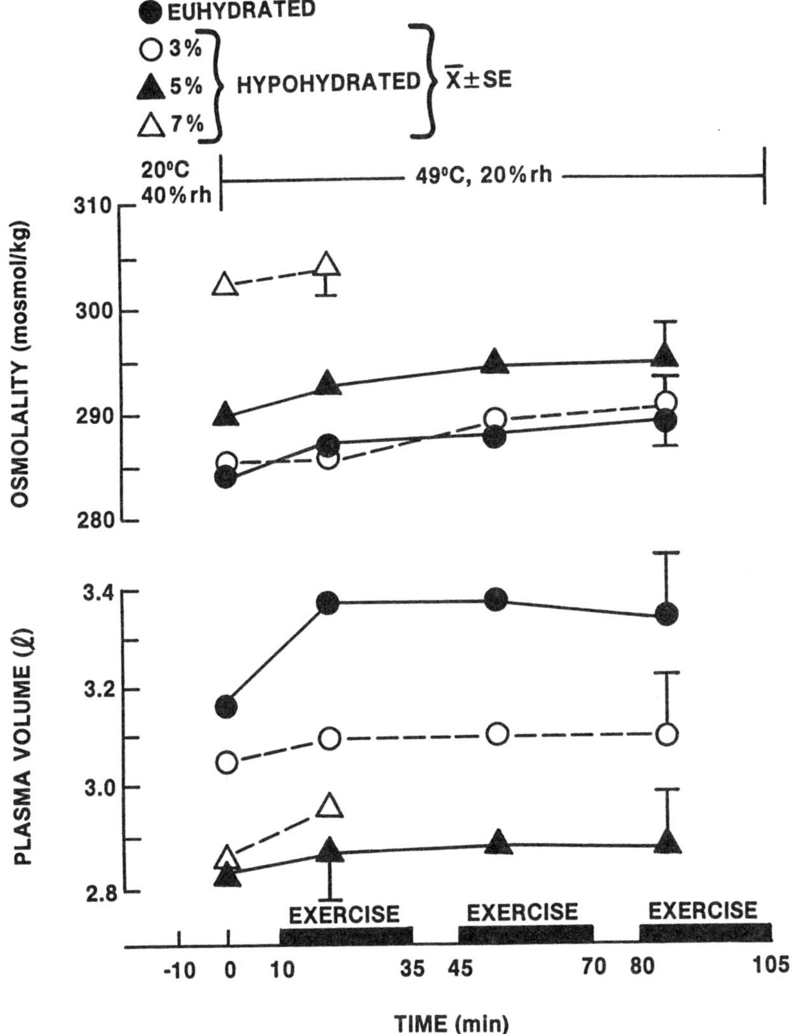

FIGURE 1-5. *Plasma osmolality and plasma volume values (+SE) at rest and exercise when euhydrated and hypohydrated (redrawn from Sawka et al., 1985).*

line). Post-acclimation, the subjects had a smaller plasma volume reduction at a given body water loss. It can be theorized that, because hypohydration was induced by exercise-heat stress, a more hypotonic sweat secretion in heat-acclimated subjects resulted in a greater amount of solute remaining in the plasma to redistribute fluid from the intracellular space. Therefore, an individual's state of heat acclimation probably alters the magnitude of hypovolemia associated with hypohydration.

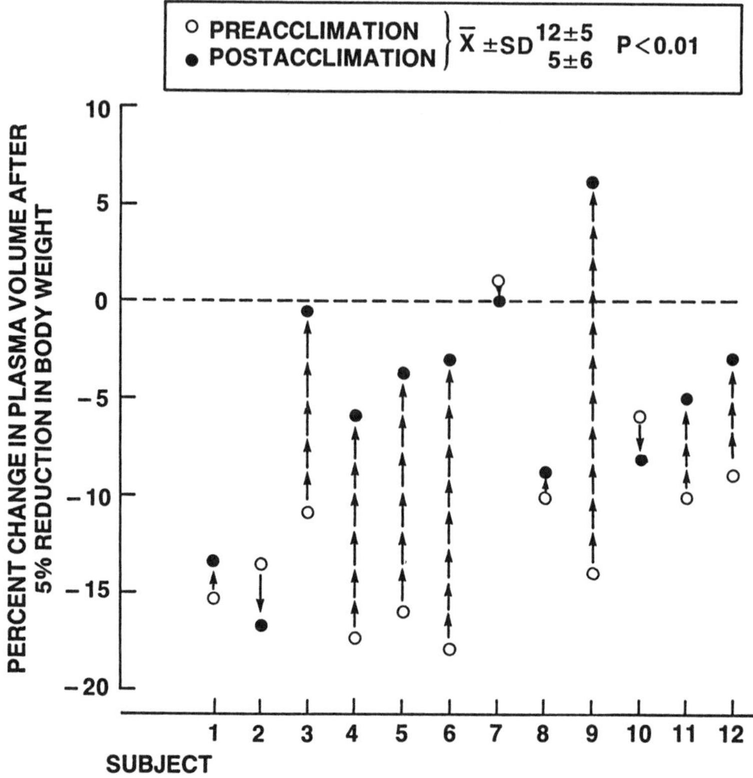

FIGURE 1-6. *The magnitude of plasma volume reduction, while at rest, associated with a hypohydration of 5% body weight both before and after a heat acclimation program (Sawka, 1988a).*

The plasma volume responses of heat acclimated subjects when euhydrated and hypohydrated by 3%, 5%, and 7% of their body weight are presented on the bottom of Figure 1-5 (Sawka et al., 1985). Dehydration procedures were identical to those previously described. Note that plasma volumes were generally reduced with increased hypohydration, although there was some evidence of a plasma volume defense during the 7% hypohydration. The most important point from this figure is that the hypohydration-mediated plasma volume reduction that occurs at rest continues throughout the subsequent moderate intensity (30% $\dot{V}O_2$max exercise. In fact, the differences between the euhydration and hypohydration plasma volume values are greater during exercise than rest because of the small exercise hemodilution that occurs when subjects are euhydrated but not when hypohydrated (Sawka et al., 1984a, 1985b, 1989b). These data clearly demonstrate that an exercise or heat-induced hypohydration results in hyperosmotic hypovolemia during both rest and exercise.

There is evidence that plasma volume can be somewhat defended despite having a progressive dehydration during intense (65–75% $\dot{V}O_2max$) running exercise (Gass et al., 1983; Kolka et al., 1982; Sawka et al., 1980). For example, Sawka and colleagues (1980) showed that during 100 min of treadmill running the plasma volume remained stable despite a 4% reduction in body weight. Likewise, Kolka et al., (1982) reported that during a competitive marathon race the plasma volume remained stable despite a 7% reduction in body weight. Reasons for the stable plasma volume during intense exercise despite progressive dehydration might include the release of water from glycogen breakdown and metabolic water (Pivarnick et al., 1984) and the redistribution of water from inactive skeletal muscle (Mellander, 1978; Sawka, 1988a). The higher the exercise intensity, the greater the use of muscle glycogen as a metabolic substrate (Conlee, 1987) and therefore water release from glycogen breakdown. Also, the greater amount of substrate oxidation, including fat, will result in a greater amount of metabolic water release.

Convertino (1987) has speculated that the endocrine system could contribute to the redistribution of water into the intravascular space during intense exercise. The plasma concentration of angiotensin and vasopressin are increased in relation to the exercise intensity (Convertino et al., 1981, 1983) and the magnitude of water deficit (Brandenberger et al., 1986; Francesconi et al., 1983, 1985). Both of these hormones are potent vasoconstrictors, and their increased circulating concentrations cause vasoconstriction in inactive tissues (Convertino, 1987). Vasoconstriction increases the ratio of pre- to post-capillary resistance, and favors fluid absorption from inactive tissues (Mellander, 1978; Sawka, 1988a). Therefore, during high intensity exercise while hypohydrated, the elevated circulating concentrations of these hormones favor additional fluid absorption from inactive tissues. Regardless of the physiological mechanisms, exercise intensity may influence the availability of water for redistribution to the intravascular space.

As previously discussed, some individuals may use diuretics to reduce their total body water. Diuretics are drugs that increase the rate of urine formation and generally result in the loss of solutes (Weiner & Mudge, 1985). The commonly used thiazide (e.g. Diuril), carbonic anhydrase inhibitors (e.g. Diamox), and furosemide (e.g. Lasix) are all diuretics that result in naturesis. Diuretic-induced hypohydration generally results in an iso-osmotic hypovolemia, with a much greater ratio of plasma loss to body water loss than either exercise- or heat-induced hypohydration (Hubbard & Armstrong, 1988). As a result, with a diuretic mediated loss of body water, solute does not accumulate in the plasma to exert an osmotic gradient for the redistribution of body water. Therefore, diuretic-induced hypohydration produces a greater loss of extracellular and thus plasma water than sweat-induced hypohydration.

EXERCISE PERFORMANCE

Individuals who incur a body water deficit may have to perform a variety of exercise tasks. For example, the exercise tasks required of a soldier in combat are different from those of competitive athletes; and the exercise tasks required of a wrestler, power lifter, and marathon runner are all dissimilar. Some of these athletes utilize primarily anaerobic metabolism and skeletal muscle strength, whereas others utilize primarily aerobic metabolism and the support of the cardiovascular and thermoregulatory systems. Because the metabolic and physiological system requirements can vary greatly, it is not surprising that hypohydration does not have homogeneous effects upon exercise performance. Environmental conditions also influence the magnitude of the performance decrement during exercise when hypohydrated.

Table 1-1 presents a summary of studies investigating the influence of hypohydration on muscular strength and muscular endurance as well as anaerobic performance. These investigations were ordered to present a continuum from the lowest to most severe water deficit. Caution should be employed when comparing the results of these different investigations (within, Tables 1-1 and 1-2) because of differences in subject populations, exercise protocols, and methods of elicit hypohydration. The arrows in the table denote the direction of a significant difference between euhydration and hypohydration.

Muscular strength was examined in 12 studies, of which four demonstrated a strength reduction after hypohydration. Of the four studies that demonstrated strength reductions, hypohydration was achieved by fluid restriction in three (Bosco and Terjung, 1968; Bosco et al., 1974; Houston et al., 1981) and by a combination of exercise and heat exposure in the fourth (Webster et al., 1988). Therefore, prolonged fluid restriction, perhaps accompanied by a caloric deficit (Bosco and Terjung, 1968; Houston et al., 1981), was the dehydration method that most often reduced muscular strength. The magnitude of water deficit appeared to influence the frequency with which muscular strength reductions were reported. Only one (Bosco and Terjung, 1968) of the five studies, employing less than a 5% reduction in body weight, reported a strength reduction; three of the seven studies employing between a 5% to 8% reduction in body weight reported strength reductions. Interestingly, the magnitude of water deficit did not appear to influence the magnitude of strength reduction, as decreases approximating 10% were reported for each study. Finally, it appears that the upper body muscle groups are more likely than the lower body muscle groups to show a strength reduction from hypohydration (Bosco & Terjung, 1968; Webster et al., 1988).

Muscular endurance was evaluated in four studies, of which two (Bijlani & Sharma, 1980; Torranin et al., 1979) demonstrated a reduction

	STUDY		n	DEHYDRATION PROCEDURE	Δ WT.	STRENGTH METHODOLOGY	RESULTS	ANAEROBIC METHODOLOGY	RESULTS
1.	AHLMAN & KARVONEN	1961	32	SAUNA & EXERCISE	-2 kg	BACK & LEG LIFTS	NC IN STRENGTH	–	–
2.	GREENLEAF et. al.	1967	12	EXERCISE IN HEAT	-3%	ISOMETRIC	NC IN STRENGTH	–	–
3.	BOSCO & TERJUNG	1968	9	FLUID RESTRICTION	-3%	ISOMETRIC	↓(11%) IN STRENGTH	–	–
4.	BIJLANI & SHARMA	1980	5	EXERCISE IN HEAT	-3%	ISOMETRIC	NC IN STRENGTH ↓ IN ENDURANCE	–	–
5.	NIELSEN et. al.	1981	6	DIURETIC	-3%	–	–	SUPRAMAXIMAL CYCLE	↓(18%)
			6	SAUNA	-3%	–	–	SUPRAMAXIMAL CYCLE	↓(35%)
			5	EXERCISE	-3%	–	–	SUPRAMAXIMAL CYCLE	↓(44%)
6.	SALTIN	1964	4	SAUNA, EXERCISE IN HEAT, EXERCISE	-4%	ISOMETRIC	NC IN STRENGTH	–	–
7.	TORRANIN et. al.	1979	20	SAUNA	-4%	ISOMETRIC	↓(31%) IN ISOMETRIC ENDURANCE	–	–
						ISOTONIC	↓(29%) IN ISOTONIC ENDURANCE	–	–
8.	MNATZAKANIAN & VACCARO	1982	?	?	-4%	ISOKINETIC	NC IN ENDURANCE	–	–
9.	TUTTLE	1943	13	EXERCISE & HEAT	-5%	ISOMETRIC	NC IN STRENGTH	–	–
10.	JACOBS	1980	11	HEAT	-5%	–	–	WINGATE TEST	NC
11.	SERFASS et. al.	1984	11	?	-5%	ISOMETRIC	NC IN STRENGTH NC IN ENDURANCE	–	–
12.	WEBSTER et. al.	1988	7	EXERCISE IN HEAT, SAUNA	-5%	ISOKINETIC	NC IN LEG STRENGTH ↓(7%) IN SHOULDER AND CHEST STRENGTH	WINGATE TEST	↓(21%) ANAEROBIC POWER ↓(10%) ANAEROBIC CAPACITY
13.	BOSCO et. al.	1974	21	FLUID RESTRICTION	-6%	ISOMETRIC	↓(10%) IN STRENGTH	–	–
14.	GREENLEAF et. al.	1966	9	FLUID RESTRICTION	-7%	ISOMETRIC	NC IN STRENGTH	–	–
15.	SINGER & WEISS	1968	10	?	-7%	ISOMETRIC	NC IN STRENGTH	–	–
16.	HOUSTON et. al.	1981	4	FLUID RESTRICTION	-8%	ISOKINETIC	↓(11%) IN STRENGTH	SUPRAMAXIMAL RUN	NC

TABLE 1-1. *Influence of Hypohydration on Muscular Strength and Endurance as well as Anaerobic Performance*

after hypohydration. The two studies that found no change in muscular endurance did not report their dehydration procedure (Mnatzakanian & Vaccaro, 1982; Serfass et al., 1984); but the other two studies used either thermal (Torranin et al., 1979) or exercise and thermal (Bijlani & Sharma, 1980) dehydration procedures. There were no systematic differences among these four studies in the magnitude of water deficit, muscle group tested, or test methodology.

Torranin et al., (1979) evaluated the isometric endurance of a small muscle group (hand grip) and the isotonic endurance of large muscle groups (arm and leg). Despite the use of the very diverse methodology, they found a consistent 30% reduction in muscular endurance when hypohydrated. Torranin et al., (1979) speculated that during the hypohydration experiements, a greater muscle temperature might have mediated the reduced muscular endurance. The muscular endurance experiments were conducted approximately 1 h after the subjects had finished dehydrating in an 80°C sauna.

Bijlani and Sharma (1980) performed their muscular endurance experiments either immediately after or within 30 min of dehydrating their subjects in a 41°C environment. In addition, it appeared that all of their muscular testing (when eu- and hypohydrated) was conducted in a warm (30–35°) environment. They present a figure demonstrating an inverse relationship between the control (euhydration) muscular endurance values and the dry bulb temperature. Therefore, in that study (Bijlani & Sharma, 1980) an elevated muscle temperature could have mediated the reduced muscular endurance during the hypohydration experiments (Clarke et al., 1958; Edwards & Lippold, 1972; Petrofsky & Lind, 1975).

Anaerobic exercise performance was evaluated in four studies, of which two employed Wingate type tests (Jacobs, 1980; Webster et al., 1988) and two employed supramaximal endurance tests (Houston et al., 1981; Nielsen et al., 1981). Jacobs (1980) performed a comprehensive evaluation of anaerobic exercise performance (Wingate test) in subjects when they are euhydrated and when they were hypohydrated by 2%, 4%, and 5% of their body weight. This investigator found that hypohydration did not alter anaerobic exercise performance or post-exercise blood lactate values. On the other hand, Webster and colleagues (1988) found a 21% reduction in anaerobic power and a 10% reduction in anaerobic capacity when their subjects were hypohydrated (5% body weight). Both of these studies used similar methodologies so that their disparate results are not easily explained.

Nielsen et al., (1981) had subjects perform a supramaximal (105% of VO_2max) cycle ergometer test when euhydrated and when hypohydrated (3% of body weight). The supramaximal exercise performance was decreased in subjects when they were hypohydrated by diuretics (–18%), sauna (–35%), and previous exercise (–44%). These reductions in supramaximal exercise performance were related to an elevation of plasma potassium concentration as well as an increase in skeletal muscle temperature. Houston et al., (1981) reported that hypohydration (8% of body weight) did not affect performance in a supramaximal (~1 min) treadmill run. In these experiments, dehydration was achieved by fluid and food restriction over several days, and the subjects were not exposed to any heat stress.

Table 1-2 presents a summary of studies investigating the influence of hypohydration on maximal aerobic power and physical work capacity. A body water deficit of less than 3% body weight did not alter maximal aerobic power in a neutral environment. Maximal aerobic power was decreased (Buskirk et al., 1958; Caldwell et al., 1984; Webster et al., 1971) in three of the five studies when hypohydration equaled or exceeded 3% body weight. Therefore, a critical water deficit (3% body weight) might exist before hypohydration reduces maximal aerobic power in a neutral environment. For experiments conducted in a neutral environment, the reduction in maximal aerobic power was not related to the magnitude of body water deficit or the dehydration procedures employed. In a hot environment, Craig and Cummings (1966) demonstrated that small (2% body weight) to moderate (4% body weight) water deficits resulted in large reductions of maximal aerobic power. Likewise, their data indicate a disproportionately larger decrease in maximal aerobic power with an increased magnitude of body water deficit. It seems that environmental heat stress further reduces the fall in maximal aerobic power produced by hypohydration.

The physical work capacity for aerobic exercise was decreased by hypohydration in all of the studies presented in Table 1-2. Physical work capacity was decreased by even a marginal water deficit that did not alter maximal aerobic power (Armstrong et al., 1985; Caldwell et al., 1984). The more pronounced the water deficit, the larger the reduction in physical work capacity. In addition, the environmental temperature influenced the magnitude of reduction in physical work capacity. Hypohydration elicited a much larger reduction in physical work capacity in a hot as compared to a neutral temperature environment. Again, it appears that the thermoregulatory system, via increased body temperature, has an

INFLUENCE OF HYPOHYDRATION ON MAXIMAL AEROBIC POWER AND PHYSICAL WORK CAPACITY

	STUDY		n	DEHYDRATION PROCEDURE	ΔWT.	TEST ENVIRONMENT	EXERCISE MODE	MAXIMAL AEROBIC POWER	PHYSICAL WORK CAPACITY
1.	ARMSTRONG et. al.	1985	8	DIURETICS	-1%	NEUTRAL	TM	NC	↓(6%)
2.	CALDWELL et. al.	1984	16	EXERCISE	-2%	NEUTRAL	CY	NC	↓(7w)
			15	DIURETICS	-3%	NEUTRAL	CY	↓(8%)	↓(21w)
			16	SAUNA	-4%	NEUTRAL	CY	↓(4%)	↓(23w)
3.	SALTIN	1964	10	SAUNA, EXERCISE, HEAT, DIURETICS	-4%	NEUTRAL	CY	NC	↓(?)
4.	CRAIG & CUMMINGS	1966	9	HEAT	-2%	HOT	TM	↓(10%)	↓(22%)
					-4%	HOT	TM	↓(27%)	↓(48%)
5.	BUSKIRK et. al.	1958	13	EXERCISE, HEAT	-5%	NEUTRAL	TM	↓(-0.22 l/min)	—
6.	WEBSTER et. al.	1988	7	EXERCISE IN HEAT, SAUNA	-5%	NEUTRAL	TM	↓(7%)	↓(12%)
7.	HERBERT & RIBISL	1971	8	?	-5%	NEUTRAL	CY	—	↓(17%)
8.	HOUSTON et. al.	1981	4	FLUID RESTRICTION	-8%	NEUTRAL	TM	NC	—

TABLE 1-2. *Influence of Hypohydration on Maximal Aerobic Power and Physical Work Capacity*

important role in the reduced exercise performance mediated by a body water deficit.

One investigation has examined the effects of a body water deficit on competitive distance running. In a study by Armstrong and colleagues (1985a) individuals competed in 1,500-, 5,000-, and 10,000-meter races when euhydrated and when hypohydrated. Hypohydration was achieved by administration of a diuretic (furosemide), which decreased body weight by ~2% and plasma volume by ~11%. Remember, diuretics produce a disproportionately larger loss of plasma water relative to total body water loss than that caused by either exercise or thermally mediated hypohydration. Figure 1-7 presents a summary of the subjects' running velocities at different race distances when they were euhydrated and when they were hypohydrated. They found that running performance was reduced by hypohydration to a greater extent in the longer (5,000 and 10,000 meters) than in the shorter (1,500 meters) race. These investigators speculated that hyperthermia may have provided the physiological mechanism that caused greater performance decrements in the longer races.

PHYSIOLOGICAL FUNCTION

Generally, the loss of body water adversely influences exercise performance. The critical water deficit and magnitude of performance dec-

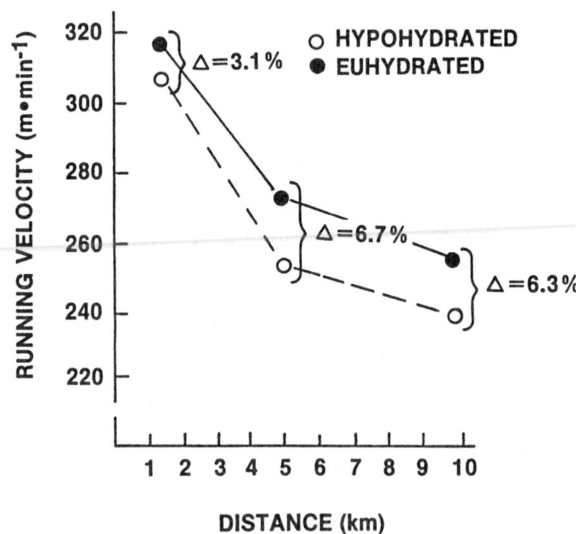

FIGURE 1-7. *Group mean running velocities of euhydrated and hypohydrated runners during outdoor track races (redrawn from Armstrong et al., 1985).*

rement are related to the exercise task and the environmental temperature. Exercise tasks that primarily require aerobic metabolism and are prolonged will more likely be adversely influenced by hypohydration than exercise tasks that primarily require anaerobic metabolism as well as muscular strength and power. In addition, the warmer the environment the greater the potential for decrements in exercise performance. There is no evidence that hypohydration can benefit exercise performance. In fact, man cannot adapt to chronic dehydration (Adolph & associates, 1947), and most of the thermoregulatory advantages conferred by high aerobic fitness and heat acclimation are negated by hypohydration during exercise in the heat (Buskirk et al., 1958; Cadarette et al., 1984; Sawka et al., 1983). It should be noted that mental performance is also adversely influenced by body water deficits (Adolph & associates, 1947; Gopinathan et al., 1988; Ladell, 1955). For many complex athletic, military and industrial tasks, both mental decision-making and physiological functions are closely related. As a result, hypohydration can have more profound effects on real-life tasks than on the solely physiological performance measures discussed in this chapter.

Hypohydration does not have consistent effects on muscular strength, but muscular endurance is often reduced by hypohydration (Table 1-1). Reduced muscular endurance is probably mediated by the dehydration procedures that cause an elevation of skeletal muscle temperature. Increased skeletal muscle temperature markedly reduces muscular endurance, but does not affect strength (Petrofsky & Lind, 1975). Clarke and colleagues (1958) found that if skeletal muscle was heated beyond 32°C there was a reduction of isometric endurance. Other laboratories (Edwards & Lippold, 1972; Petrofsky & Lind, 1975) have substantiated these findings. Possibly, the dehydration process rather than hypohydration per se is responsible for the decreased muscular endurance.

The effects of hypohydration on anaerobic performance are not clear. Hypohydration can reduce anaerobic performance; however, there does not appear to be a distinguishable critical water deficit. Rather, the dehydration procedures employed may play an important role in determining a decrement in anaerobic performance. Anaerobic performance (Table 1-1) is more likely to be reduced if the dehydration procedures of exercise and heat exposure (Nielsen et al., 1981; Webster et al., 1988) are employed as opposed to fluid restriction alone (Houston, 1981). Electrolyte imbalances and elevated body temperature encountered during hypohydration are the physiological mechanisms responsible for hypohydration reducing anaerobic performance. Nielsen et al., (1981) found that anaerobic performance was inversely related to plasma potassium concentration and muscle temperature in hypohydrated subjects. Interestingly, these investigators found no effect of hypovolemia on anaerobic performance. Because potassium is the primary intracellular cation, an increased plasma concentration may indicate an intracellular electrolyte imbalance. Sjogaard (1986) suggested that a loss of intracellular potassium might hyperpolarize the membrane electrochemical potential and reduce muscle contractability. Finally, high muscle temperatures may elevate hydrogen ion concentration which would inhibit phosphofructokinase activity and therefore anaerobic performance (Faulkner, 1980).

Hypohydration decreases maximal aerobic power with the critical water deficit and magnitude of reduction dependent upon the presence of environmental heat stress. In a neutral environment, a 4–8% decrease in maximal aerobic power occurs after hypohydration by ~3% body weight. In hot environments, a marginal water deficit (2% body weight) will decrease maximal aerobic power by a substantial amount (10%), and this performance decrement is amplified at greater hypohydration levels. Maximal aerobic power is dependent upon both central circulatory (oxygen delivery) and peripheral (oxygen extraction) factors; cardiac output and arteriovenous oxygen difference serve as indices of these central and peripheral factors, respectively.

A reduced maximal cardiac output might be the physiological mechanism by which hypohydration decreases maximal aerobic power. Remember, hypohydration is associated with a decreased blood (plasma) volume during both rest and exercise. A decreased blood (plasma) volume can increase blood viscosity (Vanderwalle et al., 1988) and possibly reduce venous return. During maximal exercise, a viscosity-mediated increased resistance and a reduced cardiac filling pressure could both decrease stroke volume and cardiac output. Several investigators (Allen et al., 1977; Sproles et al., 1976) have reported a tendency for hypohydrated subjects to have a reduced cardiac output during short-term, moderate-intensity exercise in a neutral environment.

It is not surprising that environmental heat stress potentiates the hypohydration-mediated reduction in maximal aerobic power. For euhydrated individuals, environmental heat stress alone decreases (~7%) maximal aerobic power (Sawka et al., 1985a). In the heat, the superficial skin veins reflexly dilate to increase cutaneous blood flow and blood volume. This displacement of blood to the cutaneous vasculature could decrease maximal aerobic power by: (a) reducing the portion of cardiac output perfusing the contracting musculature or, (b) decreasing the effective central blood volume and thus reducing venous return and cardiac output. If an individual was hypohydrated and encountered environmental heat stress, he/she would be hypovolemic and still have to simultaneously perfuse the cutaneous vasculature and contracting skeletal muscles. As a result, both environmental heat stress and hypohydration could act independently to limit cardiac output and therefore oxygen delivery during maximal exercise.

Hypohydration has its most adverse effects on the performance of prolonged aerobic exercise (Table 1-2, Figure 1-7). Not surprisingly, prolonged aerobic exercise is reduced by thermoregulatory and cardiovascular impairment due to hypohydration. Hypohydration has little effect on respiratory and acid-base responses during rest and exercise in the heat (Sawka et al., 1980; Senay & Christensen, 1967). In comparison to euhydration, hypohydration increases core temperature during exercise in a comfortable (Cadarette et al., 1984; Grande et al., 1959; Neufer et al., 1989a; Sawka et al., 1980); as well as in a hot (Claremont et a., 1976; Pearcy et al., 1956; Pitts et al., 1956; Sawka et al., 1988b; Senay, 1968; Smith et al., 1952) environment. The critical water deficit of 1% body weight elevates core temperature during exercise (Ekblom et al., 1970). As the magnitude of water deficit increases, there is a concomitant gradation in the elevation of core temperature during exercise. A comparison of results from investigators who examined a single level of body water deficit during exercise-heat stress, however, does not support this concept of graded core temperature responses with hypohydration (Sawka et al., 1984b). But conclusions based on inter-investigation comparisons can be tenuous because of differences in subject populations, environmental conditions, exercise intensities, and test methodologies (Sawka et al., 1984b).

Two studies examined core temperature responses to exercise while hypohydration levels were varied during independent tests in the same subjects. Strydom and Holdsworth (1968) studied two miners at two hypohydration levels (low—3%-5%, and high—5%-8% weight loss) and found higher core temperatures at the greater hypohydration level. Sawka et al., (1985b) reported that hypohydration linearly increased the core temperature by ~0.15°C during exercise in the heat for each percent decrease in body weight. Other investigators, reporting a gradation of elevated core temperature with increased water deficits, have interpolated from a single hypohydration level (Greenleaf & Castle, 1971) and/or employed prolonged exercise-heat exposure to elicit a progressive dehydration (Adolph & associates, 1947; Gisolfi & Copping, 1974). Reanalyzing the data of Adolph and associates (1947), we find that their subjects had an elevated core temperature of ~0.20°C for each percent decrease in body weight. Their data represents progressive dehydration under a variety of field and laboratory conditions. Greenleaf and Castle (1971) reported that core temperature rose 0.10°C for each percent decrease in body weight during exercise (49% $\dot{V}O_2max$) in a moderate environment. This relationship was based on interpolation from a single hypohydration (5% body weight loss) level. Gisolfi and Copping (1974) reported that core temperature is elevated by 0.40°C for each percent decrease in body weight after a weight loss of greater than 2% during intense exercise (74% $\dot{V}O_2max$) in a hot environment. Figure 1-8 pre-

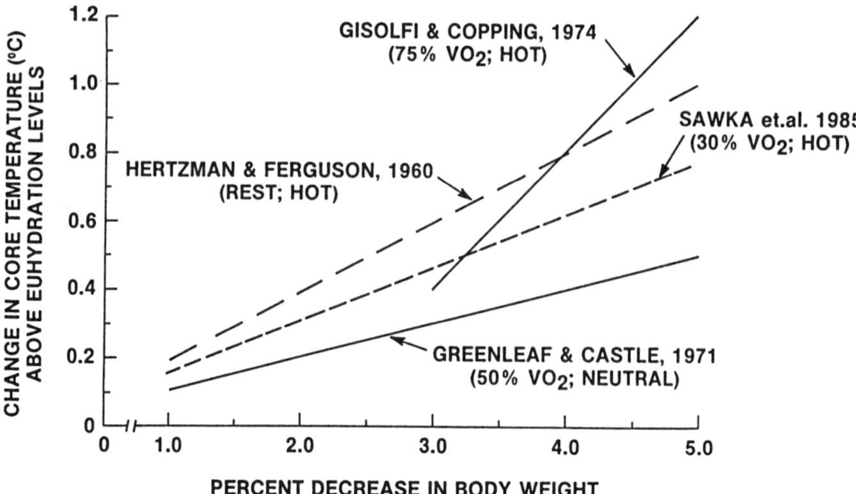

FIGURE 1-8. *Relationships for the elevation in core temperature (about euhydration) at a given magnitude of water deficit during rest and exercise conditions in different environments.*

sents the relationships between hypohydration and the elevation in core temperature (above euhydration levels) from several investigations (Gisolfi & Copping, 1974; Greenleaf & Castle, 1971; Hertzman & Ferguson, 1960; Sawka et al., 1985b). Clearly, exercise intensity and environmental conditions modify the magnitude of core temperature elevation associated with hypohydration.

Body heat storage occurs from either an increase in metabolic heat production or a decrease in heat loss. Hypohydration probably does not influence the rate of aerobic or anaerobic metabolism during exercise (Greenleaf & Castle, 1971; Saltin, 1964b; Sawka et al., 1979, 1983, 1985b, 1989b) and as a result does not cause greater metabolic heat production. It should be noted, however, that an increased aerobic (Pitts et al., 1956) and anaerobic (Neufer et al., 1989c) metabolism during exercise when hypohydrated have been reported. Because most studies indicate that metabolic heat production is not increased, the hypohydration-mediated increase in heat storage during exercise must be attributed to decreased heat dissipation. The relative contributions of evaporative and dry heat exchange during exercise depend on the specific environmental conditions, but both avenues of heat loss are adversely affected by hypohydration (Sawka et al., 1984b).

Hypohydration is associated with reduced or unchanged sweating rates at a given metabolic rate during rest (Hertzman & Ferguson, 1960) and exercise (Sawka et al., 1984b) in the heat. Investigators who report no change in sweating rate, usually still observe an elevated core temperature. Therefore, during hypohydration the sweating rate is lower for a given core temperature, and the potential for heat dissipation through sweat evaporation is reduced. Figure 1-9 presents data showing a systematically reduced sweating rate with increased hypohydration levels during exercise in the heat (Sawka et al., 1985b).

The physiological mechanisms mediating the reduced sweating rate during hypohydration are not clearly defined. Both the singular and combined effects of plasma hyperosmolality (Candas et al., 1986; Fortney et al., 1984; Harrison et al., 1978; Senay, 1979) and hypovolemia (Fortney et al., 1981b; Hertzman & Ferguson, 1960; Sawka et al., 1985b) have been suggested as mediating this reduced sweating response. Figure 1-10 presents individual data for the reduction (from euhydration) in sweating rate plotted against the change in osmolality and plasma volume (Sawka, 1985b). Plasma osmolality changes may relate to tonicity changes in the extracellular fluid bathing the hypothlamic neurons (Kozlowski et al., 1980; Nielsen et al., 1971). Silva and Boulant (1984) demonstrated that in rat brain slices, there are preoptic-anterior hypothalamic neurons that are both thermosensitive and osmosensitive. Nakashima and colleagues (1984) reported similar results for preoptic medial hypothalamic neurons in rats. Such data suggests a central interaction be-

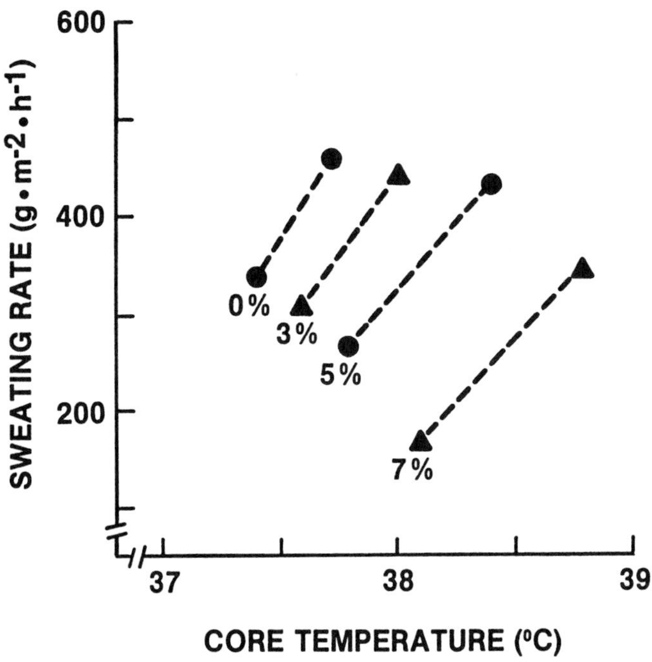

FIGURE 1-9. *Plot of mean total body sweating rate and final exercise core temperature when euhydrated (0%) and hypohydrated by 3%, 5%, and 7% of body weight (redrawn from Sawka et al., 1985).*

tween thermoregulation and body water regulation. Numerous other animal studies show that intravascular (Baker & Doris, 1982; Baker et al., 1983; Greenleaf et al., 1976; Kozlowski et al., 1980) or intracranial (Doris, 1983; Turlejska & Baker, 1986) infusion of hypertonic solutions will elevate core temperature during rest and exercise in the heat. Tonicity could also exert a peripheral effect via a high interstitial osmotic pressure inhibiting the fluid availability to the eccrine sweat gland (Greenleaf & Castle, 1971; Nielson et al., 1971).

Several human studies show that ingesting hypertonic fluid elevates core temperature in the heat, despite the maintenance of euhydration (Harrison et al., 1978; Nielsen, 1974; Nielsen et al., 1971). Consistent with this observation in humans, there is a significant relationship (r = 0.62 to 0.85) between the change in plasma osmolality and the change in thermoregulatory sweating during exercise-heat exposure (Sawka et al., 1985b, 1989a; Senay, 1979). Likewise, Fortney et al., (1984) have reported that hyperosmolality increases the threshold temperatures for sweating and cutaneous vasodilation even without a fall in blood volume, during exercise in the heat. The combined results of these studies indicate that plasma hyperosmolality exerts a powerful influence on thermoregulatory sweating and body temperature during exercise and heat stress.

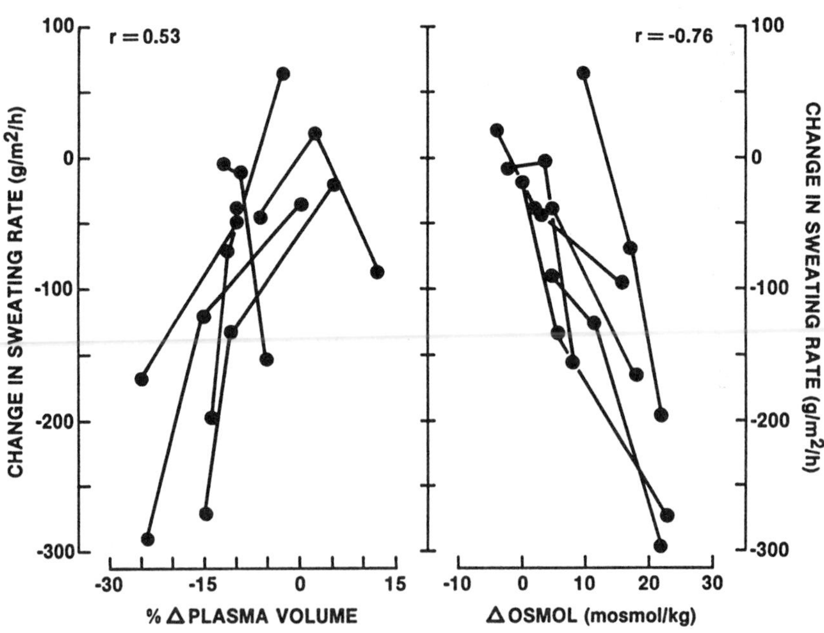

FIGURE 1-10. *Individual relationships for the change in exercise sweating rate from euhydration with changes in plasma volume and changes in osmolality from euhydration (Sawka et al., 1985).*

Hypovolemia can also mediate a decreased sweating rate during exercise in the heat (Fortney et al., 1981b, 1984; Sawka et al., 1985b, 1989a). The thermoregulatory disadvantages of hypohydration can also be partially reversed by the re-establishment of the normal blood volume during exercise in the heat (Stephenson et al., 1983). Fortney et al., (1981b) provide strong evidence that an iso-osmotic hypovolemia reduces sweating rate and elevates core temperature during exercise. They theorize that hypovolemia may alter the activity of atrial baroreceptors with afferent input to the hypothalamus. Therefore, a reduced atrial filling pressure might modify neural information to the hypothalamic thermoregulatory centers that control sweating rate. Consistent with these findings, a significant relationship (r = 0.53 to 0.75) between changes in blood (or plasma) volume and changes in thermoregulatory sweating during exercise-heat exposure have been reported (Sawka et al., 1985b, 1989a).

The effects of hypohydration on cardiovascular responses to exercise have been investigated (Allen et al., 1977; Nadel et al., 1980; Saltin, 1964b; Sawka et al., 1979; Sproles et al., 1976). During submaximal exercise with little thermal strain, hypohydration elicits an increase in heart rate and decrease in stroke volume, and usually no change in cardiac output relative to euhydration levels (Allen et al., 1977; Saltin, 1964b; Sproles et al., 1976). Apparently, during hypohydration, a decreased blood volume reduces central venous pressure (Kirsch et al., 1981) and cardiac filling pressure. As a consequence, stroke volume falls, requiring a compensatory increase of heart rate.

Figure 1-11 shows the relationship between stroke volume and the reduction in plasma volume for eu- and hypohydrated subjects during exercise-heat stress (Nadel et al., 1980). During submaximal exercise with moderate (Nadel et al., 1980) or severe (Sawka et al., 1979) thermal strain, hypohydration (3%–4% body weight) elicits an increase in heart rate, decrease in stroke volume, and a decrease in cardiac output relative to euhydration levels. Note that the increased heart rate does not compensate for the decreased stroke volume and results in a decreased cardiac output. Likewise, Sproles et al. (1976) demonstrated that a severe water deficit (7% body weight) in the absence of thermal strain can also reduce cardiac output during submaximal exercise.

The combination of exercise and heat strain results in competition between the central and peripheral circulation for a limited blood volume (Rowell, 1983). As body temperature rises during exercise, cutaneous vasodilation occurs and the superficial veins become more compliant, thus decreasing venous resistance and pressure. As a result of decreased blood volume and increased blood displacement to cutaneous vascular beds, venous return, and thus cardiac output, fall below that for euhydration (Nadel et al., 1980; Sawka et al., 1979). Several investigators (Fort-

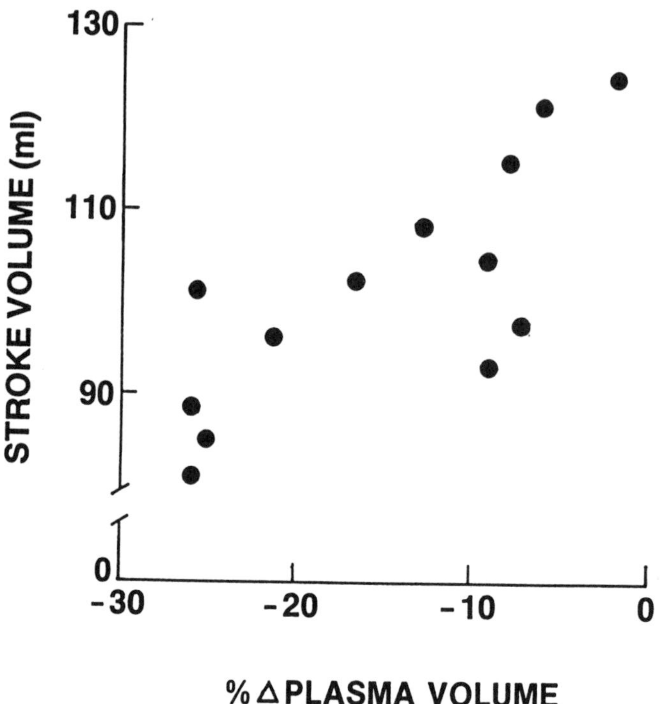

FIGURE 1-11. *Relationship between cardiac stroke volume and reduction in plasma volume for eu- and hypohydrated subjects during exercise-heat stress (redrawn from Nadel et al., 1980).*

ney et al., 1981a, 1984; Nadel et al., 1980) report that these conditions also reduce cutaneous blood flow for a given core temperature and therefore the potential for dry heat exchange. Figure 1-12 presents forearm (cutaneous) blood flow for eu- and hypohydrated individuals during exercise-heat stress (Nadel et al., 1980). The diuretic-induced hypohydration (3% body weight) delayed the onset and reduced the maximal cutaneous blood flow. Likewise, hyperosmolality, in the absence of hypovolemia, can also reduce the cutaneous blood flow response during exercise-heat stress (Fortney et al., 1981a).

Another physiological mechanism by which hypohydration might limit submaximal exercise performance is by altering skeletal muscle metabolism. Skeletal muscle glycogen concentration has been demonstrated to be related to submaximal exercise performance (Conlee, 1987). In preliminary work, Neufer et al. (1989c) found no significant difference in muscle glycogen use during 1 h of cycling exercise (50% $\dot{V}O_2max$, 18°C, 30% rh) with subjects hypohydrated (−5% body weight) or euhydrated. Although muscle glycogen depletion did not differ between the experiments, evaluation and interpretation of this data are not conclusive due to subnormal muscle glycogen and hydration levels before exercise in the

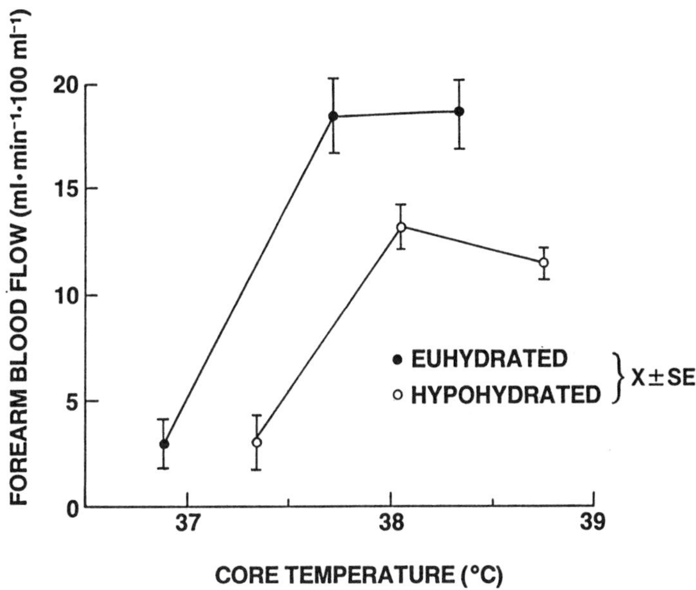

FIGURE 1-12. *Forearm blood flow as a function of core temperature for eu- and hypohydrated subjects during exercise-heat stress (redrawn from Nadel et al., 1980).*

control "euhydration" experiments. Because 3–4 g of water are bound to each gram of glycogen, as much as 400–500 mL of water might be needed for glycogen resynthesis after heavy exercise. Neufer and colleagues (1989b) also hypothesized that hypohydration might reduce glycogen resynthesis because of water nonavailability, despite the intake of an adequate carbohydrate diet. Preliminary findings by Neufer et al. (1989b) indicate that, despite reduced muscle and body water availability, muscle glycogen resynthesis is not altered by hypohydration for the first 15 h after heavy exercise.

SUMMARY

Individuals in athletic, occupational, and military settings may have to perform physical exercise while incurring a body water deficit. Usually, the individual dehydrates because of fluid nonavailability or a mismatch between thirst and body water requirements. This fluid deficit comprises water loss from both the intracellular and extracellular fluid spaces, and results in a decreased plasma volume and increased plasma osmolality. If diuretics are employed to dehydrate an individual, a relatively greater loss of extracellular and therefore plasma water occurs, but tonicity is not increased as high as compared to dehydration elicited from exercise-heat exposure.

Generally, the loss of body water adversely influences exercise performance. There is absolutely no evidence that hypohydration can benefit exercise performance; in addition, man cannot adapt to chronic dehydration. Prolonged exercise tasks that primarily require aerobic metabolism are more likely to be adversely influenced by hypohydration than short-term exercise tasks requiring anaerobic metabolism as well as muscular strength and power. Likewise, the warmer the environmental temperature, the greater the potential for decrements in exercise performance.

Hypohydration will reduce exercise performance by primarily acting through the thermoregulatory and cardiovascular systems; however, intracellular electrolyte imbalances might also contribute to performance decrements. Hypohydration causes greater body heat storage (elevated core temperature) during exercise in neutral or hot environments. The greater the water deficit, the greater the elevation in core temperature during exercise; but exercise intensity and environmental conditions modify the rise in core temperature. The greater heat storage is attributed to a decreased sweating rate as well as decreased cutaneous blood flow. These thermoregulatory impairments are attributed to both plasma hyperosmolality and decreased blood volume. The latter together with the displacement of blood to the cutaneous vasculature make it more difficult to maintain cardiac output during exercise. The inability to maintain cardiac output during exercise in the heat when hypohydrated can result in reduced oxygen delivery to the active muscles and perhaps syncope. Ladell (1955) summarized that during exercise in the heat, "Fatigue, usually sudden in onset, was more pronounced when the water debt was high."

BIBLIOGRAPHY

Adolph, E.F. and associates. *Physiology of Man in the Desert.* New York: Interscience, 1947.

Ahlman, K. and M.J. Karvonen. Weight reduction by sweating in wrestlers, and its effect on physical fitness. *J. Sports Med. Phys. Fitness* 1:58–62, 1961.

Allan, J.R. and C.G. Wilson. Influence of acclimatization on sweat sodium concentration. *J. Appl. Physiol.* 30:708–712, 1971.

Allen, T.E., D.P. Smith and D.K. Miller. Hemodynamic response to submaximal exercise after dehydration and rehydration in high school wrestlers. *Med. Sci. Sports Exerc.* 9:159–163, 1977.

Armstrong, L.E., D.L. Costill and W.J. Fink. Influence of diuretic-induced dehydration on competitive running performance. *Med. Sci. Sports Exerc.* 17:456–461, 1985a.

Armstrong, L.E., R.W. Hubbard, B.H. Jones and J.T. Daniels. Preparing Alberto Salazar for the Heat of the 1984 Olympic Marathon. *Physician Sportsmed.* 14:73–81, 1986.

Armstrong, L.E., R.W. Hubbard, P.C. Szlyk, W.T. Matthew and I.V. Sills. Voluntary dehydration and electrolyte losses during prolonged exercise in the heat. *Aviat. Space. Environ. Med.* 56:765–770, 1985b.

Baker, M.A. and P.A. Doris. Control of evaporative heat loss during changes in plasma osmolality in the cat. *J. Physiol. (Lond.).* 328:535–545, 1982.

Baker, M.A., P.A. Doreis and M.J. Hawkins. Effect of dehydration and hyperosmolality on thermoregulatory water loss in exercising dogs. *Am. J. Physiol.* 244:R516–R521, 1983.

Bar-Or, O., R. Dothan, O. Inbar, A. Rotshtein and H. Zonder. Voluntary hypohydration in 10- to 12-year old boys. *J. Appl. Physiol.* 48:104–108, 1980.

Bijlani, R.L. and K.N. Sharma. Effect of dehydration and a few regimes of rehydration on human performance. *Indian J. Physiol. Pharmacol.* 24:255–266, 1980.

Bosco, J.S., J.E. Greenleaf, E.M. Bernauer and D.H. Card. Effects of acute dehydration and starvation on muscular strength and endurance. *Acta Physiol. Pol.* 25:411–421, 1974.
Bosco, J.S. and R.L. Terjung. Effects of progressive hypohydration on maximal isometric muscular strength. *J. Sports Med. Phys. Fitness* 8:81–86, 1968.
Brandenberger, G., V. Candas, M. Follenius, J.P. Libert and J.M. Kahn. Vascular fluid shifts and endocrine responses to exercise in the heat. *Eur. J. Appl. Physiol.* 55:123–129, 1986.
Buskirk, E.R. and W.P. Beetham. Dehydration and body temperature as a result of marathon running. *Med. Sport.* 37:493–506, 1960.
Buskirk, E.R., P.F. Iampietro and D.E. Bass. Work performance after dehydration: effects of physical conditioning and heat acclimation. *J. Appl. Physiol.* 12:189–194, 1958.
Cadarette, B.S., M.N. Sawka, M.M. Toner and K.B. Pandolf. Aerobic fitness and the hypohydration response to exercise-heat stress. *Aviat. Space Environ. Med.* 55:507–512, 1984.
Caldwell, J.E., E. Ahonen and U. Nousiainen. Differential effects of sauna-, diuretic-, and exercise-induced hypohydration. *J. Appl. Physiol.* 57:1018–1023, 1984.
Candas, V., J.P. Libert, G. Brandenberger, J.C. Sagot, C. Amoros and J.M. Kahn. Hydration during exercise: effects on thermal and cardiovascular adjustments. *Eur. J. Appl. Physiol.* 55:113–122, 1986.
Claremont, A.D., D.L. Costill, W. Fink and P. Van Handel. Heat tolerance following diuretic induced dehydration. *Med. Sci. Sports* 8:239–243, 1976.
Clarke, R.S.J., R.F. Hellon and A.R. Lind. The duration of sustained contractions of the human forearm at different muscle temperatures. *J. Physiol. (Lond).* 143:454–473, 1958.
Commonwealth of Massachusetts. *The Report of the Investigation of Attorney General James M. Shannon of the Class 12 Experience at the Edward W. Connelly Criminal Justice Training Center, Agawam, Massachusetts.* Department of the Attorney General, October 28, 1988.
Conlee, R.K. Muscle glycogen and exercise endurance: a twenty year perspective. In: K.B. Pandolf (ed.). *Exercise and Sport Sciences Reviews*, Vol. 15. New York: Macmillan Publishing Co., 1987, pp. 1–28.
Convertino, V.A. Fluid shifts and hydration state: effects of long-term exercise. *Can. J. Sports Sci.* 12:1365–1395, 1987.
Convertino, V.A., L.C. Keil, E.M. Bernauer and J.E. Greenleaf. Plasma volume, osmolality, vasopressin, and renin activity during graded exercise in man. *J. Appl. Physiol.* 50:123–128, 1981.
Convertino, V.A., L.C. Keil and J.E. Greenleaf. Plasma volume, renin and vasopressin responses to graded exercise after training. *J. Appl. Physiol.* 54:508–514, 1983.
Costill, D.L., R. Cote' and W. Fink. Muscle water and electrolytes following varied levels of dehydration in man. *J. Appl. Physiol.* 40:6–11, 1976.
Costill, D.L., R. Cote', W.J. Fink and P. Van Handel. Muscle water and electrolyte distribution during prolonged exercise. *Int. J. Sports Med.* 2:130–134, 1981.
Costill, D.L. and B. Saltin. Muscle glycogen and electrolytes following exercise and thermal dehydration. In: H. Howald and J.R. Poortmans (eds.). *Metabolic Adaptation to Prolonged Physical Exercise.* Basel: Birkhauser Verlag 1975, pp. 352–360.
Craig, F.N. and E.G. Cummings. Dehydration and muscular work. *J. Appl Physiol.* 21:670–674, 1966.
Doris, P.A. Osmotic regulation of evaporative water loss and body temperature by intracranial receptors in the heat-stressed cat. *Pflugers Arch.* 398:337–340, 1983.
Draper, E.S. and J.J. Lombardi. *Combined Arms in a Nuclear/Chemical Environment: Force Development Testing and Experimentation. Summary Evaluation Report Phase I.* Ft. McClellan, AL: U.S. Army Chemical School, 1986.
Durkot, M.J., O. Martinez, D. McQuade and R. Francesconi. Simultaneous determination of fluid shifts during thermal stress in a small-animal model. *J. Appl. Physiol.* 61:1031–1034, 1986.
Edwards, R.H.T. and O.C.J. Lippold. Effect of temperature on muscle energy metabolism and endurance during successive isometric contractions sustained to fatigue of the quadriceps muscle in man. *J. Physiol. (Lond.)* 220:335–352, 1972.
Eichna, L.W., W.B. Bean, W.F. Ashe and N. Nelson. Performance in relation to environmental temperature. *Bull, Johns Hopkins Hosp.* 76:25–58, 1945.
Ekblom, B., C.J. Greenleaf, J.E. Greenleaf and L. Hermansen. Temperature regulation during exercise dehydration in man. *Acta Physiol. Scand.* 79:475–583, 1970.
Engell, D.B., O. Maller, M.N. Sawka, R.P. Francesconi, L. Drolet and A.J. Young. Thirst and fluid intake following graded hypohydration levels in humans. *Physiol. Behav.* 40:226–236, 1987.
Faulkner, J.A. Heat and contractile properties of skeletal muscle. In: S.M. Horvath and M.K. Yousf (eds.). *Environmental Physiology: Aging, Heat and Altitude.* New York: Elsevier/North Holland, 1980, pp. 191–203.
Fortney, S.M., E.R. Nadel, C.B. Wenger and J.R. Bove. Effect of acute alterations of blood volume on circulatory performance in humans. *J. Appl. Physiol.* 50:292–298, 1981a.
Fortney, S.M., E.R. Nadel, C.B. Wenger and J.R. Bove. Effect of blood volume on sweating rate and body fluids in exercising humans. *J. Appl. Physiol.* 51:1594–1600, 1981b.
Fortney, S.M., C.B. Wenger, J.R. Bove and E.R. Nadel. Effect of hyperosmolality on control of blood flow and sweating. *J. Appl. Physiol.* 57:1688–1695, 1984.
Francesconi, R.F., R. Byrom and M. Mager. United States Army Research Institute of Environmental Medicine: First Quarter Century. *The Physiologist.* 29:58–62, 1986.

Francesconi, R.P., M.N. Sawka and K.B. Pandolf. Hypohydration and heat acclimation: plasma renin and aldosterone during exercise. *J. Appl. Physiol.* 55:1790–1794, 1983.
Francesconi, R.P., M.N. Sawka, K.B. Pandolf, R.W. Hubbard, A.J. Young and S. Muza. Plasma hormonal responses at graded hypohydration levels during exercise-heat stress. *J. Appl. Physiol.* 59:1855–1860, 1985.
Gass, G.C., E.M. Camp, J. Watson, D. Eager, L. Wicks and A. Ng. Prolonged exercise in highly trained female endurance runners. *Int. J. Sports Med.* 4:241–246, 1983.
Gisolfi, C.V. and J.R. Copping. Thermal effects of prolonged treadmill exercise in the heat. *Med. Sci. Sports* 6:108–113, 1974.
Gopinathan, P.M., G. Pichan and V.M. Sharma. Role of dehydration in heat stress-induced variations in mental performance. *Arch. Environ. Health.* 43:15–17, 1988.
Grande, F., J.E. Monagle, E.R. Buskirk and H.L. Taylor. Body temperature responses to exercise in man on restricted food and water intake. *J. Appl. Physiol.* 14:194–198, 1959.
Greenleaf, J.E., P.J. Brock, L.C. Keil and J.T. Morse. Drinking and water balance during exercise and heat acclimation. *J. Appl. Physiol.* 54:414–419, 1983.
Greenleaf, J.E. and B.L. Castle. Exercise temperature regulation in man during hypohydration and hyperhydration. *J. Appl. Physiol.* 30:847–853, 1971.
Greenleaf, J.E., S. Kozlowski, K. Nazar, H. Kaciuba-Uscilko, Z. Brzezinska and A. Ziemba. Ion-osmotic hyperthermia during exercise in dogs. *Am. J. Physiol.* 230:74–79, 1976.
Greenleaf, J.E., M. Matter, J.S. Bosco, L.G. Douglas and E.G. Averkin. Effects of hypohydration on tolerance to $+G_z$ acceleration in man. *Aerospace Med.* 37:34–39, 1966.
Greenleaf, J.E., E.M. Prange and E.G. Averkin. Physical performance of women following heat-exercise hypohydration. *J. Appl. Physiol.* 22:55–60, 1967.
Harrison, M.H., R.J. Edwards and P.A. Fennessy. Intravascular volume and tonicity as factors in the regulation of body temperature. *J. Appl. Physiol.* 44:69–75, 1978.
Herbert, W.G. and P.M. Ribisl. Effects of dehydration upon physical working capacity of wrestlers under competitive conditions. *Res. Quart.* 43:416–422, 1971.
Hertzman, A.B. and I.D. Ferguson. Failure in temperature regulation during progressive dehydration. *U.S. Armed Forces Med. J.* 11:542–560, 1960.
Horvath, S.M. and E.C. Horvath. *The Harvard Fatigue Laboratory: Its History and Contributions.* Englewood Cliffs, NJ: Prentice-Hall Inc., 1973.
Houston, M.E., D.A. Marrin, H.J. Green and J.A. Thomson. The effect of rapid weight loss on physiological functions in wrestlers. *Physician Sportsmed.* 9:73–78, 1981.
Hubbard, R.W. and L.E. Armstrong. The heat illnesses: biochemical, ultrastructural, and fluid-electrolyte considerations. In: K.B. Pandolf, M.N. Sawka and R.R. Gonzalez, (eds). *Human Performance Physiology and Environmental Medicine at Terrestrial Extremes.* Indianapolis: Benchmark Press, 1988, pp. 305–359.
Hubbard, R., M. Mager and M. Kerstein. Water as a tactical weapon: A doctrine for preventing heat casualties. *Army Sci. Conf. Proc.* 125–139, 1982.
Hubbard, R.W., B.L. Sandick, W.T. Matthew, R.P. Francesconi, J.B. Sampson, M.J. Durkot, O. Maller and D.B. Engell. Voluntary dehydration and alliesthesia for water. *J. Appl. Physiol.* 57:868–875, 1984.
Jacobs, I. The effects of thermal dehydration on performance of the Wingate Anaerobic Test. *Int. J. Sports Med.* 1:21–24, 1980.
Kirby, C.R. and V.A. Convertino. Plasma aldosterone and sweat sodium concentrations after exercise and heat acclimation. *J. Appl. Physiol.* 61:967–970, 1986.
Kirsch, K.A., H. von Ameln and H.J. Wicke. Fluid control mechanisms after exercise dehydration. *Eur. J. Appl. Physiol.* 47:191–196, 1981.
Knochel, J.P. Dog days and Siriasis: How to kill a football player. *J.A.M.A.* 233:513–515, 1975.
Kolka, M.A., L.A. Stephenson and J.E. Wilkerson. Erythrocyte indices during a competitive marathon. *J. Appl. Physiol.* 52:168–172, 1982.
Kozlowski, S., J.E. Greenleaf, E. Turlejska and K. Nazar. Extracellular hyperosmolality and body temperature during physical exercise in dogs. *Am. J. Physiol.* 239 R180–R183, 1980.
Kozlowski, S. and B. Saltin. Effect of sweat loss on body fluids. *J. Appl. Physiol.* 19:1119–1124, 1964.
Kristal-Boneh, E., J.G. Glusman, C. Chaemovitz and Y. Cassuto. Improved thermoregulation caused by forced water intake in human desert dwellers. *Eur. J. Appl. Physiol.* 57:220–224, 1988.
Kubica, R., B. Nielsen, A. Bonnesen, I.B. Rasmussen, J. Stoklosa and B. Wilk. Relationship between plasma volume reduction and plasma electrolyte changes after prolonged bicycle exercise, passive heating and diuretic dehydration. *Acta. Physiol. Pol.* 34:569–579, 1983.
Ladell, W.S.S. The effects of water and salt intake upon the performance of men working in hot and humid environments. *J. Physiol. (Lond.)* 127:11–46, 1955.
Mellander, S. On the control of capillary fluid transfer by precapillary and postcapillary vascular adjustments. *Microvasc. Res.* 15:319–330, 1978.
Mnatzakanian, P.A. and P. Vaccaro. Effects of 4% dehydration and rehydration on hematological profiles, urinary profiles and muscular endurance of college wrestlers. *Med. Sci. Sports Exerc.* (Abst.) 14:117, 1982.

Molnar, G.W., E.J. Towbin, R.E. Gosselin, A.H. Brown and E.F. Adolph. A comparative study of water, salt and heat exchanges of men in tropical and desert environments. *Am. J. Hyg.* 44:411–433, 1946.
Morimoto, T.K., K. Miki, H. Nose, S. Yamada, K. Hirakawa and C. Matsubara. Changes in body fluid volume and its composition during heavy sweating and the effects of fluid and electrolyte replacement. *Jpn. J. Biometeorol.* 18:31–39, 1981.
Nadel, E.R., S.M. Fortney and C.B. Wenger. Effect of hydration on circulatory and thermal regulation. *J. Appl. Physiol.* 49:715–721, 1980.
Nakashima, T., T. Hori, T. Kiyohara and M. Shibata. Effects of local osmolality changes on medial preoptic thermosensitive neurons in hypothalamic slices In Vitro. *Thermal Physiology* 9:133–137, 1984.
Neufer, P.D., A.J. Young and M.N. Sawka. Gastric emptying during exercise: effects of heat stress and hypohydration. *Eur. J. Appl. Physiol.* 58:433–439, 1989a.
Neufer, P.D., A.J. Young, M.N. Sawka, M.D. Quigley, L. Levine and W.A. Latzka. Hypohydration and muscle glycogen resynthesis. *Med. Sci. Sports Exerc.* (Abstract), 21:S19, 1989b.
Neufer, P.D., A.J. Young, M.N. Sawka, M.D. Quigley, L. Levine and W.A. Latzka. Substrate levels and muscle metabolism while hypohydrated. *FASEB Journal* (Abstract), 3:A990, 1989c.
Nielsen, B. Effects of changes in plasma volume and osmolality on thermoregulation during exercise. *Acta Physiol. Scand.* 90:725–730, 1974.
Nielsen, B., G. Hansen, S.O. Jorgensen and E. Nielsen. Thermoregulation in exercising man during dehydration and hyperhydration with water and saline. *Int. J. Biometerol.* 15:195–200, 1971.
Nielsen, B., R. Kubica, A. Bonnesen, I.B. Rassmussen, J. Stoklosa and B. Wilk. Physical work capacity after dehydration and hyperthermia: a comparison of the effect of exercise versus passive heating and sauna and diuretic dehydration. *Scand. J. Sport Sci.* 3:2–10, 1981.
Nielsen, M. Die Regulation der Korpertemperatur bei Muskelarbeit. *Scand. Arch. Physiol.* 79:193–230, 1938.
Nose, H., G.W. Mack, X. Shi and E.R. Nadel. Shift in body fluid compartments after dehydration in humans. *J. Appl. Physiol.* 65:318–324, 1988.
Nose, H., T. Morimoto and K. Ogura. Distribution of water losses among fluid compartments of tissues under thermal dehydration in the rat. *Jpn. J. Physiol.* 33:1019–1029, 1983.
Olsson, K.-E. and B. Saltin. Variation in total body water with muscle glycogen changes in man. *Acta Physiol. Scand.* 80:11–18, 1970.
Pearcy, M., S. Robinson, D.I. Miller, J.T. Thomas and J. De Brota. Effects of dehydration, salt depletion and pitressin on sweat rate and urine flow. *J. Appl. Physiol.* 8:621–626, 1956.
Petrofsky, J.S. and A.R. Lind. The relationship of body fat content to deep muscle temperature and isometric endurance in man. *Clin. Sci. Mol. Med.* 48:405–412, 1975.
Phillips, P.A., B.J. Rolls, J.G.G. Ledingham, M.I. Forsling, J.J. Morton, M.J. Crowe and L. Wollner. Reduced thirst after water deprivation in healthy elderly men. *N. Engl. J. Med.* 311:753–759, 1984.
Pitts, G.C., R.E. Johnson and F.C. Consolazio. Work in the heat as affected by intake of water, salt and glucose. *Am. J. Physiol.* 142:253–259, 1956.
Pivarnik, J.M., E.M. Leeds and J.E. Wilkerson. Effects of endurance exercise on metabolic water production and plasma volume. *J. Appl. Physiol.* 56:613–618, 1984.
Pugh, L.G.C.E., J.L. Corbett and R.H. Johnson. Rectal temperatures, weight losses and sweat rates in marathon running. *J. Appl. Physiol.* 23:347–352, 1967.
Rowell, L.B. Cardiovascular aspects of human thermoregulation. *Circ. Res.* 52:367–379, 1983.
Saltin, B. Aerobic and anaerobic work capacity after dehydration. *J. Appl. Physiol.* 19:1114–1118, 1964a.
Saltin, B. Circulatory response to submaximal and maximal exercise after thermal dehydration. *J. Appl. Physiol.* 19:1125–1132, 1964b.
Sawka, M.N. Body fluid responses and hypohydration during exercise-heat stress. In: K.B. Pandolf, M.N. Sawka and R.R. Gonzalez, (eds). *Human Performance Physiology and Environmental Medicine at Terrestrial Extremes.* Indianapolis: Benchmark Press, 1988a, pp. 227–266.
Sawka, M.N., R.P. Francesconi, N.A. Pimental and K.B. Pandolf. Hydration and vascular fluid shifts during exercise in the heat. *J. Appl. Physiol.* 56:91–96, 1984a.
Sawka, M.N., R.P. Francesconi, A.J. Young and K.B. Pandolf. Influence of hydration level and body fluids on exercise performance in the heat. *J.A.M.A.* 252:1165–1169, 1984b.
Sawka, M.N., R.R. Gonzalez, A.J. Young, R.C. Dennis, C.R. Valeri and K.B. Pandolf. Control of thermoregulatory sweating during exercise in the heat. *Am. J. Physiol.* 257:R311–R316, 1989a.
Sawka, M.N., R.R. Gonzalez, A.J. Young, S.R. Muza, K.B. Pandolf, W.A. Latzka, R.C. Dennis and C.R. Valeri. Polycythemia and hydration: effects on thermoregulation and blood volume during exercise-heat stress. *Am. J. Physiol.* 255:R456–R463, 1988b.
Sawka, M.N., R.G. Knowlton and J.B. Critz. Thermal and circulatory responses to repeated bouts of prolonged running. *Med. Sci. Sports.* 11:177–180, 1979.
Sawka, M.N., R.G. Knowlton and R.G. Glaser. Body temperature, respiration and acid-base equilibrium during prolonged running. *Med. Sci. Sports Exerc.* 12:370–374, 1980.
Sawka, M.N., M.M. Toner, R.P. Francesconi and K.B. Pandolf. Hypohydration and exercise: effects of heat acclimation, gender and environment. *J. Appl. Physiol.* 55:1147–1153, 1983.

Sawka, M.N., A.J. Young, B.S. Cadarette, L. Levine and K.B. Pandolf. Influence of heat stress and acclimation on maximal aerobic power. *Eur. J. Appl. Physiol.* 53:294–298, 1985a.

Sawka, M.N., A.J. Young, R.C. Dennis, R.R. Gonzalez, K.B. Pandolf and C.R. Valeri. Human intravascular immunoglobulin responses to exercise-heat and hypohydration. *Aviat. Space Environ. Med.* 60:634-638, 1989b.

Sawka, M.N., A.J. Young, R.P. Francesconi, S.R. Muza and K.B. Pandolf. Thermoregulatory and blood responses during exercise at graded hypohydration levels. *J. Appl. Physiol.* 59:1394–1401, 1985b.

Senay, L.C. Relationship of evaporative rates to serum Na^+, K^+ and osmolarity in acute heat stress. *J. Appl. Physiol.* 25:149–152, 1968.

Senay, L.C. Temperature regulation and hypohydration: a singular view. *J. Appl Physiol.* 47:1–7, 1979.

Senay, L.C. and M.L. Christensen. Changes in blood plasma during progressive dehydration. *J. Appl. Physiol.* 20:1136–1140, 1965.

Senay, L.C. and M.L. Christensen. Respiration of dehydrating men undergoing heat stress. *J. Appl. Physiol.* 22:282–286, 1967.

Serfass, R.C., G.A. Stull, J.F. Alexander and J.L. Ewing. The effects of rapid weight loss and attempted rehydration on strength and endurance of the handgripping muscles in college wrestlers. *Res. Quart.* 55:46–52, 1984.

Shapiro, Y., K.B. Pandolf, R.F. Goldman. Predicting sweat loss response to exercise, environment and clothing. *Eur. J. Appl. Physiol.* 48:83–96, 1982.

Sherman, W.M., M.J. Plyley, R.L. Sharp, P.J. Van Handle, R.M. McAllister, W.J. Fink and D.L. Costill. Muscle glycogen storage and its relationship with water. *Int. J. Sports Med.* 3:22–24, 1982.

Singer, R.N. and S.A. Weiss. Effects of weight reduction on selected anthropometric, physical, and performance measures in wrestlers. *Res. Quart.* 39:361–369, 1968.

Silva, N.L. and J.A. Boulant. Effects of osmotic pressure, glucose and temperature on neurons in preoptic tissue slices. *Am. J. Physiol.* 247 R335–R345, 1984.

Sjogaard, G. Water and electrolyte fluxes during exercise and their relation to muscle fatigue. *Acta Physiol. Scand.* 128 (Suppl. 556):129–136, 1986.

Smith, J.H., S. Robinson and M. Pearcy. Renal responses to exercise, heat and dehydration. *J. Appl. Physiol.* 4:659–665, 1952.

Sproles, C.B., D.P. Smith, R.J. Byrd and T.E. Allen. Circulatory responses to submaximal exercise after dehydration and rehydration. *J. Sports Med. Phys. Fit.* 16:98–105, 1976.

Stephenson, L.A., A. Tripathi, C.B. Wenger, J.R. Bove and E.R. Nadel. Plasma volume expansion during hypovolemic exercise (Abst.). *Fed. Proc.* 42:585, 1983.

Strauss, R.H., J.E. Wright, G.A.M. Finerman and D.H. Catlin. Side effects of anabolic steroids in weight-trained men. *Physician Sportsmed.* 11:87–96, 1983.

Strydom, N.B. and L.D. Holdsworth. The effects at different levels of water deficit on physiological responses during heat stress. *Int. Z. Angew. Physiol.* 26:95–102, 1968.

Strydom, N.B. and C.H. Wyndham and C.H. van Graan et al. The influence of water restriction on the performance of men during a prolonged march. *S. Afr. Med. J.* 40:539–544, 1966.

Tipton, C.M. and T.K. Tcheng, Iowa wrestling study: weight loss in high school students. *J.A.M.A.* 214:1269–1274, 1970.

Torranin, C., D.P. Smith and R.J. Byrd. The effect of acute thermal dehydration and rapid rehydration on isometric and isotonic endurance. *J. Sports Med. Phys. Fitness* 19:1–9, 1979.

Turlejska, E. and M.A. Baker. Elevated CSF osmolality inhibits thermoregulatory heat loss responses. *Am. J. Physiol.* 251:R749–R754, 1986.

Tuttle, W.W. The effect of weight loss by dehydration and the withholding of food on the physiologic responses of wrestlers. *Res. Quart.* 14:158–166, 1943.

Vanderwalle, H., C. Lacombe, J.C. Lelie'vre and C. Poirot. Blood viscosity after a 1-h submaximal exercise with and without drinking. *Int. J. Sports Med.* 9:104–107, 1988.

Webster, S.F., R.A. Rutt and A. Weltman. Effects of typical dehydration practices on performance. *Med. Sci. Spt. Exerc.* (Abst.) 20:S 20, 1988.

Weiner, I.M. and G.H. Mudge. Diuretics and other agents employed in the mobilization of edema fluid. In: A.G. Gilman, L.S. Goodman, T.W. Rall and F. Murad (eds.) *The Pharmacological Basis of Terapeutics.* New York: MacMillan Publishing Co., 1985, pp. 887–907.

Wenger, C.B. Heat evaporation of sweat: thermodynamic considerations. *J. Appl. Physiol.* 32:456–459, 1972.

Zambraski, E.J., D.T. Foster, P.M. Gross and C.M. Tipton. Iowa wrestling study: weight loss and urinary profiles of collegiate wrestlers. *Med. Sci. Sports* 8:105–108, 1976.

ACKNOWLEDGMENTS

The authors gratefully acknowledge Ms. Patricia DeMusis for preparing the manuscript.

The views, opinions and findings in this report are those of the authors and should not be construed as an official Department of the Army position, policy or decision, unless so designated by other official documentation. Approved for public release; distribution is unlimited.

DISCUSSION

BUSKIRK: I think that one comment that could be made is that for a number of years, we've been thinking about the matter of euhydration and exactly what it is. A number of years ago, Ladell described euhrdration as varying within 2 L, called a labile fluid volume. When we get into appraisals of what is going on, one has to measure things very precisely in terms of establishing initial water balance, and particularly if interested in exercise capacity and strength, strength endurance, anaerobic capacity, aerobic capacity, and other variables. If one considers an elevated body temperature along with hypovolemia within 2 L, one is perhaps straining our ability for detection of significant effects. There are probably subtle differences within such a frame of reference, but I wonder, are our techniques really good enough to say that significant physiological effects can be identified within labile fluid volume.

SAWKA: I think that with current technology, the measurement resolution could be better and more reproducible.

BUSKIRK: What about the availability of water when it comes from different sources? You took a look at fluid distribution in terms of the breakdown of intravascular, extravascular, and intracellular fluid, but what about release of water bound to glycogen in muscle or with water made available by various metabolic processes that perhaps would be available in most metabolically active tissues and perhaps not available in most tissues that are not as metabolically active. I don't think we've really worked out these relationships for extra water availability very well. Can you comment on this?

SAWKA: It may be that with exercise of particularly high intensity with glycogen breakdown and metabolic water release, there would be more intracellular water release. The literature comparing exercise as opposed to thermal dehydration as to the amount of extracellular water loss is, at best, inconclusive. One study showed a difference, and one study from Costill's lab showed no difference. I've thought about this and I think that perhaps more important than whether the water is lost from intracellular or extracellular space might be the amount of inactive skeletal muscle available, which can act as a fluid reservoir. With the current trend towards resistance training and skeletal muscle hypertrophy, perhaps it might be an advantage to do running activities with a little bit of extra skeletal muscle in the upper body so that you have this water reservoir to draw from. I know that Lundvall showed that if you perfused hypertonic solution into an exercising animal, the inactive muscle will give up fluids from those tissues.

COSTILL: In the mid 1970s, we did muscle biopsies on both active and inactive muscle and examined their water contents. The water content of the inactive muscles decreased during prolonged effort. So the inactive tissue does serve as a reservoir, providing fluids to maintain plasma volume. Plasma volume doesn't drop as dramatically because water can be drawn from the less active areas.

HUBBARD: It seems to me that one avoidable consequence of a long, slow dehydration is for a more defined equilibration to occur in the more severely dehydrated conditions. It would be reasonable to look at the change in plasma volume with time in the shorter, more intensive dehydration. Does this preclude the possibility that there would be shorter periods of dehydration if equilibration is not complete? I'm not sure you can control an experiment like that. You would need a time constant as you follow the change in plasma volume with time. Can you make sure you reach the minimum value? It is very difficult to especially graph water as it equilibrates in soluble fluid.

SAWKA: We recently did a study where we dehydrated subjects and then measured plasma volume 1 h and 16 h postdehydration. We found that after 1 h plasma volume was essentially the same as it was 16 h later. Thus, you may be correct, but most of those changes might occur in that first hour.

NADEL: That is a good point, Mike, because you probably remember in Nose's paper published last year about this time, we followed the changes after dehydration in both the plasma volume and the volumes in the other body fluid compartments. After only one half hour, the body fluid compartments had stabilized.

GISOLFI: How important is the water that is bound to glycogen in thermoregulation during prolonged exercise?

SAWKA: It's of some importance because if you do the calculations, approximately 400 mL of water can be made available. Regarding its relative importance to thermoregulation in exercise, I can't really comment.

CONVERTINO: This is a follow-up to Dr. Gisolfi's question. How much of that water stays in the muscle and how much of it reaches the vasculature? I'm interested in a comment that you brought up in your chapter regarding the fluid within the muscle and how might that act, particularly in a dehydration state, as a buffer to acid changes, particularly during high-intensity exercise. Does it help to protect the intracellular muscle environment, or does it pass into the vasculature to help with cardiovascular stability? Or does this fluid shift leave a smaller volume within muscle cells and a lower reservoir for buffering hydrogen?

SAWKA: I don't know that answer. There are two things concerning your question that I'd like to comment on. One is, I did not address the idea of acid-base balance with dehydration. We find no additional metabolic acidosis as indicated by blood lactate concentration with dehydration. Most of our work was low-intensity work, but we did perform one study at 70% VO_2max with prolonged dehydration. In that study we found no additional increase in blood lactate; and if anything, a slightly greater respirator alkalosis with exercise dehydration. It may be that the hyperthermia slightly increases the hyperpnea of exercise. The second is, Darrell Neufer looked at the effects of dehydration on muscle glycogen levels. First he examined the effects of exercise on glycogen utilization when subjects were dehydrated. Those experiments were inconclusive. They suggested no difference in glycogen usage during exercise when subjects were dehydrated. What was more interesting was that when subjects continued to be dehydrated at rest with adequate carbohydrate intake, there was no effect on glycogen synthesis compared to euhydration conditions.

CONVERTINO: Maybe we need to talk about or define what we mean by hypohydration or dehydration. We conduct bed-rest studies and decrease plasma volume on the order of 10–15% and then exercise individuals before and after to examine the effect of this dehydration. In one study, we found that at the same work rate after 10 days of bed-rest-induced dehydration, there was a significant increase in blood lactate. But the interesting thing is that if we corrected for the plasma volume loss due to the bed rest, and the plasma volume shift due to the exercise bout that we had the subjects performing, there was no difference in the accumulated total circulating lactate, suggesting that an absence of fluid in a dehydration state may contribute to decreases in buffer reservoir. It may put the individual at somewhat of a disadvantage in terms of high-intensity exercise.

SAWKA: It is surprising that most investigators don't see higher lactates with dehydration, although I'm sure there are studies that do that I'm not aware of. If you look at exercise in heat as opposed to a comfortable environment, with exercise in the heat there is generally a greater lactate accumulation and perhaps greater glycogen breakdown. If you do an experiment in a comfortable to hot environment, you get a much higher body core temperature when dehydrated. But you do not get the extra accumulation of plasma lactate.

NADEL: Your original question, Carl, had to do with the importance of water production associated with glycogenolysis. One of my students did a calculation for some experiments that are currently in progress. He figured that at 120 min of moderate exercise, using the respiratory exchange ratio to partition the use of glucose and free fatty acids, and assuming all the glucose oxidation was from muscle glycogen (which is not quite true), he calculated the production of muscle water from glycogen was about 300 g. The total body water loss in that 2-hour period was about 3% of body weight, so in a 70-kg person that would have been about 2 kg of body water loss. Therefore, about 300 g of water was released within the muscle tissue. He also calculated, based on glucose oxidation and free fatty acid oxidation, that there was about another 200–300 g of water produced as a byproduct of metabolism. So the question then becomes, does this water serve any function? I'm not sure, because water follows solute movement in any case. It may help to replace some of the water lost by evaporation.

SCHEDL: I was interested in the possible correlation between where the water is lost, that is the organs from which the water is lost during stress and the temperature of the particular organ. Would the liver lose less water because its temperature does not rise with the exercise? Is there some effect of increasing organ temperature on increasing membrane fluidity, and increasing fluid loss? Temperature alters membrane enzymes. Can you correlate organ temperature and water movement?

SAWKA: The only experiments that really looked at that, to my knowledge, are those by Nose and colleagues. In those experiments, they examined the water content of the liver and brain. They may have looked at the heart tissue also. In those experiments, they did wait until the animals were back to normal temperature before sacrifice. So they would have controlled any changes in body temperature. They showed that there was a defense of water in those organs and postulated the mechanisms responsible for water conservation in each organ.

SHERMAN: Concerning the glycogen and water issue, you acknowledged in your paper that the presumed constant relationship of 3–4 mL H_2O/g glycogen may not be true. The amount of water released by the active muscle tissue over a prolonged exercise period is not very much relative to the total volume of water loss due to dehydration. When Mike Plyley was at Dave Costill's laboratory, he performed a study in which people were glycogen supercompensated compared to a nonsupercompenated condition in which they exercised in heat for 90 min at 75% $\dot{V}O_2max$. He examined thermoregulation and other responses. The results suggest that if the water released from glycogen breakdown in the supercompensated stage were significant, that didn't significantly alter thermoregulation during exercise.

SAWKA: I think that with exercise, you would be at more of a disadvantage with water loss because it's important that you thermoregulate.

HARVEY: I'd like to go back to your first slide about the wrestlers losing weight. The past couple of years, we have worked with a lot of our lead wrestlers, and I can tell you that they routinely lose 2–3 kilos. On occasion, I've seen them lose 10–12 kilos within a couple of days before a match. Certainly when they're this desperate, they're using caloric deprivation as well as fluid restriction. The athletes who routinely lose 2–3 kilos wrestle very successfully, so it's not surprising that your data on strength and anaerobic performance says that there's not much of a detriment. The problem that we get into is that we tend to lose credibility with our athletes when we tell them things that aren't true. Typically, the line is, don't dehydrate, you won't perform well. Yet, the young wrestlers see the elite athletes do it all the time. Have any of the prehydration studies looked at isotonic vs. hypotonic solution and what kind of realistic timeframe since they do have 10–12 hours to do this?

SAWKA: First, I want to compliment you for making a very good point. Remember, for those of muscular strength and power activities, it wasn't necessarily the water loss that influenced how they performed. If wrestlers lose weight in the sauna or a rubber suit and go into competition, they may be at a disadvantage. But if they lose weight and live at that weight for several hours and cool down, they probably perform OK. There are studies that have looked at replacement of hypertonic and isotonic solutions. Two studies from Bodil Nielson's laboratory and one study from Michael Harrison's laboratory showed that if an individual rehydrates with a hypertonic solution, they have a higher core temperature than when they rehydrate with an isotonic solution. Again, it comes back to a point that I'd like to emphasize; we need to pay attention to plasma hyperosmolality. That's a very key factor.

COYLE: My question relates to fluid shifts. The studies of Costill and Durkot and Nose had subjects exercise to dehydrate and then they'd look at their fluid balances when they were back in a resting state. Do we know much about fluid shifts during exercise, rather than when you recover from exercise and are resting?

SAWKA: In terms of the various fluid containing compartments? Not to my knowledge; those would be very difficult experiments, although Dr. Costill's measurements were made immediately post exercise. As a result, his data might provide better insight into exercise fluid shifts than the studies of Durkot and Nose. Those, I think, would be more of an equilibrium condition. In my opinion, however, both those groups of experiments essentially showed the same thing.

GREENLEAF: I have one comment on Ed Coyle's comment in that the Austrians have now been working out a method to do a continuous estimation of changes in plasma volume using changes in the density of the plasma. I think this technique has great application for use during exercise. Ordinarily, if one utilizes Evans blue, you have one measurement at the beginning and one possibly at the end of exercise, and all we know is what happens at either end. It would be nice to know the time course of changes in plasma volume over the exercise period. This is possibly a new way to look at that. What I really was interested to ask is, do you have data indicating an increase in internal body temperature at rest in dehydrated subjects?

SAWKA: Good question. That is something that we should discuss because some of our recent studies show some thermoregulatory set point changes in dehydration. I always thought that if dehydration affects the thermoregulatory set point, you might expect resting temperature to be higher. I found the answer in looking at Mary Ann Baker's work and maybe some of Nielson's research. If you are dehydrated in a neutral environment, you have a normal core temperature at rest. When you are exposed to thermal stress or perform exercise, you start to see core temperature differences. I believe that osmolality changes are of greater influence on threshold changes and that volume changes are more important on slope changes of thermoregulatory effector responses. If you look at Suzanne Fortney's studies of iso-osmotic hypovolemia, the changes are in slope. If you look at some of her research, the osmolality changes are near threshold; and the same with our data.

NADEL: I think Sue Fortney's studies are instructive because she tried to separate the effects of increased plasma osmolality from the effects of reduced plasma volume by using an isosmotic hypovolemia and an isovolemic hypertonicity which simulate the changes in the effector responses. The other good point you made was that the changes in temperature regulation and the ability to distribute blood flow during exercise when dehydrated are really tied very closely together. I'd like to ask what you think are the primary reasons for the reduced cardiac output when dehydrated.

SAWKA: I think it's a combination of two factors. One is the reduced blood volume, or hypovolemia, and the second is the displacement of central blood volume to the cutaneous vasculature. The second factor may be more important in contributing to cardiovascular drift. The experiments that Larry Rowell did where he looked at several exercise intensities with hyperthermia might provide insight. In those experiments, the individuals were euhydrated as they increased exercise intensity, and more importantly as they had a greater thermal load they saw the reduction in cardiac output. I think that reduction in cardiac output though, is more likely to be seen in an environment where dry heat exchange is of great importance. There is another point that I wanted to make. That is, when you get into an environment where you depend on dry heat exchange, you have more blood displaced to the skin, so you are more likely to see cardiovascular instability. It may be that you'll see more syncopy and more cardiovascular instability.

NADEL: Can I follow up that question a little bit? Mine was a leading question because the question of whether a reduced cardiac output occurs when dehydrated is debatable. Rowell showed that there was a reduction of cardiac output during upright walking exercise, when the hydrostatic effects of gravity reduce the filling pressure of heart. In a study we published in 1980, we showed that in semirecumbent cycle exercise, the individuals had a lower cardiac output when hypovolemic than when normovolemic. The hypovolemia induced a similar reduction in cardiac preload as during upright exercise in the heat.

SAWKA: Good point; I agree. I think that the cardiovascular responses to cycle exercise are not the same as for treadmill exercise in the heat. During cycle exercise, you do not experience the full effects of gravity.

Cycle exercise is probably not a good model to look at central cardiovascular changes over time in the heat.

NADEL: I think Mike has answered the basic question correctly, and your question is why does the body allow this to occur. I think the answer lies in the fact that the body's two regulatory mechanisms are competing with each other. Cutaneous vasodilation acts to increase blood flow to the skin for thermoregulatory purposes. As a consequence, there is increased pooling of blood in the periphery and a reduced ability to maintain the same cardiac output in steady-state submaximal exercise. During maximal exercise, the sympathetic drive increases markedly and the cutaneous vasculature constricts. Temperature regulation is effectively shut down, and at least a part of that circulatory reserve that resides in the skin is mobilized to maintain the same maximum cardiac count. That would be at least in keeping with Rowell's concept that the maximal potential cardiac output is on the order of 60 to 70 L/min, but we can never obtain this because the filling pressure cannot be elevated to the level necessary.

LAMB: I'd like to respond to Jack Harvey's question about wrestlers. When I was at Purdue, we took a group of Purdue wrestlers and had them cycle at 40% of the maximal anaerobic power of the legs. Simultaneously, they were cycling with 25% of the maximal aerobic power of the arms. We had them do this at 60 rpm. This leads to exhaustion in about 3 minutes. We had them do this in a euhydrated state and then had them lose 5% of their body weight in a 24-hour period after which they repeated this cycling test. Out of 30 subjects, at least 29 of them had a 30–40% reduction in their high-power endurance. Then we tried rehydrating them. We tried water, glucose electrolyte beverages, and glucose polymers. We did this for five hours and endurance did not return to normal. Even after 10 hours, endurance was not normal. After 10 hours of rehydration, my guess is that the plasma volume had pretty well returned to normal. My opinion is that it's probably not the reduced plasma volume that impairs this type of performance, and I think that Vic Convertino's idea about the buffers is a good one. Finally, my son, Jason, is a high school wrestler, and I've seen him avoid dehydration and go up against opponents who look like monsters. He's almost always more successful when he dehydrates. So, my opinion is that whatever disadvangage acute dehydration causes for high-power exercise in terms of reduced physiological capacity, wrestling a smaller person who has less leverage probably outweighs the physiological disadvantages of dehydration.

HARVEY: Did you train these people prior to the cycling with their arms and legs? Were they trained in that type of exercise?

LAMB: No.

HARVEY: One of the really hard things with wrestling is that it's hard to have a standard test for wrestlers. Sometimes wrestling is an endurance event, sometimes it turns out to be isometric, sometimes it's certainly anaerobic power. So this may have been a type of exercise that was really unfamiliar to the wrestlers' systems.

LAMB: The wrestlers claimed that at the end of the exercise task, they felt as though they had just finished an exhaustive wrestling bout.

CONVERTINO: To add to that, when we did our study, we did conduct repeat tests and it is very reproducible. So even if the subjects are not accustomed to the test, they were certainly able to produce their control values.

HUBBARD: Those of us who work with experimental heat models tend to accept the proposition that there are some individuals who do not tolerate hyperthermia well and apear to suffer a decline in blood pressure as peripheral blood flow increases. These individuals tend to have heat exhaustion whereas others who are more resistant to a fall in pressure sometimes go on to extraordinary levels of hyperthermia and unfortunately suffer from heat stroke. I think in some people it involves their state of training and, perhaps, even the type of training may affect the adequacy of the shift in available cardiac output. You might appear to have very good maximum oxygen uptake, but still not be that heat tolerant.

SAWKA: Roger brought up a good point that I should have commented on. That is, when you are dehydrated, what advantage do you gain from high aerobic fitness or being heat acclimated? When Elsworth Buskirk was an investigator at our research institute, he did a study, and we did a subsequent study in 1982, that looked at the effects of heat acclimation and the dehydration response. Dehydration appears to negate the thermoregulatory advantages gained from heat acclimation and high aerobic fitness. Both Buskirk's data and my data support this. Neither study, however, advanced the question of whether either of these factors allow improved exercise endurance. It is well known that competitive marathon runners compete at very high internal temperatures that most normal people could not tolerate.

2

Influence of Thirst and Fluid Palatability on Fluid Ingestion During Exercise

ROGER W. HUBBARD, PH.D.

PATRICIA C. SZLYK, PH.D.

LAWRENCE E. ARMSTRONG, PH.D.

INTRODUCTION

The prior chapter addressed the question of what magnitude of body water deficit would adversely affect exercise performance. It exposed the complex interrelationship between hydration status (euhydration, hypohydration, and dehydration), environmental heat stress, thermoregulation, and physiological strain. Although a great deal of experimental evidence was presented on the consequences of hypohydration, the causes were described generally as either the nonavailability of fluids (involuntary dehydration) or the commonly observed mismatch between water deficit and intake (voluntary dehydration).

Most physiologists would agree that repaying the water debt incurred through evaporative cooling is part of the physiological cost of work in the heat. Pitts and coworkers (1944) emphasized that during work in the heat, men never voluntarily drink as much water as they lose and usually replace only two thirds of the net water loss. Rothstein et al. (1947) observed that this occurred even when water was available, and called this phenomenon "voluntary dehydration." Explaining why this occurs draws upon knowledge within the domains of behavioral psychologists, biologists, physiologists, biochemists, endocrinologists, physical chemists, and even evolutionists and will occupy a major portion of this chapter. Some physiologists feel that voluntary dehydration occurs "because thirst is an 'inadequate stimulus' to drinking" (Ladell, 1965). On the other hand, Vokes (1987) contends "One of the best examples of a perfectly functioning homeostatic system is water balance." One of our goals is to reconcile the fact that under certain conditions, both of these statements are correct.

We will also try to switch the reader's interest from water to salt for, without an understanding of water and salt balance, we cannot appreciate the essential nature of our reservoir within, the *milieu interieur* of Claude Bernard. It is almost intuitive that the body "leaks," primarily water as sweat (approximately 98.8% water by weight). It is not as obvious that as cells "leak" sodium (Na^+) and potassium (K^+) across the cell membrane (down their electrochemical gradients), and the rates of this leakage can alter cellular energy demand (level?) and, potentially, cellular volume. It is this fact that may, in part, account for such diverse phenomena as hormone release, behavioral change, physiological strain, and heat stroke mortality (Hubbard and Armstrong, 1988; Hubbard et al., 1987). For, although man may drink, "water cannot be held until the missing osmoles are made good" (Ladell, 1965). This may emerge as one explanation as to why "thirst is inadequate."

The first chapter has provided clear examples of "as the level of body water loss increases, a proportionately greater percentage of the water deficit comes from the intracellular space" (Sawka and Pandolf, 1990). Is this true or an artifact of sampling times? Does it suggest that more solute is lost from the intracellular space, also? It is certainly difficult to equate with the fact that water distributes across cell membranes according to the amount of impermeant solute within each compartment (Peters, 1944; MacKnight and Leaf, 1977).

There is also good evidence to claim that increased muscle temperature reduces muscular endurance and is inversely related to anaerobic performance (Chapter 1). Increases in core temperature, along with Na^+ concentration and other physical factors such as ultra violet light (Cook, 1965) or viruses (Knutton et al., 1976), increase the permeability of cells to Na^+ (MacKnight and Leaf, 1977). The Na^+ pump adjusts its activity and, therefore, the metabolism of the cell to balance the rate of entry. This pump accounts for a substantial percentage of the oxygen consumption (Whittam, 1962) of the cell (~30%). Thus, it is difficult to understand how hypohydration "does not influence the rate of aerobic or anaerobic metabolism during exercise" (Chapter 1). These apparent inconsistencies are sure to stimulate a "thirst" for further inquiry but, first, what is thirst?

THIRST AND FLUID CONSUMPTION

Thirst As A Drive To Drink: The Water Demand

Common sense would dictate that it is quite useless to estimate a "normal" fluid intake because we are dealing with a homeostatic system designed to equate water requirements with the various losses (respiratory, urinary, skin, and sweat). Let us look briefly at these as a partial inventory of our water demand. The evaporative loss by a non-sweating man comprises the respiratory water loss and the insensible perspiration and is called the insensible water loss (Ladell, 1965). It is not really possible to give a firm figure for either the respiratory water loss or for the insensible perspiration, because the lower the atmospheric water-vapor pressure, the greater the loss. Although the temperature and humidity of the expired air does not vary greatly (Osborne, 1913), the increased water (90% saturated) content (Burch, 1945; McCutchan and Taylor, 1951) relative to the inspired air represents an inevitable loss. Under normal conditions, respiratory water loss is about 200 mL per day but may be around 350 mL per day for men working in a dry climate. It may approach 1500 mL per day for men working at altitude in cold air (Ladell, 1965). Insensible water loss may be as low as 600 mL per day in a temperate climate. With a minimum urine volume (800 mL/day), a minimum fluid intake of about 1700 mL/day is required to maintain water balance (Guyton, 1986).

Obligatory urine volume varies with diet. It is high on a high protein diet and low on a high carbohydrate diet. A reasonable figure for urine volume represents a maximum of 1.4 osmoles of metabolic end-products (mostly urea and surplus electrolytes) per liter of urine on a mixed European-style diet. This, the greatest rate of water loss, by far, is represented in a healthy individual by eccrine sweating which most physiologists would agree can be sustained at something over 1L/h under certain environmental/exercise conditions. This rate of water loss is sustainable in principle because gastric emptying, the limiting factor in intake, has been estimated between 15 to 20 mL/min or 900 to 1200 mL/h[1] (Davenport, 1982).

Thus, for soldiers working hard in a hot climate, a logistical planning factor of 13 quarts of drinking water per man per day (TB Med 507, 1980) is not unreasonable. Since one cannot be "trained" to get by on decreasing amounts of water (Johnson, 1964), how does thirst insure an adequate water intake? According to Ladell (1965), "thirst is primarily a sensation, which often serves as a drive to drink, but the drive and the sensations are not necessarily identical." Let us first examine the notion of a "drive" which could simply mean the body's ability to titrate the net gain or loss of some substance necessary for life. Table 2-1 provides our concept of some common drives, such as the drives for oxygen, carbohydrate or food, water, and salt as Na^+ and K^+ chlorides.

We hypothesize that the strength or intensity of a drive like thirst is inversely proportional to the rate of disappearance ($Rate_{DIS}$) of the factor or substance in question. Thus, the drive to breathe is very strong because oxygen in the blood stream is reduced so rapidly (3.3-3.4 min?) when breathing ceases. (This scenario ignores the obvious role of hyper-

TABLE 2-1. *Common Drives*

Substance	Drive	Disappearance Rate	Clinical Threshold	Symptoms
Oxygen	Breathing	258 mL/min	Minutes	Fainting
Glucose	Hunger	11 Kcal/min	90-180 min	Hypoglycemia
(Glycogen)			at 70% VO^2_{max}	Fatigue
Water	Thirst	1422 mL/h_{Urine}	2-3% BW loss	Hypohydration
		1-1.5 L/h_{Sweat}	in 90-180 min	
Sodium	Hunger	80-560$mmol/d_{Urine}$	Hours-days	Hypotension
		7-70mEq/L_{Sweat}	(~500 mEq ? 8h?)	
Potassium	?Hunger	40 mEq/h_{Urine}	~500mEq?	Fatigue
		3-4 mEq/L_{Sweat}	Hours-days?	

capnia in producing hyperventilation.) From this perspective, the drive to replace carbohydrate in the form of blood glucose or muscle glycogen could be imagined as, at least, 1 to 2 orders of magnitude less (e.g. 90-180 min at an exercise rate of 70% $\dot{V}O_2$max) than for breathing (1-3 min).

Interestingly, the drive to replace water (given a 2–3% body weight loss threshold at a 1.0 L/h sweat rate) would be roughly equivalent to the drive to replace carbohydrates. This may establish some basis for man's well known custom of replacing most of his water deficit at mealtime (Figure 2-1). Note how well the current estimate for gastric empyting agrees with the kidneys' ability to excrete excess fluid (1200 mL/h intake

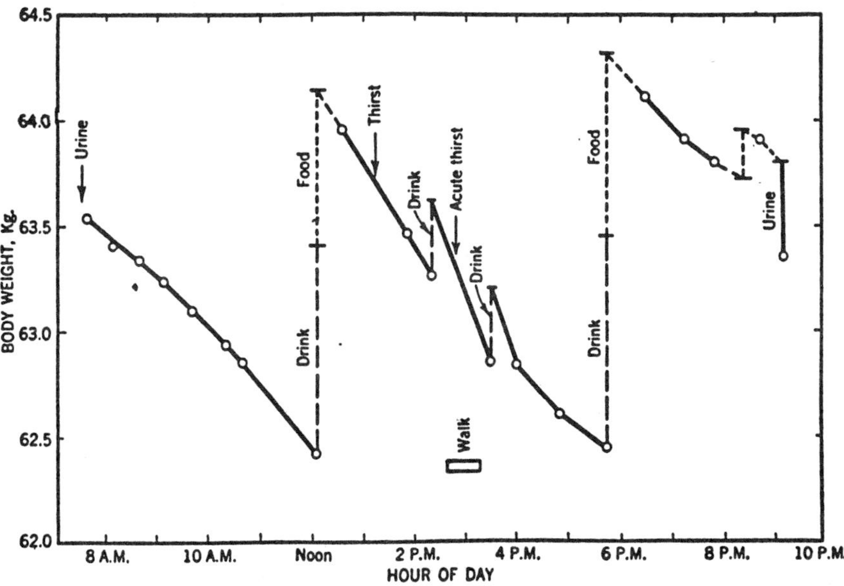

FIGURE 2-1. *Changes in body weight of one man during one day in the desert, August 19, 1942. Routine camp activities, with brief walk in the afternoon, were performed. (Reprinted with permission from Adolph, E.F. Heat exchanges, sweat formation, and water turnover,* Physiology of Man in the Desert.)

vs 1422 mL/h urine production). The maximum rate of water loss by the kidneys in overdrinking is directly correlated with the glomerular filtration rate and the solute load (Kleeman et al., 1956). In the absence of antidiuretic hormone (ADH), as in overdrinking, nearly all of the urine that reaches the distal tubules is excreted (Welt and Nelson, 1952). This is the maximum rate of water loss by the kidneys no matter how much water is drunk. In Kleeman's (1956) subjects, this rate was equivalent to 23.7 mL/min or 1422 mL/h.

Thirst and Voluntary Dehydration

Several classical studies (Pitts et al., 1944; Rothstein et al., 1947; Sohar et al., 1962) have reported that, when working in desert heat, men do not voluntarily replace all of the water losses incurred due to sweating. Adolph and coworkers (1947) called this phenomenon voluntary dehydration, and reported that many factors can modify the intensity of voluntary dehydration. For example, dehydration (process of water loss) or hypohydration (body water loss) increase with elevated sweat rates induced by high ambient temperatures or work level, inadequate time allowed for rehydration, and the effort involved in acquiring water (Adolph, 1947; Rothstein et al., 1947).

Thirst and Fluid Palatability

The palatability of drinking beverages also significantly contributes to rehydration, because the quality, flavor, and temperature are important factors determining consumption (Adolph, 1947; Armstrong et al., 1985; Boulze et al., 1983; Hubbard et al., 1984; Rothstein et al., 1947; Sohar et al., 1962; Szlyk et al., 1987; Szlyk et al., 1989; Szlyk et al., 1989b). Organoleptic characteristics of water such as turbidity, color, odor, temperature, and taste affect human senses, and therefore, are critical to palatability and intake. Prevalence of one or more of these less desirable characteristics can result in beverages so offensive that individuals refuse to drink. Of primary concern are the effects of palatability of drinking water on fluid consumption during physical work in temperate and hot climates because of the physiological decrements and increased risk of heat injury associated with body water loss (Adolph, 1947).

Thirst, Fluid Temperature, and Consumption

The significant impact of water temperature on drinking behavior is depicted in Figure 2-2. Data from our studies (Armstrong et al., 1985; Hubbard et al., 1984; Szlyk et al., 1989; Szlyk et al., 1989b) show that increasing water temperature dramatically reduced intake (upper panel) and that the primary effect occurred during the first 2 (2 h) of a series of 6 work/rest cycles (lower panel). We interpret these findings to mean that as the heat/exercise trial continues, physiological factors (e.g. sweating, solute loss, change in plasma osmolality) may eventually override behavioral preferences, particularly when only warm water is available (Armstrong et al., 1987).

Boulze and colleagues (1983) observed that when rating the preference for water ranging in temperature from 0° to 50°C, maximum intake for 15 sec of drinking occurred between 15°–22°C, while consumption of cooler and warmer water was reduced. While very cold water (0°C) was rated as the most pleasurable, cool water (15°C) was consumed in greater quantities. Their results concur with earlier findings (Adolph, 1947; Sohar et al., 1962) that 15°C is the preferred temperature for consumption, particularly when large quantities must be drunk to reduce dehydration. In comparison, our data (Figure 2-2) show that for periods of up to 6 h, maximum consumption occurred at 22°C.

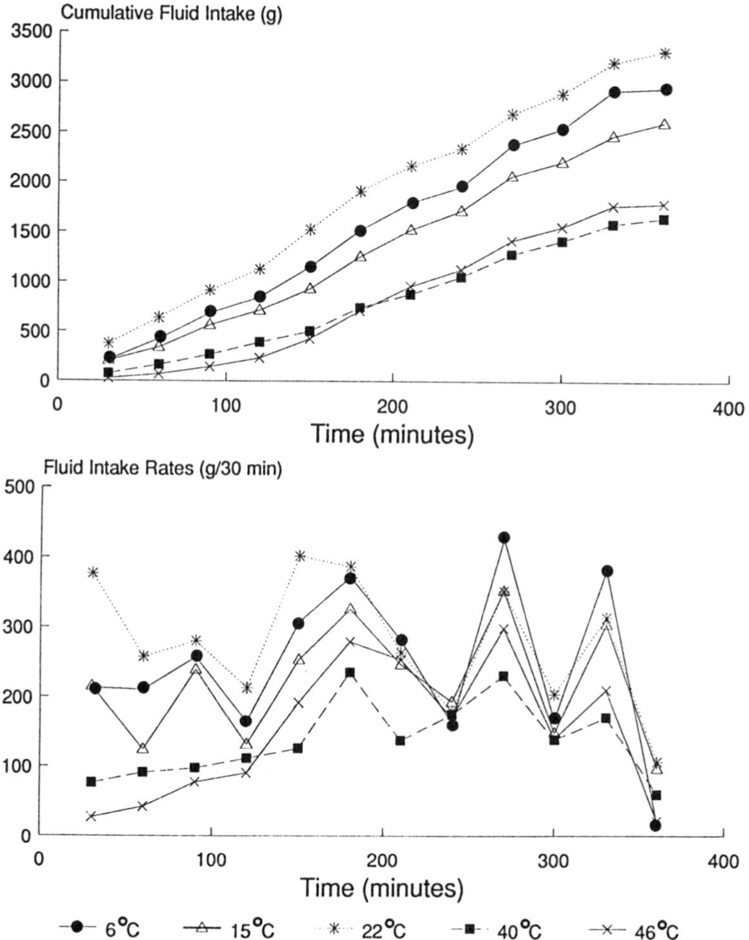

FIGURE 2-2. *Cumulative water consumption (upper panel) and intake rate (lower panel) of groups drinkings 6° (n=8), 15° (n=33), 22° (n=8), 40° (n=33), and 46°C (n=8) water. For cumulative intake: 6°=15°≠22°≠40°=46°C during all work and rest periods.*

Dehydration, Beverage Temperature Preference, and The Consumption Paradox

Sandick and coworkers (1984) observed that subjects tend to perceive extreme water temperatures (5° and 38°C) as colder and hotter following exercise than when sedentary. After exercise, cool water temperatures received even higher preference ratings while a greater dislike was reported for hot water, and preference ratings tracked fluid intake during rest and exercise. Cabanac (1971) demonstrated that a stimulus could be perceived as pleasant or unpleasant, depending upon the internal status of an individual. Boulze (1983) and Hubbard et al. (1984) reported that when subjects were dehydrated, they manifested an increased pleasure for drinking cold water and an increased displeasure for drinking hot water. Thus, greater intake in subjects consuming cool water was explained by an increased preference for cold water, whereas *the apparent paradox* of reduced consumption in dehydrated and hyperthermic individuals was attributed to increased displeasure for warm/hot water.

If thirst is mediated predominantly by receptors responding to changes in either osmolaltiy or an increased Na^+ concentration or even extracellular fluid volume, why do exercising subjects drink less warm water when dehydrated and more cool water when not dehydrated? Perhaps this paradox could be explained if the cellular energy state in some way impacted thirst. For example, behaviors that would improve the cellular energy state (drinking cool water when exercising in the heat) would be reinforced and behaviors that are thought to increase the energy demand (drinking hot water when exercising in the heat; Q_{10} effect) would be inhibited. This intriguing speculation suggests a research pathway to be explored.

Fluid Flavoring and Consumption

Increased fluid intake has been elicited by flavoring (cherry, raspberry, citrus) both cool and warm water (Hubbard et al., 1984; Sohar et al., 1962; Szlyk et al., 1987; Szlyk et al., 1989). Rothstein (1947) reported that some flavors (grape, lemon, orange) were popular when small weight deficits had been incurred, particularly when warm or salted, unpalatable water was available. However, as judged by intake, none of the flavorings was more palatable than cool, pure water (Rothstein et al., 1947). Sohar and colleagues (1962) reported that soldiers marching in the desert heat preferred cold flavored drinks when large quantities of fluid had to be rapidly (15–20 min) consumed. Although these investigators (Sohar et al., 1962) observed that flavoring may enhance intake for short periods of time, beverages (e.g., milk, beer, carbonated drinks) typically consumed with meals or at leisure (recreational drinks) were unacceptable during exercise, or when large quantities had to be consumed. We observed that, during 6 h of intermittent treadmill walking, subjects consumed more flavored than plain water (Hubbard et al., 1984; Szlyk et al., 1989). In these experiments, fluid consumption of both cool (15°C) and warm (40°C) water was enhanced about 50% when flavoring was introduced. In addition, in a scenario of 6 consecutive walk/rest cycles (30/30 min each), flavoring encouraged a greater fluid consumption during the walks, particularly when the beverage was warm (Szlyk et al., 1989). It should be noted, however, that "flavoring" is synonomous, in most cases, with carbohydrate as an energy source.

Predicted Preference Versus Measured Intake

Sohar and colleagues (1962) concluded that what men actually drink when working in hot climates is not always what they originally believed they would drink. Zellner and colleagues (1988) recently reported that individuals' expectations and concepts of appropriateness influence their preference for drinks at certain temperatures. In addition, the sensory perception of beverages can be affected by modifying expectations. For example, although we expect beverages at inappropriate temperatures to be unpalatable, and may rate them as such, following consumption we rate them more favorably. Potable water is generally disinfected by chlorine or iodine, making it suitable for human consumption but contributing to nonpalatability. Hubbard et al. (1984) suggested that availability of such water would reduce fluid intake during hot weather events and increase the risk of dehydration. Surprisingly, although subjects complained about the poor taste and irritating odor of disinfected water, no statistical difference in intake of plain water versus chlorinated (Armstrong et al., 1985) or iodinated (Hubbard et al., 1984) water was observed, when water temperatures ranged from 6° to 46°C during 6 hours of intermittent exercise.

Sohar and colleagues (1962) had earlier hypothesized that dehydration during work in the heat would be reduced if pleasant-tasting drinks were provided. However, under conditions of high sweat and electrolyte loss, Ladell (1965) suggested that *water cannot be retained and rehydration is incomplete, until the solute lost in sweat is replaced.* Although our studies did not specifically address Ladell's hypothesis, Figure 2-3 shows that food consumption (lunch) elicited increase in fluid intake rates for most water temperatures relative to pre-lunch levels especially where a prior temperature-induced water deficit has accrued (Szlyk et al., 1989b). Following lunch, average fluid consumption rate moderated, but remained 4–133% higher than pre-lunch levels. While food consumption has been encouraged to replace electrolytes lost in sweat during work in the heat, our results also indicate that food consumption, with its attendant osmolar and caloric load, may also provide further impetus to fluid consumption (Szlyk et al., 1989b).

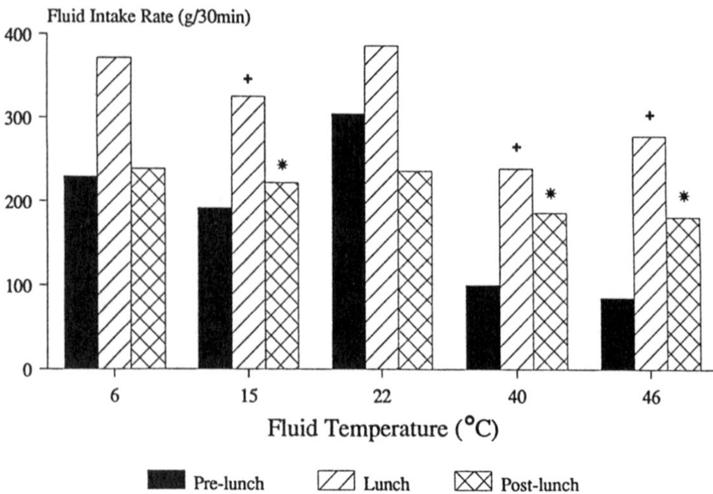

FIGURE 2-3. *Fluid intake rate (g/30 min) during pre-lunch, lunch, and post-lunch during the 5 water temperature trials. Significant differences ($p < 0.05$) between pre-lunch and lunch are indicated by +; between pre-lunch and post-lunch by **

Influence of Exercise on Drinking Behavior

When humans exercise, they must deal with several factors that are not present at rest. These factors (e.g. mental distractions, coordination, internal fluid shifts) indicate that exercise *per se* may change drinking behavior. Despite this fact, the literature involving drinking behavior during exercise is minimal and often inconclusive.

Considering the effect of continuous exercise and/or rest on drinking behavior, Adolph and colleagues (1947) were pioneers during their desert studies of 1941–42. They reported the fluid intakes of eight soldiers at work in the desert sun (maximum temperature 105°F), noting that they ingested 7.5 L of fluid per day and formed less than 1 L of urine of normal specific gravity. Interestingly, these men replaced lost fluids more adequately during meals and rest periods than during field exercises (Figure 2-1). However, no systematic observations were undertaken, in the field or in the laboratory, to clarify the effect of exercise *per se* on drinking behavior and thirst.

Thirst—Independent of The Rate of Water Loss?

Greenleaf and colleagues (1965) have conducted subsequent observations, including the *ad libitum* drinking data that we have redrawn in Figure 2-4. This figure indicates a curious finding in that rest trials (square symbols) involved a more positive water balance than exercise trials (circular symbols), during both the hydrated phase (open symbols) and the dehydrated phase (closed symbols). Although these data agree in

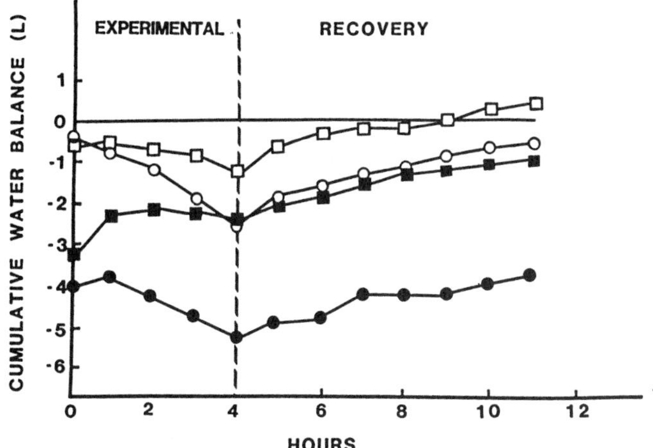

FIGURE 2-4. *Cumulative water balance (L) during 4-hour* ad libitum *water trials in a hot environment (49°C, 25% rh), and recovery in a cool environment (24°C, 25% rh). Exercise involved treadmill walking at 6.4 km/h, 0% grade. Redrawn from Greenleaf* et al., *1965.*

principle with the findings of Adolph (1947), the rate of sweat loss during exercise was not balanced by consumption. This suggests that thirst is independent of the *rate* of water loss. Further, the rate of rehydration during recovery appears to be independent of the *magnitude of the deficit* (greatest in the exercise-dehydrated condition). These curious results could be explained if a factor necessary to stimulate thirst (solute in sweat) had been lost at a greater rate during the exercise trials than at rest.

Thirst, Exercise, and Gastric Emptying

Gastric distention may play a role in drinking behavior during continuous exercise. Gastric emptying during exercise varies among subjects and may result in differences in the "fullness" sensation emanating from the stomach. Figure 2-5, published by Neufer et al. (1986), presents the differences in gastric emptying for runners who drank equal volumes of three solutions: water, 3% maltodextrin + 2% glucose (MG5.0), and 4.5% maltodextrin + 2.6% fructose (MF7.1). After ingesting 1 solution, subjects either sat quietly for 15 min or ran continuously on a treadmill for 15 min (at 50 to 70% $\dot{V}O_2$max). Clearly, the amount of fluid leaving the stomach was greater during exercise than at rest for all solutions. The authors hypothesized that this may have been due to an increased

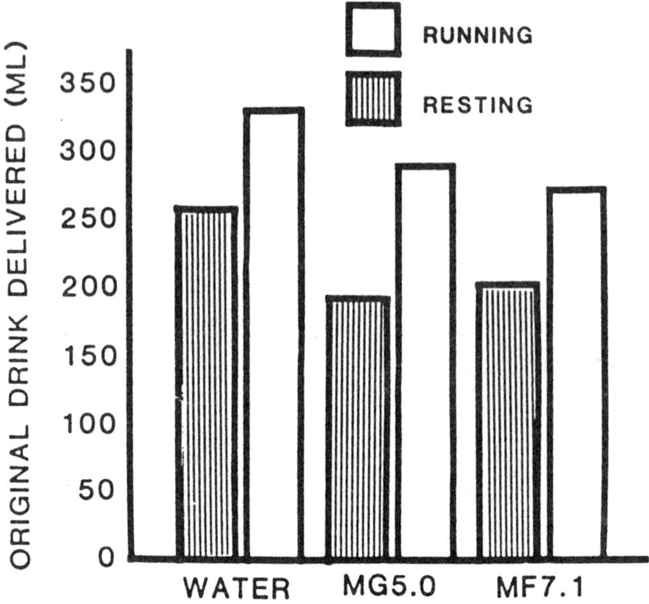

FIGURE 2-5. *Mean volumes (mL) of original drink delivered from the stomach to the system for 3 test drinks, following 15 min seated rest or 15 min running (50 to 70% VO_2max). All values for running are significantly greater ($p<0.05$) than values for seated rest. The phrase "original drink delivered" is equivalent to gastric emptying rate. Redrawn from Neufer, 1986.*

mechanical movement of fluid within the stomach during the continuous running trials.

Water Intake: Continuous vs Intermittent Exercise

In considering the impact of intermittent exercise, Figure 2-6 offers a unique presentation of the data from 2 investigations presented in Figure 2-2 (Armstrong et al., 1985; Szlyk et al., 1989). Each bar represents the mean (± SE) water intake of at least 8 trials conducted during 6-h simulated desert marches (4.82 km/h, 5% grade, 14.5 km total distance, 724 m climbed in 6 h). These simulated marches involved 30 min of exercise and 30 min of rest per hour. The total water consumed during all exercise and rest periods have been plotted separately. In contrast to the Greenleaf and Sargent (1965) data presented in Figure 2-4, the *ad libitum* rate of water intake during successive 30-min exercise periods was greater than during rest periods. This illustrates a primary difference between continuous experiments that involve either rest or exercise for a short duration, and experiments that include intermittent exercise for longer durations. In addition, the interaction between water tempera-

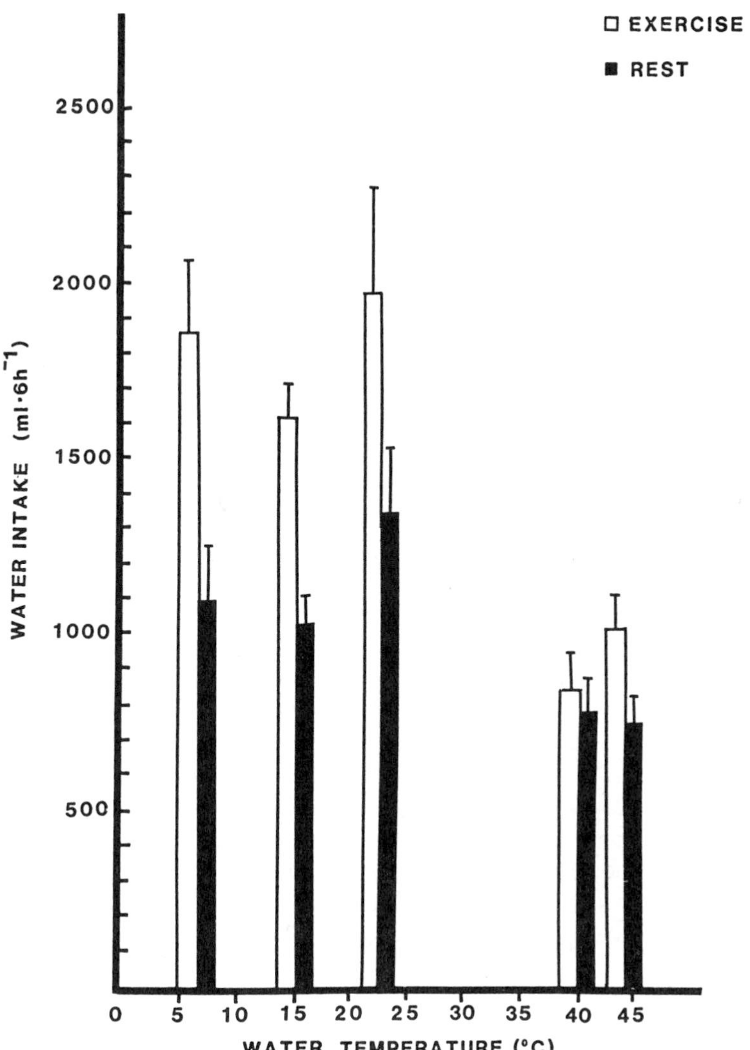

FIGURE 2-6. *Effect of rest versus exercise on total water intake (mL) during 30-min rest and exercise periods. Total trial duration was 6 hours. Redrawn from Figure 2-2.*

ture and water consumption during intermittent exercise is illustrated in Figure 2-6. Clearly, cooler water temperatures (<25°C) increased the rate of water intake during successive exercise bouts. This reinforces the concept (alliesthesia) that a stimulus can be perceived as pleasant or unpleasant depending on the intensity of the stimulus and the internal state of the individual (Cabanac, 1971). Thus, the higher consumption of cool water during walks compared to rest periods probably resulted from a greater preference for cool water during exercise (Hubbard et al., 1984; Szlyk et al., 1989b). The subjects who received 40° and 46°C water drank much less water than those who received cooler water. Although cooler temperature water (e.g. 6°, 15°, and 22°C) resulted in relatively large differences between exercise and rest periods, the 40° and 46°C water decreased the difference in water intake between exercise and rest periods probably as a result of the negative alliesthesia for warm water (Cabanac, 1971; Hubbard et al., 1984; Szlyk et al., 1989b).

Thirst and Rehydration: A Search For Mechanisms

Regarding the mechanism that controls drinking behavior, Greenleaf and colleagues published a report in 1966 (Greenleaf et al., 1966) that statistically evaluated the stimuli to an immediate drinking response during exercise. In this study, a statistical analysis of 22 physiological variables was performed using 87 young soldiers undergoing 6 days of basic training in a warm, humid environment. Mean daily water intake (range: 1.950 to 5.850 L/d^{-1}) during exercise was more strongly related to variables associated with water deficit (i.e. sweat rate, mean daily urine volume) and solute loss (i.e. mean daily urinary K^+ or Cl^-) than to variables associated with the osmotic concentration of the body fluids (i.e. serum osmolarity, serum Na^+). A stepwise multiple linear regression analysis also suggested that the body's osmoreceptors reacted to the osmotic concentration of the blood rather than to the concentrations of the major serum ions (e.g. Na^+, K^+, Cl^-). Sweat rate (total body weight change per 24 h) was the only variable that was directly correlated ($p<0.05$) to mean daily water intake in this study (Greenleaf et al., 1966), but because a complete data base was not published, it is not clear which of four possible interpretations (e.g., the rate of water loss, the rate of solute loss, the total volume deficit, or the total solute deficit) was related to rehydration.

Rehydration: Osmolality as a Primary Factor

These data prompted Greenleaf, in a 1982 review, to conclude that satiation of drinking behavior is not strongly influenced by plasma dipsogenic factors. These dipsogenic factors may, however, *initiate* drinking. Our investigation of fluid intake during the heat acclimation of running subjects (Armstrong et al., 1989; Armstrong et al., 1986) (described below) supports this concept. Multiple linear regression correlations indicated that sweat rate ($r^2 = 0.40$), defined as total body weight change per 100 min trial, and final plasma osmolality ($r^2 = 0.46$) were the variables that were most strongly (but not significantly) correlated with water intake. Other factors (i.e. body weight, $r^2 = 0.15$; VO_2max, $r^2 = 0.19$; final serum K^+, $r^2 = 0.15$; change in plasma osmolality, $r^2 = 0.14$) were weakly correlated with water intake. It is interesting that the sweat rate per 100 min. and the sweat rate per 24 h (see above, Greenleaf et al., 1966), both were strongly correlated with water intake over those periods; this great difference in elapsed time (100 min vs 24 h) suggests that the mechanism that stimulates drinking behavior is the same in both short-term and long-term situations.

Rehydration: Acclimation and Hormonal Influences

In 1983, Greenleaf et al. introduced their data by noting that animal research has identified two general systems that regulate drinking: a sodium ion-osmotic-vasopressin (SOV) pathway and a renin-angiotensin II-aldosterone (RAA) pathway; these pathways suggest primary water loss, and primary salt loss respectively. Both of these systems respond to changes in plasma volume and Na^+ concentration. Measuring hormonal influences on drinking behavior in a group of 5 men who underwent eight days of heat acclimation (39.8°C, 50% rh), they observed that plasma Na^+ and osmolality were negatively correlated with fluid intake; the greater the drinking, the lower the concentrations. This observation argued against hypernatremia or hyperosmotemia being major stimuli for total fluid intake. In contrast, plasma renin activity increased greatly throughout the heat acclimation exposures, in conjunction with reductions in total body water deficits and extracellular volume, and appeared to be the predominant mechanism for the control of fluid intake. This was an obvious departure from the generally accepted theoretical mechanism explaining drinking behavior, and may indicate that this experimental design did not allow investigators to observe the true relationships between total water deficit and rehydration.

In a prior publicaton, Greenleaf et al. (1967) indicated that 7 days of heat acclimation resulted in subjects drinking more during daily exercise-heat exposures than when they were unacclimated. As far as water balance was concerned, however, the heat acclimated subjects were no better off than unacclimated subjects. This apparent paradox (increased drinking; no change in water balance) is because heat acclimated subjects produced sweat at a higher rate, and their increased water intake merely balanced the increased losses in sweat. In a later study, Greenleaf et al. (1983) similarly demonstrated that water intake increased, subsequent to eight days of heat acclimation, from 450 to approximately 1000 mL/hr. This was due to an increase in the number of drinks per trial (4 vs 9) and the time for subjects to take their first drink (26 vs 11 min).

Figure 2-7 presents previously unpublished drinking data from a heat acclimation investigation conducted in our laboratory (Armstrong et al., 1989; Armstrong et al., 1986). Not only did the mean volume consumed (960 vs 1215 mL) increase from day 1 to day 8, but the mean number of drinks taken per trial also increased (6 vs 7). However, the subjects in this investigation exercised intermittently on a treadmill, during nine work/rest periods of 5–10 min duration; they ran or jogged at

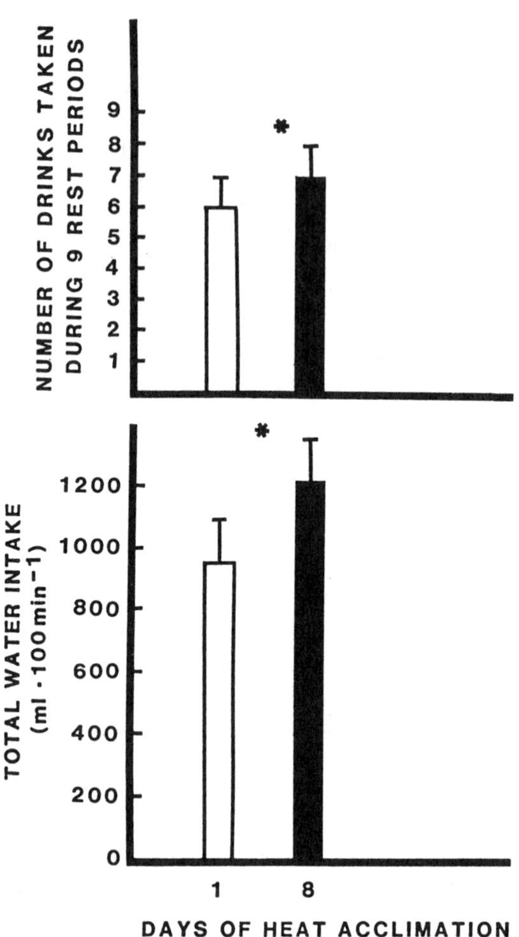

FIGURE 2-7. *Effect of intense, intermittent exercise (100 min duration) in a hot environment on total water intake (mL/100 min) and number of drinks taken.*

self-selected speeds (63.0–71.8% $\dot{V}O_2max$) and drank cool water during the nine rest periods only. In contrast, Greenleaf's heat acclimation exercise trials (Greenleaf et al., 1983; Greenleaf et al., 1967) involved either continuous treadmill walkng or ergometry for 120 min (no rest periods). This suggests that differences in the type of exercise (i.e. walking versus intermittent running) may not influence the increase in water consumption that results from successive days of exercise in a hot environment (heat acclimation).

SODIUM: THE MAJOR EXTRACELLULAR CATION

Total exchangeable Na^+ in a 70-kg man averages 41 mEq/kg (2870 mEq, total) or roughly 168 g of NaCl. About 70% of body Na^+ is exchangeable and, with its anions, accounts for over 90% of the osmolality of the extracellular fluid (ECF). The non-exchangeable portion is bound in long bones. The bones of a 70-kg man contain 35 g of pure Na^+. There may even be a relationship between Na^+ appetite and some forms of cannibalism (Denton, 1986). Cannibalism and salt depletion are common factors in the equatorial belt suggesting that cannibalism may be a means of satisfying extreme salt hunger. The clinically normal range for the concentration of serum Na^+ is 136–145 mEq/L (Marcus, 1962).

Sodium Concentration May Not Reflect Sodium Stores

During dehydration, the dynamic state of water and salt losses, a Na^+ deficit often develops, which results in hyponatremia. Since the actual concentration of Na^+ in the ECF depends on the relative losses of salt and water versus their intakes, a normal serum Na^+ or even hypernatremia can occur in Na^+ deficient states. Thus, hyponatremia and Na^+ deficiency are not synonymous terms because many hyponatremic states are of the dilutional variety associated with normal or even excessive body Na^+ stores (Vaamonde, 1982).

Sodium Deficiency: Clinical Signs

Na^+ deficiency is estimated clinically by evaluating the signs of ECF volume loss such as circulatory status, orthostatic hypotension, and tachycardia. The hemodynamic consequences are dependent on the extent and rapidity of the developing deficit (Vaamonde, 1982). For example, in acute severe Na^+ deficiency (Elkinton et al., 1946), with deficits producing a 20–40% contraction in the ECF Na^+ concentration or ECF volume (300–500 mEq Na^+), there are significant reductions in mean blood pressure (30–80%) and cardiac output (60–80%), with concomitant increases (50–200%) in total peripheral vascular resistance (PVR). The rapid loss of Na^+ results in a rapid decline in ECF osmolality, the movement of ECF water into cells to balance the osmolalities of the extracellular compartments, and a decline in plasma volume. Because of systemic peripheral vasoconstriction, there is a decreased renal function, oliguria, and possibly azotemia.

In contrast, when marked Na^+ depletion (500–600 mEq) occurs chronically over days (McCance, 1936), the hemodynamic changes are less impressive with tachycardia and a modest decline in orthostatic tolerance. Thus, mild orthostatic intolerance can represent either a moderate (<200 mEq) acute Na^+ loss or a severe, chronic deficit (600 mEq). The renin-angiotensin system, especially angiotensin II, plays a key role in blood pressure support, as indicated by inhibitor studies in animals and man with saralasin (Johnson and Davis, 1973; Posternak et al., 1977; Samuels et al., 1976). There is also considerable evidence that the adrenergic system is activated in Na^+ depletion with increased plasma levels and urinary excretion of nonrepinephrine (Alexander et al., 1974; Cuche et al., 1972; Kelsch et al., 1971).

Sodium Intake: Hedonic and Geographical Variables

In humans, the hedonic desire for salt exceeds need, as most fast-food providers are aware. The stimulus for Na^+ appetite is probably humoral, perhaps aldosterone and angiotensin acting synergistically (Stricker and Verbalis, 1988). Salt intake varies markedly among cultures and geographic locations from as little as 2–3 g/day in Indonesia up to 20 g/day in the United States of America (Hubbard et al., 1986). A 6 g intake of sodium chloride (NaCl, 102 mEq of Na^+) would be very similar to the average K^+ intake (110 mEq/day) (Geigy Scientific Tables, 1981). The average excretion rate for Na^+ derived from data on 106 normal American males was 224 mEq/day suggesting an intake of at least 14.2 g of NaCl. This was calculated on the assumption that about 90–95% of the Na^+ ingested is excreted in the urine (Forbes, 1962). A salt craving in humans has been associated with Addison's disease (Wilkins and Richter, 1940) and a lack of adrenal cortical cells with the loss of the ability to retain salt.

Sodium Deficiency and Heat Exhaustion

Heat exhaustion due to salt and water depletion is caused by the inadequate replacement of NaCl losses during prolonged sweating. The symptoms (Hubbard and Armstrong, 1988) include fatigue, profound weariness, muscular weakness, nausea, vomiting, giddiness, muscle cramps, and in the later stages, circulatory failure. Marriott (1950) divided the salt-depletion syndrome into three clinical grades. The first or "early" grade represented a deficit of 0.5 g NaCl/kg of body weight. This would be roughly equivalent to a 35-g deficit (~600 mEq) in a 70-kg man (Table 2-2, adapted from 64,65) or approximately equal to 4 L of isotonic saline (approximately 28% of the extracellular volume). A loss of Na^+ in excess of 500 mEq (approximately 23% of the extracellular volume) is now considered as a moderately severe to severe Na^+ deficiency (Vaamonde, 1982).

TABLE 2-2. *Sweat Volumes and Sodium Concentrations Producing a 500mEq Sodium Deficit*

Physiological State	Sweat Sodium Conc. (mEq/L)	Sweat Volume Equivalent to a 500 mEq Deficit (L)
Unacclimatized	75	6-7
Acclimatized	30	16-17

The 60% reduction in sweat Na^+ (75–30 mEq) is a typical decrease following repeated bouts of heat exposure over 8–10 days (Armstrong et al., 1987; Conn, 1949). Although renal Na^+ conservation begins early in the course of Na^+ depletion (Leaf and Couter, 1949; McCance and Widdowson, 1937), due primarily to an increased aldosterone release (Crabbe et al., 1958; Lipsett and Pearson, 1958), the reduced sweat concentrations of Na^+ in the acclimatized individual represent a considerable buffer against extrarenal salt losses and is one of the fundamental manifestations of the physiological phenomenon of heat acclimation. It has been reported (Richter, 1942–1943) that Na^+ deficits stimulate a salt hunger. It should be noted (Table 2-2) that a severe Na^+ deficit is theoretically achievable in the unacclimatized state with a 6–7 L sweat loss. This assumes no Na^+ intake and indicates the importance of *meal eating* in preventing this illness! Fasting, acclimatized individuals could be ill in two days of heavy sweating (16–17 L), if salt losses are not replaced.

POTASSIUM: THE MAJOR INTRACELLULAR CATION

Nearly all of body K^+ is exchangeable K^+ (45 mEq/kg or 3150 mEq in a 70 kg man). Note in Table 2-1 that the kidneys can excrete K^+ at a rate of 35–40 mmol/h (Kaplan, 1969) which is a very high percentage of the daily intake (45–110 mmol/day). Normally, about 90% of the dietary intake is excreted in the urine. The serum K^+ is normally around 4.2 (3.1–5.4) mEq/L and must be regulated across a very narrow range because the heart is possibly injured below 3 mEq/L. If intracellular K^+ is depleted, then excitable tissues show depressed function, cardiac rhythm abnormalities, muscular weakness, and impaired nerve condition. If plasma K^+ rises to 7–8 mEq/L, as in renal disease, abnormalities of cardiac electrical condition and rhythm are often seen along with reduced chronotropic and inotropic responses (Guyton, 1986). If K^+ rises above 8 mEq/L, resting membrane potentials cannot be maintained by the ion pump mechanism and ventricular fibrillation and cardiac arrest may occur (Pitts, 1968).

Potassium: Deficiency and Polyuria

The high excretion rate (Table 2-1) could help buffer any rise in K^+ due to meal eating (30–45 mEq/meal). This amount of K^+, if confined to the extracellar space, would elevate plasma levels by 2–3 mEq/L. Renal conservation of K^+ is poor in comparison with that of Na^+ (Peters, 1953) and even worse if there is a concomitant high salt intake (Squires and Huth, 1959). Knochel (1961) has suggested that K^+ depletion ($>$500 mEq deficit) is entirely consistent with some of the features of the heat disorders, notably weakness and lethargy and pitressin-resistant polyuria. Note that this is about the same magnitude ($>$500 mEq) that produces symptoms of Na^+ deficiency.

Potassium Deficiency and Acid-Base Balance

There is also a metabolic acidosis in K^+ deficiency because intracellular K^+ is replaced by Na^+ and hydrogen ions (Huth et al., 1959) which would produce an extracellular alkalosis. Christensen (1963) suggests that as Na^+ replaces cellular K^+, approximately 1 proton accompanied 2 Na^+ ions in replacing 3 K^+ ions, thereby acidifying the intracellular and alkalizing the extracellular water. A persistent extracellular alkalosis is, thus, a possible clue to K^+ depletion. Men have been reported without symptoms, however, after 16 days on 1 mEq of K^+/day and a 500 mEq deficit (Huth et al., 1959).

Potassium Balance and Dehydration

Ladell (1965) has commented that in dehydration, "When the extracellular osmotic pressure rises, K^+ comes out of the cells, possibly in exchange for Na^+ that passes into the cells with water; this K^+ is promptly excreted by the kidneys and so is lost to the body" (Elkinton and Danowski, 1948; Elkinton and Winkler, 1944). This interesting observation raises three questions: 1) Does some form of solvent drag carry K^+ out of cells in response to an osmotic challenge?; 2) If this is possible, could an osmotic stimulus such as hypertonic sucrose ever be used to clearly distinguish between an osmoreceptor and a Na^+ receptor if it facilitates a movement of Na^+ into cells? Solute diuresis is the most common cause of extrinsic renal Na^+ wasting (Vaamonde, 1982); and 3) Could the body adjust its available solute load to the existing water content by losing K^+ between meals? Since the K^+ could be replaced at the next meal more readily than Na^+ (in potatoes and peas, the K^+;Na^+ ratios are 88 and 667, respectively), the loss of K^+ could help sustain a more adequate plasma volume by increasing the plasma solute while decreasing the intracellular solute. This should facilitate the shift of water from the intracellular space while keeping the total body Na^+ to K^+ ratio more constant following salt losses in sweat. There is about a 32-fold difference between intra- and extracellular K^+ concentrations. Our short-term experiments suggest that K^+ excretion is increased in the urine during exercise in the heat (Armstrong et al., 1987).

Potassium Hunger?

As quoted in Ladell (1965), the "potash eaters" of Africa suggest the existence of a drive or hunger for K^+ (Porteres, 1950). Although K^+ is vitally important for glucose transport across membranes, glycogen storage, enzyme regulation, and muscle vasodilation, the losses of K^+ in 5-6 hours of sweating (between meals) are low compared to total body stores. It is significant to note that both hypernatremia and hypokalemia (K^+ deficiency) both stimulate thirst and both appear to cause Na^+ to enter cells.

THE CONTROL OF THIRST

Potassium Deficiency Stimulates ADH and Thirst

K^+ deficiency and hypokalemia stimulate ADH and thirst (Fourman and Leeson, 1959). It should be noted (Vokes and Robertson, 1985) that vasopressin deficiency manifests itself as polyuria. The most common clincial cause is diabetes mellitus due to glucosuria. Solute diuresis is characterized by a total daily solute excretion above 1500 mosmol/kg. If the solute diuresis is below this level and the urine is dilute ($<$250 mosmol/kg), polyuria is due to water diuresis and is referred to as diabetes insipidus. The latter comes from one of three defects: 1) Neurogenic diabetes insipidus due to decreased or absent production of ADH; 2) Dipsogenic diabetes insipidus due to suppression of ADH by high fluid intake; or 3) Nephrogenic diabetes insipidus due to a decreased or absent renal response to ADH. This suggests that the pitressin-resistant polyuria of K^+ deficiency and in a certain variant of heat exhaustion described by Horne and Mole (1949) and Ladell and colleagues (1944) is a form of nephrogenic or vasopressin-resistant diabetes insipidus (Robertson, 1987; Robertson and Berl, 1985; Vokes and Robertson, 1985).

Hypoglycemia Stimulates ADH and Thirst

It is also interesting to note that hypoglycemia stimulates the release of many hormones including vasopressin in both rats (Baylis and Robertson, 1980) and humans (Baylis et al., 1981). According to Vokes (Vokes, 1987), the mechanism is secondary to an intracellular glucopenia because a similar effect can be induced with 2-deoxyglucose (Robertson and Berl, 1985; Vokes and Robertson, 1985).

Body Solute and the Hypertonic State

Although the solute composition of the extracellular compartment is markedly different from the intracellular space, total osmolality (solute concentration, not content) is very similar (Conway and McCormack, 1953). This is because most cell membranes are freely permeable to water. The major intracellular osmotic solutes are K^+, Mg^{++}, organic phosphates, and protein. The major osmotic solutes in extracellular fluid are normally Na^+ and its anions, Cl^- and HCO_3^-. They are referred to as impermeant, but are kept on the proper side of the membrane by molecular size, electrical charge, or active pumps. Net movement of water is determined by the osmolalities of the intra- and extracellular compartments (Peters, 1944).

The osmolal concentration or osmolality (usually in milliosmol/kg water) is an indiscriminating summation of all the particles, ions, and molecules present in a solution. It is usually measured by freezing point depression or change in vapor pressure. Measured osmolality should be differentiated from effective osmolality, i.e., the concentration of solutes that will create an osmotic force *in vivo*. For example, Na^+ is the major determinant of the effective osmolality of the extracellular fluid because its concentration is high and *acts as if restricted* from entering cells (Guyton, 1986). In contrast, urea permeates cells freely and will not exert an osmotic force if elevated in either compartment. The addition of an impermeant solute to the extracellular space causes a net intracellular fluid volume depletion and creates, by definition, a hypertonic state (Feig and McCurdy, 1977). Freezing point depression does not distinguish between permeant and impermeant solutes by measuring osmolality. Thus an elevated plasma osmolality must be checked by calculation of tonicity before it is interpreted as hypertonicity. For example: 2 [plasma Na^+ (mEq/L)] + [Plasma glucose (mg/dL/18)] = approximate tonicity.

Body Water Tracks Body Solute

Normally, intracellular fluid contains about 2/3 of total body solute and the extracellular fluid contains about 1/3. Because water distributes according to the amount of impermeant solute in each compartment, the intracellular fluid contains 2/3 of total body water (TBW) and extracellular fluid 1/3 of TBW. If extracellular fluid osmolality decreases, water must enter cells and cellular volume increases; conversely, if extracellular fluid osmolality increases, due to the addition of solutes that penetrate cell membranes poorly, water must leave cells and cellular volume decreases. Thus, the basic physiological mechanisms that control the osmolality of the extracellular fluid affect cell volume.

Hypertonicity, ADH, and Thirst

In 1937, Gilman demonstrated that intravenous infusions of hyperosmotic NaCl would elicit drinking, but that equally hyperosmotic solutions of urea stimulated thirst poorly. Because urea could diffuse into cells but Na^+ would produce shrinkage, *an osmotic basis for thirst* was established. Other solutes that cause withdrawal of water from cells, such as sucrose and sorbital, were equally effective in producing thirst when infused intravenously (Holmes and Gregersen, 1950; 1950b). These observations reinforced the important role of cellular dehydration in triggering thirst and drinking behavior. The classic work of Verney (1947) demonstrated that water diuresis in dogs could be inhibited by intracarotid infusions of hypertonic NaCl and, therefore, *both thirst and antidiuresis were linked to the osmotic withdrawal of water from cells*. Verney deduced that the inhibition of water diuresis resulted from neurohypophyseal secretion of vasopressin which later work confirmed (Wade et al., 1982). According to Andersson (1978), the most potent stimulators of ADH release and thirst are absolute and relative dehydration. Although ADH is released as a function of body osmolality (Robertson and Athar, 1976; Robertson and Mahr, 1972), it is equally well correlated with plasma Na^+ (Olsson et al., 1978).

NEW HYPOTHESIS

Is The Osmoreceptor a Sodium Receptor?

Andersson (1978) suggests that Na^+ itself is the crucial factor in the osmotic control of water balance and has proposed that the centrally located osmoreceptors are responding to specific changes in the CSF Na^+ concentration subsequent to perturbations in the extracellular fluid osmolality. This was supported by the observation that hypertonic sucrose did not stimulate thirst and ADH when infused into the third cerebral ventricle (Olsson, 1969). Intracerebral infusions of hypertonic sucrose can inhibit ADH release by dilution-reduction of CSF Na^+ concentration, which argues against a receptor location outside of the blood-brain barrier. Andersson (1978) recognized that there is the possibility that both elevated Na^+ and cellular dehydration trigger a "biochemical process" involved in the receptor-excitation mechanism.

Cellular Volume and Energy Metabolism

The maintenance of cellular volume also depends upon the energy metabolism of the cell (Robinson, 1953). Tissues incubated in a medium similar to extracellular fluid maintained a normal volume while respiring, but swelled when metabolism was inhibited (MacKnight and Leaf, 1977). Swelling was associated not only with the uptake of water, but of extracellular solutes as well (Mudge, 1951). Thus, two factors can cause or contribute to an increase in cellular volume: a decrease in extracellular osmolality and/or a decrease in the energy metabolism of the cell. These two factors must be borne in mind when interpreting factors that elicit thirst or appear to inhibit it.

Gibbs-Donnan Equilibrium

Water itself crosses cell membranes very rapidly. The gain in water and solute when metabolism is depressed is expected from a Gibbs-Donnan system with the presence of nonpermeant polyvalent macromolecules restricted to one side of the membrane (MacKnight and Leaf, 1977). Calculations show that there is an excess of osmotic pressure in that compartment contributed by the polyvalent macromolecule itself and its associated counterions. Only if the excess osmotic pressure is counterbalanced by some additional solute restricted to the opposite compartment will a steady state be achieved. It is the active extrusion of Na^+ in metabolizing tissues that allows stabilization of cellular volume. Since this transport of Na^+ out of the cell takes place against an electrochemical gradient, work or active transport is required. The energy comes from the metabolism of the cell, and any inhibition of metabolism will result in the accumulation of Na^+ in cells of the kidney (Leaf and Couter, 1949; MacKnight and Leaf, 1977; Mudge, 1951), the liver (Elshove and VanRossum, 1963; Heckmann and Parsons, 1959), skeletal muscle (Kleinzeller and Knotkova, 1964; Rixon and Stevenson, 1956), cardiac muscle (Page et al., 1964), and the brain (Bourke and Tower, 1966; Franck et al., 1968).

The Pump-Leak Hypothesis

As discussed by MacKnight and Leaf (1977), a central question confronting physiologists in the mid-1950s was not "why did cells swell when their metabolism was inhibited?", but was restated (Manery, 1954) as "why didn't cells swell, given their high content of intracellular proteins and other macromolecules exerting an osmotic pressure?". As recognized by Leaf (1956) and as explained by MacKnight (1968), "So long as the rate at which a substance crossed the membrane from the extracellular fluid into the cell was equaled by the rate at which it was passed from the cell to the extracellular fluid, that substance in effect would be held in the extracellular compartment and could offset the intracellular swelling force. They postulated that the active extrusion of Na^+ from the cells allowed stabilization of cellular volume in metabolizing tissues". It follows from this that Na^+ is leaking into cells at all times, and therefore, its transport is accounting for a substantial amount of their basal metabolic rate (Astrup, 1982; Siesjo and Wielock, 1985; Whittam, 1962; Whittam and Willis, 1963).

Sodium Receptor as an Energy Receptor

The impact of energy depletion upon cellular volume and Na^+ content is demonstrated in this classic example (Figure 2-8) adapted from Leaf (1959) by MacKnight and Leaf (1977). Note that some K^+ was lost and this may be a characteristic symptom of a low-energy state. The large gain in Na^+ equalled the K^+ lost plus the chloride required to preserve electroneutrality. The double arrows signify that the process is reversible. This model is often referred to as a "double-Donnan system" (Leaf, 1959). Erythrocytes have been used widely for the study of volume regulation and active and passive ion movements across cell membranes in these "double-Donnan systems" (Post and Jolly, 1975; Tosteson and Hoffman, 1960). This is sometimes called the "**pump-leak hypothesis**" as shown in Figure 2-9, adapted from Leaf (1956).

This model suggests that, over a range of extracellular Na^+ concentrations and rates of Na^+ entry into the cell, the Na^+ pump adjusts its activity to balance (Garay and Garrahan, 1973; Post and Jolly, 1975) Na^+ entry (maximum pumping rate occurs at an intracellular Na^+ concentration between 35–40 mM). In the pump-leak model, cellular volume and metabolism depend not only on the rate of active ion transport but also on the rate at which ions "leak" into the cells. Increased permeability to Na^+ ions can be brought about by physical factors such as temperature (Hubbard et al., 1987), Na^+ concentration (Hubbard and Armstrong, 1988) in the medium (hypohydration), ultraviolet light (Cook, 1965), or

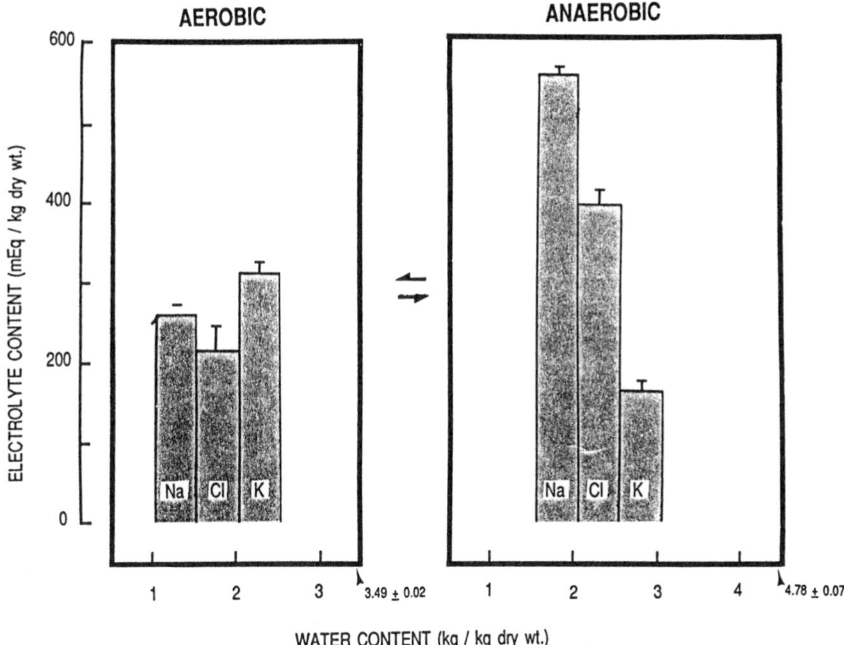

FIGURE 2-8. *Changes in content of tissue water, sodium, chloride, and potassium of guinea pig renal cortical slices resulting from 30 min of anaerobic incubation; control tissue content is shown on left and values after 30 min of anaerobic metabolism are on right. Blank area is water content and hatched columns are electrolyte values of sodium, chloride, and potassium, all expressed per kg of dry tissue weight (from MacKnight and Leaf, 1977).*

by viruses (Knutton et al., 1976). When animals are depleted of K^+, there can be a large loss of K^+ with an equivalent gain in Na^+, without an increase in cellular water or Cl^- content (Heppel, 1939). Cardiac glycosides that inhibit the pump-ATPase (ouabain) produce a similar effect; i.e. K^+-loss with Na^+-gain but without cell swelling (MacKnight and Leaf, 1977).

Heat, Sodium Permeability, Energy Depletion, and Thirst

We have recently attempted to identify the cellular site or location where the physical effects of heat are translated into the physiological manifestations of heat strain (Hubbard et al., 1987). A list of the hypothetical characteristics of such a site are compiled in Table 2-3.

The key factors in this list all relate in some way to the Na^+ pump, a change in membrane permeability to Na^+, a stimulation of metabolism (especially glycolysis), and a resultant energy drain upon the cell. For example, consider factors in Table 2-4, which tend to increase intracellular Na^+ and to drive the Na^+ pump in a hyperthermic person.

Thus, all of these factors that stimulate the influx of Na^+ into the cell will increase ATP utilization, heat production, and lactate formation, and produce an energy drain upon the cell. We have referred to this concept

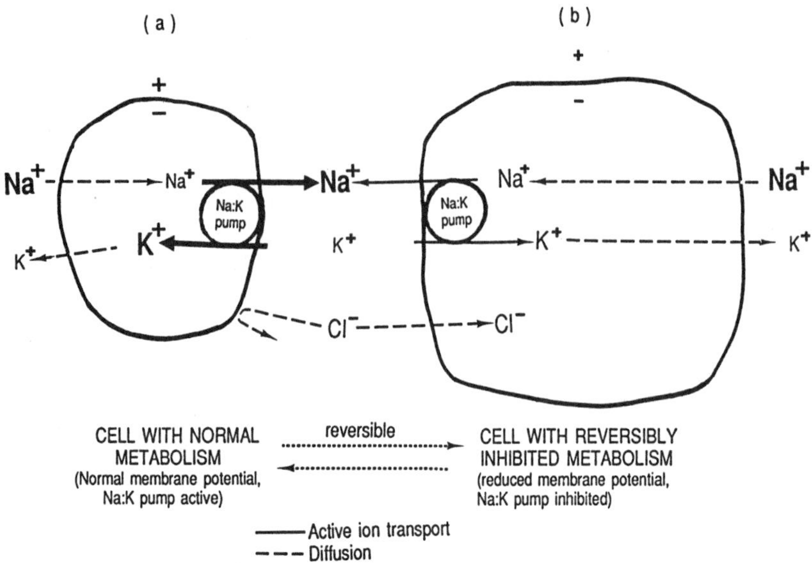

FIGURE 2-9. *(a) "In the normally metabolizing cell Na^+ diffuses into the cell and K^+ out. However, active ion transport extrudes Na^+ and causes K^+ uptake sufficient to maintain high intracellular K^+ content and low intracellular Na^+ content, respectively, in the steady-state. The membrane potential is depicted as preventing entry of chloride into the cell. (b) The situation in a swollen cell is depicted. Inhibition of metabolism slows or stops the ion pump so that the Na^+ entering the cell by diffusion cannot be extruded and the K^+ lost from the cell cannot be replaced. The cell membrane potential diminishes and chloride now enters the cell. This requires further entry of Na^+ into the cell to preserve electric neutrality. The increased solute content of the cell results in secondary entry of water and the cell becomes swollen." (from Leaf, 1959).*

as the Energy Depletion Model of heat stroke pathophysiology (Hubbard and Armstrong, 1988; Hubbard et al., 1987). As mentioned earlier, both hypoglycemia and 2-deoxyglucose treatment stimulate ADH release. Therefore, if the mechanisms operating in the Energy Depletion Model produce an intracellular effect similar to hypoglycemia, intracellular glucopenia, or a metabolic consequence related to it, this could account for part of the increased ADH and thirst associated with hyperthermia. In this regard, it is also interesting to note that Andersson (1978) suggests that the "thirst" receptors are also sensitive to temperature and that local warming of the preoptic region will elicit drinking in the water-fed goat, whereas preoptic cooling will inhibit it. This adds tremendous significance to the observation that thirst can be induced by brain heating and inhibited by brain cooling. This is exactly the behavior we would expect from a Na^+ pump-mediated process. For example, membrane leakage of Na^+ and K^+ ions and the resultant active transport may account for nearly half of the basal metabolism of the brain (Astrup, 1982; Whittam, 1962). Hypothermia provides clinical protection from circulatory arrest by thermally restricting Na^+ channels, delaying energy depletion, delaying K^+ efflux, and stabilizing the cell membrane (Astrup et al., 1981).

TABLE 2-3. *Cellular Site of Heat Stroke Injury: Hypothetical Characteristics*

* Function of the site is related to changes in cell volume
* Function of the site adapts during endurance training
* Function of the site is related to heat tolerance and fatigue during exercise
* Structure and function of the site may be irreversibly changed

It also follows that if the thirst receptor was a Na^+ receptor, then it **could interpret an increase in Na^+** concentration and leak rate as an increase **in energy demand.** If this were true, it would lead to a further profound insight; i.e., **Thirst could be sensing energy demand and therefore, could be intimately related to metabolism and hunger!** Remember, hypothermia delays energy depletion (Astrup, 1982). A metabolic component in ADH release is evident because hypoglycemia simulates ADH release (Baylis et al., 1981). The mechanism appears to be intracellular glucopenia because it is reproduced with 2-deoxyglucose (Robertson and Berl, 1985; Vokes and Robertson, 1985). This could suggest that elevated intracellular glucose might inhibit thirst apart from any osmotic effects.

Thirst and Sodium Pump Activity

Andersson (1978) has further suggested that angiotensin ll might be an activator of a cationic transporting enzyme. Angiotensin ll (Gutman et al., 1972), L-norepinephrine (Desaiah and Ho, 1977) and PGE, (Limas and Cohn, 1974) interact with Na^+, possibly at the level of Na-K-ATPase, in stimulating ADH and thirst. For example, in 1963, Gutman injected hydrochlorothiazide, an inhibitor of active Na^+ transport, and observed *reduced drinking* in response to a load of hypertonic saline in nephrectomized rats. Injections of ouabain had a similar effect (Bergman et al., 1967; Bergman et al., 1967b; Gutman et al., 1971). Ouabain apparently inhibits ADH release (Gutman et al., 1971). It was also very interesting to note that glycerol (Albers and Koval, 1972) and deuterium (D_2O) (Ahmed and Foster, 1974) are two weaker inhibitors of Na-K-ATPase. D_2O had the same inhibitory effects when used as the solvent for hypertonic saline in goats (Leksell et al., 1976; Rundgren et al., 1977). Infusions of glycerol (Olsson et al., 1978; Olsson et al., 1976) were found to suppress dehydra-

TABLE 2-4. *Factors that Increase Sodium Permeability and Energy Demand*

* Active transport hydrolyzes 1 ATP/3 Na^+ ions translocated for 2 K^+
* Heat increases kinetic energy and ion diffusion stimulating Na^+ permeability
* Heat increases intracellular acidity (glycolysis) and a Na^+-H^+ exchange
* Heat storage results in hypohydration and increased extracellular (Na^+)
* Increased extracellular Na^+ increases Na^+ permeability
* Hypohydration results in hyperthermia via increased basal metabolism
* Heat increases the required neural stimulation frequency to maintain force
* Each molecule of ACh stimulates a 50,000 cation flux at the receptor
* Increased neural stimulation increases Na^+ flux in nerves and muscles
* Heat and exercise produce regional ischemia (early splanchnic; late cerebral)
* Regional ischemia induces regional acidosis and increased Na^+ flux
* A doubling of cellular Na^+ results in an 8-fold increase in ATP hydrolysis

tive thirst and ADH secretion "much more effectively than corresponding glucose infusions." This could suggest that thirst is more easily attenuated by inhibiting the activity of the Na-K-ATPase than by raising the glucose levels within the cell.

For example, if Na^+ were leaking into the cell at a higher rate than normal, there would be a greater turnover of available ATP producing more ADP and Pi to stimulate metabolism, possibly via glycolysis in the vicinity of the cell membrane. Inhibiting the Na-K-ATPase would likely reduce this source of metabolic stimulation, ATP demand would fall, and concentrations would increase. Thus, low thirst would correlate with low pump activity and higher energy (ATP) levels within the cell. High thirst would correlate with high rates of Na^+ entrance, high rates of ATP hydrolysis, lower ATP levels, higher ADP and Pi levels, and stimulated glycolysis. In this model, *high thirst correlates with high pump activity and a lowering of steady-state ATP levels.* If the cellular trigger for thirst was related to ATP levels (energy depletion), then this might explain the analogous condition of high ADH release (Baylis and Robertson, 1980; Baylis et al., 1981) with either introcellular glucopenia or 2-dG. If glucose were either unavailable (glucopenia) or unable (2-dG) to fuel glycolysis, then steady-ATP levels would fall (energy depletion), thereby stimulating ADH release and thirst. Depending upon the situation (glucose concentrtion, insulin etc.), elevated glucose levels might elevate the ATP levels and inhibit thirst but even higher levels might deplete ATP levels by producing excess hexose phosphates. This difficult concept is summarized in Table 2-5.

Table 2-5 suggests that *thirst and ADH release can both be defined/regulated in terms of energy balance,* rather than the more common approach using water deficits and elevated osmolalities. This concept is hypothetical yet potentially useful because it tends to unify a number of observations that, on the surface, are either unrelated or difficult to interpret by the existing model (hyperosmolality). The table also provides an interesting perspective on the potential for unravelling physiological regulation by stimulating **metabolic** demand or by **reducing the substrate availability** fueling it. Selective inhibition studies then tend to identify key enzymes/regulators in the system or switching points. For example, reducing the activity of the pump enzymes with ouabain might make more ATP available for other uses such as muscular contractility. For example, this model could **predict** that a reduction in blood volume/flow and attendant reductions in substrate availability/use would stimulate thirst. This could explain the apparently inappropriate thirst found in salt depletion which tends to confound the hyperosmolality model.

Other recent experiments (Thrasher et al., 1980) infused equally hyperosmotic solutions of Na^+, sucrose, urea, and glucose intravenously. All solutions appeared to raise CSF osmolality **and** Na^+ concentrations but only saline and sucrose stimulated thirst. These results appear to

TABLE 2-5. *Effects of Cellular Energy Levels on Thirst and ADH Release*

HIGH THIRST/HIGH ADH RELEASE	LOW THIRST/LOW ADH RELEASE
Increased metabolic demand and lower energy levels	**Low/normal metabolic demand and higher energy levels**
Elevated plasma Na/Increased Na"leaks"/ hypertermia	Low plasma Na/ Low "leaks"/cold
Increased pumping/lower ATP levels/ Increased glycolysis/lactate	Decreased pumping/elevated ATP levels/elevated glucose
Inhibited metabolism and lower energy levels	**Inhibited Na-K-ATPase and higher energy levels**
Intracellular glucopenia/2dG lower ATP levels	Ouabain/hydrochlorothiazide/ glycerol/deuterium elevated ATP levels
Reduced blood volume/flow/ substrate/oxygen availability	

question the specificity of the receptor for Na^+ but are compatible with centrally located osmoreceptors since urea and glucose do not cause cellular dehydration. These results, do not rule out the possibility that either glucose or urea is interfering with some biochemical event in the receptor-response pathway. Nor is it clear, if a proper equilibrium had been established, why glucose or urea should raise CSF Na^+ in the first place. It is likely that this interesting debate will continue.

PRACTICAL CONSIDERATIONS

Physiology of ADH Release

The ADH of humans and most other mammals is arginine vasopressin produced by the neurohypophysis. Under physiological conditions, ADH release is apparently controlled primarily by plasma osmolality (Robertson and Athar, 1976; Robertson and Berl, 1985). The osmoregulatory system appears to display large individual differences in both sensitivity and threshold (Robertson, 1977; Robertson et al., 1976). However, this could be analogous to the apparent differences in the onset of sweating, which depends on an acclimation response to repeated exposures. Within any one individual, the plasma vasopressin response (ADH release) is linearly related to plasma osmolality across the same range with which thirst is stimulated (Robertson et al., 1976). Generally, the range of body fluid osmolality in health is between 280–295 mOsm/kg of water (Feig and McCurdy, 1977). At a plasma osmolality of 280 mOsm/kg water, ADH release is completely inhibited (Feig and McCurdy, 1977) and the urine osmolality is minimal (<100 mOsm/kg of water).

According to Robertson and Berl (1985), the full range of urinary concentrations can be achieved by changing the plasma ADH concentration between 0.5–5.0 pg/ml. The most important action of ADH is to conserve body water by increasing the renal reabsorption of solute-free water which increases urine concentration and decreases flow. Although there is wide variation in the individual thirst threshold, Vokes (1987) estimates its average value at 295 mOsm/kg of water. Thus, at the thirst threshold (the highest plasma osmolality that occurs normally) the increased ADH concentration elicits maximum urinary concentration ($U_{osm} > 800$–1000 mOsm/kg of water).

According to Feig and McCurdy (1977), the mathematical relation between variables across this physiologic range can be expressed by the equations:

$$0.34 \times \text{change in plasma}_{osm} = \text{change in plasma ADH (pg/ml)}$$

and

$$\text{change in urine}_{osm} = 95 \times \text{change in plasma}_{osm}$$

Thus, a 1 mOsm plasma change increases urine osmolality by almost 100 mOsm and, at the thirst threshold (295 mOsm/kg of water), urine volume is reduced 10- to 20-fold. Therefore, it can be appreciated that ADH and thirst play key roles in maintaining water balance primarily by regulating the plamsa osmolality over a very narrow range bounded on the lower end by the osmotic threshold for ADH release and on the upper end by the osmotic threshold for thirst.

Adolph (1947) contended that **voluntary dehydration** occurred because thirst is an inadequate stimulus to drinking. This is entirely true and consistent with the observation that the threshold for ADH release and renal water conserving mechanisms occurs at lower osmolalities than thirst. This lack of complete parity between an increase in osmolality and the behavior of thirst (seeking water, drinking water, ceasing to drink and absorption and distribution) (Adolph et al., 1954) could represent an important adaptation which frees the animal from "the bother of repeated thirst or drinking bouts in response to minor increases in osmolality" (Stricker and Verbalis, 1988). Thus, thirst does not become prominent until the osmotic dehydration exceeds the renal capacity to deal with it physiologically. From this perspective, it would seem more appropriate to refer to thirst as a **delayed response** to evolving dehydration (a dynamic state of change) as opposed to "inadequate."

Evidence for Volume Control

Andersson (1978)suggests that thirst may develop when the fluid volume of the body is reduced without any appreciable change in the extracellular Na^+ concentration or tonicity. An example of this could be thirst following hemorrhage. A very old concept (Gregersen, 1932) is that food causes an isosmotic reduction of the body fluids by increased secretion of gastric and intestinal juices. The fact that thirst can develop in the absence of an osmotic stimulus is taken as evidence of this. The osmometric mechanism cannot convincingly explain thirst in a Na^+ depleted individual with a reduced plasma Na^+, a contracted ECF and, if anything, swollen cells.

A baroreceptor mechanism comprised of stretch receptors in the cardiac atria, aortic arch, and carotid sinuses responds to changes in blood volume or pressure by altering the tonic inhibition of ADH release (interruption of the inhibitory signal causes increased ADH release). These receptors influence the release of ADH via the vagal nerves (Gauer et al., 1970; Gauer et al., 1951). In contrast to the linear relationship between plasma osmolality and ADH relase, the baroreceptor response appears to be exponential (Dunn et al., 1973), and thus is not sensitive to small hemodynamic changes and is not useful in fine-tuning water balance (Vokes, 1987).

The impact of reduced blood volume compromising to some extent the delivery of substrate and oxygen to tissues could be a mechanism whereby the energy depletion model could explain thirst, due to metabolic inhibition rather than increased demand (Table 2-5).

Renal Factors in Thirst

Restriction of renal blood flow stimulates renin release and thirst without change in overall water and salt balance (Fitzsimons, 1969). Injection of angiotensin causes drinking (Fitzsimons and Simons, 1969) and ADH release (Bonjour and Malvin, 1970). Although angiotensin is a potent dipsogen in experimental animals when injected systemically (Fitzsimons and Simons, 1969) or intracerebroventricularly (Epstein et al., 1970), the evidence with humans is less clear because most patients with high levels of renin and angiotensin have no apparent abnormality in thirst (Robertson, 1984). Andersson (1978) has proposed that the interaction between angiotensin and Na^+ makes the Na^+ receptors more sensitive in some way. This could be accomplished if angiotensin made the receptor more permeable to Na^+ or stimulated the Na^+ pump directly (Gutman et al., 1972). Thus, a volumetric mechanism mediated by the renal renin-angiotensin system could still have its final link in the Na^+ receptors.

Ladell's Free Circulating Water Concept

Ladell (1965) has introduced a concept of "free circulating water" equivalent to some 2 liters which does not appear to participate in the osmotic balance of the body. This suggests that the "drive" to drink would not come into play until this "free circulating water" had been expended. We have reasoned that this interesting notion actually delivered two important ideas. First, there is an inherent "delay" in the onset or drive of thirst. If this could be explained, it would then be more accurate to describe thirst as "delayed" rather than "inadequate." Second, the delay is a manifestation of the body's osmotic control.

Let us examine Ladell's concept in light of the current theory of thirst stimulation. For ease of calculation, we shall assume that the average 70-kg adult is 60% water (TBW = 42 L), that 2/3 of this water (28 L) is intracellular and 1/3 (14 L) is extracellular (3.5 L of plasma and 10.5 L of interstitial fluid). By calculation (Feig and McCurdy, 1977), the intravascular or plasma volume is equivalent to 1/12 of the total body water (42 L TBW/12 = 3.5 L plasma volume). Furthermore, the plasma volume is 1/4 the extracellular volume (14 L/4 = 3.5 L, plasma volume). Thus, by definition, if a pure water loss occurs (no salt loss), we would expect 2/3 of the loss from the intracellular water and 1/3 from the extracellular water (Feig and McCurdy, 1977). In practice, usually less than 1/12 of the water loss comes from the plasma space because of its increased plasma protein oncotic pressure (Feig and McCurdy, 1977). Since the plasma volume represents 1/4 of the total extracellular volume and if the extracellular space lost 4 L of isotonic solution, approximately 1 L would be lost from the plasma fluid. If we further assume that a pure water deficit does not alter the total body solute, then hypertonicity will be proportional to the volume of water lost (Feig and McCurdy, 1977). We will also assume parity between 1 L and 1 kg of water:

$$(\text{normal TBW}) \times (\text{normal plasma}_{osm}) = (\text{present TBW}) \times (\text{present plasma}_{osm})$$

If a man begins to lose insensible water (70 hours at 24°C) at normally the lowest fully hydrated plasma osmolality of 280 mOsm/kg water (Feig and McCurdy, 1977), we can calculate about how much water will be lost before the average threshold for thirst (Vokes, 1987) is reached (295 mOsm/kg water).

$$(\text{normal TBW}) \times (\text{normal plasma}_{osm}) = (\text{thirst TBW}) \times (\text{thirst plasma}_{osm})$$

$$(42\text{ L}) \times (280\text{ mOsm/kg}) = (?\text{ L}) \times (295\text{ mOsm/kg})$$

$$(11{,}760\text{ mOsm} / 295\text{ mOsm/kg}) = ?\text{ L} = 39.9\text{ L} = \text{TBW at the thirst threshold}$$

$$(42\text{ L} - 39.9\text{ L}) = 2.1\text{ L} = \text{TBW deficit}$$

This calculation suggests that, on the average, 2.1 L of water would be lost before reaching the thirst threshold. This assumes that one is fully hydrated before losing water, which is a more common practice in research than other activities. This value appears to confirm the prior observation by Ladell (1965) that there is **"free circulating water"** equivalent to approximately 2 L which does not **appear** to participate in the osmotic balance of the body. This calucation provides further support to two arguments: 1) that thirst is "delayed" rather than inadequate, and 2) that the delay is a manifestation of the body's osmotic control.

Six Sample Calculations

This section illustrates the calculations performed to derive the values in Table 2-6. Examples are presented which also illustrate key principles in understanding the role of fluid-electrolyte balance on thirst and body hydration status.

EXAMPLE 1. A PURE WATER DEFICIT IN THE HYDRATED STATE: IMPACT ON REHYDRATION

Let us examine the impact of the thirst threshold on **rehydration** in the situation of a pure body water deficit in the hydrated state (TBW loss = 6% of body weight or 4.2 L). First, let us calculate to what point the plasma osmolality would be driven without fluid intake (dehydration):

DEHYDRATION

$$(\text{normal TBW}) \times (\text{normal plasma}_{osm}) =$$
$$(\text{dehydrated TBW}) \times (\text{dehydrated plasma}_{osm})$$
$$(42\text{ L}) \times (280\text{ mOsm/kg}) = (42\text{ L} - 4.2\text{ L}) \times (?\text{ mOsm/kg})$$
$$(11{,}760\text{ mOsm}/37.8\text{ L} = 311.1\text{ mOsm/kg}) = \text{the dehydrated plasma}_{osm}$$

In losing 4.2 L of pure water (~1500 mL/day at altitude; Table 2-6), the plasma osmolality will rise to 311 mOsm/kg water, or 16 mOsm/kg of water above the thirst threshold (295 mOsm/kg of water). The extracellular fluid volume would contribute 1/3 of this deficit (4.2 L/3 = 1.4 L) and the plasma volume would contribute 350 mL (4200 mL/12) as shown in Table 2-6. How much fluid would be consumed in returning the plasma osmolality to the thirst threshold (rehydration)?

REHYDRATION

$$(\text{dehydrated TBW}) \times (\text{dehydrated plasma}_{osm} =$$
$$(\text{thirst TBW}) \times (\text{thirst plasma}_{osm})$$
$$(37.8\text{ L}) \times (311.1\text{ mOsm/kg}) = (295\text{ mOsm/kg}) \times (?\text{ L})$$
$$(11{,}760\text{ mOsm} / 295\text{ mOsm/kg}) = 39.9\text{ L} = \text{rehydrated TBW}$$

Thus, in returning to the thirst threshold (a plasma osmolality of 295 mOsm/kg), a rehydrated TBW of 39.9 L is theoretically achieved. Since the prior, dehydrated TBW was 37.8 L, there was a net gain in TBW of 2.1 L (39.9 L - 37.8 L). This suggests that only **50%** (2.1 L × 100/4.2 L) of the fluid deficit would be **rehydrated** before the thirst threshold is reached. Under these conditions, thirst is not "inadequate." The rehydration deficit is an inherent feature of the "offset" between the thirst "set point" and the renal diuresis "set point," in the fully hydrated condition. For example, it is not uncommon to assess a fully hydrated condition by having test subjects consume water until urine specific gravity declines to some target end-point. Thus, fully hydrated test subjects will rarely fully rehydrate. This calculation appears to confirm the early assertion of Pitts (1944) that subjects rarely consume sufficient water to replace the deficit. Since only 1/12 of this pure water deficit (2.1 L/12 = 175 mL) will come from plasma (3.5 L:42 L as 1:12) there may be very little impact on cardiovascular performance.

EXAMPLE 2. CLINICAL SHOCK VIA PRIMARY WATER DEPLETION

Clinical shock from pure water loss generally requires a Na^+ above 170 mEq/L (Feig and McCurdy, 1977). This water deficit can be calculated using the following formula (Yarbrough and Hubbard, 1988):

Water deficit (L) = TBW (0.6 × wt in kg) – [TBW × (desired plasma Na^+/ measured plasma Na^+)]
Water deficit = 42 L – [(42 L) × (140 mEq Na^+/L / 170 mEq Na^+/L)]
= 42 L – 34.6 L = 7.4 L

Thus, in a pure water deficit sufficient to produce shock, one might estimate a minimum loss of some 7.4 L of body water or 10.6% (7.4 L × 100/70 kg) of body weight. Since 1/12 of this pure water deficit comes from the plasma (7400 mL/12 = 616 mL), there is a decline in plasma volume of about 18% (616 mL/3500 mL). The extracellular fluid volume would contribute 2.47 L (7.4 L/3) of this deficit. One rarely sees a pure water deficit since salt is usually lost as well.

EXAMPLE 3. A PURE WATER DEFICIT IN THE HYPOHYDRATED STATE—IMPACT ON REHYDRATION

If a subject begins losing water in a hypohydrated state, at the thirst threshold (–2.1 L), with a thirst plasma osmolality of 295 mOsm/kg water (thirst TBW = 39.9 L), and then loses 4.2 L (6% of initial body weight), the plasma osmolality could rise to:

DEHYDRATION

$$(\text{thirst TBW}) \times (\text{thirst plasma}_{osm}) = (\text{dehydrated TBW}) \times (\text{dehydrated plasma}_{osm})$$
$$(295\ \text{mOsm/kg}) \times (39.9\ \text{L}) = (39.9\ \text{L} - 4.2\ \text{L}) \times (?\ \text{mOsm/kg})$$
$$(11{,}770\ \text{mOsm} / 35.7\ \text{L}) = 330\ \text{mOsm/kg water}$$

The dehydrated plasma volume could be 330 mOm/kg and the dehydrated TBW could be 35.7 L.

REHYDRATION

If the subject rehydrates until the starting thirst threshold is reached, he should consume:

$$(\text{dehydrated TBW}) \times (\text{dehydrated plasma}_{osm}) = (\text{thirst TBW}) \times (\text{thirst plasma}_{osm})$$
$$(35.7\ \text{L}) \times (330\ \text{mOsm/kg}) = (?\ \text{L}) \times (295\ \text{mOsm/kg})$$
$$(11{,}781\ \text{mOsm} / 295\ \text{mOsm/kg}) = 39.9\ \text{L (the thirst TBW)}$$

Thus, at the thirst threshold (a plasma osmolality of 295 mOsm/kg), a TBW of 39.9 L would be achieved. Since the dehydrated TBW was 35.7 L, an intake of 4.2 L was required to reach the thirst threshold. This suggests that, by beginning the dehydration in the hypohydrated state at the thirst threshold, a nearly 100% rehydration of the dehydration deficit, but only 66.7% (4.2 L/6.3 L) of the fully hydrated state could be expected. **This would be an important consideration for studies in which the initial hydration statuses of the subjects were not known, because the resultant rehydration value could be 50, 66.7, or 100% of the experimental body weight change.** Thus, rehydration results will depend upon whether test subjects arrive in a hydrated or hypohydrated state, for an experiment producing a 6% loss in body weight.

EXAMPLE 4. A HYPOTONIC WATER DEFICIT IN THE HYDRATED, NON-HEAT ACCLIMATIZED STATE

Assume that the subject is not heat acclimatized and produces a hypotonic sweat (0.43% NaCl = 0.5 isotonic saline) as the source of body water deficit. He begins exercise in the heat in a fully-hydrated, normal condition (plasma osmolaity = 280 mOsm/kg of water) and then loses 6% of body weight (4.2 L) as sweat.

SOLUTE DEFICIT

We first compute the impact of the solute loss (sweat NaCl) on the total solute content of the body. The total mOsmoles will be reduced from 11,760 mOsmoles (280 mOsm/kg × 42 L) by an amount equivalent to the solute content of the lost sweat. Assume that 0.5 isotonic saline is equivalent to an osmolality of 140 mOsm/kg (0.5 × 280 mOsm/kg), then:

(140 mOsm/kg sweat) × (4.2 L) = **588 mOsmoles of lost solute.**
This is equivalent to 294 mEq (588 mOsm/2) of NaCl.

The new salt-depleted total solute content will be 11,172 mOsmoles (11,760 mOsm - 588 mOsm).

DEHYDRATION

The new salt-depleted TBW will be 37.8 L (42.0 L - 4.2 L). The new salt-depleted, dehydrated plasma osmolality will be 295.6 mOsm/kg (11,172 mOsmoles/37.8 L). Assume 1/2 of the fluid loss is pure water (2.1 L) and the other 1/2 is isotonic saline. The extracellular space could lose 700 mL due to the pure water loss (2100 mL/3) plus the loss of isotonic saline (2100 mL) for a total deficit of 2800 mL. The plasma would contribute 1/12 of the pure water deficit or 175 mL. The extracellular space would lose 2.1 L of isotonic saline, of which the **plasma contributes** 25% (3.5:14 as 1:4), or 525 mL. If we add the 175 mL from the pure water portion of the total loss (525 mL + 175 mL = **700 mL**), we see that the plasma could lose **20%** of its volume (700 mL/3500 mL) which is close to the shock threshold (example 2 above). **Thus, a 4.2 L sweat loss has theoretically as much impact on the plasma volume (-20%) as a much greater volume (7.4 L) of pure water loss (-18%).**

REHYDRATION

If the subject drinks pure water until the plasma osmolality reaches the thirst threshold (295 mOsm/kg), he would reach a thirst TBW of: (dehydrated TBW) × (dehydrated $plasma_{osm}$) = (thirst TBW) × (thirst $plasma_{osm}$)

The assumptions are: (a) the dehydrated condition involves a TBW of 37.8 L and a salt-depleted, dehydrated plasma osmolality of 295.6 mOsm/kg of water, and (b) the plasma osmolality is 295 mOsm/kg at the thirst threshold.

(37.8 L) × (295.6 mOsm/kg) = (? L) × (295 mOsm/kg)
(11,172 mOsmoles / 295 mOsm/kg) = 37.88 L of TBW

This subject would increase his TBW by only 80 mL (37.88 L - 37.8 L) before the thirst threshold was reached. This is equivalent to only 1.9% of the initial water deficit (80 mL/4200 mL). **In contrast to a similar volume of pure water loss from a hydrated starting point, a hypotonic fluid loss reduces the percent rehydration from 50% to 1.9%** of the deficit. This example serves to illustrate the impact of solute loss on rehydration. Under these conditions, thirst is not inadequate. The missing solute is problematic, and fluid intake under these conditions would probably be stimulated by the volume deficit.

EXAMPLE 5. A HYPOTONIC WATER DEFICIT IN THE HYDRATED, HEAT ACCLIMATIZED STATE

Assume that a subject was producing very hypotonic sweat of minimum Na^+ concentration (0.17% NaCl = 0.2 isotonic saline), subsequent to heat acclimatization and a low salt diet (high aldosterone levels). If he loses 6% of his body weight (4.2 L) after beginning work in the heat **fully hydrated**, then:

SOLUTE DEFICIT

His total solute content would be 11,760 mOsmoles (280 mOsm/kg × 42 L) and his solute loss would be equivalent to the sweat solute concentration (280 mOsm/kg × 0.2 = 56 mOsm/kg) multiplied by the sweat volume (4.2 L), or 235 mOsmoles. His salt depleted total solute content would be 11,525 mOsmoles (11,760 mOsmoles - 235 mOsmoles).

DEHYDRATION

His salt-depleted, dehydrated TBW would be 37.8 L and, therefore, the plasma osmolality would be (11,525 mOsmoles / 37.8 L) 305 mOsm/kg of water. If we assume that istonic saline is equivalent to an osmolality of 280 mOsm/kg, then this deficit is equivalent to 839 mL (1000 mL × 235/280) of isotonic saline (0.84 L) lost from the extracellular space. The plasma contributes 25% (210 mL) of this deficit (839 mL/4). The remaining deficit is pure water (4200 mL - 839 ml = 3361 mL), of which the intracellular volume contributed 2/3 (2241 mL) and the extracellular 1/3 (1120 mL). The plasma portion of the pure water deficit would be 280 mL (3361 mL/12). The total extracellular fluid deficit would be the sum (1959 mL) of the pure water (1120 mL) and saline deficits (839 mL). The total plasma deficit would be 490 mL (280 ml + 210 mL) or 14% (490 mL/3500) of the plasma volume.

REHYDRATION

If the subject drank until the plasma osmolality reached the thirst threshold, then he would rehydrate as follows:

$$(\text{dehydrated TBW}) \times (\text{dehydrated plasma}_{osm}) = (\text{thirst TBW}) \times (\text{thirst plasma}_{osm})$$

$$(37.8 \text{ L}) \times (305 \text{ mOsm/kg}) = (? \text{ L}) \times (295 \text{ mOsm/kg})$$

$$(11{,}525 \text{ mOsmoles} / 295 \text{ mOsm/kg}) = 39.07 \text{ L}$$

The subject would consume 1.27 L (39.07 L - 37.8 L) in reaching the thirst threshold. This represents a **30.2** % replacement of the total fluid deficit (1.2 L/4.2 L). Approximately 100 mL of this 1.27 L would be returned to the plasma (1.27 L/12 L) and would reduce the plasma volume deficit to 11% (390/3500 mL).

Thus, comparing example 5 to example 6, heat acclimatization coupled with a low-salt diet (to insure low sweat Na^+ concentrations), could be expected to improve cardiovascular stability (at equivalent sweat volume losses) by reducing the solute loss and preserving some plasma volume (390 mL vs 750 mL deficits). Moreover, heat acclimatization should have a pronounced impact on rehydration (**30.2% vs 1.9%**).

EXAMPLE 6. HYPOTONIC WATER DEFICIT IN THE HYPOHYDRATED, HEAT ACCLIMATIZED STATE

If the **same** subject began exercise slighty **hypohydrated**, at the thirst threshold, at a plasma osmolality of 295 mOsm/kg, he would have a TBW of 39.9 L (2.1 L deficit).

SOLUTE DEFICIT

His total solute content would be 11,760 mOsmoles (295 mOsm/kg × 39.9 L). His solute loss would be equivalent to the sweat solute concentration (56 mOsm/kg) multipled by the sweat volume (4.2 L), or 235 mOsmoles. The salt-depleted total solute content would be 11,525 mOsmoles.

DEHYDRATION

After losing 4.2 L of sweat (39.9 L - 4.2 L = 35.7 L), the salt-depleted plasma osmolality would be 323 mOsm/kg [11,525 mOsmoles = (35.7 L)

$\times$ (? mOsm/kg)]. The extracellular fluid deficit due to salt loss would be equivalent to 0.84 L of saline (235/280 mL of isotonic saline) of which the plasma would contribute 1/4 (210 mL). The pure water deficit would equal 5460 mL ([4200 mL - 840 mL] + 2100 mL) of which the intracellular volume contributed 2/3 (3640 mL) and the extracellular 1/3 (1820 mL). The plasma would contribute 665 mL (455 mL + 210 mL). Thus, without drinking there would be a 19% deficit (668 mL/3500 mL) in plasma volume. The total extracellular fluid deficit would total 2.66 L (1820 mL + 840 mL).

REHYDRATION

If the subject drank until the thirst threshold was reached, then he would rehydrate as follows: (dehydrated TBW) $\times$ (dehydrated plasma_{osm}) = (thirst TBW) $\times$ (thirst plasma_{osm})

$$(35.7 \text{ L}) \times (323 \text{ mOsm/kg}) = (? \text{ L}) \times (295 \text{ mOsm/kg})$$
$$(11{,}531 \text{ mOsmoles} \,/\, 295 \text{ mOsm/kg}) = 39.09 \text{ L}$$

The subject would consume 3.39 L (39.09 L - 35.7 L) in returning to the thirst threshold. This volume (3.39 L) represents 81% (3.39/4.2 L) of the dehydration deficit, but only 54% of the total deficit (3.39/6.3 L). **This again would be an important consideration, in studies where the initial hydration status of a subject was not known. The resultant rehydration value could be either 54 or 81% of the experimental body weight change**.

With drinking, the subject would consume 3.39 L, of which the plasma would receive 1/12 (282 mL). This would reduce the plasma deficit from **-19%** (close to the shock threshold) to **-11%** (386 mL/3500 mL).

It is clear from the examples in Table 2-6 that the dessication producing a relatively pure water loss is a slow process. For example, even at minimum water losses per day (1500 mL/24 h), it would take nearly 5 days to reproduce the situation in Table 2-6 (Example 2). Note the large increase in plasma osmolality or Na^+ (170 mEq/L) in this case and the enormous loss of fluid necessary to produce an 18% deficit in plasma volume. For these reasons, shock from primary water depletion is relatively rare.

A pure water deficit producing a 6% loss in body weight (Example 1) primarily through non-sweating means would probably have to occur through work in the cold at altitude. The large respiratory water loss (~1500 mL/day) would make this another unlikely scenario. Even more unlikely is the 6% loss in body weight superimposed upon a preexisting deficit (-3%) at the thirst threshold (9% total; Example 3). Even if these examples overestimate the times required to produce this form of primary water depletion, they serve to illustrate the highly unlikely prospect of ever being relevant.

The first hypotonic sweat losses calculated (Example 4) for non-acclimatized individuals are striking for several reasons. First, it takes a

TABLE 2-6. *Scenarios Illustrating Fluid Shifts and Water/Salt Losses*

Condition/ Example	Water Loss (L) / % BW loss	Salt Loss (mOsm or mEq)	PV Loss (mL)/ ECF loss	%PV	P_{Osm} (mOsm)	% Re-hydration Estimated	Incidence
Voluntary dehydration euhydrated (Example 1)	4.2 L 6.0%	—	350 mL 1.4 L	−10%	311	50% 2.1 L	~3 days work cold/altitude
Shock/ Involuntary dehydration (Example 2)	7.4 L 10.6%	—	616 mL 2.47 L	−18%	350	—	Life raft/ confinement/ 5 days
Voluntary dehydration hypohydrated (Example 3)	6.3 L 9.0%	—	525 mL 2.1 L	−15%	330	66.7% 4.2 L	~4 days cold/altitude
Voluntary dehydration non-acclimated euhydrated (Example 4)	4.2 L 6.0%	588/ 294	700 mL 2.8 L	−20%	295.6	1.9% 80 mL	~4 hrs work heat
Voluntary dehydration acclimated euhydrated (Example 5)	4.2 L 6.0%	235/ 118	490 mL 1.96 L	−14%	305	30.2% 1.3 L	~4 hrs work heat
Voluntary dehydration acclimated hypohydrated (Example 6)	6.3 L 9.0%	235/ 118	665 mL 2.66 L	−19%	323	54% 3.39 L	~4 hrs work heat

relatively short time to produce a severe loss in plasma volume (–20%, 4h) versus a similar deficit via pure water routes (–18%, 5 days, Example 2). The calculated values are at equilibrium concentrations, and plasma osmolality (and therefore, thirst) would be greater before the extracellular water debt was paid by intracellular losses. This indicates why thirst and rehydration experiments should not be started until the equlibrium state has been achieved. Second, the equilibrium plasma osmolality reflects a solute concentration but does not reflect the volume loss because of the concurrent salt losses. It is assumed that the kidneys would eliminate "excess water." In these conditions, the only inclination to drink at equlibrium times would be due to volume-depletion signals. Third, the percent change in the extracellular fluid volume (2.8 L × 100/14 L) equals the percent change in plasma volume (–20%). Finally, this model assumes no gain in solute from a prior meal. This strongly reenforces the concept of skipped meals in the etiology of this condition and further lends support for electrolyte replacement as soon as even one meal is missed.

The advantages conferred by heat acclimation on reducing electrolyte losses are seen (Example 5) if one assumes equivalent volume losses. In actuality, either the time to achieve a 4.2 L deficit would be shorter or the volume lost would be greater. The 50% reduction in sweat Na^+ losses (294 vs 118 mEq/L) reduces the plasma volume deficit from severe to moderate levels and, at the same time improves the osmotic drive for thirst (70 vs 1270 mL). The impact of sweat Na^+ reduction is further appreciated when one estimates that a 9% body weight loss in the acclimatized state (Example 6) is roughly equivalent to a 6% loss in the non-acclimatized condition (Example 4).

Thirst and Other Homeostatic Challenges

Let us examine thirst from the perspective of how a few other homeostatic challenges are met (Table 2-7). This table serves to highlight the apparent fact that thirst is a homeostatic challenge that cannot be satisfied by a simple detector/message/effector type-response by a particular effector-organ. This suggests that it is a reasonably recent phylogenetic phenomenon requiring a set of complicated and integrated actions. This does not preclude that a similar functional problem (hypohydration or salt imbalance) did not confront a more primitive organism and was not ultimately dealt with by very similar or analogous measures. How salt became so fundamental to our metabolism is hidden in the phylogenetic past but may relate to the chemistry of the late-Cambrian seas. This might explain why the blood sera of such diverse species as lizards, platypuses, sheep, and humans are so similar. Therefore, it is instructive to explore, as an intellectual exercise, such problems in a hypothetical single-cell organism. Appendix A presents this hypothesis.

TABLE 2-7. *Ways in Which Man Meets Homeostatic Challenges*

Homeostatic challenge	Message origin	Signal	Message destination	Effector	Function/ destination
Too cold	brain	sympathetic	skin	arterioles	vasoconstriction/ save heat
Too cold	brain	cholinergic	muscle	end plate	shiver/make heat
Too hot	brain	sympathetic	skin	arterioles; superficial cutaneous veins	vasodilate/lose heat
Too hot	brain	cholinergic	skin	sweat glands	secrete/lose heat, water, salt
Hypohydrated	brain	ADH	kidney	nephron	reabsorb water/thirst
Hyperhydrated	brain	ADH	kidney	nephron	diuresis
Na depleted	?	aldosterone; Na^+/K^+ ratio?	adrenals	nephron	Na^+ reabsorption
K depleted	?	Na^+/K^+ ratio?	?	nephron	thirst/drinking?
Thirsty	brain	behavior	integrated	organism	1. Find water 2. Drink 3. Absorption 4. Stop drinking

SUMMARY AND IMPLICATIONS FOR FUTURE RESEARCH DESIGN

Our calculations and review of the research involving thirst suggest that: a) thirst is delayed rather than inadequate; b) the delay is a manifestation of the body's osmotic control; c) thirst does not become prominent until the osmotic dehydration exceeds the renal capacity to deal with it physiologically; d) the rehydration deficit, secondary to water loss, is an inherent feature of the offset between the thirst set point relative to the renal set point in the fully hydrated condition; e) if test subjects appear to rehydrate fully it is likely that they began the dehydration test hypohydrated at or near the thirst threshold; f) a 4.2 L sweat loss can have as great an impact on plasma volume (shock threshold) as a much greater volume of pure water loss (7.4 L); g) hypotonic sweat losses produce solute deficits having a profound impact on potential rehydration rates; h) heat acclimatization, by reducing solute losses at equivalent sweat volumes, could be expected to improve cardiovascular stability by conserving plasma solute and should have a pronounced positive impact on rehydration volumes, and i) the osmoreceptor might function as an energy receptor. Our analysis of fluid palatability and exercise effects on fluid consumptions raises two important questions regarding future research design.

First, several studies published by Greenleaf and others do not fit the current osmotic model for the control of thirst. This could represent either an inadequacy in the theory of osmotic control or an inadequacy in an experimental design which allows rehydration before dehydration-induced perturbations are equilibrated.

Second, the initial chapter in this book provides data to suggest that water does not equilibrate in proportion to the solute content of intra- and extracellular compartments. We believe that this is an artifact of sampling time, and again strongly suggests that rehydration be delayed until dehydration-induced perturbations in fluid compartments are equilibrated. Otherwise, a major dipsogenic response could peak prematurely or appear out of phase with the dehydration/rehydration response. From this perspective, it is not surprising that the literature results are contradictory and difficult to analyze. To correctly identify the major independent variables in any future study, adequate equilibration time must be allowed after dehydration, or dehydration and rehydration overlap and measurements are obscured. Further studies should explore the apparent relationship between thirst and cell energy levels.

BIBLIOGRAPHY

Adolph, E.F. *Physiology of Man in the Desert*. New York: Interscience Publishers Inc., 1947, pp. 1–357.

Adolph, E.F., J.P. Barker and P.A. Hoy. Multiple factors in thirst. *Am. J. Physiol.* 178:538–562, 1954.

Ahmed, K., and D. Foster. Studies on effect of $^2H_2$ on Na-K ATPase. *Annals N.Y. Acad Sci.* 242:280–292, 1974.

Albers, R.W. and G.J. Koval. Sodium-potassium-activated adenosine triphosphate. *J. Biol. Chem.* 247:3088–3902, 1972.

Alexander, R.W., J.R. Gill, H. Yamobe, W. Lovenberg, and H.R. Keiser. Effects of dietary sodium and of acute saline infusion on the interrelationship between dopamine excretion and adrenergic activity in man. *J. Clin. Invest.* 54:194–200, 1974.

Andersson, B. Regulation of water intake. *Physiol. Rev.* 58:582–603, 1978.

Armstrong, L.E., D.L. Costill, and W.J. Fink. Changes in body water and electrolytes during heat acclimation: Effects of dietary sodium. *Avait. Space Environ. Med.* 58:143–148, 1987.

Armstrong, L.E., R.P. Francesconi, W.J. Kraemer, N. Leva, J.P. DeLuca, and R.W. Hubbard. Plasma cortisol, renin and aldosterone during an intense heat acclimation program. *Int. J. Sports Med.* 10:38–42, 1989.

Armstrong, L.E., R.W. Hubbard, J.P. DeLuca, and E.L. Christensen. Self-paced heat acclimation procedures. Natick, MA: U.S. Army Research Institute of Environmental Medicine, Technical Report No. T8–86, 1986, pp. 1–28.

Armstrong, L.E., R.W. Hubbard, P.C. Szlyk, W.T. Matthew, and I.V. Sils. Voluntary dehydration and electrolyte losses during prolonged exercise in the heat. *Avait. Space Environ. Med.* 56:765–770, 1985.

Astrup, J. Energy-requiring cell functions in the ischemic brain: Their critical supply and possible inhibition in protective therapy. *J. Neurosurg.* 56:482–487, 1982.

Astrup, J., P.M. Sorensen, and H.R. Sorensen. Oxygen and glucose consumption related to Na-K transport in the canine brain. *Stroke* 12:726–730, 1981.

Baylis, P.H. and G.L. Robertson. Rat vasopressin response to insulin-induced hypoglycemia. *Endocrinol.* 107:1975–1979, 1980.

Baylis, P.H., R.L. Zerbe, and G.L. Robertson. Arginine vasopressin response to insulin-induced hypoglycemia in man. *J. Clin. Endocrinol. Metab.* 53:935–940, 1981.

Bergman, F., M. Chaimovitz, A. Costin, Y. Gutman, and Y. Ginath. Water intake of rats after implantation of ouabain into the hypothalamus. *Am. J. Physiol.* 213:328–332, 1967.

Bergman, F., A. Costin, M. Chaimovitz, and F. Banzakein. The effect of ouabain on water consumption in the rat. *Experentia* 22:700–71, 1967b.

Bonjour, J.P. and R.L. Malvin. Stimulation of ADH release by the renin-angiotensin system. *Am. J. Physiol.* 218:1555–1559, 1970.

Boulze, D., P. Montastruc, and M. Cabanac. Water intake, pleasure and water temperature in humans. *Physiol, and Behav.* 30:97–102, 1983.

Bourke, R.S. and D.B. Tower. Fluid compartmentation and electrolytes of cat cerebral cortex in vitro-l. Swelling and solute distribution in mature cerebral cortex. *J. Neurochem.* 13:1071–1097, 1966.

Burch, G.E. Rate of water and heat loss from respiratory tract of normal subjects in subtropical climate. *Arch. Intern. Med.* 76:315–327, 1945.

Cabanac, M. Physiological role of pleasure. *Science* 173:1103–1107, 1971.

Christensen, H.N. *Body Fluids and Their Neutrality*. New York: Oxford University Press, pp. 1–197, 1963.

Conn, J.W. The mechanism of acclimatization to heat. In: *Advances in Internal Medicine. Volume 3*. New York: Interscience, pp. 377, 1949.

Conway, J.E. and J.I. McCormack. The total intracellular concentration of mammalian tissues compared with that of the extracellular fluid. *J. Physiol.* 120:1–14, 1953.

Cook, J.S. The quantitative interrelationships between ion fluxes, cell swelling, and radiation dose in ultraviolet hemolysis. *J. Gen. Physiol.* 48:719–734, 1965.

Crabbe, J.E., J. Ross, and G.W. Thorn. The significance of excretion of aldosterone during dietary sodium deprivation in normal man. *J. Clin. Endocrinol. Metab.* 18:1159–1177, 1958.

Cuche, J.L., O. Kuchel, A. Barbeau, R. Beucher, and J. Genest. Relationship between the adrenergic nervous system and renin during upright posture: A possible role for 3,4-dehydroxyphenethylamine. *Clin. Sci.*, 43:481–491, 1972.

Davenport, H.W. *Physiology of the digestive tract*. 5th ed., Chicago: Yearbook Medical Publishers, 1982.

Denton, D. The most-craved crystal: Why humans consume salt in such excess. *The Sciences*, Nov/-Dec:29–34, 1986.

Desaiah, D. and I.K. Ho. Kinetics of catecholamine sensitive Na-K-ATPase activity in mouse brain synaptosomes. *Biochem. Pharmacol.* 26:2029–2035, 1977.

Dunn, F.L., T.J. Brennan, A.E. Nelson, and G.L. Robertson. The role of blood osmolality and volume in regulating vasopressin secretion in the rat. *J. Clin. Invest.* 52:3212–3219, 1973.

Elkinton, J.R. and T.S. Danowski. Transfers of cell sodium and potassium in experimental and clinical conditions. *J. Clin. Invest.* 27:74–81, 1948.

Elkinton, J.R., T.S. Danowski, and A.W. Winkler. Hemodynamic changes in salt depletion and in dehydration. *J. Clin. Invest.* 25:120–129, 1946.
Elkinton, J.R. and A.W. Winkler. Transfer of intracellular potassium in experimental dehydration. *J. Clin. Invest.* 23:93–101, 1944.
Elshove, A. and G.D.V. Van Rossum. Net movements of sodium and potassium, and their relation to respiration, in slices of rat liver incubated in vitro. *J. Physiol. (London)* 168:531–553, 1963.
Epstein, A.N., J.T. Fitzsimons, and B.J. Rolls. Drinking induced by injection of angiotensin into the brain of the rat. *J. Physiol.* 210:457–474, 1970.
Feig, P.U. and D.K McCurdy. The hypertonic state. *N. Eng. J. Med.* 297:1444–1454, 1977.
Fitzsimons, J.T. The role of a renal thirst factor in drinking induced by extracellular stimuli. *J. Physiol (London)* 201:349–68, 1969.
Fitzsimons, J.T. and G.J. Simons. The effect on drinking in the rat of intravenous infusion of angiotensin, given alone or in combination with other thirst stimuli. *J. Physiol. (London)* 203:45–57, 1969.
Forbes, G.B. In: *Mineral Metabolism*, Vol. 2, part B. C.L. Comar and F. Bronner, eds., New York: Academic Press, p. 1, 1962.
Fourman, P. and P.M. Leeson. Thirst and polyuria, with a note on the effects of K^+ deficiency and Ca^{+2} excess. *Lancet* 1:268–271, 1959.
Franck, G., M. Cornette and E. Schoffeniels. The catonic composition of incubated cerebral cortex slices. *J. Neurochem.* 15:843-857, 1968.
Garay, R.P. and P.J. Garrahan. The interaction of sodium and potassium with the sodium pump in red cells. *J. Physiol. (London)* 231:297–325, 1973.
Gauer, O.H., J.P. Henry, and C. Behn. The regulation of extracellular fluid volume. *Ann. Rev. Physiol.* 32:547–595, 1970.
Gauer, O.H., J.P. Henry, H.O. Sicker, and W.E. Wendt. Heart and lungs as a receptor region controlling blood volume. *Amer. J. Physiol.* 167:786–787, 1951.
Geigy Scientific Tables. Volume 1. West Caldwell, NJ: Ciba-Geigy Inc., pp. 58–62, 1981.
Gilman, A. The relation between blood osmotic pressure, fluid distribution and voluntry water intake. *Am. J. Physiol.* 120:323-328, 1937.
Greenleaf, J.E. Dehydration-induced drinking in humans. *Federation Proceedings* 41:2509–2514, 1982.
Greenleaf, J.E., E.G. Averkin, and F. Sargent. Water consumption by man in a warm environment: a statistical analysis. *J. Appl. Physiol.* 21:93–98, 1966.
Greenleaf, J.E., P.J. Brock, L.C. Keil, and J.T. Morse. Drinking and water balance during exercise and heat acclimation. *J. Appl. Physiol.* 54:414- 419, 1983.
Greenleaf, J.E., L.G. Douglas, J.S. Bosco, M. Matter, and J.R. Blackaby. Thirst and artificial heat acclimatization in man. *Int. J. Biometeorol.* 11:311–327, 1967.
Greenleaf, J.E. and F. Sargent. Voluntary dehydration in man. *J. Appl. Physiol.* 20:719–724, 1965.
Gregersen, M.I. The physiological mechanism of thirst. *Amer. J. Physiol.* 101:44–45, 1932.
Gutman, J. An extrarenal effect of hydrochlorothiazide. *Experientia* 19:544–545, 1963.
Gutman, Y., F. Bergmann, and A. Zerachia. Influence of hypothalamic deposits of antidipsic drugs on renal excretion. *European J. Pharmacol.* 13:326–329, 1971.
Gutman, Y., D. Shamir, D. Glushevitzky, and S. Hochman. Angiotensin increases microsomal (Na-K)-ATPase activity in several tissues. *Biochim. Biophys. Acta* 273:401–405, 1972.
Guyton, A.C. *Textbook of Medical Physiology*, A.C. Guyton, ed. Philadelphia: Saunders, 7th ed., pp. 382–392, 1986.
Heckmann, K.D. and D.S. Parsons. Changes in the water and electrolyte content of rat-liver slices in vitro. *Biochim. Biophys. Acta.* 36:203–213, 1959.
Heppel, L.A. The electrolytes of muscle and liver in potassium-depleted rats. *Am. J. Physiol.* 127:385–392, 1939.
Holmes, J.H. and M.I. Gregersen. Role of sodium and chloride in thirst. *Am. J. Physiol.* 162:338–347, 1950.
Holmes, J.H. and M.I. Gregersen. Observations on drinking induced by hypertonic solutions. *Am. J. Physiol.* 162:326–337, 1950b.
Horne, G.O. and R.H. Mole. The effect of water and salt intake in prickly heat. *Lancet* 2:279–281, 1949.
Hubbard, R.W. Diet and physical performance: Water and salt. *Activities Report of the R and D Associates for Military Food and Packaging Systems.* 34:90–94, 1982.
Hubbard, R. W. and L.E. Armstrong. The heat illnesses: biochemical, ultrastructural, and fluid-electrolyte considerations. In: *Human Performance Physiology and Environmental Medicine at Terrestrial Extremes.* K.B. Pandolph, M.N. Sawka, and R.R. Gonzalez, eds., Indianapolis: Benchmark Press, pp. 305–359, 1988.
Hubbard, R.W., L.E. Armstrong, P.K. Evans, and J.P. DeLuca. Long term water and salt deficits: A military perspective. In: *Predicting Decrements in Military Performance Due to Inadequate Nutrition.* Washington, D.C., National Academy Press, pp. 29–48, 1986.
Hubbard, R.W., C.B. Matthew, M.J. Durkot, and R.P. Francesconi. Novel approaches to the pathophysiology of heatstroke: The energy depletion model. *Ann. Emerg. Med.* 16:1066–1075, 1987.
Hubbard, R.W., B.L. Sandick, W.T.Matthew, R.P. Francesconi, J.B. Sampson, M.J. Durkot, O. Maller, and D.B. Engell. Voluntary dehydration and alliesthesia for water. *J. Appl. Physiol.: Respirat. Environ. Exercise Physiol.* 57:868–875, 1984.

Huth, E.J., R.D. Squires, and J.R. Elkinton. Experimental potassium depletion in normal human subjects. II. Renal and hormonal factors in the development of extracellular alkalosis during depletion. *J. Clin. Invest.* 38:1149–1165, 1959.
Johnson, J.A. and J.O. Davis. Effect of a specific antagonist of angiotensin II on arterial pressure and adrenal steroid secretion in the dog. *Circ. Res.* 32 (Suppl. 1), 159–168, 1973.
Johnson, R.E. Water and osmotic economy of survival rations. *J. Am. Dietetic Assoc.* 45:124–129, 1964.
Kaplan, N.M. *Ann. Intern. Med.* Suicide by oral ingestion of a potassium preparation. 71:363–364, 1969.
Kelsch, R.C., G.S. Light, J.R. Luciano, and W.J. Oliver. The effect of prednisone on plasma norepinephrine concentration and renin activity in salt-depleted man. *J. Lab. Clin. Med.* 77:267–277, 1971.
Kleeman, C.R., F.H. Epstein, and C. White. Effect of variations in solute excretion and glomerular filtration on water diuresis. *J. Clin. Invest.* 35:749–756, 1956.
Kleinzeller, A. and A. Knotkova. Electrolyte transport in rat diaphragm. *Physiol. Bohemoslov.* 13:317–326, 1964.
Knochel, J.P., W.R. Beisel, E.G. Herndon, E.S. Gerard, and K.G. Barry. The renal, cardiovascular, hematologic and serum electrolyte abnormalities of heat stroke. *Amer. J. Med.* 30:299–309, 1961.
Knutton, S., D. Jackson, J.M. Graham, K.J. Micklem, and C.A. Pasternak. Microvilli and cell swelling. *Nature* 262:52–54, 1976.
Ladell, W.S.S. Water and salt (sodium chloride) intakes. In: *The Physiology of Human Survival*, O. Edholm and A. Bacharach, eds., New York: Academic Press, 1965, pp. 235–299.
Ladell, W.S.S., J.C. Waterlow, and M.F. Hudson. Desert climate: Physiological and clinical observations. *Lancet* 2:491, 1944.
Leaf, A. On the mechanism of fluid exchange of tissues in vitro. *Biochem. J.* 62:241–248, 1956.
Leaf, A. Maintenance of concentration gradients and regulation of cell volume. *Ann. N.Y. Acad. Sci.* 72:396–404, 1959.
Leaf, A. and W.T. Couter. Evidence that renal sodium excretion by normal human subjects is regulated by adrenal cortical activity. *J. Clin. Invest.* 28:1067–1081, 1949.
Leksell, L.G., F. Lishajko, and M. Rundgren. Negative water balance induced by intracerebroventricular infusion of deuterium. *Acta Physiol. Scand.* 97:142–144, 1976.
Limas, C.J. and J.N. Cohn. Stimulation of vascular smooth muscle Na-K-ATPase by vasodilators. *Circulation Res.* 35:601–607, 1974.
Lipsett, M.B. and O.H. Pearson. Sodium depletion in adrenalectomized humans. *J. Clin. Invest.* 37:1395–1402, 1958.
MacKnight, A.D.C. Water and electrolyte contents of rat renal cortical slices incubated in potassium-free media and media containing ouabain. *Biochim. Biophys. Acta* 150:263–270, 1968.
MacKnight, A.D.C. and A. Leaf. Regulation of cellular volume. *Physiol. Rev.* 57:510–573, 1977.
Manery, J.F. Water and electrolyte metabolism. *Physiol. Rev.* 34:334–417, 1954.
Marcus, E. Problems in fluid and electrolyte imbalance and their management. *The Surgical Clinics of North America.* 42:35–54, 1962.
Marriott, H.L. *Water and salt depletion.* Springfield, IL: Charles C. Thomas, pp. 1–80, 1950.
McCance, R.A. Experimental sodium deficiency in man. *Proc. Royal Soc. London* 119:245–268, 1936.
McCance, R.A. and E.M. Widdowson. Secretion of urine in man during experimental salt deficiency. *J. Physiol. London* 91:222–231, 1937.
McCutchan, J.W. and G.L. Taylor. Respiratory heat exchange with varying temperature and humidity of inspired air. *J. Appl. Physiol.* 4:121–135, 1951.
Mudge, G.H. Studies on potassium accumulation by rabbit kidney slices: Effect on metabolic activity. *Am. J. Physiol.* 165:113–127, 1951.
Neufer, P.D., D.L. Costill, W.J. Fink, J.P. Kirwan, R.A. Fielding, and M.G. Flynn. Effects of exercise and carbohydrate composition on gastric emptying. *Med. Sci. Sports Exer.* 18:658–662, 1986.
Olsson, K. Studies on central regulation of secretion of antidiuretic hormone (ADH) in the goat. *Acta Physiol Scand.* 77:465–474, 1969.
Olsson, K., F. Fyhrquist, B. Larsson, and L. Eriksson. Inhibition of vasopressin-release during developing hypernatremia and plasma hyperosmolality: an effect of intracerebroventricular glycerol. *Acta Physiol Scand.* 102:399–409, 1978.
Olsson, K., B. Larsson, and E. Liljekvist. Intracerebroventricular glycerol: a potent inhibitor of ADH-release and thirst. *Acta Physiol. Scand.* 98:470–477, 1976.
Osborne, W.A. Water in expired air. *J. Physiol.* 47:12, 1913.
Page, E.R., J. Goerke, and S.R. Storm. Cat heart muscle in vitro. IV. Inhibition of transport in quiescent muscles. *J. Gen. Physiol.* 47:531–543, 1964.
Peters, J.P. Water exchange. *Physiol. Rev.* 24:491–531, 1944.
Peters, J.P. Physiology of renal excretion. *Lancet* 73:180–182, 1953.
Pitts, R.F. *Physiology of the Kidney and Body Fluids.* (2nd ed.), Chicago: Yearbook Medical Publishers, 1968.
Pitts, G.C., R.E. Johnson, and F.C. Consolazio. Work in the heat as affected by intake of water, salt and glucose. *Am. J. Physiol.* 142:253–259, 1944.
Post, R.L. and P.C. Jolly. The linkage of sodium, potassium and ammonium active transport across the human erythrocyte membrane. *Biochim. Biophys. Acta* 25:118–128, 1975.
Posternak, L., H.R. Brunner, H. Gavras, and D.B. Brunner. Angiotensin II blockade in normal man:

Interaction of renin and sodium in maintaining blood pressure. *Kidney Int.* 11:197-203, 1977.
Porteres, R. "Les Sels Alimentaires: Cendres D'Origine Vegetale." Gouvern. Gen de PA O.F., Dakar, 1950.
Richter, C.P. Total self-regulatory functions in animals and human beings. *Harvey Lect.* 38:63-103, 1942-1943.
Rixon, R.H. and J.A.F. Stevenson. The water and electrolyte metabolism of rat diaphragm in vitro. *Can. J. Bichem. Physiol.* 34:1069-1083, 1956.
Robertson, G.L. The regulation of vasopressin function in health and disease. *Rec. Prog. Horm. Res.* 33:333-385, 1977.
Robertson, G.L. Abnormalities of thirst regulation. *Kidney Int.* 25:460- 469, 1984.
Robertson, G.L. Posterior pituitary. In: *Endocrinology and Metabolism.* P. Felig, J. Baxter, A.E. Broadus, and L.A. Frohman, eds., New York: McGraw-Hill, 2nd ed., pp. 339-386, 1987.
Robertson, G.L. and S. Athar. The interaction of blood osmolality and blood volume in regulating plasma vasopressin in man. *J. Clin. Endocrinol. Metab.* 42:613-620, 1976.
Robertson, G.L. and T. Berl. Water metabolism. In: *The Kidney.* B.M. Brenner and F.C. Rector, eds., Philadel: Saunders, 3rd ed. pp. 385-432, 1985.
Robertson, G.L. and E.A. Mahr. The importance of plasma osmolality in regulating antidiuretic hormone in man. *J. Clin. Invest.* 51:79a, 1972.
Robertson, G.L., R.L. Shelton, and S. Athar. The osmoregulation of vasopressin. *Kidney Int.* 10:25-37, 1976.
Robinson, J.R. The active transport of water in living systems. *Biol. Rev.* 28:158-194, 1953.
Rothstein, A., E.F. Adolph, and J.H. Wills. Voluntary dehydration. In: *Physiology of Man in the Desert.* New York: Interscience, 1947, p. 254-270.
Rundgren, M., L.G. Leksell, F. Lishajko, and B. Anderson. Deuterium-induced extinction of ADH release in response to intracerebroventricular infusions of hypertonic NaCl and angiotensin. *Acta Physiol. Scand.* 100:45-50, 1977.
Samuels, A.I., E.D. Miller, J.C. Fray, E. Haber, and A.C. Barger. Renin-angiotensin antagonists and the regulation of blood pressure. *Fed. Proc.* 35:2512, 1976.
Sandick, B.L., D.B. Engell, and O. Maller. Perception of drinking water temperature and effects for humans after exercise. *Physiol. and Behav.* 32:851-855, 1984.
Sawka, M.N. and K.B. Pandolf. Effects of body water loss on exercise performance and physiological function. In: *Perspectives in Exercise Science and Sports Medicine: Volume 3. Fluid Homeostasis During Exercise.* Chapter 1, 1990.
Siesjo, B.K. and T. Wielock. Cerebral metabolism in ischemia: Neurochemical basis for therapy. *Br. J. Anesth.* 57:47-62, 1985.
Sohar, E., J. Kaly, and R. Adar. The prevention of voluntary dehydration. *UNESCO/India Symp. Environ. Physiol. Psychol. Lucknow.* 7-12 Dec. 1962, pp. 129-135.
Squires, R.D. and E.J. Huth. Experimental potassium depletion in normal human subjects. I. Relation of ionic intakes to the renal conservation of potassium. *J. Clin. Invest.* 38:1134-1148, 1959.
Stricker, E.M. and J.G. Verbalis. Hormones and behavior: The biology of thirst and sodium appetite. *Am. Scientist* 76:261-267, 1988.
Szlyk, P.C., R.W. Hubbard, W.T. Matthew, L.E. Armstrong, and M.D. Kerstein. Mechanisms of voluntary dehydration among troops in the field. *Mil. Med.* 152:405-407, 1987.
Szlyk, P.C., I.V. Sils, R.P. Francesconi, R.W. Hubbard, and L.E. Armstrong. Effects of water temperature and flavoring on voluntary dehydration in men. *Physiol. and Behav.* 45:639-647, 1989.
Szlyk, P.C., I.V. Sils, R.P. Francesconi, and R.W. Hubbard. Patterns of human drinking: Effects of exercise, water temperature and food consumption. *Aviat. Space Environ. Med.*, in press, 1989b.
TB MED 507 (1980). *Prevention, treatment and control of heat injury.* Department of the Army Technical Bulletin, Washington, DC: US Government Printing Office.
Thrasher, T.N., C.J. Brown, L.K. Keil, and D.J. Ramsay. Thirst and vasopressin release in the dog: an osmoreceptor or sodium receptor mechanism? *Am J. Physiol.* 238:R 333-339, 1980.
Tosteson, D.C. and J.F. Hoffman. Regulation of cell volume by active cation transport in high and low potassium sheep red cells. *J. Gen. Physiol.* 44:169-194, 1960.
Vaamonde, C.A. Sodium depletion. In: *Sodium: Its biological significance.* S. Papper, ed., Boca Raton: CRC Press, 207-234, 1982.
Verney, E.B. The antidiuretic hormone and factors which determine its release. *Proc Roy. Soc., London.* Ser B, 135:25-106, 1947.
Vokes, T. Water homeostasis. *Ann. Rev. Nutr.* 7:383-406, 1987.
Vokes, T. and G.L. Robertson. Physiology and secretion of vasopressin. *Front Horm. Res.* 13:127-155, 1987.
Vokes, T. and G.L. Robertson. Clinical effects of altered vasopressin secretion. In: *Neuroendocrine Perspectives.* E.E. Muller, R.M. MacLeod, and A. Frohmam, eds., Amsterdam: Elseveir Science, 4:pp. 1-41, 1985.
Wade, C.E., P. Bie, L.C. Keil, and D.J. Ramsay. Effect of hypertonic intracarotid infusions on plasma vasopressin concentration. *Am. J. Physiol.* 243: (Endocrinol. Metab. 6) E522-E526, 1982.
Welt, L.G. and W.P. Nelson. Excretion of water by normal subjects. *J. Appl. Physiol.* 4:709-714, 1952.

Whittam, R. The dependence of the respiration of brain cortex on active cation transport. *Biochem. J.* 82:205–212, 1962.
Whittam, R. and J.S. Willis. Ion movements and oxygen consumption in kidney cortex slices. *J. Physiol (London)* 168:158–177, 1963.
Wilkins, L. and C.P. Richter. A great craving for salt by a child with cortico-adrenal insufficiency. *J. Am. Med. Assoc.* 114:866–868, 1940.
Yarbrough, B.E. and R.W. Hubbard. Heat-related illness. In: *Management of Wilderness and Environmental Emergencies. Sec. ed.* St. Louis: C.V. Mosby Co., pp. 119–143, 1989.
Zellner, D.A., W.F. Stewart, P. Rozin, and J.M. Brown. Effect of temperature and liking for beverages. *Physiol. and Behavior.* 44:61–68, 1988.

ACKNOWLEDGMENTS

The authors wish to express their sincere thanks to Dr. Ralph Francesconi for his scholarly review and to Mrs. Diane Danielski, Ms. JoAnn DeLuca and Ms. Ingrid Sils for their efforts in the preparation of this manuscript.

- APPENDIX A -

ION PUMPING, BEHAVIORAL THERMOREGULATION, MOBILITY AND THIRST:

THE BOUYANT CELL-HYPOTHESIS

A primitive cell suspended near the surface of some primordial sea would a) probably lack mechanisms for mobility (cilia), b) be limited to primitive photosynthetic or anaerobic mechanisms for making chemical energy (ATP), and c) probably possess some primitive ion pumping capability. Surface evaporation, lack of rainfall, and thermal inversions could produce a tendency toward hypersalinity, analogous to thirst (cell shrinkage), in the microenvironment and make ion pumping necessary. Given some thermal stratification in the aqueous environment, and depending upon its depth from the surface and the time of day, this cell's metabolic rate would be driven by the surrounding water temperature (Q_{10} effect) and the effect of temperature on membrane permeability to Na^+ (leaks). For example, cooling would slow the Na^+ leak rate and lower the metabolic rate.

If the cell could move vertically within the aqueous environment, it could adjust its thermal environment with the time of day and take advantage of lateral currents (three-dimensional movement). This would represent a primitive connection between thermoregulation, carbohydrate metabolism and mobility. If the cell could exchange K^{35} for Na^{23}, it could alter its density without affecting its total osmolality. This alteration in density would alter the bouyancy of the cell, thus allowing it to rise or sink in its aqueous milieu.

Interesting aspects of this simple hypothesis are: a) Mobility (achieved by altering the cell density/bouyancy) is linked to the Na^+/K^+ ratio, perhaps the precursor to the membrane potential. b) A Na^+ leakage rate and, thereby, the energy demand is linked to the solar day. c) The thermal lag inherent in the heating and cooling of water coupled with changes in membrane permeability, related control mechanisms, and metabolic rate establishes the basis for circadian periodicity or a biological clock. d) The ability to move away from an aversive stimulus (heat) suggests behavioral thermoregulation as a basic feature of even single cells. e) Behavioral thermoregulation (movement) and chemical thermoregulation (metabolic heat production) become linked at the site of greatest energy utilization (Na-K-ATPase). f) Thirst, manifested either as a loss of water, an increase in the external Na^+ content, or an increase in the Na^+ "leak" rate of the extracellular fluid, can be seen as a problem confronting even unicellular organisms. g) A loss of K^+ as a response to an increased permeability to Na^+ could be seen as a fundamental homeostatic mechanism and should be explored in higher systems. h) The causes and consequences of the breakdown and resynthesis of ATP around a 24-hour day establishes a pattern for evolution to follow.

DISCUSSION

HARVEY: I'd just like to comment about something that is somewhat practical, relating to 10 years of providing medical care to bicycle racers. I was interested that your data showed you are more likely to drink twice the volume if the water is cold. It seems that we have a very archaic way of delivering fluids to a cyclist. If you're a triathlete, your water bottle basks in the sun for 20–40 minutes while you're getting your swim done, it continues to warm while fastened on the down tube where it is exposed to radiant and convective heat, riding in an 80°F day at 27 mph. By the time you're ready to drink, you have a fluid that is very warm and unpalatable. I'm certainly stimulated to take a thermometer on my next ride and measure everyone's water bottle temperature. It would seem to me that no matter how scientific a fluid we formulate, we need to find a better way of keeping it cool to enhance palatability.
HUBBARD: You're absolutely right. In the military, this is also a very significant problem. Clearly, the obvious response to that is to deliver cooled water to the subject as opposed to letting it sit in a 500-gallon water trailer at 120°F like it was in arid regions during World War II. The water is now delivered to the soldiers cooled through a small mobile chiller and an insulated canteen keeps it reasonably cool and palatable. I would think that a simpler solution for sports would be possible. You've put your finger on a very simple and obvious problem, but one that has profound impact on performance decrements and illness rates with large numbers of people.
SCHEDL: In Figure 2-6, you compare water consumption under conditions of rest and exercise in relation to temperature. At rest, you drink about the same amount of water regardless of water temperature. Look-

ing at the scatter, there doesn't seem to be a statistical difference. During exercise, the water temperature determines consumption. Is this related to the higher body temperatures during exercise?

HUBBARD: We originally offered a behavioral explanation for why warm drinks were consumed at a lower rate than cool drinks (negative and positive alliesthesia). We are currently seeking a cellular mechanism for explaining the aversion to warm water in hyperthermic, dehydrated subjects. We're thinking conceptually that heat increases sodium permeability into the cell and this stimulates sodium pumping and energy demand. So during exercise, we envision hot water was worsening the cellular energy status and being avoided. In contrast, cool water, by lowering sodium permeability, would improve the energy state and the drinking behavior is reinforced. At rest, the elevated state of energy consumption is not there, and you're right, there doesn't seem to be any effect of temperature on the resting consumption.

SCHEDL: Just one other point that I was thinking about. In the 1950s we did some studies with anabolic steroids in normal young women. During a period of a few days, we noticed that their body weights increased by about 1 or 2 kg before there was any effect on nitrogen balance. Is it characteristic that people on anabolic steroids start out with a greater total body water, and would this be a factor in relation to the response to exercise?

HUBBARD: That is an excellent question. It suggests that the total body water content of people taking anabolic steroids, because of their sodium retention qualities, start off with a higher reservoir. If our model is correct, this would have an impact on what one would find for a relative deficit in terms of rehydration. It depends, again, on the total solute content in the body at that point and depends, also, on what kind of sweat sodium one finds in a subject taking anabolic steroids. If the response at the sweat gland were similar to the response at the kidney, one would expect less solute loss and, therefore, a tendency for a higher rehydration rate. As a starting point, at least hypothetically, I would look to sodium retention in subjects that were consuming anabolic steroids; they might have a larger content of total exchangeable sodium. The question leads to the difficulty of how one addresses the very vexing question, "What is the change, if any, in total solute content?" How do we approximate that, short of doing some very expensive and risky studies with radioactive tracers? One of the things that we are hoping is that there is a development of stable isotope technology that would allow use of some of the stable isotopes of potassium or rubidium for potassium, and tracking sodium with, say, bromine. Knockel and Schline, for example, showed an enormous increase in intracellular sodium levels in potassium depleted dogs. What is the trend in transmembrane equilibration of sodium and potassium in hypohydrated states and in exercise training states, and in other states where hormones might be affecting the leakiness of cells as opposed to the activities of pump enzymes themselves? I think these are basic questions that must be addressed by measuring where the solutes are and what their mixes or proportions are in future experiments. The problem is that we don't have a very useful technology for addressing these questions now.

WADE: I think we should make a distinction between thirst and satiation of thirst. I think that thirst drive is affected via a possible oral pharyngeal reflex. However, as ingested fluids are absorbed into the system when the drinking stops, there's a difference in osmotic drive. The osmotic drive is still there when people have finished their drinking.

HUBBARD: You are absolutely right. The reason we present these calculations is not to suggest that they are absolutely correct and that they will serve to distinguish between thirst and the ultimate amount of water consumed, but simply to point out something that is intrinsic in the studies that Ethan has done, i.e., that one should allow time for a proper equilibration to occur before even setting out to measure what the rehydration rate or total volume consumed would be. In other words, it's hard to make sense out of what is occurring when things are going in 2 different directions at once. We are just now taking to heart what we are doing from a design point of view. This has somewhat compromised even our ability to clearly look at some of these factors, and you have adequately pointed out one. On the other hand, can you be sure that the oral pharyngeal reflex does not have a local, osmotic or temperature component?

WADE: Which brings up a second point. When you look at the osmotic drive for thirst from a psychological point of view, it matches the basic osmotic drive for vasopressin in terms of threshold. Threshold, you must remember, is the resting osmolality. This is because, in the basal state, you have no drive for thirst or stimulation of vasopressin. It doesn't take much change to elicit a response. The other problem is that you have looked at humans who have other inputs modulating thirst and satiation.

HUBBARD: Let me just address your initial point. Again, my only comment is that we rarely know what the resting osmolality is for our subjects when we start an experiment. We have gone back and looked at them, and they're never really close to the hydrated threshold (280 mOsm/kg. I would agree with you that our subjects tend to start out at a variety of inter-individual levels and consistently tend to be hypohydrated. As I mentioned in the beginning, Kristal-Bonet has just looked at the Negev desert residents, and their resting osmolality is 294 mOsm/kg. Well, they're going to lose just a little bit of water, and one or two things will happen: 1) they will get thirsty, and 2), subsequent to the dehydration, if it was a hypotonic water loss in a well acclimatized subject, they will have an enormous increase in plasma osmolality as compared to what we see. Just to make a final comment, it is extremely important to know what your starting levels are.

WADE: My final comment is that I do not understand your emphasis on energy in the system. I think if you look at osmotic drive, it's still there in the systems you are looking at, but you have secondary influences on top of that osmotic drive. If you altered the osmolality, you would still see a proportional change. It may shift the intercept, but the osmotic drive is still a primary factor. I don't understand how you could say that it is energy-related because other osmotic substances besides sodium do elicit that drive.

HUBBARD: Well that's true as far as we know. On the other hand, it is difficult to suggest why something like 2-deoxyglucose could stimulate thirst.

SUMMERS: In the slide where you looked at the drinking behavior before, during, and after a meal, you concluded that the osmotic drive was the factor which stimulated the most drinking during the meal. If that were the case, wouldn't one expect the solute load to have its greatest effect after the meal? Don't you also think that there are very important cultural factors and dietary habits which cause people to drink during the meal, such as dry or spicy food?

HUBBARD: Absolutely. I don't disregard the excellent point that Wade made that it may be oral pharyngeal input to the system. I'm only trying to define the simplest explanation for why the subjects drank more after or during a meal. I would agree with you; it's hard to explain why they drank more during the meal if they weren't responding to something other than solute load, because the solute hasn't presented itself to the thirst receptor at that point. It's a very complex situation. My only point is that if we do not begin to sort some of these things out by allowing the system to re-equilibrate before we look at such factors as thirst, then we're not going to make a lot of progress.

SUTTON: I would be interested to know if there is any differences between males and females in the response to an exercise test in terms of water intake and rehydration, particularly in the 2 phases of the menstrual cycle when presumably the females are starting with a different core temperature and a different hormonal profile.

HUBBARD: That's a good question. I don't know of any data, personally, that would support any suggestion that there are differences. Those of you who work in that field might be able to address the question. I would think that if the dehydrated female tended to have a higher working or resting core temperature, then from our experience, presenting that subject with cool water might stimulate intake greater than we would see in a male at the same relative water loss. There is an enormous behavioral component to female rehydration, at least in the military where I have observed it, and in the field. Generally, females tend to remain more hypohydrated than males at a given time of day. They tend to have a higher incidence, for example, of heat exhaustion for the percentage of their population within the total population. I don't know whether this is just related to their reluctance to drink a lot when there are limited facilities for urination, which is a common explanation, or that there is something more profoundly and physiologically different in females. Clearly, they tend to have a higher incidence of hypohydration-induced disorders.

SAWKA: I have 2 questions. The first is practical and the second is physiological. I was interested in your slides showing the effects of varying water temperature preference as indicated by consumption stayed relatively constant over time. Subjects liked 15° or 22° C water depending on the experiment. I assume that over time, core temperature was rising. When I think of palatability, I think of temperature and taste. What does the literature tell us about the effect of sweetness? Does consumption of different fluids vary with sweetness? How does that change as body temperature rises? As you get hotter, do you desire a less sweet beverage?

HUBBARD: We haven't done a controlled study on that except that in our initial long term studies with Kool-Aid, it became obvious within the first 5 subjects that the subject would not drink cherry Kool-Aid for 6 hours at the normal sugar content recommended by the manufacturer. In those studies we reduced the carbohydrate concentration to about half the recommended value. At that point, we see the so-called flavoring effects on temperature-induced intake. They are quite dramatic with more intake of cool water. Clearly, there was some indication in the preliminary studies that if the carbohydrate content was too high, after about 3 hours, and we did some tests where the subjects were not eating, the subjects refused to consume it; they got nauseous, some said it made them sick. Perhaps that relates to gastric emptying.

SAWKA: The second question had to do with that 295 milliosmal threshold for thirst. I know Engell did a study, you're familiar with, that looked at thirst and different levels of dehydration. They showed thirst occurring, at fairly low osmolalities, 285 milliosmal and slightly higher. Do you think any differences might be due to something like an osmolality threshold due to a core body temperature difference or perhaps a change in regional blood flow affecting the osmo-receptors?

HUBBARD: I think all of the above, and perhaps even acclimatization. We would like to look at inter-individual variation with regard to the renal diuresis threshold as well as the thirst threshold and see what the biological variability within the population suggests and, whether those thresholds change with some kind of chronic behavior of acclimatization. Clearly, something is happening with these Negev residents, long term desert dwellers where they maintain a resting osmolality of 294 mOsm/kg, compared to what one would expect to find in the American population, probably 283-287 on average in our studies.

JOHNSON: I wanted to touch on this concept of "voluntary dehydration" and the concepts of thirst vs. sodium appetite. I want to discuss this from the standpoint of what has become reasonably well accepted and what is based on an animal appetitive behavior literature that has existed for the past 20-25 years. That is, by the late 1960s there was ample evidence that drinking behavior would be induced by either dehydration of the intracellular compartment or the extracellular space. In the case of pure intracellular dehydration, animals behave as if they are perfect osmometers. In other words, when pure water is the only fluid available there is no impairment in rehydration. However, in the case of extracellular depletion, animals will not drink to repletion if the only fluid they have access to is pure water. Animals will not drink themselves into a state of severe hyponatremia. At the point where water intake ceases, but the animal is still hypovolemic, presentation of a hypertonic NaCl solution (2-3%) to the animal will provide evidence that the animal displays a "sodium appetite." That is, the animal will consume a normally adversive concentration of NaCl along with pure water so that he, in effect, creates an "isotonic cocktail' that permits a restoration of the extracellular fluid compartment to homeostasis. In order to understand the mechanisms involved in the restoration of fluid homeostasis it is necessary to understand the neurobiology of both the drinking of water (i.e., thirst) and the ingestion of sodium (i.e., sodium appetite) when the animal is operating under conditions of deficits to both substances.

HUBBARD: I couldn't agree with you more. There is clearly good evidence that low pressure receptors and baroreceptors and the renin-angiotensin systems, as well as other experiments with portal ligation, suggest that there are non-osmotic or extracellular causes of thirst behavior. My only point is that to get clearly at those factors, one should at least know where you are vis-a-vis the osmotic theory. I don't see myself doing that as an investigator and I don't see a lot of other people doing it either in terms of controlling those situations prior to any circumstance where we're looking at some of these other factors. Clearly, the response you are attempting to study will vary with either primary water depletion or salt depletion dehydration. You may find additive situations where you're then trading off between osmotic and pressure signals for thirst. Perhaps there are volume depletion thresholds. I don't know whether it's a linear relationship, for example, relating ADH release or thirst relative to plasma deficit. What I've read suggests that the volume response tends to be non-linear and logarithmic. And as a matter of fact, Vokes has recently suggested that volume-dependent regulation is probably not as fine-tuned a phenomenon in humans as is the ADH mechanism. I tended to discount it in the review, but only because it's a very different form of thirst regulation that I'll readily admit I have little or no experience with and didn't really care to get terribly involved with (i.e. hypovolemic shock). But I don't discount its existence.

JOHNSON: In terms of developing the methodology looking at behavioral responses to dehydration, it is apparent to me that the human studies need to look at the response to various solutions. Subjects must be allowed to choose water vs. solutions containing solute (e.g., NaCl). Animals clearly show a preference for water under a state of pure cellular dehydration. Whereas in the case of hypovolemia, animals titrate their ingestion of water and saline to basically drink an isotonic solution.

HUBBARD: Many of those animal experiments depend on how the volume-depletion occurred. If you're injecting something intraperitoneally and it's pulling fluid out of the vascular space, that's not something that we're doing readily with humans, but the tendency to consider glycerol as a substance that might enhance or maintain volume during exercise may well start to produce some data on those theories.

COYLE: Tying energy metabolism to thirst is intriguing. It triggers a question. As you exercise more intensely, you might be lowering the energy status at least of the musculature, raising ADP levels. According to your model, that would trigger thirst to a greater extent. Is there any data that fits that suggestion? For a given level of bodily dehydration, that exercise of a higher intensity stimulates greater thirst.

HUBBARD: I haven't seen that data. I think that's the trend in terms of what we would try to design to get at some of the questions. Not only that, perhaps I might even perform those experiments where hypertonic saline was infused and then study the effects of that on exercise and thirst. We know, for example, that during exercise with hypertonic saline infusions, the exercising core temperature tends to stay higher. With a given sweat rate, this suggests a greater heat production at some point. That basically fits our idea, but we have yet to design our experiments to do that.

COYLE: So the cell where thirst is sensed is muscle? Is that a correct assumption?

HUBBARD: Well, I'm not sure how the thirst receptor corresponds to what is going on in the muscle. That's a difficult question. That's why we have tended to focus attention on temperature as being one of the covariables that could likely affect a remote sensor such as the thirst receptor, at the same time some event was happening metabolically in another tissue.

PHILLIPS: I want to raise a couple of points. First, a long time ago we found that whenever animals drink, their blood pressure goes up (Hoffman, W.E., Phillips, M.I. et al Proc. Soc. Exp. Biol. Med. 154:1212-1214, 1977). We've worked on this to find out exactly what is going on, and it seems to be an oral reflex. I don't actually know what the effects of different temperature would be, but this reflex has now been seen in dogs, sheep, lambs, and humans. So there are reflexes activated as soon as you have the water in the mouth. Second, if you have cold water in the mouth, as I said, I don't know specifically what happens to the reflex, but you could get cooling of the hypothalamus just a few mm away. There is still a possibility that temperature in the mouth might have a direct effect on the brain. In your studies, you're mixing the need to keep temperature down and the need to replace water altogether. This brings me back to the point that was raised about extracellular dehydration. A way you can do that, very simply, is to hemorrhage. Then you take away the need to reduce temperature, you still get the thirst and then you can see if there are differences in relationship to the temperature of the water.

HUBBARD: That's an excellent idea. Another one that we found intriguing, although we don't do thermode research, would be in those situations where you're stimulating or inhibiting thirst with a thermode, why not change the temperature of the water you're presenting to the animal? If our concept is correct, then stimulating thirst with a warm thermode might not produce the same response with room temperature water as with water at 46°C.

COSTILL: In the process of listening to your discussions, I think one topic has been overlooked. That is, the question of palatability. Certainly there is a difference in what you want to drink when you're sitting at rest versus when you're exercising. That becomes very clear when you deal with athletes or individuals who are performing hours of exercise. Over the time of exercise, there is a change in our taste preference. Lars Hermansen and I studied a group of cyclists who exercised nonstop from Troudheim in Oslo, taking about 20 hours. When they started out, they all preferred a very sweet drink. Even though they were accumulating a considerable dehydration, they still did not prefer the sweetness that you suggested might be a stimulus for additional drinking. They got to the point where they lost their thirst. I think we should be aware of the fact that what seems to be a nice model in a very controlled environment may not be the case that we see during prolonged exercise dehydrations.

HUBBARD: I'd like to address another aspect of Costill's excellent comment. You bring out another effect of flavor or sweetness on consumption. One could make a similar case for volume of intake over time. For example, in a situation where an athlete may be losing 3 quarts of water an hour as we've seen in marathoners and find that attempting to maintain water balance, even by forcing that kind of fluid intake, would be unsuccessful because you're then titrating some other threshold that is not a factor in a short-term experiment. We would say that the first thing to look at would then be the cumulative intake effects on gastric distention and whatever that subject's vomiting threshold happened to be; literature suggests it is around a 3-quart capacity. But we just can't have run away enhancement of thirst intake by flavoring or forced hydration and not take into account what the affect of accumulating an increased stomach volume is over time. That may well be a factor.

TIPTON: Where does calcium fit into your model? In hypertension, there is a debate concerning whether sodium changes are mediated by calcium shifts. I noticed that there was no mention of whether calcium plays a role in the movement and exchange of sodium in your model.

HUBBARD: Let me try to address the first question in terms of why we are not talking about calcium. We are addressing it, at least theoretically in our own minds, under conditions where the transmembrane sodium gradient tends to be reduced. The reason we think that intracellular calcium might be increased in those situations goes back to what happens in the digitalized heart during congestive heart failure. At some dose of digitalis, there is an inotropic response in the heart of the patient suffering congestive heart failure. One of the models is that by reducing the activity of the sodium pump, one is, in effect, reducing the transmembrane electrochemical gradient for sodium. Under those conditions, by the model that was suggested, the potential energy available to countertransport calcium out of the cell is reduced. As a result, myocardial calcium levels tend to increase and its a steady-rate increase in calcium levels that accounts for the improved contractility in the congestive heart. Thus, in any situation where the transmembrane sodium gradient is reduced, we are indirectly suggesting that there is an obligate increase in intracellular calcium levels. How this affects performance and heat production is a very interesting question. In response to Block's recent findings looking at heat production in the brains and eyes of Bill fish, for example, they've shown that an eye muscle is involved in an energy producing cycle involving calcium, magnesium, and ATPase, which is directly related to sodium influx. In other words, sodium influx stimulates this process and produces heat for the brains and eyes of the animal. It suggests that calcium is involved in all these processes and it takes quite a bit of figuring to find out exactly how or why, but clearly that is an important question.

MURRAY: I'd like to return briefly to the issue of palatability–an often overlooked and extremely important area, because anything we can do to increase the voluntary consumption of fluids during exercise in the heat is a good thing. The palatability of a fluid certainly is one of the factors that will determine voluntary fluid intake along with availability of the fluid, coolness, and so on. Anything we can do to understand how beverage palatability influences fluid consumption is important. Part of the research that we've recently undertaken is to look just at that relationship. One of our very basic findings is that when people are hot, sweaty, and thirsty they will initially drink just about anything to remove their initial thirst. Thereafter, their fluid consumption pattern varies quite nicely with their ratings of beverage palatability. I was just wondering if you could very briefly comment based on your experiences with feeding beverages to troops in the field.

HUBBARD: That's a good question, and it's the second part of Costill's question that I didn't answer and it addresses this question: If our model is correct and people are increasing their initial fluid consumption when it contains "flavoring" or carbohydrate, why is it that they stop drinking it after a while? It suggests, for example, that people will regulate their energy state faster than they'll regulate their hydration state. If that's the case, then our paradigm would suggest that thirst would continue in the flavored, artificial sweetened situation if energy was not a function in the equation. And that's probably why I would market artificial drinks because if part of people's intake is based on their energy state, then you're not solving that by giving them artificial sweeteners, and they'll keep on drinking your product. If part of their ingestion of fluid is related to their energy state and they're satisfying that with a carbohydrate-rich drink, unfortunately they are going to stop drinking it after awhile, perhaps even in spite of a continuing water deficit. I think those paradigms could be addressed in chronic, long-term intake studies comparing flavoring plus carbohydrate or no carbohydrate, and knowing the fact that some things will tend to reduce performance. Explosive gastric emptying being one, energy depletion being another.

3

Gastric Emptying of Fluids During Exercise

David L. Costill, Ph.D.

INTRODUCTION

The metabolic demands of prolonged exercise in warm environments place severe demands on sweat production and evaporation to minimize body heat storage. During endurance events such as distance running, athletes have been found to lose more than 4 kg of body weight, resulting in a body water deficit in excess of 6% (Costill et al., 1970; Pugh et al., 1957). Previous studies have shown that dehydration of more than 2% can significantly lower one's exercise capacity and heat tolerance (Armstrong et al., 1985; Buskirk et al., 1958; Saltin, 1964). Fluid intake during exercise can, however, reduce the degree of dehydration, thereby minimizing the risk of hyperthermia (Costill et al., 1970; Pitts et al., 1944).

In addition to dehydration and hyperthermia, limited availability of carbohydrates (i.e., blood glucose and muscle glycogen) are factors known to limit one's endurance capacity. Studies conducted early in this century noted the occurrence of low blood glucose during exhaustive long-distance running and cycling. In events lasting for more than 2 h, blood glucose has been seen to drop from normal levels of 5.0 mM to less than 2.5 mM in 30 to 40% of the subjects (Levine et al., 1924). These low blood glucose values have been associated with fatigue and exhaustion, but a direct cause and effect relationship has not been repeatedly documented (Felig et al., 1982). Several studies, however, have noted improvements in performance when the subjects were given carbohydrate feedings during exercise lasting 1–4 h (Costill et al., 1978; Costill, 1970; Hargreaves et al., 1984).

Thus, the intake of fluids containing carbohydrate (CHO) can reduce the risk of dehydration, minimize the risk of hyperthermia, and provide an alternate source of CHO, thereby enhancing endurance performance. The replacement of water and CHO during exercise is, however, limited by the rate of gastric emptying (Costill & Saltin, 1974). Marathon runners, for example, have been reported to lose 21 to 33 mL of sweat per min during competition (Costill et al., 1970; Noakes, 1988); efforts to offset these body fluid losses by ingesting fluids are only partially effective because the maximal rates of gastric emptying generally range from 12–14 mL/min (Mitchell et al., 1988; Neufer et al., 1986).

There are several review articles that thoroughly describe the past century of research on the regulation of gastric emptying in resting humans and animals (Hollander & Penner, 1939; Hunt and Knox, 1969a; Marbaix, 1898; Thomas, 1957). Although studies have been conducted concerning gastric function during exercise, only limited attempts have been made to summarize these findings (Murray, 1987; Sherman & Lamb, 1988). The present review, therefore, will describe the factors that influence gastric function during short- and long-term exercise with special attention given to solute composition, volume, and frequency of ingestion.

MEASUREMENT OF GASTRIC EMPTYING

Much of our early knowledge of gastric function can be credited to the careful studies of William Beaumont in 1833. His observations were based on a single patient who possessed a permanent gastric fistula as a consequence of a musket wound. Since that time other studies on patients with gastric fistula have been made (Carlson, 1923; Wolf & Wolff, 1943). In more recent times a variety of techniques has been used to assess the rate at which foods and fluids leave the stomach. These include gastric aspiration and the use of x-ray, radioisotopic, and tomographic techniques. These procedures have been previously described in considerable detail by Hunt and Knox (1969a), and Hollander and Penner (1939).

Serial x-rays and feedings containing barium sulfate have been used to follow the movement of meals within the stomach (Minami & McCallum, 1984). This non-quantitative method is limited by the density of the marker substance (i.e., barium sulfate) which rapidly falls to the lowest part of the stomach unless it is finely dispersed as a stable suspension in water. This fact, plus the risk of repeated x-ray exposures, makes this method undesirable.

As noted by Murray (1987), the non-invasive radioisotopic methods employ indium or 99m technetium to follow the movement of materials within the gastrointestinal tract. An external scanner is used to count the radiation emitted from the stomach, thereby sensing the relative degree of movement of materials out of the stomach. Although this method offers an index of gastric emptying, it fails to provide specific information relative to gastric secretion and a quantitative rate of emptying.

Tomography, using skin electrodes placed over the stomach, has recently been used to study gastric emptying. Changes in resistance resulting from a small electric current passing among electrodes are used to produce a computer-generated image of stomach contents. Serial analysis of such images can be used to assess gastric emptying. Although this procedure offers a non-invasive method with no risk to the subject, measurements are limited to a relative index of gastric emptying, and the method does not offer an opportunity to sample the stomach's contents (Barber & Brown, 1984).

The majority of our knowledge of gastric emptying has been obtained using the "aspiration" technique. This procedure employs a 10 to 14 French gauge tube that is passed through the nasal passage to the stomach. Because most studies have used tubes that are not radiopaque, the locations of the tube tip within the stomach have not been clearly described. It is common practice to perform gastric analysis in the morning after an overnight fast by the subjects. After positioning the gastric tube, the subject's stomach is emptied of all residue using a 50 mL syringe. The subject then ingests a volume of test solution. After a predetermined period, often 15–30 min, the residue in the stomach is aspirated and the rate of emptying determined by subtracting the volume of the residue from the volume of the original solution consumed. Because the gastric residue also contains the secretions from the mucosa, a nonabsorbable marker such as phenol red or polyethylene glycol is added to the original solution to permit determination of the amount of gastric secretion (Fordtran, 1966; Schedl et al., 1966). Because there is little absorption directly from the stomach, measurements of the gastric residue and secretion are used to estimate the net volume of the original solution that was delivered to the duodenum (Minami & McCallum, 1984). Although the position of the tube may cause some discomfort, studies have shown that the presence of the tube does not alter normal gastric function (Mitchell et al., 1989; Muller-Lissner et al., 1982).

Unless otherwise noted, the studies reported in this review have used only the aspiration technique. The reliability of this method has been determined by repeated trials with 400 mL of a glucose solution (Costill & Saltin, 1974). The standard error of the mean for 16 trials was 6.7 mL, with a mean gastric residue (15 min after ingestion) of 190 mL. Because the location of the gastric tube within the stomach is unknown, a single aspiration of the stomach may not remove all of the residue. In an effort to determine whether all fluids have been removed during the first aspiration of the stomach, subjects are given an additional 50 to 200 mL drink of distilled water immediately after the initial aspiration. The stomach is again aspirated, and this second residue is analyzed to determine if any of the original drink remained in the stomach. Mitchell, et al., (1989), using a 200 mL wash, noted that a single aspiration would, on the average, have missed only 7.3 mL of the original solution.

Methodological differences and means of calculation make it difficult to compare the results of various studies. The elapsed time from ingestion to aspiration, for example, has varied for some investigations from 5 min to several hours (Costill & Saltin, 1974; Mitchell et al., 1989). The rate of gastric emptying varies over time and is affected by the volume of the feeding. Nevertheless, most studies have reported the absolute volume of gastric residue as an index of emptying rate (Costill & Saltin, 1974; Hunt & MacDonald, 1954). In an effort to compare findings from studies that used similar feeding volumes and test durations, other investigators have expressed gastric emptying in mL/min (Mitchell et al., 1988; Neufer et al., 1986).

Finally, it should be noted that there are wide individual variations in rates of gastric emptying. In each group of subjects, there are frequently those who show little or no gastric emptying 20–30 min after a feeding, whereas others may empty 90–95% of a feeding within this time (Costill, unpublished). Despite these wide variations in response, most individuals show a similar pattern of gastric emptying when studied on successive days. Thus, the mean data reported in most investigations show trends that may be considerably different when examined in another group of subjects.

PHYSIOLOGICAL CONTROLS OF GASTRIC EMPTYING

Before the turn of the century, Marbaix (1898) demonstrated that when fluid leaving the stomach was allowed to run out through a duodenal fistula close to the pylorus, the stomach emptied rapidly. However, when the fluid was allowed to pass into the small intestine, gastric emptying was much slower. It was also known that the composition of the gastric contents emptying into the small intestine exerted some influence on the rate of emptying. Acid solutions, for example, were found to empty more slowly than alkaline drinks.

Marbaix (1898) and others (Costill & Saltin, 1974; Hunt & MacDonald, 1954; Minami & McCallum, 1984) have demonstrated that larger ingested volumes empty more rapidly from the stomach than smaller ones. Working with men and dogs, Marbaix (1898) showed that the stimulus for increased emptying was the stomach's distention rather than the weight of the ingested fluid. He also noted that opening of the pylorus was not the sole condition for gastric emptying. Placing an open tube through the pylorus into the duodenum, for example, does not accelerate gastric emptying. Rather, the rate of emptying is proportional to the rate of gastric motility, which is regulated by both sympathetic and parasympathetic activity (Davenport, 1969). In general, sympathetic stimulation reduces the strength of peristalsis, and parasympathetic stimulation enhances it.

On the other hand, Spurrell (1935) has noted that distension of the duodenum will diminish the gastric outflow by reflexly increasing the tone of the pylorus, whereas lowering the pressure in the duodenum increases the rate of gastric outflow. Such reflexes are induced by both mechanical and chemical stimulation of the intestine (Christensen, 1981; Kewenteer, 1970; Mei, 1985).

Early in the 1900s Carnot and Chassevant (1905) demonstrated that the osmotic pressure of the gastric contents influences the rate of emptying. They observed that isotonic saline left the stomach more rapidly than weaker or stronger solutions, leading them to conclude that there were receptors in the walls of the duodenum that controlled the rate of emptying. Additional evidence has been provided which implicates other chemosensitive receptors in the duodenal regulation of gastric motility, specifically after the ingestion of salts of fatty acids (Marbaix, 1898; Quigley & Meschan, 1941).

Fat in any digestible form (triglycerides or phospholipids) in the presence of bile and pancreatic juice is the most powerful of the chemical agents that slow gastric motility (Davenport, 1969). In the first 15 min after ingesting a meal containing 100 g of fat, strong antral contractions are entirely absent, and thereafter their frequency and strength are about half those observed after a carbohydrate feeding. If the fatty meal is removed from the stomach, its inhibitory influence disappears in 3–5 min.

Gastrointestinal hormones and related peptides are located in endocrine cells scattered throughout the gastrointestinal mucosa from the stomach through the colon (Johnson, 1977). Specific stimuli evoke the release of gastrin, cholecystokinin, secretin, and pancreozymin, for example, causing the pancreas to excrete neutralizing and digestive secretions into the duodenum (Wang & Grossman, 1951). Since secretin and pancreozymin tend to inhibit gastric activity, they appear to play an important role in the regulation of gastric emptying (Johnson et al., 1966).

Although the nervous and hormonal regulation of gastric emptying is not fully understood, it is clear that there is a wide variety of stimuli that control the rate at which materials pass through the stomach. Through feedback mechanisms the receptors in the duodenum exert considerable control on the composition of the effluent from the stomach. When gastric emptying is slowed, materials in the stomach are made more dilute by gastric secretions, which add water and minerals to the stomach contents. This point is illustrated in Table 3-1, which illustrates the analysis of gastric residue for water and carbohydrate (CHO) solutions. While both feedings show a gain in electrolytes, the CHO feedings tend to elicit a greater amount of gastric secretion. The importance of these changes should not be overlooked because they can drastically alter the composition of ingested materials. In summary, all solutions and/or solid feedings are modified by the stomach before being delivered to the intestine for absorption.

EFFECTS OF SOLUTE CHARACTERISTICS ON THE RATE OF GASTRIC EMPTYING DURING REST

Patterns of Emptying

An examination of the composition of gastric residue and volume might lead one to believe that the stomach holds its ingesta until it has been made suitable for acceptance by the duodenum. This is not the case. Marbaix (1898) first described the pattern of gastric emptying as being exponential as illustrated by plotting the volume of gastric residue against the time of recovery. Hunt and MacDonald (1954), on the other hand, observed that gastric emptying of meals was exponential only at the beginning and at the end of the digestive period. The initial rate of emptying of effluent from the stomach may be as high as 20–30 mL/min

TABLE 3-1. *Composition of water and glucose (glu) solutions before and 20 min after ingestion (Costill, unpublished; Foster et al., 1980). Gastric secretion denotes the volume of secretion calculated to be present in the residue. Ingested volume was 400 mL.*

Variables	Water Before	Water Residue	5 g glu/100 mL Before	5 g glu/100 mL Residue	10 g glu/100 mL Before	10 g glu/100 mL Residue
Osmolality (mOsm/L)	23	87	266	245	532	434
Sodium (mEq/L)	0.7	7.9	1.5	18.6	1.9	14.5
Potassium (mEq/L)	0.1	4.11	0.11	5.21	0.10	3.63
Glucose (g/100 mL)	0.0	0.0	5.0	3.3	10.0	6.5
pH	4.76	2.05	3.50	2.29	3.46	2.40
Gastric Secretion (mL)	—	32	—	52	—	65

immediately after fluid ingestion, then slows to 5–15 mL/min as the gastric volume decreases. The rapid initial movement of materials out of the stomach might be explained as a volume effect, since large fluid volumes leave the stomach more rapidly than small ones. As the volume within the stomach becomes progressively smaller, the stimulus for emptying appears to diminish (Hunt & Knox, 1969a; Hunt & Spurrell, 1951).

Wilson et al. (1929) first reported that food began to leave the stomach 2–3 min after it was swallowed. When 5% solutions of glucose or fructose were tagged with ^{14}C-glucose and ^{14}C-fructose, respectively, radioactivity was initially noted in the venous blood 5–7 min after ingestion (Costill et al., 1973). As shown in Figure 3-1, there was no difference between the fructose and glucose trials in the accumulation in the blood of glucose that was derived from the beverages as calculated from the ^{14}C radioactivity in the blood. Although these data do not enable us to calculate the rate of gastric emptying, they suggest that ingested materials are initially delayed by the stomach, then empty at a relatively rapid, exponential rate, depending on the volume within the stomach.

Gastric Volume

As has been mentioned at several points in the preceding discussion, gastric volume is one of the strongest regulators of gastric emptying, i.e., the greater the volume of the contents, the greater the rate of emptying. Marbaix (1898) reported that distending the stomach with 250 mL of air

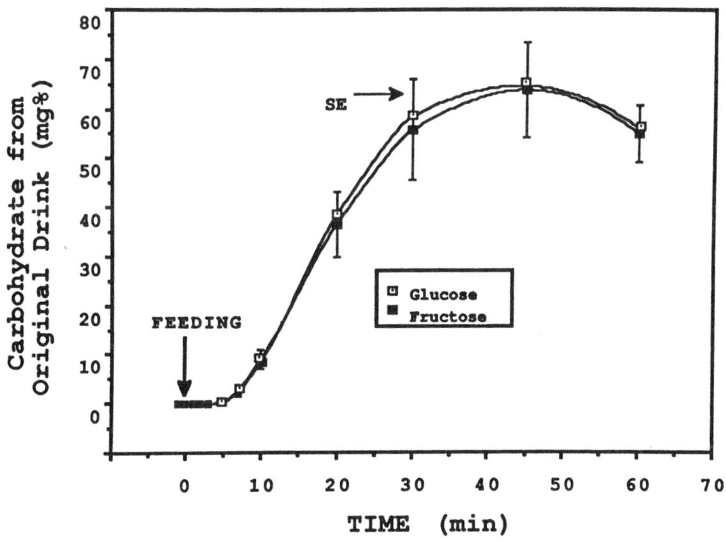

FIGURE 3-1. *Calculated accumulation in blood of glucose derived from ingested 5% solutions of glucose or fructose labelled with ^{14}C-glucose or ^{14}C-fructose, respectively (Costill et al., 1973).*

after putting 250 mL of water in the stomach increased the rate of emptying to the same level as if the subject had consumed 500 mL of water, demonstrating that the stimulus was distention rather than the weight of the stomach's contents. Subsequent studies have shown that receptors in the gastric musculature respond to increasing distension and pressure by increasing the rate of emptying (Hunt & MacDonald, 1954; Minami & McCallum, 1984).

Costill and Saltin (1974) reported that gastric emptying increased in proportion to the volume ingested, up to a volume of 600 mL. Above that level a further increase was absent in most subjects. The maximal rate of gastric emptying observed in this study was 25.3 mL/min with an ingested volume of 600 mL. When a liter of fluid was ingested, the mean rate of emptying was only 19.3 mL/min. The ingestion of 200 mL, on the other hand, resulted in an emptying rate of only 6.6 mL/min. Though this suggests that it is important to maintain a sizable volume of fluid in the stomach (e.g., 400–600 mL) to promote gastric emptying, excessive distension may retard emptying.

Solute Osmolality

The influence of solute osmolality on the rate of gastric emptying was first noted by Carnot and Chassevant in 1905. They contended that the osmotic pressure of the stomach's contents was gauged by receptors in the walls of the duodenum. Solutions of salts or glucose that were hypertonic to tap water were found to slow gastric emptying. Subsequent studies by Hunt and Pathak (1960) examined the effect on gastric emptying of osmotic pressure in test meals containing various electrolytes. They observed that a number of solutes had similar effects per osmole in slowing gastric emptying. As noted in Figure 3-2, Hunt and Knox (1969a) showed that a 500 mOsm/L solution of sodium chloride emptied at about the same rate as water, i.e., about 27 mL/min, whereas an increased rate of gastric emptying occurred with test meals containing 250 mOsm/L sodium chloride. Hunt and Knox concluded that sodium chloride exerts an osmotic effect in speeding gastric emptying at concentrations below 500 mOsm/L; this finding was not confirmed by later studies of Costill and Saltin (1974).

Hunt (1960) also observed that isocaloric solutions of starch and glucose left the stomach at almost the same rate, despite marked differences in their osmotic pressures. This was interpreted by Hunt to demonstrate that the starch solution stimulated the osmoreceptors after being hydrolyzed by amylase and maltase in the duodenum, since there was no hydrolysis of starch in the stomach. It was, therefore, argued that the osmoreceptors concerned with the regulation of gastric emptying are not within the stomach, but at some point in the duodenum. It might, however, be argued that the rate of emptying of these solutions was regu-

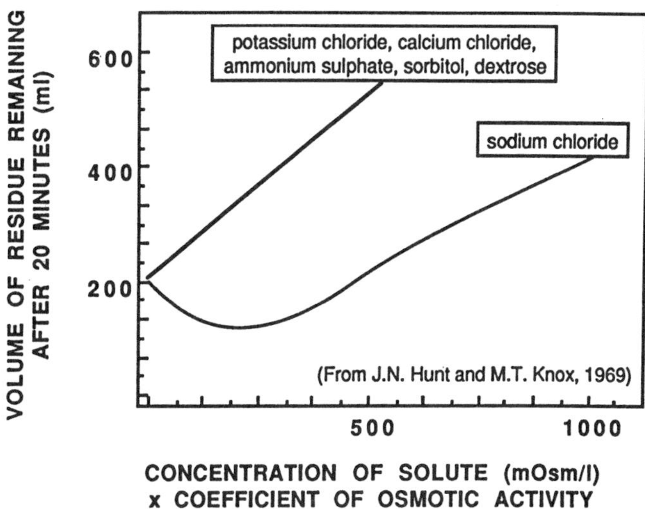

FIGURE 3-2. *Effect of osmotic pressure of test solutions on gastric emptying of a 750 mL feeding recovered 20 min after ingestion (Hunt & Knox, 1969 a).*

lated by their caloric contents, which were similar, rather than by their solute osmolality.

Murray (1987) has suggested that solutions of maltodextrins (maltodextrins) offer a convenient method for studying the effects of solute osmolality on gastric emptying because they have a significantly lower osmolality than isocaloric solutions of glucose or fructose. This, of course, assumes that maltodextrins are not hydrolyzed in the stomach or in the duodenum before reaching the osmoreceptors in the small intestine. There is only limited evidence to substantiate this assumption. However, analysis of gastric residue following the ingestion of maltodextrin drinks revealed that there was no measurable hydrolysis within the stomach (Costill, unpublished). A 5% solution of a maltodextrin, for example, was found to have 1.91 g of free glucose per 100 mL. Fifteen minutes after ingesting 400 mL of this solution, the gastric residue contained 1.86 g free glucose per 100 mL.

Studies using various mixtures of glucose, fructose, and maltodextrin solutions have shown only a modest relationship between gastric emptying (mL/min) and solution osmolality (Mitchell et al., 1988; Neufer et al., 1986). The data in Figure 3-3 illustrate an exponential relationship ($R = 0.73$) between these two variables, though there is a wide individual variation in the rate of emptying at each level of solute osmolality. Though these data are consistent with the theory that osmolality of the stomach's contents may influence gastric function, especially when hypertonic solutions are ingested, they also suggest that caloric content and carbohydrate form may likewise influence the rate of emptying.

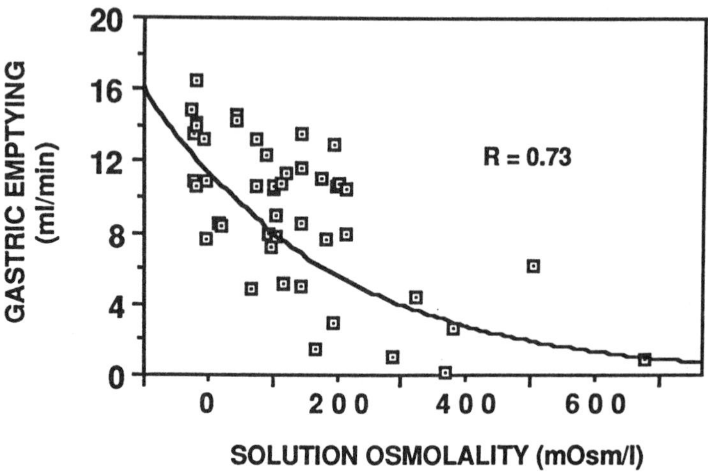

FIGURE 3-3. *Effects of osmolality of ingested solutions on the rate of gastric emptying. Data points represent mean values from five different studies conducted in the author's laboratory, two of which are published (Mitchell et al., 1988; Neufer et al., 1986).*

Caloric Content

It is generally agreed that progressively more concentrated carbohydrate solutions empty progressively more slowly from the stomach than does water or a weak NaCl solution (Coyle et al., 1978; Fordtran & Saltin, 1967; Costill & Saltin, 1974). As illustrated in Figure 3-4, the rate of gastric emptying was inversely related to the glucose concentration of the test solution. However, there was no significant difference between the emptying rate for water and a 139 mM (2.5 g/100 mL) glucose solution. Likewise, when gastric emptying was studied at various times (5–120 min) after the ingestion of solutions containing 139 to 834 mM glucose, nearly all of the 139 mM solution was emptied from the stomach within 20 min, whereas the 834 mM solution took nearly 120 min to empty from the stomach (Costill & Saltin, 1974). Interestingly, the quantity of glucose delivered to the duodenum in the first 15 min following the feedings was similar for all the glucose concentrations. During that period approximately 550 mmol (500–567 mmol) of glucose was aspirated from the stomach; this constituted about 92% of the glucose ingested in the 139 mM drink but only 16% of the glucose contained in the 834 mM solution. Similar findings have been reported by Brener et al., (1983), who examined the gastric emptying rates of 400 mL of isotonic saline and of solutions containing 5.0, 12.5, and 25 g/100 mL glucose. Although the gastric emptying rate is inversely related to the glucose concentration of the drinks, the rate at which calories were emptied from the stomach (kcal/ min) was similar (2.13 kcal/min) for all of the glucose solutions.

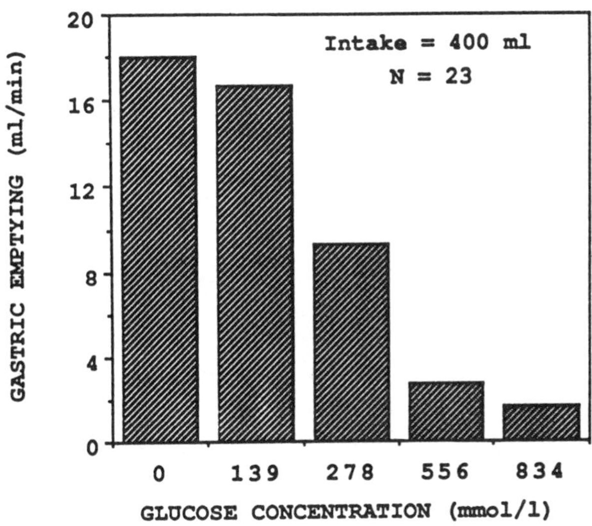

FIGURE 3-4. *Relationship between the glucose concentration of a test solution (400 mL) and the rate of gastric emptying (mL/min). Gastric residue was removed from the stomach 15 min after ingestion (modified from Costill & Saltin, 1974).*

Additional studies of the role of caloric content in the regulation of gastric emptying have been conducted by Hunt et al. (1985). By varying both ingested volume (300, 400, and 600 mL) and glucose (polymer) content (12.5, 17.5, 25.0, 32.5, 37.5, and 50 g/100 mL) they observed that the rate of caloric emptying from the stomach was most rapid during the first 30 min after the feeding (4.5 kcal/min). From 30 to 120 min after ingestion, the emptying rate slowed to an average of 2.6 kcal/min. Based on these data, Murray (1987) has concluded that ". . . the control mechanisms governing the delivery of calories to the absorptive surface of the small intestine can be over-ridden by substantially increasing the volume and energy content of the ingested fluid."

It has also been observed that isocaloric meals of other nutrients (i.e., carbohydrate, fat, and protein) empty from the stomach at similar rates (Hunt & Stubbs, 1975; McHugh & Moran, 1979). These findings, however, have not been confirmed by other investigators. Foster et al. (1980), for example, compared the gastric emptying and caloric delivery rates of solutions containing glucose or maltodextrins. Gastric contents were aspirated 30 min after ingesting 400 mL of various glucose and maltodextrin drinks (5, 10, 20, and 40 g/100 mL). As noted in Table 3-2, they observed that the delivery of carboydrate to the intestine increased with solute concentration.

Although these findings confirm the fact that gastric emptying is controlled more by caloric content than solute osmolality, it appears that

TABLE 3-2. *A comparison of gastric emptying and caloric emptying rates for glucose (G) and maltodextrin (GP) solutions (modified from Foster et al., 1980)*

	5 g/100 mL		10 g/100 mL		20 g/100 mL		40 g/100 mL	
Variable	G	GP	G	GP	G	GP	G	GP
Osmolality (mOsm/L)	266	75	532	150	1064	300	2128	600
Emptying (mL/min)	9.2	10.2	6.9	7.3	4.5	4.7	2.6	2.8
Caloric Delivery (kcal/min)	2.0	2.6	3.8	2.9	7.5	7.5	11.3	13.9

the caloric delivery to the small intestine can be increased by increasing the caloric content of the carbohydrate solution. Based on the volume of residue remaining in the stomach, these investigators reported that the 5% maltodextrin solution emptied faster than did the glucose solution. However, when gastric secretion was subtracted from the residue volume, the rates of emptying for isocaloric glucose and maltodextrin drinks were not statistically different.

Despite the inhibiting influence of carbohydrate solutions on the rate of gastric emptying, more glucose and/or maltodextrin is delivered to the duodenum following the ingestion of strong rather than weak carbohydrate solutions. There is no evidence that maltodextrin solutions empty from the stomach more rapidly than glucose solutions of similar concentration.

Elias et al. (1968), on the other hand, provided some evidence that fructose may empty faster from the stomach than other monosaccharides and disaccharides. When fructose alone was given in a test meal, it had little or no slowing action on gastric emptying in some subjects until the concentration in the feeding had reached 200 mOsm/L. There was some suggestion that fructose in low concentrations actually increased the rate of gastric emptying in a manner similar to hypotonic solutions of sodium chloride, urea, and glycerol. Unfortunately, this finding has not been confirmed. We have, however, observed that solutions containing 5–10 g fructose/100 mL (322 to 622 mOsm/L, respectively emptied from the stomach at about the same rates as similarly concentrated glucose and sucrose solutions (Costill, unpublished). Finally, it should be noted that sucrose, maltose, galactose, and lactose all have an inhibitory influence on gastric emptying, but not to the same degree as reported for glucose (Elias et al., 1968).

Solute Acidity

As early as 1900, acid test meals were shown to slow gastric emptying. However, most studies have used relatively high concentrations of hydrochloric acid to provide an effective stimulus. The greater the concentration of acid in the meal, the slower is gastric emptying (Hunt & Pathak, 1960; Pathak, 1959; Shay & Gershon-Cohen, 1934, Shay et al., 1939; Van Liere & Sleeth, 1940). This slower removal of acidic stomach contents is believed to depend on the stimulation of duodenal receptors. In addition to slowing gastric emptying, acids introduced into the jejunum reduce the gastric secretion of acid.

A later study by Hunt and Knox (1969b) found a rectilinear relationship between the mean concentration of acid (mEq/L) in the test meal that was required to give a gastric residue recovery of 450 mL and the square root of the acid's molecular weight. The acids with high molecular weights (e.g., citric acid) were less effective in slowing emptying than those with low molecular weights. These findings suggested that the anions determine the effectiveness of the acids in slowing gastric emptying; the large molecules apparently diffuse to the site of the receptor more slowly than smaller ones. Hunt and Knox (1972) further observed that the receptor for acid was acting as a titration apparatus to pH 6.5 rather than as an electrode detecting pH or concentration. Lin et al. (1988) recently reported that acids inhibit gastric emptying in a dose-related fashion that depends on the titratable acidity rather than on pH. They have concluded that the acid sensors are present in the proximal half of the gut, with inhibition being dependent on the titratable acidity and the length of the small intestine exposed to the acid.

Under normal conditions gastric secretions, which are already quite acid (pH ~1.0), lower the pH of ingested fluids to about 2.0–3.0 (Coyle, 1976). Thus, it is difficult to understand how test meals having pH values above 4.0 can be responsible for slowing the rate of emptying (Coyle, 1976; Foster et al., 1980). Nevertheless, studies by Hunt and Knox (1962) have shown that duodenal receptors are stimulated to inhibit gastric emptying when the duodenal contents are below pH 6.0. They observed that citric acid, commonly used as flavoring in many drinks, slowed the rate of gastric emptying when the test meal pH ranged from 2.4 to 5.0. It was concluded, however, that the receptor mechanism was so organized as to regulate the number of milliequivalents of citric acid delivered to the duodenum without reference to the concentration of acid.

Other Factors

In addition to citric acid, a number of commercially available solutions used for rehydration during and following exercise include artificial sweeteners (e.g., aspartame) to enhance their palatability while maintaining a low caloric content. A comparison of gastric emptying rates for water and a 375 ppm solution of aspartame revealed no significant differences between these two drinks (Costill, unpublished). The rates of emptying for water and the aspartame solution after 15 min of running (60% $\dot{V}O_2$ max) and 5 min of rest averaged 15.6 and 16.0 mL/min, respec-

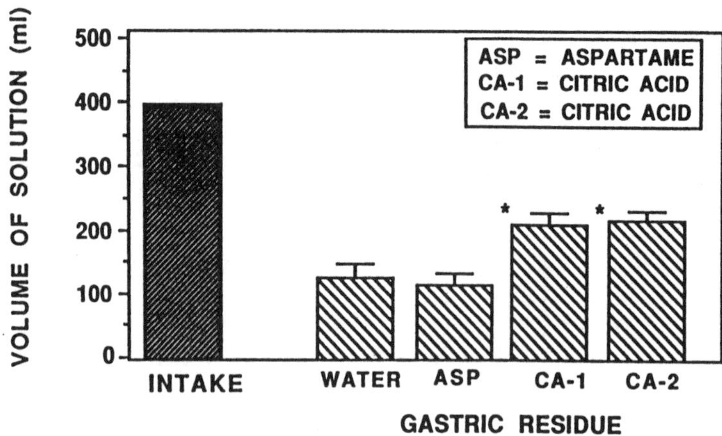

FIGURE 3-5. *The effects of aspartame and citric acid on the volume of gastric residue remaining 20 min (15 min running and 5 min rest) after ingesting 400 mL of either water, or solutions containing 375 ppm aspartame (ASP), 518 ppm aspartame plus 25 mg/100 mL citric acide (CA-1) or 375 ppm aspartame plus 25 mg/100 mL citric acide (CA-2) (Costill, unpublished).*

tively, when gastric secretion was subracted from gastric residue. As shown in Figure 3-5, the addition of a relatively small amount of citric acid to the aspartame solution, however, resulted in a significantly greater gastric residue (and a lower rate of gastric emptying, i.e., 13.1–13.3 mL/min).

Fluctuations in the stomach temperature occur daily due to the ingestion of hot and cold fluids and foods. Hepburn et al. (1933) observed that the ingestion of cold water and ice cream can reduce gastric temperature by 22.9–27°C, with an average recovery time of more than 30 min. Cooling the stomach appears to increase the rate of gastric emptying (Gershon-Cohen et al., 1940; Shapiro, 1968; Costill & Saltin, 1974). This influence of solution temperature on the amount of residue in the stomach 15 min after a 400 mL glucose feeding (139 mM) is illustrated in Figure 3-6.

It appears that the factors listed in this section are not the only ones that influence gastric function. Limited data are available which suggest that caffeine, emotional distress, diurnal variations, environmental conditions, and the menstrual cycle may also influence gastric emptying (Owen et al., 1986; Wald et al., 1981; Dickinson et al., 1984). Unfortunately, the mechanisms that control their influence on antral motility and emptying are not understood, nor in most cases have these findings been replicated.

GASTRIC EMPTYING DURING EXERCISE

Although there is a wealth of information concerning the influence of solution characteristics on the rate of gastric emptying, nearly all pre-

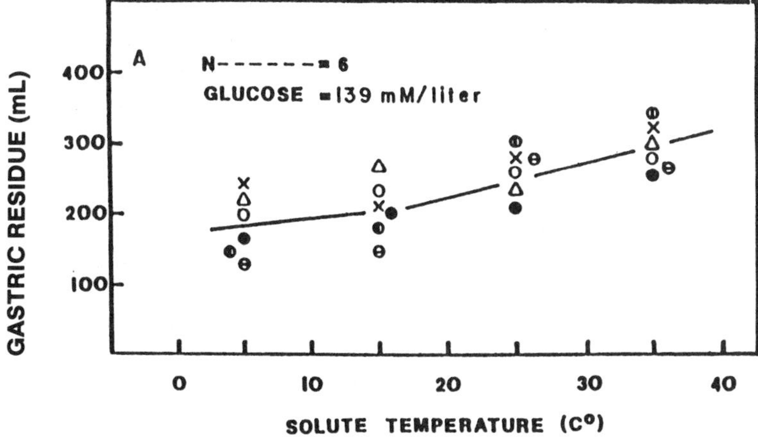

FIGURE 3-6. *The effects of solution temperature on the volume of gastric residue in the stomach 15 min after a 400 mL feeding (Costill & Saltin, 1974).*

viously mentioned findings were conducted with resting men and women. Since physical activity after a full meal has long been considered prejudicial to digestion (Beaumont, 1833; Graham, 1851; Campbell et al., 1928), one might question the applicability of these results to active subjects. In the following discussion, attention will be given to the effects of exercise intensity and duration on the rate of gastric emptying.

As early as 1833, Beaumont noted that severe and fatiguing exercise retarded digestion. Nearly a century later, Campbell, et al. (1928) reported that in young men moderate exercise such as running 2 or 3 miles after a light meal slowed gastric emptying while reducing gastric secretion. Lighter activity such as walking, however, did not effectively delay gastric secretion, but increased the rate of emptying. He even noted that, "Walking with a friend and talking caused more rapid emptying than walking alone, and this showed the importance of psychological factors."

The level of exercise needed to impair gastric emptying has been suggested to vary in accordance with the subject's fitness (Campbell et al., 1928). Thus, in one subject, walking quickly was enough to slow emptying, whereas in another man who trained regularly, running 2 miles had no effect on gastric function. Campbell et al. (1928) observed that, "Exercise which produced no discomfort helped on digestion, and exercise which produced discomfort delayed it."

These early findings were later confirmed by other investigators (Costill & Saltin, 1974; Feldman & Nixon, 1982), who reported that exercise had no effect on gastric emptying (~13 mL/min) until the exercise intensity exceeded 65–80% of the subject's maximal oxygen uptake ($\dot{V}O_2$ max). In addition, Costill and Saltin (1974) examined the rate of gastric emptying at 4 intervals during 2 h of cycling to determine the effects of exercise duration. Despite the fatiguing effects of the exercise, there was no change in the rate of gastric emptying from the beginning of the activity (0–30 min) until the end (90–120 min). As a consequence of these studies, it has been assumed that data on gastric emptying measured at rest would be applicable during prolonged activities (e.g., > 2 h), which are generally performed at intensities below 80% $\dot{V}O_2max$.

On the other hand, recent studies by Neufer et al. (1986, 1989b) have confirmed the early observations by Campbell (1928), finding that mild to moderate exercise (i.e., walking and slow running) may accelerate the rate of gastric emptying. It has also been shown that water and 5–7% solutions of carbohydrate emptied 38% faster during treadmill exercise (15 min at 50 and 70% $\dot{V}O_2max$) than when the subjects remained inactive (i.e., seated) for 20 min after the feeding (Neufer et al., 1986). Submaximal cycling may also increase the rate of gastric emptying, though the findings of recent investigations have often presented conflicting results (Costill, unpublished, Mitchell et al., 1989; Neufer et al. 1986; Cammack et al., 1982).

Campbell et al. (1928) also suggested that gastric emptying might be increased when exercise was performed in intermittent bouts. One subject ". . . took very gentle exercise in the laboratory, running a quarter of a mile slowly four times in the hour, showing that the rate of emptying had increased, but the secretion of gastric juice had been rather diminished . . ." A recent study by Mitchell et al. (1989), however, reported that intermittent exercise provides no significant advantage as a means of enhancing gastric emptying.

Mitchell et al. (1988, 1989) observed that 96–98% of all fluid ingested (0.0–7.5 g CHO/100 mL) was emptied in 2 h of submaximal intermittent and continuous cycling. However, stronger carbohydrate solutions (12 and 18 g/100 mL) significantly reduced the emptying rate to 85% and 72% of the ingested volume during the 2 h of exercise. Table 3-3 illustrates that the rate of gastric emptying during prolonged exercise (i.e., 2-h cycling) is not appreciably affected by the caloric content of the solution until the concentration of carbohydrate (e.g., glucose, fructose, and/or maltodextrin) in the beverage is greater than 10 g/100 mL. Ingesting larger volumes, however, may increase the rate of emptying. Costill et al. (1970) fed their subjects (4.4 g CHO/100 mL) at a rate of 16.7 mL/min during 2 h of treadmill running and observed a gastric emptying of 13.6 mL/min. This rate of emptying may, however, have approached the subjects' maximal rate because they all became uncomfortably full and had great difficulty ingesting the final feedings during the experiments. It was also noted that one of the subjects developed diarrhea when water was administered at the same rate during the 2-h treadmill run.

In an effort to compare the influence of exercise mode on the rates of gastric emptying, carbohydrate solutions (6 and 10 g/100 mL) were stud-

TABLE 3-3. *Effects of carbohydrate concentration of ingested beverages on the rate of gastric emptying during 2 h of continuous cycling at 70% $\dot{V}O_2$max Modified from Mitchell et al. (1988, 1989) and Costill (unpublished). An asterisk (*) denotes a significant mean difference from the water trial*

CHO (g/100 mL)	Rate of Intake (mL/min)	Rate of Emptying (mL/min)	% Intake Emptied
0	10.9	10.6	97.2
5.0	10.9	10.3	94.5
6.0	10.3	9.9	96.1
7.5	10.9	10.4	95.7
10.0	10.9	9.8	89.9
12.0	10.3	8.8*	85.4*
18.0	10.3	7.4*	71.7*

ied during 20 and 120 min of rest, cycling, and running (Costill, unpublished; Mitchell et al., 1989). A faster rate of emptying was consistently experienced during running (70% $\dot{V}O_2$max) than cycling (70% $\dot{V}O_2$max) trials (Figure 3-7). Although both running and cycling induced a higher rate of gastric emptying of the 10% solution during 20 min of exercise than under resting conditions, only running caused a greater rate of gastric emptying of the 6% solution compared to rest during the 120-min trial. Costill and Saltin (1974) also noted no time-related effects on gastric emptying during cycling or rest for 15–120 min. Although the influence of cycling on gastric emptying is not clear, it appears that moderately intense running and/or walking may facilitate gastric emptying. Although anecdotal evidence has been presented to suggest that cross-

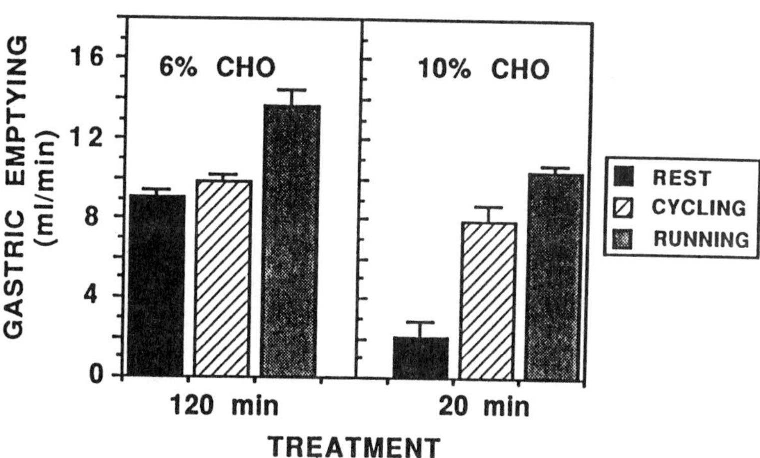

FIGURE 3-7. *A comparison of gastric emptying (mL/min) during 20 and 120 min of rest, cycling, and running following the ingestion of solutions containing 6 and 10% glucose and maltodextrins. Both forms of exercise were performed at 70% $\dot{V}O_2$max. The subjects were given 150 mL of the 6% solution every 15 min during the 120-min trials, whereas a single feeding of the 10% solution was administered immediately before the 20-min treatment. (From Costill, unpublished).*

country skiing may also accelerate gastric emptying, little information is available concerning the influence of other modes of exercise.

The mechanisms responsible for the faster rate of gastric emptying observed during moderately intense running exercise have not been defined. It has been suggested, however, that body motion involved during the activity may aid in shifting the stomach's contents toward the antrum, thereby facilitating the delivery of chyme to the duodenum (Neufer et al., 1986). Slowing of gastric emptying during more intense exercise (> 75–80% $\dot{V}O_2$max), on the other hand, has been attributed to the potential inhibitory effects of increased catecholamine and endogenous opiod levels on splanchnic blood flow and gastric motility (Neufer et al., 1989a; Murray, 1987).

Exercise vs Resting Values for Gastric Emptying

Based on the study by Costill and Saltin (1974) it was concluded that the optimal fluid for rehydration during exercise should be one that was hypotonic (< 300 mOsm/L) and contained less than 2.5 g of carbohydrate per 100 mL. These conclusions were, for the most part, based on gastric emptying data that had been obtained under resting conditions using a single feeding and a digestive interval of only 15 min. Since that study demonstrated that there was no influence of moderately intense cycling (⩽ 70% $\dot{V}O_2$max), it appeared valid to apply the resting data for gastric emptying to exercise conditions. There is recent evidence, however, which suggests that frequent feedings over a 2–4 h period may not be comparable to the single, 15–20 min trials conducted in the early investigations (Mitchell et al., 1988, 1989). There are several reasons why brief (i.e., 15–20 min), single feeding (i.e., 400 mL) trials present a different picture than is now seen with smaller feedings (e.g., 120 mL) taken at 15-min intervals during 2 h of exercise.

In addition to the mechanical movement of fluids within the stomach, smaller, frequent feedings appear to result in a constant emptying (e.g., 9–10 mL/min) throughout the exercise, with only a small residue remaining in the stomach at the time of each subsequent feeding. This point is illustrated in Figure 3-8, which shows the theoretical ingested and residual volumes in the stomach after a single 400 mL feeding, and after serial 120 mL (120 mL/15 min) feedings. In contrast to the single feeding, serial feedings of ~150 mL are mostly emptied prior to each subsequent drink. As a result, the total residue in the stomach immediately after each feeding may only increase by 10–15 mL per feeding. Consequently, by the end of 120 min, the residue may be relatively small. Thus, the ability to consume fluids throughout the exercise period without becoming unduly full is a function of constant emptying with partial filling, rather than an exercise-induced acceleration of gastric emptying. This point is supported by recent findings of Mitchell et al. (1989), who have

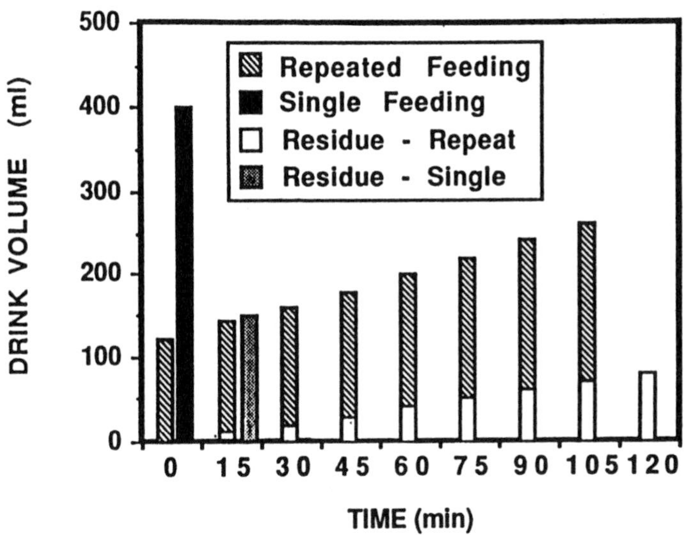

FIGURE 3-8. *Theoretical comparison of gastric residue at various times after a single 400 mL feeding and after repeated 120 mL feedings.*

shown that small serial feedings (150 mL/ 15 min) resulted in similar rates of gastric emptying during 120 min of exercise and rest.

Calculated gastric emptying rates are, in fact, faster during the single, 400 mL, 15–20 min trials, than during the serial feedings (120–150 mL) taken over a 120-min period. A single 400 mL feeding of water may result in a mean emptying rate of 13–18 mL/min, whereas taking repeated drinks during longer periods of rest or exercise will produce an average emptying of only 8–11 mL/min (Neufer et al., 1986; Mitchell et al., 1988, 1989). The difference in emptying rates appears to be a function of the gastric volume, which is greater after the single feeding than at any time during the serial drink administration.

In light of recent evidence that gastric emptying may be faster during some forms of exercise (e.g., running) and may result in less risk of gastric fullness with smaller serial feedings, one might be led to believe that the studies performed under resting conditions are not applicable to the conditions of prolonged exercise. As noted earlier, this may hold true with regard to the tolerable concentration of carbohydrate in the drink. The caloric content of the solution does not appear to have a detrimental effect on the rate of gastric emptying during exercise until the concentration exceeds 10 g/100mL, whereas solutions above 2.5 g/100 mL have shown a reduction in gastric emptying under resting conditions (Costill & Saltin, 1974; Mitchell et al., 1988, 1989). Unfortunately, other factors known to influence gastric emptying at rest (e.g., solute temperature, electrolytes, etc.) have not been studied during physical activity.

Effects of Environmental Stress

The need to maintain a fluid balance during prolonged exercise has been well documented (Pitts et al., 1944; Pugh et al., 1957; Noakes et al., 1988; Costill et al., 1970). However, the ability to consume fluid at the same rate that it is lost in sweat during exercise in the heat is limited by the relatively slow rate of gastric emptying (Fordtran & Saltin, 1967; Costill et al., 1970). Sweat rates, for example, have been reported to exceed 25 mL/min, which is substantially greater than the highest gastric emptying rates of only 16 mL/min in men working in warm conditions (Owen et al., 1986; Pugh et al., 1957; Mitchell et al., 1988, 1989). In fact, exposure to a hot environment may compromise the rate of gastric emptying, thereby making it more difficult to maintain a body water balance.

In 1928, Campbell et al. observed that the rate of gastric emptying was reduced when subjects sat in a hot bath (39.0–41.5°C) for 1 h. Owen et al. (1986) measured gastric residue following 2 h of treadmill running at 65% $\dot{V}O_2max$ in the heat (35°C) and in a cooler environment (25°C). Each subject consumed 200 mL of water every 20 min during the activity. Gastric emptying was significantly slower during exercise in the heat compared to the cooler environment, averaging 4.9 and 6.6 mL/min, respectively.

Similar findings have been reported by Neufer et al. (1989a), who studied subjects during 15 min of exercise (~50% $\dot{V}O_2max$) in hot (49°C), warm (35°C) and neutral (18°C) environments, following a 400-mL water feeding. They observed a 34% decrease in gastric emptying during exercise in the heat (13.9 mL/min) compared to neutral conditions (21.0 mL/min). The higher rates of emptying seen in this study than in the investigation by Owen et al. (1986) were probably due to differences in fluid volume, exercise intensity, and the duration of the activity used in these two studies.

Neufer et al. (1989a) also examined the influence of hydration and heat acclimation on gastric emptying. Using the same protocol described above, subjects were studied before and after heat acclimation and dehydration. The authors observed that heat acclimation did not significantly influence the rate of gastric emptying during exercise in a warm (35°C) environment. Hypohydration, on the other hand, reduced gastric emptying and stomach secretion during exercise in the warm environment. The authors concluded that the gastric emptying rate is influenced adversely by the severity of the thermal strain induced by both exercise and heat stress. The cause for this change in stomach function has been postulated to be a reduction in splanchnic blood flow and/or an increase in plasma β-endorphin levels.

SUMMARY

This review of early and recent studies on gastric function has emphasized the variety of factors that are known to influence the rate of gastric emptying. The factors identified in Figure 3-9 represent those that have been shown to stimulate or retard the movement of ingested materials from the stomach into the deodenum. Although it is difficult to establish the magnitude of control exerted by each variable, there appear to be two factors that have unusually strong influences on the rate of gastric motility and emptying.

First, larger volumes tend to empty faster than small ones. Consequently, gastric emptying rate is fastest immediately after fluid ingestion, diminishing exponentially as the volume remaining in the stomach becomes small. It has been shown that antral motility and pyloric relaxation are stimulated by intragastric pressure. Unusually large fluid volumes (>500 or 600 mL), however, tend to retard emptying, though there is limited information concerning excessive intragastric pressure and its inhibitory influence on emptying. Although this point has not been confirmed during exercise, current data suggest that this factor exerts the same controls during rest and submaximal exercise, at least during activities requiring less than 70–80% $\dot{V}O_2max$.

A second major influence on gastric emptying appears to be the solution's energy content, i.e., energy rich materials are emptied from the

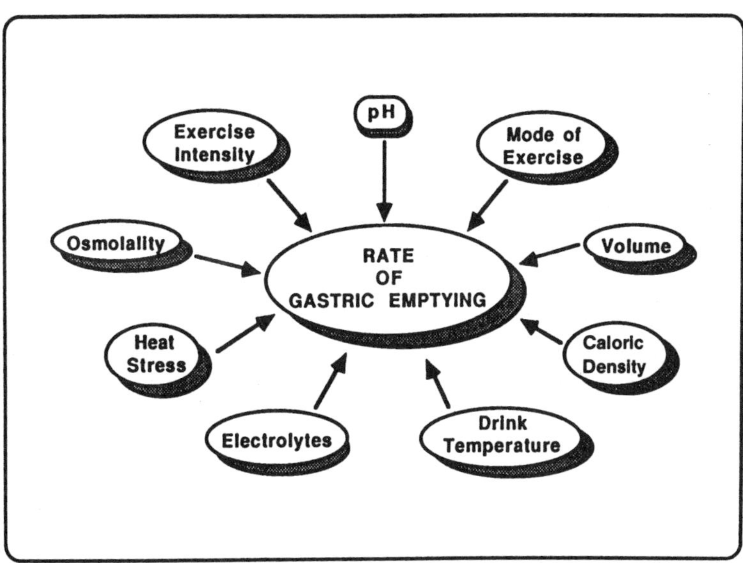

FIGURE 3-9. *Selected factors that have been shown to influence the rate of gastric emptying.*

stomach more slowly than solutions with little energy content. This effect is experienced both at rest and during exercise, though the rate of emptying appears to be somewhat faster during light to moderate activity. Although some studies have shown only a small gastric residue when subjects were given frequent (4 feedings/h), small feedings (~120–150 mL/feeding), the rate of gastric emptying is still somewhat slower with carbohydrate solutions than with water.

Although early studies by Hunt and Pathak (1960) suggested that beverage osmolality controlled the rate of gastric emptying, more recent studies do not fully support this concept (Neufer et al., 1986; 1988; Mitchell et al., 1988, 1989; Costill & Saltin, 1974). Fluids having similar CHO contents but different osmolalities have been found to empty from the stomach at about the same rate, supporting the concept that the caloric content of a solution is a stronger regulator of gastric emptying than osmolality.

As noted earlier, gastric emptying is significantly faster during moderate, submaximal exercise, especially during running, than when the subjects remain inactive. Evidence suggests that activities of low to moderate intensity may speed the movement of materials out of the stomach, but exhaustive, distressful activity slows gastric motility and emptying.

From a practical point of view, it should be noted that there are wide individual variations in the response to each of the variables known to affect gastric emptying. Whereas some subjects may empty 80–90% of an ingested solution in 15–20 min, others may empty less than 10% of the test drink. To date we have no explanation for this individual difference in response.

The primary reasons for taking fluids during prolonged exercise are to (1) minimize dehydration and (2) provide an energy supplement, thereby enhancing performance. Any factor that slows gastric emptying will, therefore, reduce the benefits of fluid ingestion. Thus, we are left with the question of what carbohydrate concentration will provide the best opportunity for both water and carbohydrate delivery during long term exercise. Studies by Mitchell et al. (1988 & 1989) showed that both water and carbohydrate delivery to the duodenum were at near maximal rates when the carbohydrate concentration of the drink was in the range of 8–10 g/100 mL. This point is illustrated in Figure 3-10 and is based on data obtained during 2 h of exercise with repeated feedings (120 mL/15 min). It should be noted that this response is unaffected by the form of carbohydrate used in the drink.

Finally, though the mechanisms which regulate gastric emptying are not fully understood, a variety of stimuli have been identified that control gastric motility and delivery of materials into the duodenum, where they can be absorbed. Additional information concerning the optimal volume and frequency for feedings during exercise would be helpful for

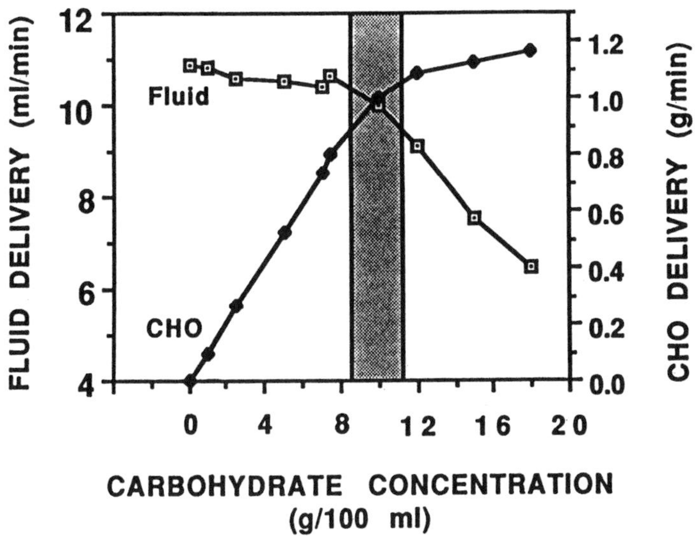

FIGURE 3-10. *Influence of beverage carbohydrate concentration on the rate of delivery of water (fluid) and carbohydrate to the duodenum. The gray vertical column represents the range of carbohydrate concentrations in beverages that permitted the highest rates for both fluid and carbohydrate delivery (Mitchell et al., 1988 & 1989).*

prescribing fluid therapy during prolonged exercise in the heat to maximize work tolerance and enhance physical performance.

BIBLIOGRAPHY

Armstrong, L.E., D.L. Costill, A. Katz, and W.J. Fink. Influence of diuretic-induced dehydration on competitive running performance. *Med. Sci. Sports Exer.* 17:456–460, 1985.

Barber, D.C. and B.H. Brown. Applied potential tomography. *J. Physics E: Scientific Instruments* 17:723–733, 1984.

Beaumont, W. *Experiments and Observations on the Gastric Juice and the Physiology of Digestion.* Dover Publ.: New York, pp. 279, 1833.

Brener, W., T.R. Hendrix, and P.R. McHugh. Regulation of gastric emptying of glucose. *Gastroent.* 85: 76–82, 1983.

Buskirk, E., P.F. Iampietro, and D.E. Bass. Work performance after dehydration: effects of physical conditioning and heat acclimatization. *J. Appl. Physiol.* 12:189–194, 1958.

Cammack, J., N.W. Read, P.A. Cann, B. Greenwood, and A.M. Holgate. Effect of prolonged exercise on the passage of a solid meal through the stomach and small intestine. *Gut* 23:957–961, 1982.

Campbell, J.M.H., M.B. Mitchell, and A.T.W. Powell. The influence of exercise on digestion. *Guy's Hosp. Rep.* 78:279–293. 1928.

Carlson, A.J. The secretion of gastric juice in health and disease. *Physiol. Rev.*, 1923, 3, 1.

Carnot, P. and A. Chassevant. Modifications subies dans l'estomac et le duodenum par les solutions salines suivant leu concentration moleculaire. Le reflex regulateur de sphincter pylorue. *Compt. Rend. Soc. Biol.* 58:173–176, 1905.

Christensen, J. Motility of the colon. In: *Physiology of the Gastrointestinal Tract*, ed. by L.R. Johnson. New York: Raven, 1981, p. 445–471.

Costill, D.L. and B. Saltin. Factors limiting gastric emptying during rest and exercise. *J. Appl. Physiol.* 37:679-683. 1974.

Costill, D.L. A. Bennett, G. Branam, and D. Eddy. Glucose ingestion at rest and during prolonged exercise. *J. Appl. Physiol*, 34:764–769, 1973.

Costill, D.L. G.P. Dalsky and W.J. Fink. Effects of caffeine ingestion on metabolism and exercise performance. *Med. Sci. Sports*, 10:155–158, 1978.
Costill, D.L., W.E. Kammer, and A. Fisher. Fluid ingestion during distance running. *Arch. Environ. Health.* 21:520–525, 1970.
Coyle, E.F. *A comparison of selected athletic drinks in their rates of gastric emptying.* Masters Thesis. Ball State University, Muncie, IN. p.46, 1976.
Coyle, E.F., D.L. Costill, W.J. Fink, and D.G. Hoopes. Gastric emptying rates for selected athletic drinks. *Res. Quart.* 49:119–124, 1978.,
Davenport, H.W. *Physiology of the digestive tract.* Year Book Med. Publishers, Inc.: Chicago, 1969, pp. 230.
Dickinson, A.L., E.M. Haymes, K.E. Sparks, G.P. Dalsky, and D.G. Welsh. Effects of moderate caffeine ingestion on factors contributing to the quality of endurance performance. *Med. Sci. Sports Exer.* 16: 171, 1984.
Elias, E., G.J. Gibson, L.F. Greenwood, J.N. Hunt, and J.H. Tripp. The slowing of gastric emptying by monosaccharides and disaccharides in test meals. *J. Physiol.* 194:317–326, 1968.
Feldman, M. and J.V. Nixon. Effect of exercise on postprandial gastric secretion and emptying in humans. *J. Appl. Physiol.* 53:851–854, 1982.
Felig, P., A. Cherif, A. Minagawa, and J. Wahren. Hypoglycemia during prolonged exercise in normal men. *N. Engl. J. Med.*, 306:895–900, 1982.
Fordtran, J.S. Marker profusion techniques for measuring intestinal absorption in man. *Gastroent.* 51: 1089–1093, 1966.
Fordtran, J.S., and B. Saltin. Gastric emptying and intestinal absorption during prolonged severe exercise. *J. Appl. Physiol.* 23:331–335, 1967.
Foster, C., D.L. Costill, and W.J. Fink. Gastric emptying characteristics of glucose and glucose polymer solutions *Res. Quart. Exerc. Sport*, 51:299–305, 1980.
Gershon-Cohen, J., H. Shay, and S.S. Fels. The relation of meal temperature to gastric motility and secretion. *Am. J. Roentgenol. Radium Therapy Nucl. Med.* 43:237–242, 1940.
Graham, T.J. *The Best Methods of Improving Health.* London, p. 206–291, 1851.
Hargreaves, M., D.L. Costill, A. Coggan, W.J. Fink, and I. Nishibata. Effect of carbohydrate feedings on muscle glycogen utilization and exercise performance. *Med. Sci. Sports Exer.*, 16:219–222, 1984.
Hepburn, J.S., H.M. Eberhard, R. Ricketts, and C.L.W. Rieger. Temperature of the gastrointestinal tract. The effect of hot and cold foods and physical therapeutic agents. *Arch. Intern. Med.* 52:603–615, 1933.
Hollander, F. and A. Penner. History and development of gastric analysis procedure. *Am. J. Digest. Diseases* 5:22–25, 739, 786–791, 1939.
Hunt, J.N. The site of receptors slowing gastric emptying in response to starch in test meals. *J. Physiol. London* 154:270–276, 1960.
Hunt, J.N. and M.T. Knox. The regulation of gastric emptying of meals containing citric acid and salts of citric acid. *J. Physiol.* 163:34–43, 1962.
Hunt, J.N. and M.T. Knox. Regulation of gastric emptying. In: *Handbook of Physiology IV. Alimentary Canal.* Washington D.C.: American Physiological Society, pp. 1917–1935, 1969a.
Hunt, J.N. and M.T. Knox. The slowing of gastric emptying by nine acids. *J. Physiol.* 163:161–179, 1969b.
Hunt, J.N. and M.T. Knox. The slowing of gastric emptying by four strong acids and three weak acids. *J. Physiol.* 22:187–208, 1972.
Hunt, J.N. and I. MacDonald. The influence of volume on gastric emptying. *J. Physiol.* 126:459–474, 1954.
Hunt, J.N. and J.D. Pathak. The osmotic effects of some simple molecules and ions on gastric emptying. *J. Physiol.* 154:254–269, 1960.
Hunt, J.N., J.L. Smith, and C.L. Jiang. Effect of meal volume and energy density on the gastric emptying of carbohydrates. *Gastroent.* 89:1326–1330, 1985.
Hunt, J.N. and W.R. Spurrell. The pattern of emptying of the human stomach. *J. Physiol., London* 113: 157–168, 1951.
Hunt, J.N. and D.F. Stubbs. The volume and energy content of meals as determinant of gastric emptying. *J. Physiol. London* 245:209–215, 1975.
Johnson, L.R. Gastrointestinal hormones and their functions. *Ann. Rev. Physiol.* 39:135–158, 1977.
Johnson, L.R., J.C. Brown, and D.F. Magee. Effect of secretin and cholecystokinen-pancreozymin extracts on gastric motility in man. *Gut* 7:52–57, 1966.
Kewenteer, J. The vagal control of the jejumal and ileal motility in cat. *Acta Physiol. Scand.* 80:353–359, 1970.
Levine, S.A., B. Gordon, and C.L. Drick. Some changes in the chemical constituents of the blood following a marathon race. *J. Am. Med. Assoc.* 82:1778–1779, 1924.
Lin, H.C., J.E. Doty, T.J. Reedy, and J.H. Meyer. Inhibition of gastric emptying by acids depends on titratable acidity and length of intestine exposed to acid. *Gastroent.* 95:877, 1988.
Marbaix, O. Le passage pylorique. *Cellule* 14:249–332, 1898.
McHugh, P.R. and T.H. Moran. Calories and gastric emptying: a regulatory capacity with implications for feeding. *Am. J. Physiol.* 236:R254–260, 1979.
Mei, N. Intestinal Chemosensitivity. *Physiol. Rev.* 65:211–237, 1985.
Minami, H. and R.W. McCallum. The physiology and pathophysiology of gastric emptying in humans. *Gastroent.* 86:1592–1610, 1984.

Mitchell, J.B., D.L. Costill, J.A. Houmard, M.G. Flynn, W.J. Fink, and J.D. Beltz. Effects of carbohydrate ingestion on gastric emptying and exercise performance. *Med. Sci. Sports Exer.* 20:110–115, 1988.
Mitchell, J.B., D.L. Costill, J.A. Houmard, W.J. Fink, R.A. Robergs, and J.A. Davis. Gastric emptying: influence of prolonged exercise and carbohydrate concentration. *Med. Sci. Sports Exer.* 21:269–274, 1989.
Muller-Lissner, S.A., C.J. Fimmel, N. Will, W. Muller-Duysing, and F. Heinzel. Effect of gastric emptying and transpyloric tubes on gastric emptying and duodenogastric reflux. *Gastroent.* 83:1276–1279, 1982.
Murray, R. The effects of consuming carbohydrate-electrolyte beverages on gastric emptying and fluid absorption during and following exercise. *Sports Med.* 4:322–351, 1987.
Neufer, P.D., A.J. Young, and M.N. Sawka. Gastric emptying during exercise: effects of heat stress and hypohydration. *Eur. J. App. Physiol.* 58:433–439, 1989a.
Neufer, P.D., A.J. Young, and M.N. Sawka. Gastric emptying during walking and running: effects of varied exercise intensity. *Eur. J. Appl. Physiol.* 58:440–445, 1989b.
Neufer, P.D., D.L. Costill, W.J. Fink, J.P. Kirwan, R.A. Fielding, and M.G. Flynn. Effects of exercise and carbohydrate composition on gastric emptying. *Med. Sci. Sports Exer.* 18:658–662, 1986.
Noakes, T.D., B.A. Adams, K.H. Myburgh, C. Greeff, T. Lotz, and M. Nathan. The danger of an inadequate water intake during prolonged exercise. *Euro. J. Appl. Physiol.* 57:210–219, 1988.
Owen, M.D., K.C. Kregel, P.T. Wall, and C.V. Gisolfi. Effects of ingesting carbohydrate beverages during exercise in the heat. *Med. Sci. Sports Exer.* 18:568–575, 1986.
Pathak, J.D. Some effects of introducing HCl into human stomach. *Indian J. Med. Res.* 47:325–328, 1959.
Pitts, G.C., R.E. Johnson, and F.C. Consolazio. Work in the heat as affected by intake of water, salt and glucose. *Am. J. Physiol.* 142:253–259, 1944.
Pugh, L.G.C., J.I. Corbett, and R.H. Johnson. Rectal temperatures, weight losses, and sweating rates in marathon running. *J. Appl. Physiol,* 23:347–352, 1957.
Quigley, J.P. and I. Meschan. Inhibition of the pyloric sphincter region by the digestion products of fat. *Am. J. Physiol.* 134:803–807, 1941.
Saltin, B. Circulatory responses to submaximal and maximal exercise after thermal dehydration. *J. Appl. Physiol.* 19:1125–1132, 1964.
Schedl, H.P., D. Miller, and D. White. Use of polyethylene glycol and phenol red as unabsorbed indicators for intestinal absorption studies in man. *Gut.* 7:159–163, 1966.
Shapiro, H. and E.K. Stoner. Gastric temperature adaption. *Am. J. Gastroent.* 49:391–404, 1968.
Shay, H., and J.Gershon-Cohen. Experimental studies in gastric physiology in man. II. A study of pyloric control. Role of acid and alkali. *Surg. Gynec. Obstet.* 58:935–955, 1934.
Shay, H., J.Gershon-Cohen, and S.S Fels. The role of the upper small intestine in the control of gastric secretion; The effect of neutral fat, fatty acid, and soaps; The phase of gastric secretion influenced and the relative importance of the psychic and chemical phases. *Ann. Int. Med.* 13:294–307, 1939.
Sherman, W.M. and D.R. Lamb. Nutrition and prolonged exercise. In: *Perspectives in Exercise Science and Sports Medicine: Prolonged Exercise.* D.R. Lamb and R. Murray (eds.). Indianapolis, IN: Benchmark Press, vol. 1 (1988). pp. 213–280.
Spurrell, W.R. Duodonal reflexes. *J. Physiol.* 84:4P–5P, 1935.
Thomas, J.E. Mechanics and regulation of gastric emptying. *Physiol. Reviews.* 37:453–474, 1957.
Van Liere, E.J. and C.K. Sleeth. The emptying time of the normal human stomach as influenced by acid and alkali with a review of the literature. *Am. J. Digest Disease* 7:118–123, 1940.
Wald. A., D.H. Van Thiel, L. Hoechstetter, J.S. Gavaler, and K.M. Egler. Gastrointestinal transit: The effect of the menstrual cycle. *Gastroent.* 80:1497–1500, 1981.
Wang, C.C. and M.I. Grossman. Physiological determination of release of secretin and pancreozymin from the intestine of dogs with transplanted pancreas. *Am. J. Physiol.* 164:527–545, 1951.
Wilson, M.J., W.H. Dickson, and A.C. Singleton. Rate of evacuation of various foods from the normal stomach. *Arch. Interna Med.* 44:787–796, 1929.
Wolf, S. and H.G. Wolff. *Human gastric function.* Oxford University Press, 1943.

DISCUSSION

MEYER: There are new techniques for measuring gastric emptying that don't require nasogastric intubation. For exercise physiology, probably the simplest is gastric impedance. You just have to strap electrodes around the abdomen. This impedance method has been well cross-correlated with aspiration methods and with gamma scintigraphy, which is another more cumbersome noninvasive method. The problem of pH and titratable acidity is very complicated, but it seems that the inhibition of gastric emptying at a high pH is related to titratable acidity with an end point that is somewhere above pH 4—We don't know exactly how high. Hunt thought it was about 6.5. The total number of hydrogen ions—bound and free—are titrated by the gut. Below a pH of 2, there seems to be a fail-safe mechanism; that is; below this pH there is also a direct pH response. When you take a liquid drink that has citrate in it, somewhere between pH 2 and 4, it's a very complex poblem because the volume of the drink promotes gastric secretion. The shut-off of gastric secretion is also pH dependent. If you have a buffer in a drink and a distending stomach, you get secretion of hydrochloric acid, which in turn is buffered by the citrate. Consequently, the titratable acid content increases tremendously. That's probably the mechanism that accounts for the unexpectedly large slowing of gastric emptying of citrate-containing drinks.

COSTILL: An alkaline solution empties very rapidly. I wonder if a less acid solution might be an advantage for individuals who have to drink large volumes.

MEYER: A crucial piece of information here is where the pH threshold is, and we don't know that. It was indirectly derived by Hunt; nobody has really studied it.

MURRAY: In looking at all this gastric emptying literature, it seems to me that if you were to advise an athlete as to how to achieve the greatest rate of gastric emptying, it would be to exercise at a moderate intensity in a cool environment while consuming a large quantity of isotonic saline while lying on the right side when neither menstruating nor emotionally upset. That far-fetched example is meant to illustrate how impractical some of these research results can be. We've made mistakes in the past by making extrapolations based upon gastric emptying research that haven't been born out by subsequent research.

COSTILL: Everything that goes into the stomach does not reach the intestine in the form in which it was ingested. When you ingest water, it is markedly altered by the time it reaches the intestine. To expect drinks to be absorbed as ingested is misleading. I think the stomach plays a critical role in all of this, not only as a reservoir or a dam, but also in modifying the solution.

HARVEY: There is a problem in feeding and watering the athlete and trying to mix the two. A few years ago, the East Germans were using small boluses of very concentrated carbohydrate; they drank a 40-50% carbohydrate solution and then diluted it in their stomachs by sipping water from a bottle. I have one question. What happens when we use a scientific drink of 6% carbohydrate and then we do something very unscientific like eat a granola bar or a banana? Do we significantly change the gastric emptying? I know the food that has fat is going to make a difference, but does the fact that we're putting a solid residue in the stomach make a big difference in gastric emptying rate?

COSTILL: I anticipate that it would slow emptying. Whether you mix it on the table or you mix it in your stomach doesn't make a whole lot of difference.
MEYER: Michael Horowitz has a paper in press in the American Journal of Physiology in which he looked at the effect of a calorie-or glucose-containing drink on emptying of the solid food and vice versa and their interaction with each other. The taking of solid nutrients definitely slows emptying.
SUTTON: I'd like to ask a question about the importance of fitness in this whole business of gastric emptying. People with higher endurance fitness tend to have increased vagal tone. Is there a parallel between vagal tone as it affects the heart, and vagal tone as it affects the gastrointestinal system? I suppose we know the impact of the autonomic nervous system on the rate of gastric emptying, but do we know the impact of fitness on the autonomic activity as it affects the gastrointestinal system and its impact therefore on gastric emptying and absorption of fluids from the GI tract?
COSTILL: I can't really respond to the influence on reflex action of fitness. I can only tell you that emptying rate is relative to exercise effort. People who are less fit can't empty the stomach as well at the same absolute workloads as those who are more fit. An exercise above 60% of $\dot{V}O_2$ max may not be stressful for someone who is relatively fit. At 80% $\dot{V}O_2$ max, the stomach flow is markedly reduced, and that is magnified in a person who is untrained.
SUTTON: Do you think this is an autonomic effect or is related to gastric blood flow?
COSTILL: It's probably autonomic. I'm sure that if you measured the catacholamine responses to work, you'd see that they parallel each other.
COYLE: I think that the area concerning how much carbohydrate we can get out of the stomach into the intestines has been somewhat confused for a while. Even the resting literature that suggests you can only get 2.4 kcal/min is low because if we add it up over a course of 24 h, that's only 3200 kcal/d; we can store more than that. During exercise, you suggest a levelling off in carbohydrate gain that doesn't totally agree with Foster's work or with some recent work by Mitchell. You are suggesting, from Foster's data, with the 40% carbohydrate, that you are delivering 75 g. That was 30 min as I recall or 2-1/2 g/min in the rate of gastric emptying of carbohydrates. That is substantial. I think that is an important point that could be brought out.
DAVIS: I'd just like to say that I understand the scientific value of looking at factors that influence gastric emptying by itself. As well, I understand the scientific value of looking at intestinal absorption by itself. I would urge that when one talks about influences of gastric emptying related to athletic performance, that you at least talk about the factors of

gastric emptying and intestinal absorption together as they relate to fluid replenishment. To discuss just gastric emptying and make recommendations with respect to overall fluid replenishment I think is not satisfactory. My second point is that when you put tubes into people's stomachs and intestines you have to assume there is an added stress effect. I know that you said that it perhaps would not be a big factor, but it's hard for me to assume that when you have tubes in your intestines or stomach that your body is functioning just like it would normally in an exercise session or a resting session.

COSTILL: That is why we studied the rate of gastric emptying with the tube in place and without the tube, i.e., to see if there really was a difference. I anticipated that some of our subjects wouldn't empty because they were distressed by the tube. But that didn't prove to be the case. There are other studies that show the same thing.

DAVIS: My point is that when people summarize your chapter and try to make recommendations based on it, they look just at the gastric emptying. I would encourage that we at least bring up the issue that getting it out of the stomach is one thing, but getting it absorbed in the intestine is another.

COSTILL: One problem with studies of intenstinal absosrption is that they ignore the effects of the stomach on the composition of chyme entering the duodenum. We need to examine intestinal absorption using solutions that are similar to those being delivered to the intestine.

DAVIS: As you know, we developed a methodology with deuterium oxide. I think you can get some pretty good overall fluid retention data by using that technique. You don't have to put tubes in, you don't have unnecessary stress.

COSTILL: My only suggestion to improve those studies would be to do gastric emptying (aspiration) to check the validity of the deuterium oxide method.

HUBBARD: A military commander once told me that his troops were trained to drink very large volumes of fluid by command drinking in very short periods of time. Do you have any indication of a training effect on gastric emptying or vomiting threshold?

COSTILL: No.

NADEL: How do the electrolytes affect emptying? The reason I'm asking is that in the human powered flight studies that I was involved with, it became apparent that the amount of sodium in the drinking fluid was important for rehydration during recovery. I tried to play with the amount of sodium. This was more acting as an engineer than a scientist. The idea was to get the sodium levels up high enough to replace the sodium lost. I found that I couldn't do it, because when the people were given normal and half normal saline concentrations, or even a third normal saline concentrations, they were reporting stomach stress. My assumption was that they weren't emptying from the stomach at all. I'd like to have your comments about the affects of sodium in the solution on the ability to empty.

COSTILL: Most of the literature looks at these things independent of each other. Hunt's early data looked at different ions. Sodium chloride solutions tended to empty more rapidly with small additions of sodium chloride to the solution, and then emptied more slowly as the concentration was increased. He was dealing with relatively low concentrations of sodium. Saltin and I tried to use that same concept when we did that gastric emptying study in 1972, by adding small amounts of sodium chloride to our solutions, thinking that it might speed emptying. We found that it didn't make any difference. The difference between the results of our work and that of Hunt might be due to the overriding effects of carbohydrate in the solution. A small amount of sodium chloride probably doesn't have much of an effect. We've had the same problem you described. If you try to make it too salty, they just can't stomach it. When the salt solutions get into the stomach, many subjects still have some distress.

SAWKA: I noticed that Roger talked about optimal temperature for drinking at around 15.5° C and you showed that you can increase gastric emptying as you drop the temperature. I've noticed in some of our studies that we've had occasions where people got stomach cramps and we really hadn't precisely monitored temperature of water. We've always thought it was too cold and taken some ice out. Have you noted in your experiments where there is a temperature effect on stomach cramps? And if so, about where would this occur?

COSTILL: Some of those drinks that we gave our subjects were refrigerator temperature, about 4-5 1/2° C. Studies that examined the relationship between temperature and the rate of gastric emptying were all done at rest. That may be a factor. I've never had anyone get stomach cramps in any of the studies we've done, and in nearly all of our studies, we use cold fluids.

SAWKA: I wonder if, as the body warms and the stomach muscles warm, you should drop the temperature of the fluid. It might make an interesting study.

COSTILL: We've fed some large, cold volumes to people. Even subjects who exercise for 6 h in the heat never develop stomach cramps. I'd be a little surprised if that is a problem for concern during fluid replacement.

MURRAY: Roger Hubbard mentioned the hyperuricemic response to fructose ingestion. When you infuse fructose at 1 g/kg body weight, you get a nice hyperuricemic response. We recently published a study in which we fed fructose solutions to exercising subjects. We didn't see any hyperuricemic response, but we saw a lot of other negative responses such as an increase in GI distress, poor exercise performance, and from a fluid-regulatory standpoint, a lower plasma volume. The decrease in plasma volume was greater with ingestion of the fructose solution, and we reasoned that could probably be due to the slower absorption of fructose and subsequent slower absorption of water.

SUMMERS: One of the points that you emphasized was the role of antral motility in gastric emptying. The major role of phasic antral contractions is to grind or titrate solids; they play a relatively minor role in emptying of liquids. More important in the modification of gastric emptying of liquids is fundic tone. The tonic contractions in the fundus are regulated by local reflex mechanisms. Secondly, in drinking cold liquids, we do not know what the origin of the cramp is. I suspect that they may not be motor cramps at all. Some studies were done in the esophagus of subjects drinking cold or iced liquids. They experienced "cramps", but the origin was not a spastic motor phenomenon at all. The esophagus became dilated, and there was almost no motor activity. I suspect that something similar to that may be going on in the stomach when "cramps" are experienced with cold liquids.

COSTILL: I think it has been well documented that if you give someone a cold feeding of 300–400 mL, it will cool the stomach. You'd think that it might rewarm quickly, but the stomach temperature remains colder for 0.5-1.0 h. I'd just like to make it clear that I don't think that you get that much cramping from drinking cold fluids. In all the years that I've been doing gastric emptying studies and feedings with cold fluids, I haven't seen one case.

PHILLIPS: What time does the water get into the blood? You get more rapid gastric emptying with warmer water. Does that mean it is getting into the blood faster than cold water? What happens with the cold water; does it take longer to get into the blood or warm up and then become absorbed?

COSTILL: Athletes tend to drink cooler water because it is more palatable. I don't think there is an initial physiological effect. There may be a long-term effect. Of course, cold fluids do tend to numb some of the sensory organs in the mouth; thereby altering taste. That, in part, may explain some of the reasons why we prefer to drink cold fluids. There is a variety of reasons why they may prefer cold over warm.

PHILLIPS: What happens to the plasma osmolality?

COSTILL: From a practical point of view, it's not how quickly fluids get into the bloodstream, it's how quickly the drink's constituents reach the periphery. It took about 5-7 min. It's not that rapid when it is in a carbohydrate solution. So that may not be an accurate statement, but at least it is one of the few ways we could probably look at its delivery.

NADEL: We've done some of those studies during recovery from exercise. Certainly if you're drinking fresh water with nothing in it, the plasma osmolality goes back down to baseline within 20-30 min. If you give a fluid that has some sodium chloride in it, the plasma osmolality changes less rapidly, as you might expect.

LAMB: I've been telling students that the reason that cold fluid might be important is because the cold counteracts the heat storage.

COSTILL: I think ingesting large volumes of cold fluid into the heated core of the body has a measurable effect on body heat storage. If you calculate the calories needed to raise 4° C water up to body temperature (37-39° C), there are a lot of calories involved, especially when hypothermia can result from a 0.01° C change in blood temperature. Thus, I feel that the temperature of a fluid will have a cooling effect on central core and blood temperature. It amounts to 0.3°C/L of fluid, depending on the size of the subject.

NADEL: No! That thermoregulatory apparatus is already turned on fully. A 0.3° C decline from 39.0 to 38.7° C won't turn it off. It's more complicated than that because as you cool the blood and the brain, you turn off the thermoregulatory effectors, and that allows the heat to build up, so it's a transient effect. You will come back to the same temperature.

GREENLEAF: We should remember that the temperature of an ingested cold beverage is raised as the drink passes through the warmed esophagus.

SHERMAN: Dave, relative to your conclusion that the movement during running might enhance gastic emptying compared to cycling, have you ruled out the differences in the nature of the exercise? Perhaps you have had the cyclist cycle at those intensities out of their seats so they're moving up and down?

COSTILL: No, we haven't. We've used some of the same subjects doing both running and cycling and consistently find that they empty better when they're running.

SHERMAN: Those data don't necessarily lead to the conclusion that gastric emptying differences are caused by the movement, per se. If you do cycling with and without movement, by having subjects seated and not seated, your conclusions would be much stronger.

COSTILL: That's a possibility. It's just that we see the highest rates of emptying when subjects are moving, whether it's cross-country skiing or running. That's just a wild guess, it's the only thing that seems to differ substantially in those subjects.

SHERMAN: Is there any possibility that too concentrated of a carbohydrate solution might cause a decrease in plasma volume during exercise in the heat due to dilution of the gastric content from gastric secretions, which might be detrimental to the metabolic response in exercise?

COSTILL: We have measured gastric secretion in the residue. When you do that, you find that the amount of secretion is seldom greater than about 60 mL.

4

Intestinal Absorption of Fluids During Rest and Exercise

CARL V. GISOLFI, PH.D.

ROBERT W. SUMMERS, M.D.

HAROLD P. SCHEDL, PH.D.

INTRODUCTION

Discussions of fluid homeostasis rarely include gastrointestinal (GI) function, yet these organs play a vital role in osmoregulation (Powell, 1987) and in the maintenance of plasma volume (Powell, 1987; Sjovall et al., 1986). They also contribute importantly to electrolyte and acid-base balance (Charney & Feldman, 1984). During prolonged exercise, especially in the heat, excessive sweating and fluid redistribution lead to the contraction of plasma volume. Fluid replacement, a process that is dependent upon gastric emptying and intestinal absorption, is essential to attenuate the effects of dehydration and to assure optimal performance. The contraction of plasma volume significantly increases intestinal water absorption and electrolyte absorption (Sjovall et al., 1986). Thus, GI function plays a pivotal role in fluid homeostasis, especially during exercise when we attempt to match fluid lost in sweat with fluid gained by ingestion.

The purpose of this chapter is to review the basic mechanisms of electrolyte, water, and carbohydrate absorption at rest, and then to examine the influence of exercise on these processes. A secondary objective will be to reveal what intestinal absorption studies can contribute to our understanding of how to formulate an oral hydration solution. In addition, the chapter will also consider other GI functions, such as motility and blood flow, that may be affected by exercise. These functions are closely intertwined with that of absorption. The following questions will be addressed: 1) How is absorption measured in human subjects?, 2) What is the role of glucose in facilitating water and salt absorption in the human intestine?, 3) Does exercise limit active or passive intestinal transport?, 4) Is it necessary to include electrolytes in fluid replacement solutions? and 5) What is the optimal glucose/Na^+ ratio required to maximize water absorption? Emphasis is placed on human studies and on the absorption of water, salt, and glucose in the small intestine. To our knowledge, no studies investigating how exercise affects colonic absorption have been published.

A. Enterosystemic Water Cycle

In a normal healthy individual, approximately 9 L of fluid are presented to the intestines each day, 2 L from ingested fluid, 1.5 L from saliva, and 5.5 L from gastrointestinal secretions (Figure 4-1). Of this amount, approximately 60% (5.5 L) is absorbed by the duodenojejunum, 20% (1.8 L) by the ileum, and 15% (1.3 L) by the colon. For the exercise scientist, these facts generate two important questions: 1) Do these GI secretions represent a fluid reservoir that can be mobilized under conditions of exercise and dehydration? and 2) How does dehydration affect intestinal secretion and absorption? From the limited studies available, there apparently is no consistent effect of exercise on gastrointestinal secretions (Campbell et al., 1928; Feldman and Nixon, 1982; Konturek et al., 1973).

The duodenojejunum is relatively efficient (61%) and absorbs the major portion of the volume load presented to the small bowel (Figure 4-1). The epithelial lining of this portion of the intestine is relatively leaky, and fluid is absorbed isotonically. Because this membrane leaks, this portion of the gut is not able to generate a large potential difference (PD). The ileum absorbs less fluid at approximately 60% efficiency, such that only 1500 mL of the 9 L initially presented to the small bowel is transmitted to the colon. In contrast to the small intestine, the colon absorbs a relatively small volume of water, but it does so more efficiently (81%). Of the 1500 mL presented, all but 100 to 200 mL are absorbed.

If it is assumed that the length of the small intestine is 200 cm in the living human (Gardner et al., 1967), and that fluid absorption from a carbohydrate-electrolyte solution averages 12 $mL{\cdot}cm^{-1}{\cdot}h^{-1}$ in the proximal (duodenojejunum, 100 cm) small intestine (Gisolfi et al., In Press; Wheeler & Banwell, 1986) and about 2 $mL{\cdot}cm^{-1}{\cdot}h^{-1}$ in the distal small intestine (ileum, 100 cm), the maximal absorptive capacity of the small intestine is approximately 1.4 L/h or about 33 L/d. The maximal absorptive capacity of the large intestine is about 5 L/d (Binder, 1988). Thus, diarrhea produced by small intestinal disease only occurs when the fluid load on the colon exceeds 5 L/d.

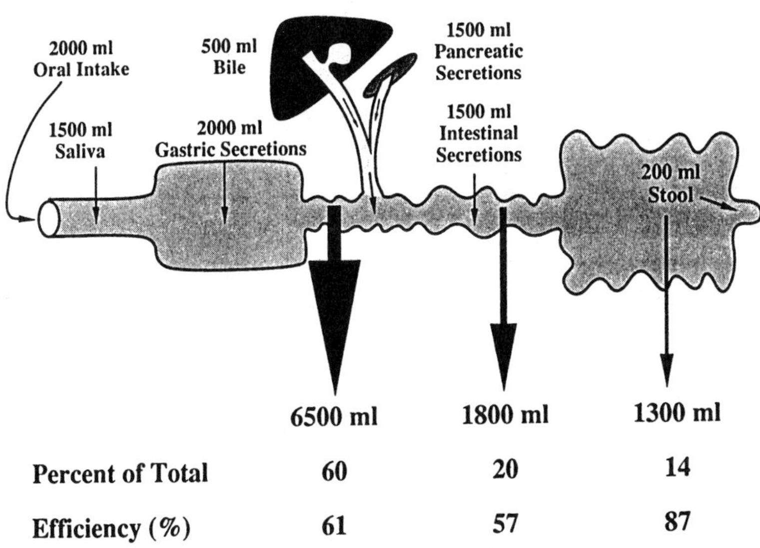

FIGURE 4-1. *Approximate values for the water load entering the intestines each day and the volumes absorbed by the small and large intestine. The relative efficiencies of the absorption process in each segment of the bowel are also shown. Efficiency is defined as the ratio of water absorbed to water entering the segment.*

METHODS FOR MEASURING INTESTINAL ABSORPTION

The different methods of studying intestinal absorption have been reviewed several times (Modigliani et al., 1973; Parsons, 1968; Sladen, 1975; Leiper & Maughan, 1989), and can be separated into direct and indirect categories. Direct methods are those that focus on the luminal compartment, whereas indirect methods focus on the plasma compartment or other compartments. The direct methods include *in vivo* luminal perfusion in human and experimental animals, *in vitro* preparations of intestinal mucosa mounted in chambers using the "short-circuit" technique (see Schultz & Curran, 1964), and, more recently, the transport of electrolytes and nutrients across membranes of mucosal cells of enterocytes. In human subjects, ingesting a solution containing xylose or 3-O-methyl glucose and monitoring the carbohydrate appearance in the plasma has been used as an indirect method of measuring passive or active glucose transport, respectively. Both direct and indirect techniques often employ the use of isotopic tracers to measure unidirectional fluxes. The short-circuit technique is an excellent method for quantifying active transport processes, but it removes the effects of extrinsic nerves, GI blood flow, motility, and hydrostatic pressure gradients (Binder, 1988). Thus it minimizes those forces that promote passive transport and solvent drag. Although the segmental perfusion technique allows for quantification of both active and passive processes, including the effects of water flow, it is not as precise as the short-circuit technique in determining active transport. Only segmental perfusion and isotopic tracer techniques will be discussed here, because these are most appropriate for use in human subjects.

A. Direct

1. Segmental Perfusion: The segmental perfusion technique was introduced by Schedl and Clifton (1963) and Cooper et al. (1966). The details of the technique have been reviewed by Modigliani et al. (1973). It is the method by choice for quantitative determinations of water and solute absorption in human subjects. The basic principle is that the net flux (Q_N) of a substance perfused through the intestine is the difference between solution concentration (C_1) times the rate of flow (V_1) entering a discrete segment (test segment) of the intestine, less the concentration (C_2) times the rate of flow leaving (V_2) that segment:

$$Q_N = V_1 \cdot C_1 - V_2 \cdot C_2.$$

If a double lumen tube is employed, one tube is used to perfuse a solution of known concentration, C_1, at a constant rate, V_1. The second tube has a lumen 25 to 40 cm distal to the site of infusion and allows the solution to be sampled for the measure of C_2. Because V_2 can not be measured, a nonabsorbable marker [such as polyethylene glycol (PEG), phenolsulphonphthalein (PSP), or bromsulphthalein (BSP)] is included in the perfusion solution to allow the determination of V_2.

$$Q_{N\,PEG} = V_1\,[PEG]_1 - V_2\,[PEG]_2$$

$Q_{N\,PEG} = 0$ (because PEG is not absorbed). Thus,

$$V_2 = V_1 \cdot \frac{[PEG]_1}{[PEG]_2}; \text{ therefore,}$$

$$Q_N = V_1 \cdot C_1 - V_1 \cdot \frac{[PEG]_1}{[PEG]_2} \cdot C_2$$

$$Q_N = V_1 \cdot \left[C_1 - C_2 \cdot \frac{[PEG]_1}{[PEG]_2}. \right]$$

Ideally, the marker should: a) not be absorbed, b) be uniformly distributed, c) not affect absorption or motility, d) be readily quantified, and e) not interfere with digestion (Modigliani et al., 1973). PEG is perhaps the most widely used marker; however it should be included in test solutions at low (1 to 2 mg/mL) concentrations to avoid the possible osmotic inhibition of water and electrolyte absorption.

The drawbacks of the double-lumen technique are: a) reflux of the perfused solution proximally, thus reducing the actual rate of perfusion, and b) contamination of the perfused solution by proximal endogenous secretions (Modigliani et al., 1973). To eliminate these problems, some investigators have included an occlusive balloon proximal to the infusion port to prevent reflux toward the stomach and to prevent the mixing of endogenous proximal secretions with the perfusate. To ensure that mixing does not occur, a second nonabsorbable dye, such as phenol red, is infused through a lumen proximal to the occlusive balloon. This second marker should not appear in the test segment. The disadvantage of this technique is that the occlusive balloon interferes with intestinal motility.

Perhaps the most widely accepted technique is to add a mixing segment to the catheter, as illustrated in Figure 4-2. Although called a triple-lumen tube (or the triple-lumen technique), it often has a fourth lumen used to temporarily inflate a balloon which, when inflated with 10–20 cc of air, facilitates movement of the tube through the intestine. The balloon also houses a mercury bag that facilitates passage of the tube through the pyloric sphincter. It is deflated when the lumens reach the desired locations in the gut, before the experiment is initiated. The mixing segment is the distance between the perfusion port and the first sampling site (usually 10–15 cm) and allows the nonabsorbable marker to

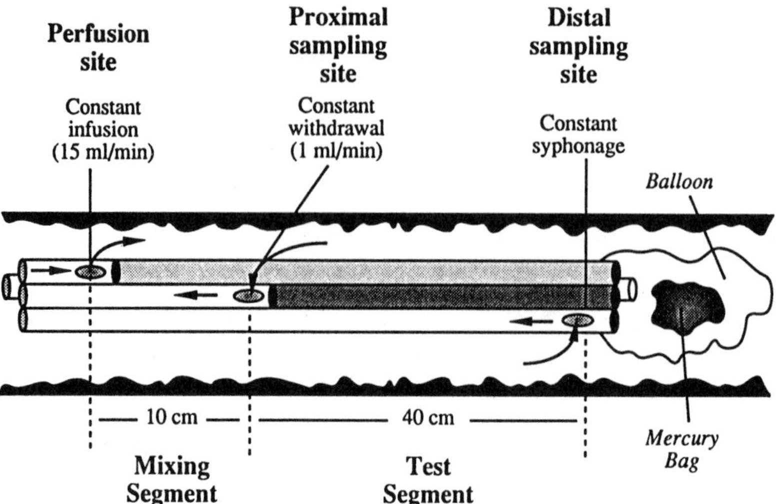

FIGURE 4-2. *Illustration of the segmental perfusion technique using a triple-lumen tube with attached balloon and mercury bag.*

form a homogenous solution with intestinal contents. A sample of this solution is aspirated at the proximal sampling site (usually 1 $mL \cdot min^{-1}$) for determination of the test substance and the marker. The fluid then traverses the test segment (usually 20-40 cm) and is collected continuously by siphonage at the distal lumen. It is not necessary to recover all of the solution. As indicated above, the flux calculations depend only on changes in concentration of the marker and test solution. Accuracy depends primarily on 2 assumptions: a) the marker is not absorbed appreciably, and b) complete mixing has occurred with endogenous secretions in both mixing and test segments. Calculations for determining net flux (Q_N) using a triple-lumen tube are as follows:

$$Q_E = I \cdot \frac{[PEG]_i}{[PEG]_p} - S_p$$

$$Q_L = Q_E \cdot \frac{[PEG]_p}{[PEG]_d}$$

$$Q_N = Q_E - Q_L ,$$

where 1 is the infusion rate in $ML \cdot min^{-1}$; Q_E and Q_L are the flow rates in $mL \cdot min^{-1}$ entering and leaving the test segment, respectively; and $[PEG]_i$, $[PEG]_p$, and $[PEG]_d$ are the concentrations of polyethylene glycol in the infusion solution (i), proximal (p) fluid sample, and distal (d) fluid sample, respectively (Cooper et al., 1966). Sp is the rate of sampling from the proximal sampling site in $mL \cdot min^{-1}$. The amounts of solute entering and leaving the test segment are obtained by multiplying solute concentrations in the fluid sampled from the proximal and distal sites ($[S]_p$ and $[S]_d$), respectively, by the flow rates entering and leaving the segment. Net soluble solute movement (S) is determined by subtraction:

$$S = Q_E \cdot [S]_p - Q_L \cdot [S]_d$$

With the equations written in this manner, Q_N will have a negative sign when secretion has taken place and a positive sign when absorption has occurred.

When using the triple-lumen technique, it is important to realize that the results from such studies only apply to the portion of gut represented by the test segment. Different results could be obtained by perfusing a longer or shorter segment or a different site in the intestine. It should also be realized that the composition of the solution tested is not the composition of the fluid perfused, but rather the composition of the fluid sampled at the proximal sampling site.

2. Endoscopic retrograde bowel insertion (ERBI): This new technique measures whole small bowel absorption (Higuchi et al., 1986) by employing a double-lumen tube with an attached balloon inserted retrograde through the colon and quantifying characteristics of a test solution and nonabsorbable marker taken orally. The discomfort of positioning the tube from above and the unknown effects of a tube throughout the bowel on small intestinal function are avoided by this technique. It is similar to earlier triple lumen techniques that located the distal lumen at the ileocecal valve.

B. Indirect

1. Tracer Technique: Isotopic tracers are either stable or unstable (radioisotopes), and generally provide good quantitative measures of unidirectional flux. They are used in *in vitro* preparations to monitor fluxes across different segments of intestinal mucosa or across membrane vesicles. They are also employed *in vivo* to quantify water, electrolyte, or nutrient movement from one compartment to another, i.e., from intestinal lumen to plasma and vice versa. To measure net flux or the movement of more than one solute, two or more isotopes are required. Stable isotopes of elements are generally considered to be excellent tracers because they respond in a similar fashion to the element in chemical reactions and exchange processes without having the risks associated with irradiation (Pinson, 1952). Deuterium (D), in the form of deuterium oxide D_2O, has been used as a common tracer for water in studies of water exchange (Pinson, 1952; Scholer & Code, 1954; Reitemeier et al., 1957; Davis et al., 1987). Unstable isotopes are less desirable because more expensive equipment is required, radioactive decay and counting efficiency must be considered, and there are potential dangers of radiation to the experimental subject (Leiper & Maughan, 1989).

In recent years, the accumulation of D_2O in the plasma after ingesting D_2O-labelled oral hydration beverages has been used as an index of rehydration, i.e., a measure of both gastric emptying and intestinal absorption (Davis et al., 1987, Leiper & Maughan, 1989). This technique is simple, non-invasive, and involves the entire intestine rather than a relatively small section of the gut employed with the segmental perfusion technique. However, the accumulation of tracer in the blood is not only determined by intestinal absorption and gastric emptying, but also by the differential rates of tracer movement out of the vascular space into the various bodily tissues and organs, including the movement of tracer from the blood back into the intestinal lumen. Based on data obtained with the segmental perfusion technique, the accumulation of D_2O in the plasma from oral hydration solutions containing D_2O appears to be inadequate as a measure of intestinal absorption (Figure 4-3; Gisolfi et al., 1990). It cannot be used to distinguish between solutions that promote net absorption or net secretion within a given segment of the intestine (Gisolfi et al., 1990).

WATER ABSORPTION

The concept that water absorption by the intestine is a passive process dependent upon net solute transport is attributed to Curran (1960), who demonstrated that net water flux is zero when net solute flux is zero, proving that the intestine cannot transport water in the absence of active solute transport. Curran (1968) is also credited with explaining how the intestinal epithelium can transport fluid against an osmotic gradient. Figure 4-4 illustrates his double membrane model (Curran & McIntosh, 1962). According to this theory, three compartments are separated by two membranes of differing permeability. Fluid can move against a concentration gradient from compartment A to compartment C, provided the osmolality in compartment B exceeds that in compartment A and the permeability of β is greater than α.

The accompanying structural diagram proposes that the basolateral membrane is α and the capillary membrane is β. Sodium is actively extruded into the intercellular space, creating an osmotic gradient for water movement. The flux of water into this space, either through the cell or through the tight junction, establishes a hydrostatic pressure gradient for water movement into the capillary. Recent studies indicate that the osmotic gradients across the brush border and basolateral membranes need only be 2.4 and 1.1 mOsm, respectively, to account for the reported flow of water from mucosa to serosa (Persson & Spring, 1982). The exact location of compartment B is controversial. Recent observations suggest

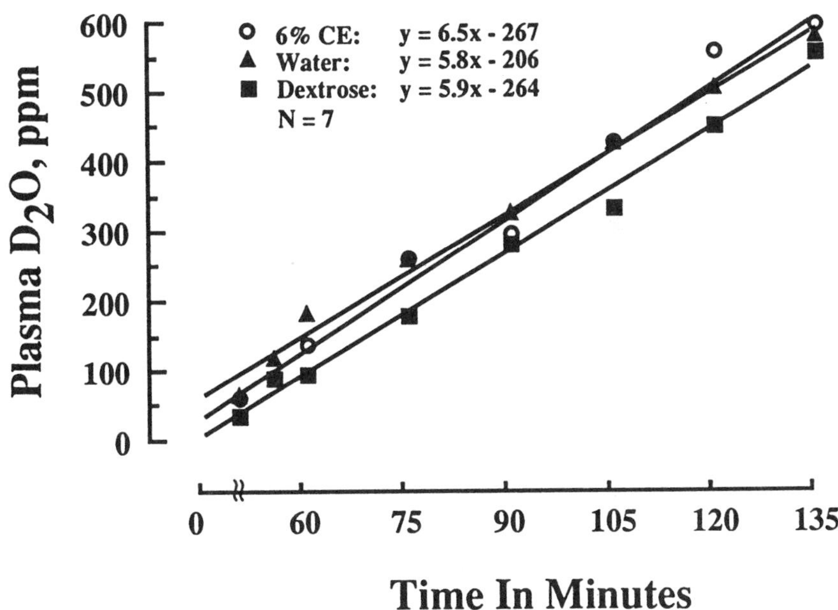

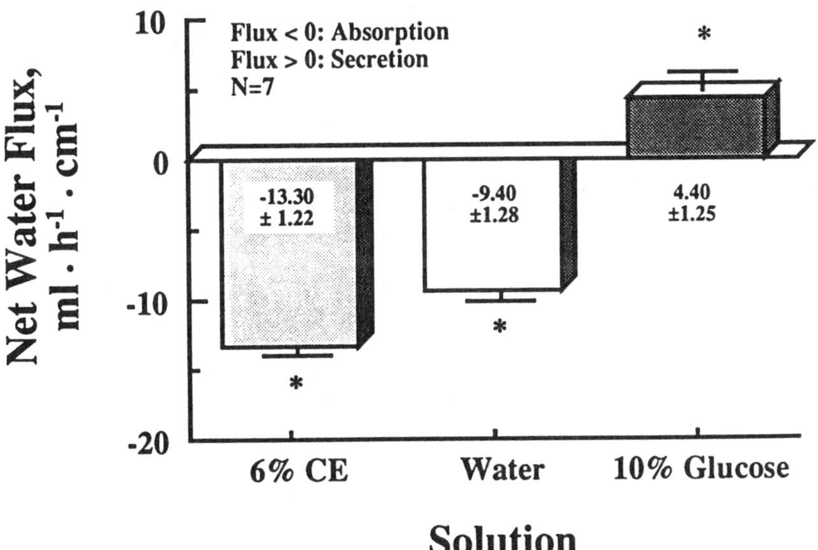

FIGURE 4-3. *Water absorption from three different solutions and the corresponding accumulation of D_2O in the plasma (Redrawn from Gisolfi et al., in press, 1990).*

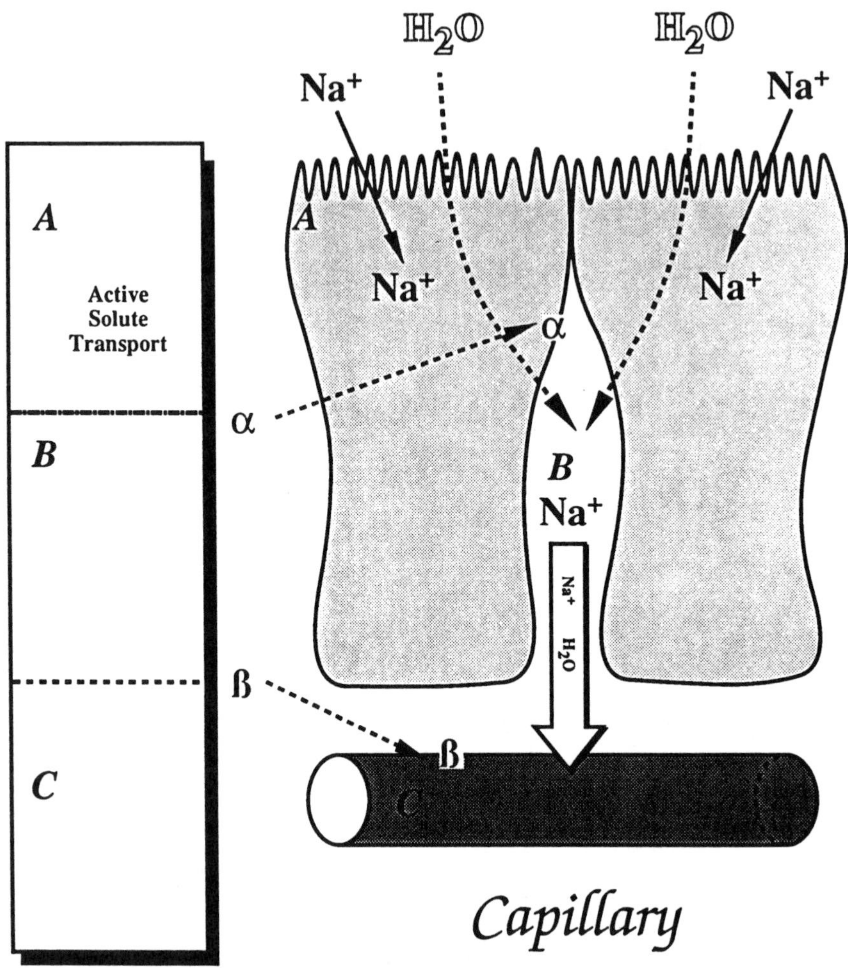

FIGURE 4-4. *The double-membrane three-compartment model for explaining water absorption. Water can move from compartment A to C against a concentration gradient. See text for explanation.*

that it is the interstitium between the basement membrane and the blood rather than the intercellular space (Bond et al., 1977; Levitt, 1977).

The proportion of water moving through the cell as opposed to across the cell junctions via solvent drag, especially in "leaky" epithelia like the duodenojejunum, is not known. Persson & Spring (1982) suggest that transcellular water movement is sufficient to account for reported water flows, but the more recent studies of Pappenheimer and his colleagues (Madara & Pappenheimer, 1987; Pappenheimer & Resiss, 1987; Pappenheimer, 1987) indicate that the paracellular pathway is the primary pathway of fluid absorption when glucose is present in luminal fluid. The rates of net water movement from the small intestines of normal healthy human subjects range from −4.4 to 13.3 $mL \cdot h^{-1} \cdot cm^{-1}$ and vary with solute absorption and the amount and form of carbohydrate in the perfusion solution (Table 4-1). The studies included in Table 4-1 are limited to those that measured absorption using the segmental perfusion technique in normal healthy subjects.

ELECTROLYTE ABSORPTION

Active and passive solute transport occurs along the entire length of the intestine, but their relative contributions vary in the small and large bowel. Most transport probably occurs across cell membranes (Persson & Spring, 1982); transport across tight junctions (intercellular or shunt pathway) is usually secondary to passive driving forces (Binder, 1988). Absorptive processes are usually located in epithelial cells of the villi, while secretory processes are usually stored in the crypt (Welsh et al., 1982). The control of absorption and secretion is extremely complex and beyond the scope of this chapter. It involves hormones, nerves, neurotransmitters, and bacterial enterotoxins that influence at least three different intracellular messengers: cAMP, cGMP, and CA^{+2} (Powell, 1987; Cooke, 1987).

A. Sodium Transport Mechanisms

Total body exchangeable Na^+ is approximately 42 mEq/kg body weight and includes all of the Na^+ in the extracellular and intracellular compartments and somewhat less than half of the Na^+ in bone (Pitts, 1963). Exchangeable Na^+ is in diffusion equilibrium with plasma Na^+ and can offset Na^+ lost in urine, sweat, vomitus, or diarrheal fluid. Plasma $[Na^+]$ is typically 138 to 142 mEq/L and generally rises during exercise due to the loss of hypotonic sweat. Sweat $[Na^+]$ ranges from 18 to 97 mEq/L (Robinson & Robinson, 1954), and increases with sweat rate (Costill, 1977).

With regard to Na^+ balance, the questions of import to exercise physiologists and sports physicians are: 1) Is the loss of Na^+ during exercise significant?; 2) Should Na^+ losses during exercise be replaced by adding Na^+ to a fluid replacement beverage, and if so, how much should be added?; 3) How important is Na^+ to intestinal absorption of water and other nutrients?; and 4) How does Na^+ affect beverage palatability?

Sodium loss via sweating during 2 to 4 h of exercise in a cool environment is approximately 200 mEq, but this loss could increase to nearly 600 mEq during a triathlon (13 h). Either of these exercise bouts could result in hyponatremia (plasma $[Na^+] < 130$ mEq/L), depending upon the volume and composition of the fluid replacement beverage ingested (Gisolfi, 1988). The effect of Na^+ on beverage palatability is discussed elsewhere in this volume, and a recommended amount of Na^+ to be added to an oral hydration solution is given later in this chapter. The

TABLE 4-1. *Rates of water, glucose, and electrolyte transport from the small intestine of human subjects during rest or exercise.*

Test Solution Intestinal Segment Technique	Intestinal Absorption H_2O	 Glucose	 Na^+	 K^+	 Cl^-	 HCO_3^-	Reference Rest/Exer
5% Glucose + 0.25% Methionine		3.18 (0.22)					Cummins, 1952 Rest
10% Glucose + 0.5% Methionine		4.72 (0.41)					
Perfusion rate: 10 ml/min ***Segment: Duodenojejunum, 45 cm*** ***Triple Lumen Tube***							
All solutions contained PEG and phenol red as indicators.							Schedl and Clifton, 1963 Rest
Soln 1: Distilled water							
Jejunal	15.30		- 2.00	- 0.09	- 2.00		
Ileal	2.40		- 2.32	- 0.11	- 2.87		
Soln 2: a Ringer's solution (Na^+ 145 mM, Cl^- 123 mM)							
Jejunal	1.80		0.41	0.01	0.64		
Ileal	0.60		- 0.06	- 0.01	- 0.05		
Soln 3: a 1% Glucose-Ringer's solution (Na^+ 118 mM, Cl^- 123 mM)							
Jejunal	15.30	2.23	2.07	0.02	2.02		
Illeal	3.00	1.12	0.04	0.02	0.73		
Perfusion Rate: 15 ml/min ***Segment: Transintestinal, 15 cm*** ***Double Lumen Tube***							
The solutions were made isotonic with appropriate amounts of NaCl. Each solution contained PEG 4000 at 5 g/L.							Holdsworth and Dawson, 1964 ** Rest
2.5% Glucose		3.22					
2.5% Glucose + 2.5% Fructose		3.22					
2.5% Glucose		3.55					
2.5% Glucose + 2.5% Galactose		3.66					
2.5% Glucose	11.40 (1.00)						
5.0% Glucose	4.60 (1.20)						
2.5% Galactose	12.00 (4.40)						
5.0% Galactose	6.00 (2.00)						
2.5% Fructose	4.00 (1.20)						
5.0% Fructose	- 1.40 (2.40)						
Perfusion Rate: 20 ml/min ***Segment: Jejunum, 30 cm*** ***Double Lumen Tube***							

** Water values interpolated from figures.

Values are Means (SE)

Units: H_2O ($ml \cdot h^{-1} \cdot cm^{-1}$), Glucose ($mM \cdot h^{-1} \cdot cm^{-1}$), Na^+, K^+, Cl^-, HCO_3^- ($mEq \cdot h^{-1} \cdot cm^{-1}$).

Positive sign (+) signifies absorption, negative sign (-) signifies secretion

TABLE 4-1. *(continued)*

Test Solution Intestinal Segment Technique	H_2O	Glucose	Na^+	K^+	Cl^-	HCO_3^-	Reference Rest/Exer
	Intestinal Absorption						
All solutions were isotonic and contained PEG.							Malawar et al., 1965 Rest
Saline	0.87	—	0.10				
Saline w/Glucose 2-10 mM	—	0.11	0.41				
Saline w/Glucose 140 mM	10.10	—	—				
Perfusion Rate: ? ***Segment: Jejunum, 30 cm*** ***Perfusion Technique ?***							
See Figure 7							Fordtran and Saltin, 1967 Rest and Exercise
Perfusion Rate: 12 or 16 ml/min ***Segment: Jejunum and Ileum, 30 cm*** ***Triple Lumen Tube***							
Each solution contained PEG. **Study 1:** To establish the chemical concentration gradient against which Na^+ can be absorbed in the **jejunum**. The rate of Na^+ movement when water movement was zero was determined for a number of different luminal Na^+ concentrations.							Fordtran et al., 1968 Rest
$[Na^+]$ (mM)							
112			- 0.16				
123			- 0.04				
127			0.01				
140			0.12				
Study 2: Solutions were isotonic, and contained Galactose (mM) at:							
Ileum							
0	0.43		0.08				
	(0.27)		(0.04)				
35	0.93		0.10				
	(0.22)		(0.03)				
57	1.20		0.13				
	(0.19)		(0.03)				
Study 3: Solutions were isotonic, components included (mM): Na^+ 140, K^+ 5, Glucose 0 and:							
Jejunum							
Cl^-	1.03		0.11		0.16	- 0.01	
	(0.32)		(0.02)		(0.03)	(0.003)	
HCO_3^- 30	1.27		0.16		0.09	0.16	
	(0.40)		(0.03)		(0.03)	(0.04)	
HCO_3^- 70	2.53		0.32		- 0.02	0.42	
	(0.60)		(0.04)		(0.06)	(0.03)	
Ileal $[Na^+]$, $[Cl^-]$, and $[HCO_3^-]$ in test segment							
111 (2.30), 100 (2.00), 8.2 (1.30)	1.60		0.15		0.21	- 0.08	
	(0.25)		(0.02)		(0.02)	(0.01)	
112 (0.9), 61.2 (1.80), 48.3 (1.80)	1.73		0.17		0.04	0.10	
	(0.34)		(0.03)		(0.01)	(0.02)	

Values are Means (SE)

Units: H_2O ($ml \cdot h^{-1} \cdot cm^{-1}$), Glucose ($mM \cdot h^{-1} \cdot cm^{-1}$), Na^+, K^+, Cl^-, HCO_3^- ($mEq \cdot h^{-1} \cdot cm^{-1}$).

Positive sign (+) signifies absorption, negative sign (-) signifies secretion

TABLE 4-1. *(continued)*

Test Solution / Intestinal Segment / Technique	H_2O	Glucose	Na^+	K^+	Cl^-	HCO_3^-	Reference Rest/Exer
	Intestinal Absorption						
Perfusion Rates: 8, 9, 12, or 16 ml/min depending on experiment. Segment: Jejunum and Ileum, 30 cm Triple Lumen Tube							
All solutions contained PEG 2.5 g/L and (mM):							Sladen and Dawson, 1968 Rest
Double Lumen Tube							
Isotonic Saline: Na^+ 150	1.10 (0.80)		0.29 (0.11)				
Isotonic Saline-Bicarbonate: Na^+ 150, HCO_3^- 30, Cl^- 120	4.20 (0.65)		0.73 (0.12)				
Isotonic Glucose-Saline: Glucose 56, and initially Na^+ and Cl^- 120	11.10 (1.1)		1.00 (0.12)				
Triple Lumen Tube							
Unbuffered Saline	0.90 (0.47)		0.20 (0.06)				
Ungassed Saline-Bicarbonate	2.67 (0.90)		0.42 (0.11)				
Buffered Saline: PO_4^{--} 24	- 1.67 (2.33)		- 0.31 (0.25)				
Gassed Saline: HCO_3^- contained 95% O_2 to 5% CO_2	3.73 (1.00)		0.63 (0.16)				
Perfusion Rate: 20 ml/min Segment: Jejunum, 30 cm Double and Triple Lumen Tubes							
All solutions contained PEG 1 g/L, pH 7. Solutions were infused at various rates. Those at 8 ml/min contained Mannitol to achieve isotonicity.							Modigliani and Bernier, 1971 Rest
Soln 1 contained (mM): Glucose 14, NaCl 60							
8 ml/min	- 3.22 (1.18)	0.26 (0.01)	- 0.68 (0.24)				
Soln 2 contained (mM): Glucose 33, NaCl 60							
8 ml/min	0.05 (0.96)	0.63 (0.04)	- 0.47 (0.23)				
Soln 3a contained (mM): Glucose 66, NaCl 60							
8 ml/min	2.45 (0.72)	1.13 (0.14)	- 0.29 (0.14)				
Soln 3b contained (mM): Glucose 66, NaCl 50, Mannitol 125							
10 ml/min	0.53 (0.96)	1.10 (0.11)	- 0.45 (0.11)				
15 ml/min	0.67 (1.54)	1.4 (0.27)	- 0.52 (0.25)				
20 ml/min	0.67 (1.42)	1.73 (0.28)	- 0.67 (0.21)				
Soln 4a contained (mM): Glucose 133, NaCl 60							
8 ml/min	4.68 (3.12)	1.75 (0.45)	- 0.17 (0.25)				

Values are Means (SE)

Units: H_2O ($ml \cdot h^{-1} \cdot cm^{-1}$), Glucose ($mM \cdot h^{-1} \cdot cm^{-1}$), Na^+, K^+, Cl^-, HCO_3^- ($mEq \cdot h^{-1} \cdot cm^{-1}$).

Positive sign (+) signifies absorption, negative sign (-) signifies secretion

TABLE 4-1. *(continued)*

Test Solution Intestinal Segment Technique	H_2O	Glucose	Na^+	K^+	Cl^-	HCO_3^-	Reference Rest/Exer
Soln 4b contained (mM): Glucose 133, NaCl 50, Mannitol 60							
10 ml/min	3.43 (1.08)	1.83 (0.31)	- 0.32 (0.09)				
15 ml/min	2.02 (2.33)	2.12 (0.63)	- 0.51 (0.21)				
20 ml/min	2.30 (1.90)	2.19 (0.39)	- 0.44 (0.22)				
Soln 5 contained (mM): Glucose 200, NaCl 50							
10 ml/min	1.75 (1.30)	2.02 (0.45)	- 0.37 (0.11)				
15 ml/min	0.79 (2.06)	2.33 (0.49)	- 0.58 (0.28)				
20 ml/min	0.79 (2.88)	2.62 (0.74)	- 0.62 (0.27)				
Soln 6 contained (mM): Glucose 260, NaCl 18							
8 ml/min	- 0.72	1.97 (0.63)	- 0.64				
10 ml/min	0.74 (1.34)	2.45 (0.39)	- 0.83 (0.26)				
15 ml/min	- 2.45 (1.80)	2.40 (0.62)	- 1.10 (0.35)				
20 ml/min	- 3.77 (1.73)	2.50 (0.63)	- 1.30 (0.35)				
Perfusion Rate: 8, 10, 15, or 20 ml/min (38°C) ***Segment: Jejunum, 25 cm*** ***Double Lumen Tube with Proximal Occlusive Balloon***							
All solutions were made isotonic with NaCl, and contained PEG 4 g/L. pH adjusted to 7.							Hellier et al., 1973 Rest
[Alanine] in mM:							
10	2.76 (1.12)						
20	3.97 (0.94)						
50	7.30 (1.02)						
Perfusion Rate: 15 ml/min ***Segment: Jejunum, 30 cm*** ***Modified Double Lumen Tube with Proximal Occlusive Balloon***							
Solutions were isotonic and contained PEG 4000, 5 g/L.							Hicks and Turnberg, 1973 Rest
Study 1 (mM)							
Control: NaCl 95, $NaHCO_3$ 45, KCl 5	4.54 (0.88)		0.61 (0.15)	0.03 (0.01)	0.32 (0.08)	0.31 (0.07)	
Study 2 (mM)							
Control: NaCl 95, $NaHCO_3$ 45, KCl 5	4.76 (1.17)		0.55 (0.01)	0.03 (0.01)	0.28 (0.10)	0.29 (0.05)	

Values are Means (SE)

Units: H_2O ($ml \cdot h^{-1} \cdot cm^{-1}$), Glucose ($mM \cdot h^{-1} \cdot cm^{-1}$), Na^+, K^+, Cl^-, HCO_3^- ($mEq \cdot h^{-1} \cdot cm^{-1}$).

Positive sign (+) signifies absorption, negative sign (-) signifies secretion

TABLE 4-1. *(continued)*

Test Solution Intestinal Segment Technique	H_2O	Glucose	Na^+	K^+	Cl^-	HCO_3^-	Reference Rest/Exer
	Intestinal Absorption						
Study 3 (mM)							
Control: NaCl 105, $NaHCO_3$ 35, KCl 5	1.64		0.19	0.01	- 0.02	0.26	
	(0.70)		(0.11)	(0.01)	(0.10)	(0.02)	
Control: NaCl 80, $NaHCO_3$ 60, KCl 5	3.40		0.46	0.02	0.13	0.33	
	(0.29)		(0.04)	(0.02)	(0.03)	(0.02)	
Study 4 (mM)							
Control: NaCl 95, $NaHCO_3$ 45, KCl 5	3.37		0.40	0.20	0.21	0.22	
	(0.48)		(0.07)	(0.004)	(0.05)	(0.03)	
Study 5: (mM)							
Control: NaCl 95, $NaHCO_3$ 45, KCl 5	2.7		0.35	0.02	0.14	0.21	
	(0.45)		(0.07)	(0.003)	(0.05)	(0.02)	
Perfusion Rate: 11 ml/min							
segment: Proximal Jejunum, 30 cm							
Triple Lumen Tube							
The different test solutions were infused at apppropriate rates so that the mean flow rate and solute concentrations would be equal in the test segment, regardless of the rate of net water absorption or secretion with the various sugars and electrolytes		**Net Sugar Abs.**					Fordtran, 1975 Rest
Study 1: Each solution contained (mM) NaCl 80 and either:							
Mannitol 130	- 2.40	0.02	- 0.37				
	(0.65)	(0.10)	(0.05)				
Glucose 130	7.15	1.75	0.21				
	(1.00)	(0.15)	(0.05)				
Fructose 130	3.40	0.95	- 0.05				
	(0.30)	(0.05)	(0.05)				
Study 2: Each solution contained (mM) NaCl 80 and either:							
Mannitol 130	- 2.50	—	- 0.42				
	(0.45)		(0.05)				
Glucose 65, Mannitol 65	4.85	1.20	0.10				
	(0.45)	(0.11)	(0.05)				
Fructose 130	3.05	1.05	- 0.10				
	(0.40)	(0.05)	(0.05)				
Study 3: Each solution contained (mM) NaCl 120 and either:							
Mannitol 40	- 0.20	—	- 0.04	- 0.05			
	(0.55)		(0.05)	(0.07)			
Glucose 30, Mannitol 10	4.40	0.34	0.45	0.46			
	(0.90)	(0.05)	(0.10)	(0.10)			
Fructose 40	4.40	0.36	0.41	0.40			
	(0.95)	(0.05)	(0.10)	(0.07)			
Study 4: Each solution contained (mM) NaCl 80, HCO_3^- 70, and either:							
Mannitol		—				0.45	
						(0.05)	
Glucose 65		0.85				0.53	
		(0.07)				(0.05)	

Values are Means (SE)

Units: H_2O ($ml \cdot h^{-1} \cdot cm^{-1}$), Glucose ($mM \cdot h^{-1} \cdot cm^{-1}$), Na^+, K^+, Cl^-, HCO_3^- ($mEq \cdot h^{-1} \cdot cm^{-1}$).

Positive sign (+) signifies absorption, negative sign (-) signifies secretion

TABLE 4-1. *(continued)*

Test Solution Intestinal Segment Technique	H_2O	Glucose	Na^+	K^+	Cl^-	HCO_3^-	Reference Rest/Exer
Fructose 130		1.05 (0.13)				0.56 (0.08)	
Study 5: Each solution contained (mM) NaCl 80, HCO_3^- 40, and either:							
Mannitol		—				0.24 (0.04)	
Glucose 65		0.90 (0.05)				0.30 (0.05)	
Fructose 130		1.05 (0.10)				0.29 (0.05)	
Study 6: This was a study of the absorptive effect of the major anion, in (mM), in the test solution. [Na^+] [Glucose] Anion							
80 65 SO_4^{--}	0.80 (0.35)		- 0.50 (0.03)				
80 65 HCO_3^-	3.20 (0.35)		- 0.10 (0.05)				
80 65 HCO_3^-/Cl^-	3.60 (0.60)		0.00 (0.07)				
80 65 Cl^-	4.85 (0.45)		0.10 (0.05)				
80 130 Cl^-	7.15 (1.00)		0.20 (0.08)				
120 30 Cl^-	4.40 (0.90)		0.45 (0.09)				
Perfusion Rate: 10-15 ml/min ***Segment: Jejunum, 20 cm*** ***Triple Lumen Tube***							
In mM: NaCl 90, K^+ 5, $NaHCO_3$ 45, Glucose 10, Xylose 10, Osmolality 280 mOsm/kg, pH 8.1, PEG 4000, 5 g/L, ^{51}Cr-EDTA 15 μCi/L, $^{22}Na^+$ 2 μCi/L, $^{42}K^+$ 3 μCi/L, $^{36}Cl^-$ 5 μCi/L.	1.85 (0.31)		2.98 (0.48)	0.09 (0.01)	0.74 (0.31)	2.04 (0.29)	Oddsson et al., 1977 Rest
Perfusion Rate: 10 ml/min (37 °C) ***Segment: Jejunum, 25 cm*** ***Modified Four Lumen Tube with Proximal Occlusive Balloon***							
In mM: Na^+ 135, K^+ 5, Cl^- 110, HCO_3^- 30, PEG 5 g/L and 1 μCi/L each of tritiated water and [^{14}C] urea for assessment of mucosal permeability.							Guenter and Fordtran, 1980 Rest
Control	5.00 (0.96)		0.62 (0.10)	0.03 (0.003)	0.43 (0.12)	0.21 (0.03)	
Control	4.10 (0.70)		0.52 (0.09)	0.03 (0.003)	0.26 (0.10)	0.23 (0.01)	
Control	5.10 (1.10)		0.74 (0.11)	0.05 (0.01)	0.50 (0.10)	0.19 (0.03)	
Control	4.60 (0.40)		0.60 (0.06)	0.03 (0.003)	0.43 (0.05)	0.19 (0.05)	
Control	4.50 (0.83)		0.57 (0.12)	0.03 (0.004)	0.35 (0.10)	0.26 (0.04)	

Values are Means (SE)

Units: H_2O ($ml \cdot h^{-1} \cdot cm^{-1}$), Glucose ($mM \cdot h^{-1} \cdot cm^{-1}$), Na^+, K^+, Cl^-, HCO_3^- ($mEq \cdot h^{-1} \cdot cm^{-1}$).

Positive sign (+) signifies absorption, negative sign (-) signifies secretion

TABLE 4-1. *(continued)*

Test Solution Intestinal Segment Technique	H_2O	Glucose	Na^+	K^+	Cl^-	HCO_3^-	Reference Rest/Exer
Control	3.80 (0.67)		0.52 (0.13)	0.03 (0.004)	0.28 (0.10)	0.25 (0.03)	
Perfusion Rate: 11 ***Segment: Jejunum, 30 cm*** ***Triple Lumen Tube***							
Soln 1: 140 mM Glucose		2.63 (0.51)	0.16 (0.05)				Jones et al., 1980 Rest
Soln 2: 70 mM Maltose		3.40 (0.49)	1.13 (0.17)				
Soln 3: 21 mM Polymer		2.54 (0.26)	1.78 (0.59)				
Perfusion Rate: ? ***Segment: Jejunum, 25 cm*** ***Double Lumen Tube with Proximal Occlusive Balloon***							
Group 1: All solutions were isotonic and contained (mM): KCl 5, $NaHCO_3$ 5, Arabinose 14, PEG 4000, 5 g/L with [^{14}C] PEG 5 µCi/L.							Brown and Ammon, 1981 Rest
Glucose 0 mM, NaCl 129 mM	2.60 (0.72)	—	0.38 (0.11)	0.02 (0.003)	0.34 (0.11)		
Glucose 14 mM, NaCl 120 mM	3.36 (0.50)	0.26 (0.01)	0.38 (0.09)	0.01 (0.004)	0.35 (0.07)		
Glucose 56 mM, NaCl 97 mM	6.70 (1.00)	0.87 (0.05)	0.48 (0.13)	0.01 (0.01)	0.42 (0.13)		
Group 2: In mM: NaCl 97, KCl 5, $NaHCO_3$ 5, Arabinose 14, and PEG 4000, 5 g/L with [^{14}C] PEG 5 µCi/L.							
Glucose 0 mM, Mannitol 56 mM	- 0.48 (0.24)	—	- 0.24 (0.05)	0.01 (0.001)	- 0.28 (0.06)		
Glucose 14 mM, Mannitol 42 mM	1.70 (0.24)	0.25 (0.07)	- 0.04 (0.03)	0.01 (0.002)	- 0.09 (0.04)		
Glucose 56 mM, Mannitol 0 mM	7.00 (0.48)	0.88 (0.07)	0.46 (0.06)	0.01 (0.004)	0.41 (0.05)		
Perfusion Rate: 9.6 ml/min (37°C) ***Segment: Jejunum, 25 cm*** ***Four Lumen Tube with Proximal Occlusive Balloon***							
All solutions contained PEG as a marker.							Sandle et al., 1982 Rest
Normal Saline: 154 mM	2.31 (2.52)		0.54 (0.36)				
Galactose-Saline: Galactose 56 mM, NaCl 122 mM	9.33 (2.01)		0.99 (0.30)				
Alanine-Saline: Alanine 56 mM, NaCl 122 mM	7.53 (2.97)		0.75 (0.33)				
Glucose-Saline **	7.56 (3.18)		0.69 (0.36)				
** Results from an earlier study by Sandle, G I et al., Scand J Gastroenterol 16:667-671, 1981.							

Values are Means (SE)

Units: H_2O ($ml \cdot h^{-1} \cdot cm^{-1}$), Glucose ($mM \cdot h^{-1} \cdot cm^{-1}$), Na^+, K^+, Cl^-, HCO_3^- ($mEq \cdot h^{-1} \cdot cm^{-1}$).

Positive sign (+) signifies absorption, negative sign (-) signifies secretion

TABLE 4-1. *(continued)*

Test Solution / Intestinal Segment / Technique	Intestinal Absorption: H_2O	Glucose	Na^+	K^+	Cl^-	HCO_3^-	Reference Rest/Exer
Perfusion Rate: 15 ml/min (37°C) ***Segment: Proximal Jejunum, 20 cm*** ***Double Lumen Tube***							
All test solutions contained PEG 4000, 5 g/L and 1 µCi/L of [^{14}C] PEG. **Bicarbonate-Saline** (mM): Na^+ 150, K^+ 5, Cl^- 130, HCO_3^- 25, pH 8.3, Osmolality 290 mOsm/kg. Solution was tested twice.							Spiller et al., 1984 Rest
1st Perfusion	2.24 (1.08)		0.50 (0.19)		0.28 (0.13)	0.29 (0.07)	
2nd Perfusion	1.82 (0.70)		0.42 (0.14)		0.18 (0.06)	0.25 (0.64)	
Lactose-Saline (mM): Lactose 15, NaCl 150	2.38 (0.83)		0.46 (0.12)				
Mannitol-Saline (mM): Mannitol 15, NaCl 145	- 0.07 (0.12)		0.15 (0.04)				
Perfusion Rate: 15 ml/min ***Segment: Jejunum, 25 cm*** ***Modified Double Lumen Tube with Proximal Occlusive Balloon***							
In mM: Na^+ 136, Cl^- 105, K^+ 5, SO_4^{--} 18, PEG 5 g/L, [^{14}C] PEG 0.5 µCi/L.	1.37 (0.29)		0.09 (0.04)	0.01 (0.002)	0.09 (0.04)		Barclay and Turnberg, 1986 Rest
Perfusion Rate: 10 ml/min ***Segment: Jejunum, 30 cm*** ***Triple Lumen Tube***							
Diorylate, a Glucose/electrolyte solution was perfused twice. It contained (mM): Glucose 222, NaCl 17.24, $NaHCO_3$ 18.52, KCl 20.27.							Leiper and Maughan, 1986 Rest
1st Perfusion	8.30 (1.07)						
2nd Perfusion	8.00 (1.01)						
Perfusion Rate: 10 ml/min (37°C) ***Segment: Jejunum, 30 cm*** ***Triple Lumen Tube***							
In mM:							Rolston et al., 1986 Rest
Saline: Na^+ 158, Cl^- 158	1.12 (0.56)		0.42 (0.10)				
Acetate (5mM): Na^+ 158, Cl^- 158	1.37 (0.47)		0.27 (0.12)				
Acetate (50 mM): Na^+ 168, Cl^- 118	3.69 (0.71)		0.83 (0.07)				
Saline: Na^+ 158, Cl^- 158	0.06 (0.54)		0.21 (0.12)				
Citrate (5 mM): Na^+ 155, Cl^- 150	2.04 (0.58)		0.61 (0.11)				
Citrate (50 mM): Na^+ 224, Cl^- 78	0.21 (0.43)		0.40 (0.13)				

Values are Means (SE)

Units: H_2O (ml•h^{-1}•cm^{-1}), Glucose (mM•h^{-1}•cm^{-1}), Na^+, K^+, Cl^-, HCO_3^- (mEq•h^{-1}•cm^{-1}).

Positive sign (+) signifies absorption, negative sign (-) signifies secretion

TABLE 4-1. *(continued)*

Test Solution Intestinal Segment Technique	Intestinal Absorption H_2O	Glucose	Na^+	K^+	Cl^-	HCO_3^-	Reference Rest/Exer
Perfusion Rate: 12 ml/min ***Segment: Jejunum, 30 cm*** ***Double Lumen Tube with Proximal Occlusive Balloon***							
In mM: NaCl 106, $NaHCO_3$ 25, KCl 4, Glucose 30, PEG 4000, 2 g/L.							Sjovall et al., 1986 Rest
Control	5.47 (0.83)		0.58 (0.15)		0.43 (0.10)		
Control	5.93 (0.60)		0.74 (0.12)		0.50 (0.10)		
Control	6.33 (1.17)		0.72 (0.13)		0.53 (0.13)		
Control	3.23 (1.00)	0.21 (0.03)					
Control	2.13 (1.10)	0.16 (0.03)					
Perfusion Rate: 12 ml/min ***Segment: Jejunum, 30 cm*** ***Triple Lumen Tube***							
All solutions contained PEG at 5 g/L. Components of each solution were (mM):							Wheeler and Banwell, 1986 Rest
Soln 1: Plain Distilled Water	10.15 (1.05)		0.10 (0.09)	0.02 (0.003)	0.04 (0.14)		
Soln 2: Glucose-Fructose Polymer (5% polymerized Glucose, 2% Fructose, Na^+ 10, K^+ 5, Cl^- 10, Mg^{++} 1.2, Ca^{++} 3.2, Osmolality 240 mOsm/kg)	9.12 (1.26)		0.04 (0.08)	0.03 (0.02)	- 0.13 (0.05)		
Soln 3: Glucose-Fructose-Sucrose Polymer (3.6% polymerized Glucose, 1.8% Fructose, 1.6% Sucrose, Na^+ 10, K^+ 5, Cl^- 10, Mg^{++} 1.2, Ca^{++} 3.2, Osmolality 260 mOsm/kg)	7.35 (0.79)		- 0.01 (0.09)	0.04 (0.01)	- 0.21 (0.11)		
Perfusion Rate: 9-11 ml/min ***segment: Jejunum, 30 cm*** ***Triple Lumen Tube***							
In mM: Na^+ 140, K^+ 5, Cl^- 110, HCO_3^- 35, PEG 3 g/L.	3.5 (0.37)		0.44 (0.06)	0.02 (0.01)	0.14 (0.14)	0.28 (0.01)	Dueno et al., 1987 Rest
Perfusion Rate: 15 ml/min ***Segment: Jejunum, 30 cm*** ***Triple Lumen Tube***							

Values are Means (SE)

Units: H_2O ($ml \cdot h^{-1} \cdot cm^{-1}$), Glucose ($mM \cdot h^{-1} \cdot cm^{-1}$), Na^+, K^+, Cl^-, HCO_3^- ($mEq \cdot h^{-1} \cdot cm^{-1}$).

Positive sign (+) signifies absorption, negative sign (-) signifies secretion

TABLE 4-1. *(continued)*

Test Solution Intestinal Segment Technique	Intestinal Absorption H_2O	Glucose	Na^+	K^+	Cl^-	HCO_3^-	Reference Rest/Exer
Modified Tyrone's solution (mM): NaCl 8.0, KCl 0.2, $NaHCO_3$ 1.0, Glucose 3.0, 10 ml of Ethanol/L, PEG 4000, 5 g/L and [^{14}C] PEG 0.25 µCi/L. ***Perfusion Rate: 10 ml/min*** ***Segment: Upper Jejunum, 30 cm*** ***Five Lumen Tube with Occlusive Balloon***	0.57 (0.02)	0.28 (0.01)	0.70 (0.16)				Ewe, 1987 Rest
All substrates were perfused at a concentration yielding 140 mM monosaccharide on complete hydrolysis. Isotonic-isocaloric sugar saline solutions (285-295 mOsm/kg) were infused. Each solution contained PEG 4000, 5 g/L and [^{14}C] PEG 1 µCi/L							Jones et al., 1987 Rest
Maltotriose Soln: 47 mM (Total Glucose 144±2 mM, Na^+ 134±1 mM)		3.40 (0.4)					
Glucose Soln: 140 mM (Total Glucose 139±2 mM, Na^+ 81±2 mM)		2.32 (0.32)					
Oligomer Soln: (Total Glucose 141±2 mM, Na^+ 141±2 mM)		3.04 (0.20)					
Sucrose Soln: 70 mM (Glucose 0 mM, Fructose 0 mM, Total monosaccharide 142±1 mM, Na^+ 111±1 mM)		1.92 (0.32)					
Glucose 70 mM & Fructose 70 mM Soln: (Glucose 70±1 mM, Fructose 69±1 mM, Total monosaccharide 140±2 mM, Na^+ 72±2 mM) ***Perfusion Rate: 20 ml/min*** ***Segment: Proximal Jejunum, 25 cm*** ***Double Lumen Tube with Proximal Occlusive Balloon***		2.12 (0.20)					
Three solutions were tested (mM):							Spiller et al., 1987 Rest
Soln 1: Glucose (free Glucose 254, Na^+ 16.2)	5.41 (1.14)	3.93 (0.50)	- 0.82 (0.06)				
Soln 2: Ensure (free Glucose 17.7, Sucrose 82.2, free Fructose 2.7, whole protein 26 g/L, unhydrolysed triglyceride 23.6 g/L, Na^+ 26.5, K^+ 25.7)	4.74 (0.65)	4.90 (0.55)	- 0.88 (0.04)				
Soln 3: NaCl 153 ***Perfusion Rate: 20 ml/min*** ***Segment: Jejunum, 25 cm*** ***Double Lumen Tube with Proximal Occlusive Balloon***	0.77 (0.47)	—	0.34 (0.07)				
In mM: Na^+ 136, Cl^- 105, K^+ 5, SO_4^{--} 18, PEG 4000, 5 g/L and [^{14}C] PEG of 0.5 µCi/L. ***Perfusion Rate: 10 ml/min*** ***Segment: Jejunum, 30 cm*** ***Triple Lumen Tube***	1.40 (0.20)		0.10 (0.03)	0.01 (0.001)	0.09 (0.03)		Barclay and Turnberg, 1988 Rest

Values are Means (SE)

Units: H_2O ($ml \cdot h^{-1} \cdot cm^{-1}$), Glucose ($mM \cdot h^{-1} \cdot cm^{-1}$), Na^+, K^+, Cl^-, HCO_3^- ($mEq \cdot h^{-1} \cdot cm^{-1}$).

Positive sign (+) signifies absorption, negative sign (-) signifies secretion

TABLE 4-1. *(continued)*

Test Solution Intestinal Segment Technique	Intestinal Absorption H_2O	Glucose	Na^+	K^+	Cl^-	HCO_3^-	Reference Rest/Exer
In mM: Na^+ 136, Cl^- 105, K^+ 5, SO_4^{--} 18, PEG 4000, 5 g/L and [^{14}C] PEG of 0.5 μCi/L.							Barclay and Turnberg, 1988 Rest vs Exercise
Control	1.28		0.10	0.01	0.08		
	(0.16)		(0.02)	(0.001)	(0.001)		
Exercise	0.65		0.02	0.0004	0.01		
	(0.24)		(0.04)	(0.002)	(0.03)		
Recovery	0.95		0.07	0.01	0.07		
	(0.17)		(0.02)	(0.001)	(0.02)		
Perfusion Rate: 10 ml/min ***Segment: Jejunum, 30 cm*** ***Triple Lumen Tube***							
All solutions contained PEG 4000, 0.5 g/L. They were isotonic and contained (mM):							Leiper and Maughan, 1988 Rest
Soln 1: Na^+ 150, K^+ 0.2, Glucose 0, Cl^- 144, pH 6.2, Osmolality 297 mOsm/kg	1.40 (0.39)	—	0.16 (0.003)	0.02 (0.004)	0.22 (0.06)		
Soln 2: Na^+ 32, K^+ 18.9, Glucose 200, Cl^- 39, Base precursor (HCO_3^-) 18, pH 7.7, Osmolality 300 mOsm/kg	7.80 (1.19)	1.45 (0.18)	0.08 (0.06)	0.13 (0.02)	0.25 (0.08)		
Soln 3: Na^+ 37, K^+ 18.2, Glucose 198, Cl^- 39, Base precursor (Citrate as citric acid 6 mM and Sodium citrate 12 mM) 17.5, pH 5.2, Osmolality 307 mOsm/kg	8.40 (0.96)	1.68 (0.16)	0.35 (0.07)	0.12 (0.01)	0.27 (0.06)		
Soln 4: Na^+ 31, K^+ 19.1, Glucose 203, Cl^- 37, Base precursor (Citrate as citric acid 12 mM and Sodium citrate 6 mM) 17.4, pH 4, Osmolality 307 mOsm/kg	6.20 (0.65)	1.20 (0.21)	0.12 (0.07)	0.11 (0.01)	0.16 (0.07)		
Soln 5: Na^+ 33, K^+ 19.2, Glucose 199, Cl^- 40, Base precursor (Acetate) 17.6, pH 7.1, Osmolality 309 mOsm/kg	7.70 (0.98)	1.31 (0.24)	0.45 (0.14)	0.09 (0.01)	0.40 (0.16)		
Soln 6: Na^+ 33, K^+ 19.1, Glucose 200, Cl^- 38, Base precursor (Lactate) 18, pH 7.3, Osmolality 305 mOsm/kg	10.4 (1.63)	1.63 (0.48)	0.54 (0.15)	0.12 (0.02)	0.57 (0.21)		
(Note- Bicarbonate concentration was not measured, but was calculated to be 18 mM in solution B and to be negligible in the other solutions.) ***Perfusion Rate: 10 ml/min (37°C)*** ***Segment: Jejunum, 30 cm*** ***Triple Lumen Tube***							

Values are Means (SE)

Units: H_2O (ml•h^{-1}•cm^{-1}), Glucose (mM•h^{-1}•cm^{-1}), Na^+, K^+, Cl^-, HCO_3^- (mEq•h^{-1}•cm^{-1}).

Positive sign (+) signifies absorption, negative sign (-) signifies secretion

TABLE 4-1. *(continued)*

Test Solution Intestinal Segment Technique	H_2O	Glucose	Na^+	K^+	Cl^-	HCO_3^-	Reference Rest/Exer
	Intestinal Absorption						
All solutions contained PEG, 1 g/L and D_2O (30 ppm/ml). the solutions contained (mM):							Gisolfi et al., 1989 Rest
Soln 1: Distilled Water (Na^+ 0, K^+ 0, Glucose 0, Osmolality 37 mOsm/kg)	9.40 (1.28)	—	- 0.07 (0.10)	0.004 (0.004)			
Soln 2: 10% Dextrose (Glucose) solution (Na^+ 0, K^+ 0, Glucose 556, Osmolality 541 mOsm/kg)	- 4.40 (1.25)	2.50 (0.18)	- 1.20 (0.09)	- 0.10 (0.01)			
Soln 3: 6% Carbohydrate-Electrolyte solution (4% Sucrose, Na^+ 23.15, K^+ 2.3, Glucose 102, Osmolality 308 mOsm/kg)	13.30 (1.22)	0.93 (0.23)	0.64 (0.11)	0.06 (0.01)			
Perfusion Rate: 15 ml/min							
Segment: Duodenojejunum, 40 cm							
Triple Lumen Tube							

Values are Means (SE)

Units: H_2O ($ml \cdot h^{-1} \cdot cm^{-1}$), Glucose ($mM \cdot h^{-1} \cdot cm^{-1}$), Na^+, K^+, Cl^-, HCO_3^- ($mEq \cdot h^{-1} \cdot cm^{-1}$).

Positive sign (+) signifies absorption, negative sign (-) signifies secretion

remainder of this section will address the importance of Na^+ in intestinal absorption.

Water transport and fluid homeostatis are highly dependent upon the movement of Na^+. Figure 4-5 illustrates the different mechanisms involved. *Transcellular* Na^+ absorption is a two-step process (Figure 4-5A): entry across the apical brush border and exit across the basolateral membrane. Mechanistically, the only means of Na^+ extrusion from the cell interior is active transport via the Na^+/K^+ ATPase pump. Thus, the exit process is relatively simple. On the other hand, there are several mechanisms of *transcellular* Na^+ entry. These include electrochemical diffusion, cotransport (symport) or exchange (antiport) with another ion, and coupled transport with an organic nonelectrolyte (sugars, amino acids). Although these Na^+-entry processes have been studied in detail, their quantitative contributions to overall Na^+ transport in different segments of the intestine are not clear. In addition to these *transcellular pathways*, Na^+ also moves across the mucosa via the *paracellular shunt pathway* (Figure 4-5B). The shunt pathway and the transcellular Na^+ entry mechanisms of electrochemical diffusion, ionic cotransport/exchange, and amino acid cotransport will be discussed below; transcellular Na^+-coupled glucose transport is discussed in a subsequent section of this chapter. The rate of Na^+ absorption in the small intestine ranges from -2.71 to 2.976 $mEq{\cdot}h^{-1}{\cdot}cm^{-1}$ (Table 4-1).

1. **Diffusion** (Figure 4-5A): The amount of Na^+ entry by diffusion down an electrochemical gradient varies with intestinal segment. It is very high in the duodenojejunum and falls to an insignificant amount in the colon (Binder, 1988; Powell, 1987). Using isolated membrane vesicles, Gunther and Wright (1983) demonstrated that simple diffusion is the primary avenue for Na^+ transport in rabbit jejunum. Only the addition of three separate Na^+/amino acid cotransport systems quantitatively approached the magnitude of Na^+ transport by simple diffusion.

2. **Luminal solution drag** (Figure 4-5B): In carrier-mediated transport by the enterocyte, individual solute ions or molecules (i.e., substrates) from the luminal solution interact with the carrier protein integrated in the brush border membrane. Substrate ions or molecules cross the brush border on this carrier to enter the enterocyte, interact with the appropriate basolateral carrier, and then exit from the enterocyte. Substrates exiting near the tight junction provide the osmotic gradient required to cause bulk flow of luminal solution through the tight junction. The tight junctions are functionally closed in the absence of luminal nutrient. Madara and Pappenheimer (1987) postulate that nutrient in the form of glucose or amino acid causes the tight junctions to open by activating the cytoskeletal system of the enterocyte, which is connected to the cytoplasmic face of the tight junction. This permits bulk absorption of

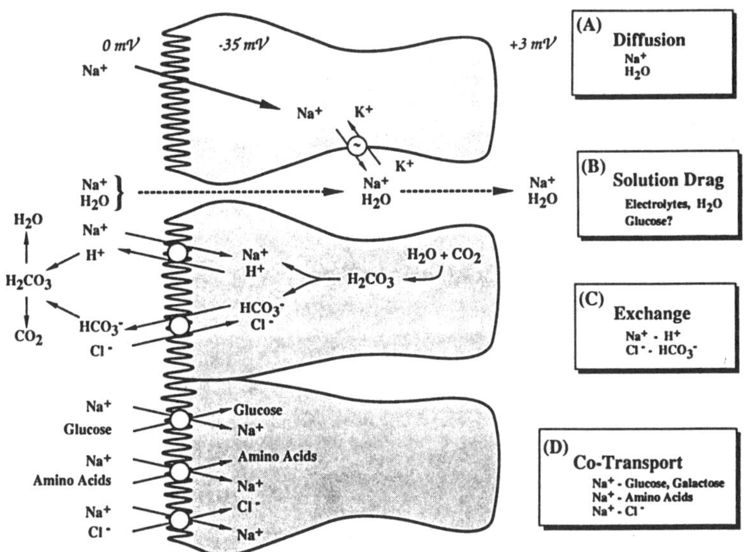

FIGURE 4-5. *Mechanisms of Na^+ transport in the small intestine.*

the luminal solution and provides the pathway for maximal absorption of substrate and water (Figure 4-6). Luminal glucose at concentrations well above that saturating the carrier is absorbed by the bulk flow of solutions. In the human jejunum, a significant portion of the glucose absorption is secondary to bulk flow of solution (Fordtran, 1975; Lewis & Fordtran, 1975; Fordtran el al., 1968; Saltzman et al., 1972; Brown & Ammon, 1981) (Figure 4-5B). Sodium-coupled glucose absorption and fructose absorption open the tight junctions.

The most compelling evidence in humans was provided by Fordtran (1975), who compared the effects of glucose, fructose, and mannitol on jejunal absorption of water, Na^+, K^+, and urea. Perfusion with mannitol provided a baseline for quantitating the effects of glucose and fructose on water and electrolyte movement; urea and K^+ served as markers for passive movement of uncharged and charged solutes, respectively. The difference between glucose and fructose absorption was used as a measure of active Na^+ absorption because fructose absorption is passive. Fructose is absorbed by carrier-mediated diffusion independent of active Na^+ transport. Figure 4-7 shows that 1 mM of fructose was almost as efficient as 1 mM of glucose in stimulating water, Na^+, and urea absorption compared with the effects of perfusing mannitol; however, to achieve these results, the perfusion solutions contained 130 mM fructose but only 65 mM glucose. Fructose and glucose had opposite effects on K^+, presumably because glucose increases the potential difference across the

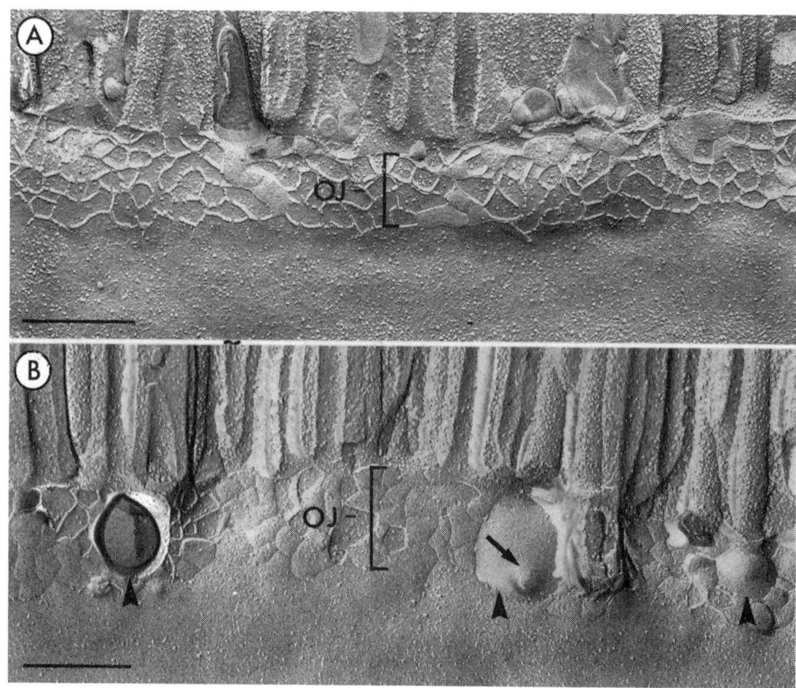

FIGURE 4-6. *Freeze-fracture electron micrographs of absorptive cell occluding junctions (OJ). (A) After perfusion in the absence of substrate, junctions consists of a net-like array of strands and/or grooves. (B) In contrast, perfusion with glucose elicits focal dilatations of interstrand compartments (arrowheads) which often have concave surfaces and which correspond to the intrajunctional dilatations seen in thin sections. Some dilatations display a secondary prominent protuberance on their fracture faces (arrow). Such dilated interstrand coompartments also distort the anatomy of the junction. For example, at sites where large dilatations exist, only two junctional strands separate the luminal from the paracellular space, whereas in the glucose-free preparation several junctional strands are always encountered separating these two compartments. Presumably this is the structural manifestation of the increased permeability to hydrophilic solutes and the decreased junctional resistance induced by glucose (Madara & Pappenheimer, 1987).*

mucosal cell due to the electrogenic transport of Na^+ with glucose. This movement of Na^+ leaves the lumen negatively charged, causing K^+ secretion. These results provide strong evidence that 60–70% of glucose-stimulated Na^+ absorption in the human jejunum is secondary to solution drag. The fact that fructose stimulated urea and K^+ absorption further supports a passive linkage between fructose and Na^+ absorption.

3. Exchange and Co-Transport Processes (Figure 4-5C and 4-5D): In the absence of sugars and amino acids, the most important step in NaCl absorption is the coupled transport of Na^+ and Cl^- across the brush border membrane (Figure 4-5D). This is an electroneutral process, and in the human ileum there is good evidence that the mechanism involved is the simultaneous exchange of Na^+ for H^+ and Cl^- for HCO_3^- (Turnberg et al., 1970a). This simultaneous exchange process is also thought to be the

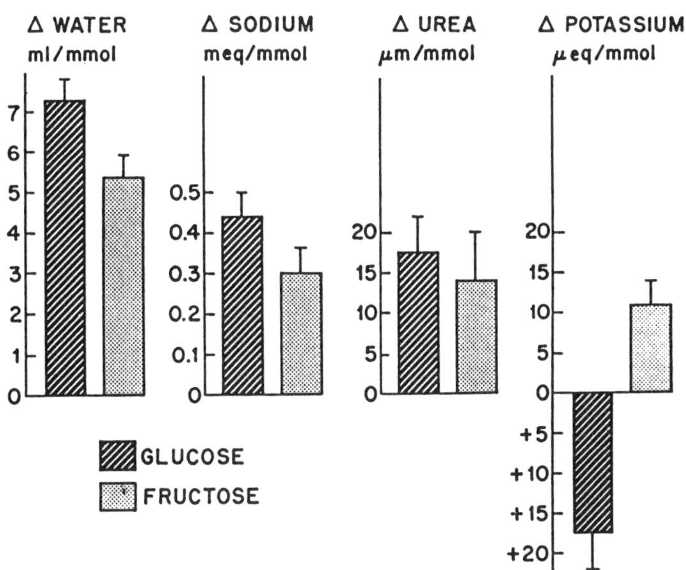

FIGURE 4-7. *Net transport of water, Na^+, urea, and K^+ per mM of glucose and fructose absorbed from the human jejunum. Baseline values represent water and solute movement with mannitol. Plus signs indicate net secretion (From Fordtran, 1975).*

mechanism responsible for HCO_3^- stimulated Na^+ absorption in the human jejunum (Turnberg et al., 1970b). Although the simultaneous exchange process seems to be the favored model, at least in humans, there is evidence to support Na^+/Cl^- (Figure 4-5D) and $Na^+/K^+/2Cl^-$ symport models (Armstrong, 1987).

4. Amino Acid-Stimulated Na^+ Transport: In addition to glucose-stimulated Na^+ transport, amino acids also stimulate Na^+ transport in mammalian species (Schultz & Curran, 1970) (Figure 4-5D). Using rabbit jejunal brush border vesicles as a model system, Stevens et al. (1982) demonstrated multiple transport pathways for neutral amino acids with a 1:1 Na^+/amino acid stoichiometry. Moreover, Patra et al. (1982b) found that a suspension of "pop-rice powder" (50 g/L) in an electrolyte (90 mM Na^+, 20 mM K^+, 80 mM Cl^-, 30 mM HCO_3^-) solution significantly reduced stool output, the duration of diarrhea, and intake of rehydration fluid compared with a 111-mM glucose solution with the same electrolyte concentrations. The protein content of "pop-rice" was 87 g/kg, and upon *in vitro* acid hydrolysis it librated 700 g/kg of glucose. Thus, the potential water absorption that would result from combining glucose and amino acids in the same rehydration solution is substantial and should be explored.

B. Potassium

Total body K^+ of a normal 70-kg man is approximately 3460 mEq (48 mEq/kg) (Shoemaker & Walker, 1974). Only 1–2% of this total resides in ECF; the remainder (98%) is intracellular. The intracellular concentration is about 140 mEq/L of intracellular water. Plasma $[K^+]$ is 3.8 to 5.0 mEq/L, and sweat $[K^+]$ ranges from 1 to 15 mEq/L, with most values ranging from 5 to 10 mEq/L (Robinson & Robinson, 1954). During exercise, plasma $[K^+]$ rises because of glycogen breakdown and increased leakage from the cells. The questions of importance to the exercise scientist and sports physician are: 1) Is the loss of K^+ during exercise significant?; 2) Should K^+ be replaced during exercise and if so, how much should be added to a fluid replacement beverage?; 3) How does K^+ affect beverage palatability?; and 4) How important is K^+ to the absorption of water and other nutrients?

Total body K^+ loss during exercise is generally not excessive (Costill, 1977), but could become significant during prolonged exercise in the heat (Knochel et al., 1972, Armstrong et al., 1985). Thus, some consideration might be given to adding K^+ to oral hydration beverages. Potassium depletion is a serious problem in diarrheal disease and requires K^+ supplementation. The symptoms of hypokalemia include disorientation, muscle weakness, hypoactive reflexes, S–T segment depression, and an inability to concentrate an acid urine (Vanatta & Fogelman, 1976). The effect of $[K^+]$ on beverage palatability is discussed elsewhere in this volume. An amount of K^+ recommended for inclusion in a fluid replacement beverage during prolonged exercise is given later in this chapter.

Intestinal mucosal cells are similar to other body cells in exhibiting a high intracellular $[K^+]$. Potassium moves down its electrochemical gradient across the basolateral membrane and apical brush border membrane (Armstrong, 1987), but it does not play a major role in the absorption of other nutrients. In the small bowel, K^+ movement is generally considered to be passive and ranges from −0.12 to 0.219 $mEq \cdot h^{-1} \cdot cm^{-1}$ (Table 4-1). In the duodenojejunum it follows changes in water movement, whereas in the ileum it follows changes in the potential difference (Binder, 1988; Powell, 1987). In the colon, there is considerable evidence that both active K^+ secretion and active K^+ absorption occur, at least in animal models.

C. Anion Transport

The major anion included in a perfusion solution can have a significant effect on water and salt absorption. Fordtran (1975) maintained Na^+ and glucose concentrations constant at 80 mEq/L and 65 mM, respectively, and varied anion composition of test solutions. Maximal water and Na^+ absorption were observed with Cl^- as the anion, followed by HCO_3^- and then SO_4^{-2} (Table 4–1). Combining Cl^- and HCO_3^- was not as effective as Cl^- alone. The organic anions, acetate (50 mM) and citrate (5 mM) have also been shown to stimulate water and Na^+ absorption in human jejunum by investigators using the double-lumen technique with a proximal occluding balloon (Table 4-1, Rolston et al., 1986). The osmolality of these solutions was adjusted to 290 mOsm/kg with NaCl, and the pH was adjusted to 6.8 with NaOH. The Na^+ and Cl^- contents of the acetate solution were 168 and 118 mEq/L, respectively. The Na^+ and Cl^- contents of the citrate solution were 155 and 150 mEq/L, respectively. A solution containing 80 mM acetate, 80 mEq/L Na^+, and 20 mEq/L K^+ with an osmolality of 300 mOsm/L was shown to significantly enhance water and Na^+ absorption in the jejunum of the anesthetized calf (Demigne et al., 1981).

CARBOHYDRATE ABSORPTION

A. Glucose

In 1958, Riklis and Quastel observed glucose-stimulated Na^+ absorption in the guinea pig small intestine, and in 1963, Schedl and Clifton reported a similar finding in humans. Today, this transport process is a firmly entrenched biological concept (Schultz & Curran, 1970). It occurs in the human jejunum, but not in the ileum (Fordtran et al., 1968), or in the colon (Binder & Sandle, 1987). Two mechanisms have been offered to explain this transport process: a) the "Na^+ gradient hypothesis" of Crane (1962), and b) solvent drag, i.e., glucose absorption stimulates the bulk flow of water, and Na^+ is transported passively. The latter process was described earlier under Na^+ transport mechanisms. According to the Na^+ gradient hypothesis, Na^+ and glucose form an obligatory ternary complex with a carrier molecule in the brush border membrane; Na^+ is transported down its electrochemical gradient, providing the energy for the uphill movement of glucose into the mucosal cell (Figure 4-5D). Active transport of Na^+ across the basolateral membrane via the Na^+/K^+ pump conserves the Na^+ gradient across the mucosal membrane. The "Na^+ gradient hypothesis" and solvent drag are not mutually exclusive mechanisms. In humans, solvent drag can account for 60 to 70% of Na^+ absorption in the jejunum (Fordtran, 1975).

What is the optimal amount of carbohydrate and Na^+ required to maximize water absorption? The addition of glucose to a perfusion solution can increase Na^+ absorption four-fold and water absorption six-fold, but the quantity of glucose required to achieve these increments is not clear. Sladen and Dawson (1969) employed a double-lumen tube and varied glucose concentrations from 1–5%, maintaining isotonicity (280 mOsm/kg) by the addition of NaCl. Their data showed a progressive increase in water absorption from 1.1 to 11.1 $mL \cdot hr^{-1} \cdot cm^{-1}$ for saline and 56-mM glucose solutions, respectively. Increasing glucose concentration to 140 mM did not further increase water absorption; however, increasing glucose concentration to 280 mM markedly reduced water absorption (3.3 mL·hr·$^{-1}$·cm^{-1}). The problem with this study is that it allowed Na^+ (Cl^-) levels to vary in order to maintain isotonicity. It also employed a double-lumen tube, which, as previously described, has several disadvantages. An ideal glucose/Na^+ ratio can not be determined from these data.

Modigliani and Bernier (1971) avoided the criticisms of using a double-lumen tube by including a proximal occluding balloon in their double-lumen perfusion studies. They infused solutions maintained isotonic (by addition of mannitol or reduction of NaCl at the highest glucose concentration) at 8 to 20 mL·min^{-1} with 50 to 60 mEq/L NaCl and 14 to 260 mM glucose. Water was secreted (−1.34 mL·min^{-1}) at the 14 mM-glucose concentration and increased to a maximum absorption of 1.95 mL·min^{-1} at a glucose concentration of 133 mM. At a glucose concentration of 200 mM, water absorption fell significantly, and at a glucose concentration of 260 mM, net water secretion occurred, but NaCl concentration in this solution was only 17 mEq/L. Thus, the optimal glucose/Na^+ ratio in this study was approximately 2:1. Malawer et al. (1965) systematically varied glucose/Na^+ ratios of isotonic solutions perfused through the jejunum and concluded that water absorption was directly proportional to net solute movement and was maximal with 140 mM glucose. The ratio of glucose to Na^+ absorbed depended upon the ratio of glucose to Na^+ perfused; however, a low initial [Na^+] ($<$90 mEq/L) in a perfusion solution can impair Na^+ and water absorption (Spiller et al., 1987).

Fordtran et al. (1968) studied the effect of glucose and galactose on Na^+ absorption in the human jejunum and ileum using the triple-lumen technique. They maintained [Na^+] in the test segment at approximately 110 mEq/L and varied net water flux. In another series of experiments they maintained [Na^+] of the test segment constant at 110 mEq/L and added 50 or 105 mM glucose to the perfusion solution. These concentrations yielded a glucose concentration in the test segment of 7.7 and 24.2 mM, respectively. In the ileum, Na^+ was absorbed independently of net water movement and against a concentration gradient of as much as 110 mEq/L. The addition of 90 mM glucose (which fell to only 22 mM in the test segment) to the perfusion solution had no effect on net sodium absorption or the osmotic gradient against which water absorption occurred. On the other hand, Na^+ absorption in the jejunum was a function of water movement. Sodium was secreted at zero water movement, absorbed against a concentration gradient when water was absorbed, and markedly secreted when net water movement was into the lumen. In contrast to the ileum, jejunal Na^+ absorption occurred against only a small (13 mEq/L) electrochemical gradient. In the human jejunum, glucose in the perfusion solution significantly enhances water and Na^+ absorption.

Spiller et al. (1987) studied the importance of intestinal Na^+ content to the absorption of different solutions containing salt, amino acids, and carbohydrate in the jejunum of human subjects using a multilumen tube with a proximal occlusive balloon. They found that perfusion solutions containing less than90 mEq/L Na^+ caused net Na^+ secretion. There was a linear relationship between net Na^+ absorption from amino acid and carbohydrate solutions and initial $[Na^+]$ of the perfusion solution. On the other hand, Saltzman et al. (1972) found that active glucose absorption was little affected by perfusing the human ileum with solutions containing a $[Na^+]$ as low as 2.5 mEq/L; however, Na^+ could be trapped in the negatively charged mucus gel adjacent to the apical membrane, making it impossible to reduce $[Na^+]$ below a given level (Smithson et al., 1981). This Na^+ could participate in glucose transport, but not be measurable. In the human jejunum, glucose absorption from perfusion solutions containing 6 mM glucose or less was reduced 50% from a Na^+ free solution. On the other hand, there was no inhibition of glucose absorption from solutions containing glucose in concentrations above those in the plasma.

In the rat duodenojejunum, Lifshitz and Wapnir (1984) found that a solution containing 111 mM glucose and 60 mEq/L Na^+ optimized both water and Na^+ absorption and concluded that the optimal molar glucose/-Na^+ ratio of an oral hydration solution was 2:1. Interestingly, intestinal fluid absorption is enhanced not only by the presence of glucose in luminal fluid, but also by elevating plasma glucose concentration (Lee, 1987).

B. Fructose

The mechanism of intestinal fructose absorption is controversial. In humans, it is slower than glucose and is thought to occur by energy-independent facilitated diffusion (Holdsworth & Dawson, 1965, Table 4-1). Absorption capacity of orally ingested fructose taken alone ranges from approximately 5 to 50 g, but when consumed in equal quantities with glucose or given as sucrose, absorption capacity is signficantly increased. The latter observation led Rumessen and Gudmand-Hoyer (1986) to suggest that glucose enhances fructose absorption in a dose-dependent fashion. This second mechanism of fructose absorption is thought to occur in addition to the transport of a saturating level of free fructose.

In the rat, fructose is absorbed by an active carrier-mediated mechanism (Gracey et al., 1972; Macrae & Neudoerffer, 1972), but infusing 60 mM sucrose with 120 mM NaCl and 20 mM KCl^- did not promote water or Na^+ absorption (Saunders & Sillery, 1985). The inhibitory influence of sucrose on water absorption has been observed in both animal and human studies (Fordtran, 1975; Newton et al., 1985; Patra et al., 1982a; Wheeler & Banwell, 1986).

C. Glucose Polymers

Wheeler and Banwell (1986) used a triple-lumen tube in human subjects to study jejunal absorption of water and minerals from solutions containing glucose polymers and fructose or glucose polymers, fructose, and sucrose. They found no differences in absorption and concluded that gastric emptying was the primary limiting factor in fluid replacement. They did not measure carbohydrate absorption. On the contrary, Jones et al. (1987) found that jejunal absorption of glucose from maltotriose and a glucose oligomer mixture (primarily maltotriose and maltohexose) exceeded that from isocaloric 140 mM glucose by 46% and 24%, respectively. They employed a double-lumen tube with a proximal occlusive balloon.

In the rat duodenojejunum, Saunders and Sillery (1985) found the greatest water absorption when a 10 mM solution of glucose polymers (equivalent to 56 mM glucose as glucose oligosaccharides) was added to 120 mM NaCl and 20 mM KCl^-. Thus, the optimal glucose/Na^+ molar ratio was approximately 1:2.

EFFECTS OF EXERCISE

Compared with the cardiorespiratory responses to exertion, little is known about the effects of exercise on gastrointestinal function. The release of catecholamines (Hartley et al., 1972a, 1972b) and endorphins (Sforzo, 1989) during exercise should theoretically enhance absorption (Powell et al., 1985), but the reduction in splanchnic blood flow (Rowell et al., 1964) may counter this effect. The effects of other circulating substances on gastrointestinal function are unknown. Numerous anecdotal accounts and some evidence indicates that overtraining and intense exercise can produce nausea, vomiting, cramps, diarrhea, and gastrointestinal bleeding (Brauns, 1987; Lorber, 1983), whereas mild exercise is frequently recommended to patients with constipation. Unfortunately, the relatively little research investigating gastrointestinal function during exercise has not been well controlled, the methods have sometimes been suspect, and the results have often been controversial. Gastric emptying has been studied most extensively and is reviewed by Costill in this volume.

A. Intestinal Absorption

Intestinal absorption during exercise has been the least studied GI process and, therefore, is the least understood. Williams et al. (1964) determined the effect of prolonged (4.5 h) treadmill exercise (3.0 mph) in a hot environment (38/27°C db/wb) on intestinal absorption of D-xylose and 3-0-methyl-D-glucose (3 MG). D-xylose is a passively absorbed carbohydrate, whereas 3 MG at the dose used in this study is an actively absorbed carbohydrate. Exercise in the heat had no effect on xylose absorption, but significantly reduced plasma levels of 3 MG for the first 2 h of exericse. These results indicate that mild exercise in the heat, sufficient to reduce splanchnic blood flow, had no effect on passive carbohydrate transport, but significantly reduced active carbohydrate transport.

Using the direct method of segmental perfusion with a triple-lumen catheter, Fordtran and Saltin (1967) found that 1 h of treadmill exercise at 64 to 78% $\dot{V}O_2$max had no consistent effect on jejunal or ileal absorption of water, Na^+, Cl^-, K^+, glucose, L-xylose, urea, or tritiated water. Although exerise has been shown to markedly reduce splanchnic blood flow (Rowell et al., 1964), Fordtran and Saltin (1967) concluded that severe exercise did not reduce intestinal blood flow enough to reduce the rate of either active or passive absorption. However, in this study of Fordtran and Saltin, five different solutions were perfused through the intestine, and most were perfused in only one or two subjects (Figure 4-8). Thus it is difficult to generalize about the effects of exercise on intestinal absorption from this investigation.

In a more recent study, Barclay and Turnberg (1988a) used the triple-lumen perfusion technique to evaluate the effects of cycle exercise at a pulse rate of 40 to 50% above mean resting heart rate (HR) on jejunal absorption of an electrolyte solution (Na^+, 136 mM; Cl^-, 105 mM; K^+, 5 mM; SO_4^{-2}, 18 mM). During exercise, HR increased from 68±4 bpm to 103±7 bpm, and absorption of water, Na^+, K^+, and Cl^- fell significantly (Table 4-1). They attributed this reduction in absorption to a "parasympathetic effect on mucosal transport."

In a study recently completed in our laboratory (Spranger et al., 1989), we used the triple-lumen technique to investigate the effects of 90 min of cycle exercise at 65% $\dot{V}O_2$max on duodenojejunal absorption of water and a carbohydrate-electrolyte (CE) solution. On separate occasions, we also determined the absorption of water and the CE solution during 1-h exercise bouts at 25, 50, and 70% $\dot{V}O_2$max. We found no effect of exercise intensity or duration on intestinal absorption of water; however, fluid absorption was significantly greater from the CE solution than from water.

The different results observed in the four studies that determined intestinal absorption during exercise may be attributed to differences in the mode of exercise, ambient temperature, method employed to measure absorption, segment of the intestine studied, or formulation of the test solution. Williams et al. (1964) utilized treadmill exercise in the heat and studied the entire bowel using an indirect method. This was unique because no other study employed heat or evaluated the entire bowel. Thus, the observed decline in absorption with treadmill exercise could have been influenced by posture, heat, or the fact that the entire bowel was being evaluated. The studies by Fordtran and Saltin (1967) and Spranger et al. (1989) were similar and arrived at the same conclusion, i.e., exercise does not influence intestinal absorption. These studies employed the triple-lumen technique and evaluated the absorption of carbohydrate-electrolyte solutions. They differed slightly in that Ford-

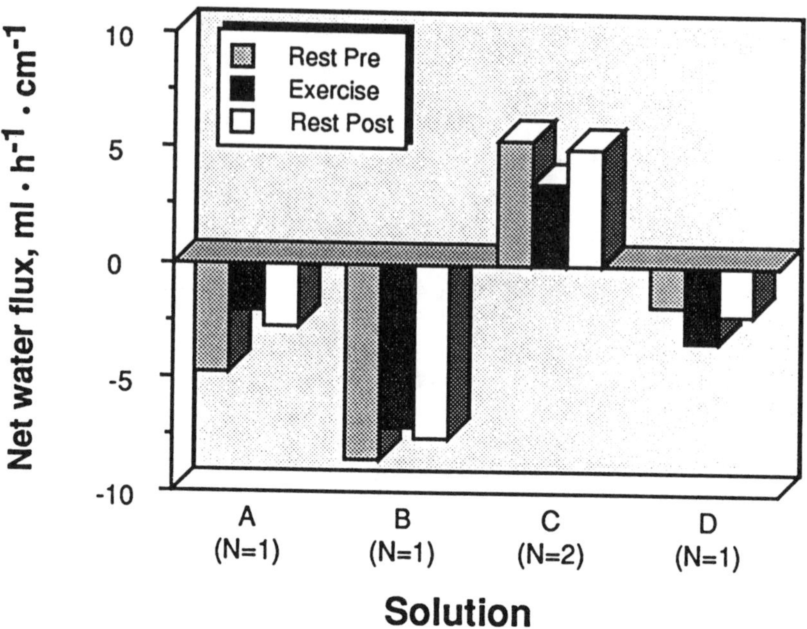

Solution Composition

	Electrolytes (mEq/l)			*Non-electrolytes (mM)*		
	Na^+	**Cl^-**	**HCO_3^-**	**Glucose**	**L-xylose**	**Urea**
A	110	50	60	55	10	10
B	95	45	50	90	10	10
	Na^+	**Cl^-**	**K^+**	**Glucose**	**L-xylose**	**Urea**
C	100	105	5	416	10	-
D	100	105	5	416	10	10

FIGURE 4-8. *Data redrawn from Fordtran and Saltin (1967) showing the effects of different glucose-electrolyte solutions on water absorption during rest, exercise, and recovery.*

tran and Saltin (1967) studied the jejunum, whereas Spranger et al. (1989) studied the duodenojejunum. The fact that absorption did not change in these studies could be attributed to the presence of glucose in the perfusion solutions. Glucose-enhanced absorption of Na^+ and water may have compensated for any decrease in absorption of water and electrolytes associated with exercise. Barclay and Turnberg (1988a) studied the jejunum and employed the triple-lumen technique during cycle exercise, but they perfused an electrolyte solution without carbohydrate. The decrease in absorption observed in their study may have been unmasked by omitting the stimulatory effect of glucose on water and salt absorption. The only data that do not fit this rationale are the absorption data obtained by Spranger et al. (1989) during the intestinal perfusion of water during light, moderate, and heavy exercise. Under all of these conditions, there was no effect of exercise compared with rest.

Other factors that can influence intestinal absorption during exercise include: a) changes in intestinal motility and transit; b) release of some humoral mediator; or c) a reduction in splanchnic blood flow secondary to increased sympathetic drive.

B. Motility and Absorption

Changes in transit and motility with exercise are controversial. In human subjects, Evans et al. (1984) used a pressure sensitive radiotelemetry capsule and reported that a tiring 12-mile walk in 4 h significantly reduced the number of Phase III activity fronts of the migrating motor complex in fasted (12 h overnight) subjects. Cammack et al. (1982), using the breath-hydrogen technique, reported that intermittent moderate (HR = 117 ± 1 bpm) exercise had no effect on small bowel transit of a solid meal. In contrast, Keeling and Martin (1987) reported a significant decrease in small bowel transit of a liquid meal using the breath-H_2 method. It must be recognized that changes in transit can be due to altered mucosal absorptive function and intraluminal fluid content as well as to altered motility.

Contractions of the bowel wall accomplish two functions—mixing and propulsion of intestinal contents. Different contractile patterns have the potential to modify intestinal absorption and secretion. Contractile activity of the gastrointestinal tract must be defined in terms of time (synchronomous vs. asynchronomous) and space (proximal vs. distal) when considering its effects on transit and mixing of intestinal or colonic contents (Summers & Dusdieker, 1981). Simple quantification of motor events does not predict or correlate with rates of transit (Scott & Summers, 1976; Ehrlein et al., 1985). In the colon, increased numbers of segmenting (non-propulsive) contractions occur in slow transmit constipation, whereas contractile activity may be nearly absent in diarrhea (Connell, 1968). The spatial orientation (pattern) of contractions is more important in determining flow of intestinal or colonic contents than simply quantifying the number or amplitude of the mechanical events occurring in those organs.

Mixing occurs as a result of contractions that propagate short distances or not at all; these waves create turbulent flow which increase and prolong exposure of intestinal contents to the absorbing mucosa and blend digestive secretions with ingested nutrients. Opiates cause this kind of contractile pattern, which partially explains why they enhance absorption and have an antidiarrheal effect. In certain disease states, reduced motor activity leads to statis, small bowel bacterial overgrowth, and malabsorption.

Propulsive motor patterns lead to rapid transit and decreased exposure of intestinal contents to the mucosal surface. They can also lead to reduced absorption of water, electrolytes, and nutrients. Certain highly propulsive contractile patterns have been associated with diarrhea; whether they actually cause diarrhea is unknown because in most situations, mucosal dysfunction is also present. Certain bacterial toxins and pharmacologic agents, such as ricinoleic acid, also induce a variety of diarrheogenic motor patterns, including migrating action potential complexes, repetitive bursts of action potentials, or ultrarapid rushes of single spike bursts (Mathias et al., 1976; Mathias et al., 1978; Burns et al., 1980; Van Trappen et al., 1986; Keeling et al., 1987). Thus it is likely that highly propulsive motor patterns can reduce the absorptive capacity of the bowel and contribute to the production of loose, watery stools and possibly crampy abdominal pain.

Extreme exercise can, in some instances, be associated with diarrhea; however, the mechanisms causing the liquid stools are unknown. The changes in small bowel absorption do not suggest that impaired mucosal function is responsible; this leaves changes in motor function as a possible cause. In fact, very little is known about the effects of exercise on motility. The only small-intestinal motility studies reported in intense exercise have been performed in dogs. In fed animals, Kenney et al. (1988) found that: a) a slow-wave frequency increased significantly during prolonged exercise, probably in association with a rise in core temperature; b) jejunal myoelectrical activity (spike-burst frequency and duration) was inhibited in recovery from exercise, even though it was unchanged or increased during exercise; and c) a migrating motor complex (MMC) took place occasionally during exercise. The latter observation essentially never occurs during the first 4 h following a meal of the size used in this study. These changes in myoelectric activity were not marked, and no highly propulsive motor activity was encountered. These changes in small bowel activity would not be expected to affect intestinal transit greatly; furthermore, the exercise did not produce diarrhea. No studies have monitored effects of exertion on colonic motor activity, and no motility studies have been published in exercising human subjects, involving either the small or large intestine. Therefore, it is currently unknown whether changes in motility patterns can explain exercise-induced symptoms. Such studies are needed to understand better the role of exercise in affecting either absorption or motility.

C. Effects of Reduced Plasma Volume

Exercise is associated with a contraction of the ECF compartment and a decrease in vascular volume. It is also associated with increased sympathetic activity, increased release of catecholamines, and stimulation of the renin-angiotensin system, all of which have been implicated in the control of intestinal hemodynamics and fluid/electrolyte transport. Convincing evidence from animal models indicates that catecholamines serve as absorptive neurotransmitters in the mammalian gut, whereas somatostatin, enkephalin, and angiotensin II serve as absorptive neuromodulators (Powell et al., 1985). Epinephrine and norepinephrine significantly enhance NaCl absorption and reduce HCO_3^- secretion in isolated rabbit ileum (Field & McColl, 1973). These effects are attributed to stimulation of alpha-adrenergic receptors because they are partially reversed by phentolamine, but not affected by propranolol. On the other hand, Morris and Turnberg (1981) demonstrated that intravenous isoproterenol significantly enhanced NaCl and water absorption in human jejunum and ileum. Intraveous propranolol reduced jejunal NaCl and K^+ absorption. In the ileum, propranolol reduced K^+ and Cl^- absorption and induced Na^+ and water secretion. These results provide evidence for beta-adrenergic control of intestinal transport in humans.

Splanchnic nerve stimulation at the preganglionic level has been shown to inhibit Cl^- secretion induced by cholera toxin (Cassuto et al., 1982) and to increase intestinal absorption of glucose solutions (Brunsson et al., 1979). This increase in absorption is not secondary to changes in blood flow (Sjovall et al., 1983). In fact, there is evidence for separate sympathetic regulation of fluid absorption and blood flow in the cat small bowel (Sjovall et al., 1984). The mechanism of noradrenergic stimulation of fluid absorption by rat jejunum is to open Ca^{+2} channels in the basolateral membrane of epithelial cells. The resulting Ca^{+2} influx stimulates ribosomal protein synthesis to produce proteins involved in fluid transport (Parsons et al., 1984). Adrenergic agonists in the intestines can be released reflexly by unloading either carotid sinus baroreceptors (Sjovall et al., 1982) or cardiac volume receptors (Sjovall et al., 1984).

The control of intestinal absorption by the renin-angiotensin system was recently reviewed by Levens (1985). All components of this system are located in the small intestine, and angiotensin II (AII) is produced in this tissue. At low plasma doses (<400 pg/mL), *in vivo* AII stimulates Na^+ and water absorption secondary to the release of norepinephrine from enteric sympathetic nerves. At high doses, AII inhibits absorption due to enteric prostaglandin production. The site of action of AII is unclear. It could enhance enteric sympathetic activity by exerting its influence centrally at sympathetic ganglia or at adrenergic nerve endings. It is also unclear whether enhanced absorption produced by endogenous AII is mediated by epithelial cells or by alterations in enteric hemodynamics. Although there is much to learn about the site and mechanism of actions of AII, this hormone plays a key role in controlling intestinal absorption under conditions of volume depletion. AII is a fluid retention hormone that contributes to the maintenance of ECF volume by stimulating thirst, aldosterone production, and ADH release (see chapters by Wade, Hubbard, and Armstrong). It also stimulates the absorption of Na^+ and water across epithelial tissues in a dose-dependent fashion (see Levens et al., 1981). Its contribution to fluid-electrolyte homeostasis in the gut is not yet known.

D. Blood Flow and Absorption

Exercise that elevates heart rate to 100 bpm can also reduce splanchnic blood flow by 30 to 35% (Rowell, 1964); however, the effects on intestinal blood flow are controversial. Some investigators show a decrease (Varro et al., 1965) and others show no effect (Brunsson et al., 1979).

Adequate mesenteric blood flow is critical to maintain mucosal structure, function, and viability. Reduced blood flow could interfere with intestinal secretion and absorption of nutrients, electrolytes, and water. If ischemia is severe enough, oxygen deprivation may cause tissue necrosis, serious morphological changes, and even more severe functional derangements. Pappenheimer (1987) demonstrated that ischemia antagonizes the absorptive effects of glucose.

Normally, absorption of nutrients is accompanied by intestinal hyperemia: not only is there an increase in total mesenteric flow in response to a meal, there is also a redistribution of flow from the muscular wall to the mucosa and submucosa. The increase in blood flow stimulated by intraluminal glucose is correlated with the rate of glucose-coupled water absorption (Norryd et al., 1975). An even closer correlation exists between oxygen uptake and intestinal absorption (Sit et al., 1980). Severe exertion can reduce mesenteric blood flow to as much as 80% of control levels (Quamer & Read, 1987; Clausen, 1977). When intestinal blood flow is reduced, movement of any passively absorbed substance from the interstitium into the blood is affected because of the changes in the concentration gradient between the interstitial fluid and vessels (Varro et al., 1965). Reduced oxygen supply from decreased blood flow and/or increased oxygen extraction may also affect the permeability characteristics of either the absorbing membrane or the capillaries of the villi. If a substance is highly diffusible (such as water), its absorption is highly dependent upon blood flow because the flowing blood carries away the substance and maintains a large concentration gradient. If blood flow is reduced greater than 50%, both glucose absorption and oxygen uptake within a segment fall linearly (Winne, 1984).Thus, glucose transport and probably other substances are affected by oxygen availability at low rates of blood flow. Further investigation is needed to explore the effects of severe exertion on the absorption of other substances. Also, because there is considerable reserve capacity of the intestine, it is unknown whether reduced segmental absorption has any significant effect on total absorption.

When blood flow and oxygen supply are reduced beyond some critical level, severe structural changes occur in the villi. The epithelium at the tips of the villi becomes detached from the basement membrane, and soon the upper portions of the villi become denuded (Robinson et al., 1981). If the process is even more severe, the entire mucosa will exhibit necrosis and diffuse inflammation accompanied by increased capillary permeability (Granger, 1980). The mechanisms of these changes are complex and multiple, but appear to include the action of proteolytic pancreatic enzymes (Bounos et al., 1970; Bounos, 1982), free radicals (Granger et al., 1981; Parks et al., 1982), and arachidonic acid metabolites (Bridenbaugh et al., 1976), as well as a number of other potential circulating substances.

It seems likely that under most exercise situations, intestinal blood flow and motility do not play a major role in altering absorption. However, under more extreme conditions, as may be experienced in a marathon or triathalon, the occurrence of certain gastrointestinal symptoms suggest more serious alterations in function. Abdominal cramps suggest abnormalities in motility or oxygen supply; diarrhea suggests abnormalities in absorption and secretion; and gastrointestinal bleeding suggests possible ischemic injury to the mucosa.

E. Exercise and Gastrointestinal Blood Studies

Over the past 10 years, numerous studies have reported that gastrointestinal bleeding is a rather common and sometimes serious complication of intense and prolonged exericse. In most situations, bleeding is occult and rather mild. Several studies have shown an increase in gastrointestinal blood loss after long-distance running with few or no serious consequences (Porter, 1983; McMahon et al., 1984; Stewart et al., 1984; Halvorsen et al., 1986; McCabe et al., 1986; Robertson et al., 1987; Selby et al., 1988). Others have documented the occurrence of iron-deficient anemia from GI blood loss in runners (Selby et al., 1988; Schoch et al., 1987; Cooper et al., 1987; Scobie, 1985; Fisher et al., 1986). There are numerous reports of hematemesis, melena, or hematachezia (Fogoros et al., 1980; Moses et al., 1988; Keeffe et al., 1984; Scobie, 1985; Fisher et al., 1986; Papaioannides et al., 1984; Cantwell, 1981; Schaub et al., 1985; Sullivan, 1987) which have occurred following running or bicycling. In one situation massive blood loss from gastritis resulted in death in a 28-year-old man following jogging (Thompson et al., 1980).

In some cases, the cause of the bleeding was identified endoscopically as erosive hemorrhagic gastritis or colitis, but in other cases no lesions were found. Similar mucosal lesions could be present in the small bowel, but adequate examination of this region has not been possible. Most clinicians suspect that acute ischemic injury is the etiology of the bleeding, and histologic examinations of biopsy material supports this hypothesis although definitive proof is not available. The use of non-steroidal anti-inflammatory drugs and the occurrence of coagulation and fibrinolytic abnormalities could play a contributing role (Moses et al., 1988).

RECOMMENDATION FOR FORMULATING AN ORAL HYDRATION SOLUTION

1. To replace Na^+ lost in sweat, improve palatability, and to assure that sufficient Na^+ is available for absorption, 20 to 30 mEq/L should be added to a replacement beverage. Unpublished data from our laboratory indicate that doubling the [Na^+] of a glucose-electrolyte solution from 25 to 50 mEq/L did not enhance water, electrolyte, or Na^+ absorption. The intestinal mucosa has a large capacity for adding Na^+ to luminal contents. Secretions from only a 10-cm segment of the duodenum can raise [Na^+] of a solution from 0 to 60 mEq/L (unpublished data); thus, the amount of Na^+ required in a fluid replacement beverage to enhance absorptive processes may be very small. On the other hand, to replace Na^+ *lost* as a result of diarrhea, the concentrations should be considerably higher because of the large volume of isotonic fluid that forms the diarrheal solution.
2. During segmental perfusion studies, maximal water absorption has been observed with glucose ranging from 100 to 150 mM. Most sport drinks contain 5 to 10% carbohydrate (278 to 556 mM) with only 20 to 30 mEq/L of Na^+. These higher concentrations of carbohydrate should be evaluated to determine the optimal amount that can be absorbed together with Na^+ without reducing water transport.
3. Determine the effectiveness of glucose polymers instead of glucose to reduce osmolality and provide for more Na^+ without reducing glucose concentration below a minimal level.
4. Include 5 to 10 mEq/L K^+ to offset the potential loss of K^+ in sweat and the K^+ secretory effect of glucose. Potassium may also help to replace ICF volume (Nielsen et al., 1986). Also, glucose-stimulated

insulin secretion facilitates K^+ uptake by cells and therefore helps to replace ICF volume (Brigs & Koechig, 1923).

5. The primary anion should be Cl^- (Fordtran, 1975); however, the organic anions acetate and citrate have also been shown to significantly enhance water and salt absorption (Rolston et al., 1986; Demigne et al., 1981). Combinations of these anions should be tested to determine if their effects are additive.
6. Consider the inclusion of a small amount of fructose because glucose causes K^+ secretion in the jejunum, while fructose causes K^+ absorption (Fordtran, 1975). Fructose is also more readily emptied from the stomach than glucose (Hunt & Knox, 1969).
7. Consider the inclusion of amino acids at low concentations. Glucose and amino acid-stimulated water absorption appear to be additive processes (Patra et al., 1982b). Moreover, different amino acids have different membrane carriers. Thus, if more than one amino acid is incorporated into a beverage, Na^+, and therefore water, absorption should be that much more enhanced (Gunther & Wright, 1983; Stevens et al., 1982).

These recommendations are based on current knowledge of the interactions between water, electrolyte, and carbohydrate absorption. They do not take into consideration factors such as palatability. Obviously, more research is required in this field before we understand how to formulate a rehydration beverage that maximizes water and carbohydrate absorption. To determine whether this same beverage can also serve as an oral hydration solution under conditions of dehydration and in the treatment of diarrheal disease also requires more research.

SUMMARY

The segmental perfusion technique utilizing a triple-lumen tube is the desired method to study intestinal absorption *in vivo*, especially if the focus of the research is to evaluate oral hydration solutions. This is because the mixing segment of the triple-lumen tube provides insight into the influence of intestinal secretions on the test solution before the absorptive characteristics of the solution are quantified in the test segment. In other words, this technique provides more insight into what would occur if the solution was taken orally. The double-lumen tube without a mixing segment and with or without a proximal occlusive balloon, does not provide this important function. Thus, if a glucose solution without Na^+ were perfused into the jejunum using a double-lumen tube, Na^+ most likely would be secreted into the test segment, and water and glucose may or may not be absorbed, depending on the length of the test segment. On the other hand, if the same solution were perfused through a triple-lumen tube with a 10-cm mixing segment, $[Na^+]$ at the end of a mixing segment would be approximately 50 to 60 mEq/L, and marked water, Na^+, and glucose absorption would occur in the same length of test segment employed with the double-lumen technique. Thus, if the objective of the study using the segmental perfusion technique is to gain insight into absorption/secretion processes of an orally ingested solution, the double-lumen technique would provide spurious information.

The second point is the importance of glucose to the absorption of water. Glucose stimulates active Na^+ transport, which in turn is responsible for opening the intercellular channels that allow for bulk absorption of solution. Thus, not only water, but Na^+ and glucose can also move across the enterocyte via the paracellular pathway, at least in the "leaky" duodenojejunum. The amount of glucose necessary to maximize water absorption is in the range of 100 to 150 mM. Most sport drinks contain considerably more carbohydrate, but not necessarily in the form of glucose. Although Na^+ is required for glucose absorption, the amount of Na^+ required in an oral hydration solution is unclear. Intestinal secretions have a remarkable ability to contribute Na^+ to luminal solutions, and the amount of Na^+ necessary in a sports drink to facilitate carbohydrate absorption may be minimal. Although the stoichiometry of the glucose/Na^+ membrane-bound carrier is 1:2, the ratio of glucose to Na^+ in a fluid replacement beverage may not be important if "solution drag" is a primary mechanism of water, electrolyte, and gluocose absorption as suggested by Fordtran (1975) for the proximal intestine and more recently by Pappenheimer and his colleagues (Madara & Pappenheimer, 1987; Pappanheimer & Reiss, 1987; Pappenheimer, 1987).

The effect of exercise on intestinal absorption remains unclear. Two of four studies show no effect of exercise on active or passive transport processes, whereas the other two studies show significant reductions in active transport. The reasons for this discrepancy are not obvious, but may relate to differences in the solution tested and the segment of the intestine studied. There is evidence that carbohydrate-electrolyte solutions are absorbed more readily than water, but the form of carbohydrate that maximizes water, electrolyte, and glucose absorption is not clear.

The diarrhea experienced by runners and cyclists remains largely unexplained. Although blood flow is undoubtedly reduced, and some changes in motility have been demonstrated with exercise, changes in small bowel absorption have not been documented. Ischemia probably contributes to gastrointestinal blood loss, which varies from inconsequential occult bleeding to massive life-threatening hemorrhage. It is possible that changes in blood flow, absorption, and motility in the colon might contribute importantly to the diarrhea and cramps that are commonly experienced, but to this point no adequate studies exist to explore this possibility.

BIBLIOGRAPHY

Armstrong, L.E., R.W. Hubbard, P.C. Szlyk, W.T. Matthew, and I.V. Sils. Voluntary dehydration and electrolyte losses during prolonged exercise in heat. *Aviat. Space Environ. Med.* 56:765–770, 1985.

Armstrong, W.M. Cellular mechanisms of ion transport in the small intestine. Ch 45: In: *Physiology of the Gastrointestinal Tract,* 2nd ed., L.R. Johnson, ed., New York: Raven Press, 1987, pp. 1251–1265.

Barclay, G.R. and L.A. Turnberg. Effect of moderate exercise on salt and water transport in the human jejunum. *Gut* 29:816–920, 1988a.

Barclay, G.R. and L.A. Turnberg. Effect of cold induced pain on salt and water transport in the human jejunum. *Gastroenterol.* 94:994–998, 1988b.

Barclay, G.R. and L.A. Turnberg. Influence of sham feeding on salt and water absorption in the human jejunum. *Gut* 27:1147–1150, 1986.

Binder, H.J. Absorption and secretion of water and electrolytes by small and large intestine. Ch. 55. In: *Gastrointestinal Disease: Pathophysiology Diagnosis and Management,* 4th edition, M.H. Sleisenger & J.F. Fordtran, eds., Philadelphia: W.B. Saunders, 1988, pp. 1022–1044.

Binder, H.J. and G.I. Sandle. Electrolyte absorption and secretion in the mammalian colon. In: *Physiology of the Gastrointestinal Tract,* 2nd ed., Ch. 49. L.R. Johnson, ed., New York: Raven Press, 1987, pp. 1389–1418.

Bond, J., D. Levitt, and M. Levitt. Quantitation of countercurrent exchange during passive absorption from the dog small intestine. *J. Clin. Invest.* 59:308–318, 1977.

Bounos, G. Acute necrosis of the intestinal mucosa. *Gastroenterol.* 82:1457–1467, 1982.

Bounos, G., D. Menard, and E. DeMedicis. Role of pancreatic proteases in the pathogenesis of ischemic enteropathy. *Gastroenterol.* 73:102–108, 1970.

Brauns, F., W.H.M. Saris, and N.J. Rehrer. Abdominal complaints and gastrointestinal function during long-lasting exercise. *Int. J. Sports Med.* 3:175–246, 1987.

Bridenbaugh, G.A., J.T. Flynn, and A.M. Lefer. Arachidonic acid in splanchnic artery occlusion shock. *Am. J. Physiol.* 231:112–118, 1976.

Brigs, A.P. and I. Koechig. Some changes in the composition of blood due to the injection of insulin. *J. Biol. Chem.* 58:721–730, 1923.

Brown, B.D. and H.V. Ammon. Effect of glucose on jejunal water and solute absorption in the presence of glycodeoxycholate and oleate in man. *Dig. Dis. Sci.* 26:710–717, 1981.

Brunsson, I., S. Eklund, M. Jodal, O.Lundgren, and H. Sjovall. The effect of vasodilation and sympathetic nerve activation on net water absorption in the cat's small intestine. *Acta Physiol. Scand.* 106:61–68, 1979.

Burns, T.W., J.R. Mathias, J.L. Martin, G.M. Carlson, and R.P. Shields. Alteration of myoelectric activity of small intestine by invasive *Escherichia coli. Am. J. Physiol.* 238:657–662, 1980.

Cammack, J., N.W. Read, P.A. Cann, B. Greenwood, and A.M. Holgate. Effect of prolonged exercise on the passage of a solid meal through the stomach and small intestine. *Gut* 23:957–961, 1982.

Campbell, J.M.H., M.B. Mitchell, and A.T.W. Powell. The influence of exercise on digestion. *Guy's Hosp. Rep.* 78:279–293, 1928.

Cantwell, J.D. Gastrointestinal disorders in runners (letter). *JAMA* 246(13):1404–1405, 1981.

Cassuto, J., H. Sjovall, M. Jodal, J. Svanvik, and O. Lundgren. The adrenergic influence on intestinal secretion in cholera. *Acta Physiol. Scand.* 115:157–158, 1982.

Charney, A.N. and G.M. Feldman. Systemic acid-base disorders and intestinal electrolyte transport. *Am. J. Physiol.* 247:G1–G12, 1984.

Clausen, J.P. Effect of physical training on cardiovascular adjustments to exercise in man. *Physiol. Rev.* 57:779–815, 1977.

Connell, A.M. Motor action of the large bowel, Ch.101. In: *Handbook of Physiology, Section G: Alimentary Canal, Volume IV: Motility,* C.F. Code, ed., Washington, D.C.: American Physiological Society, 1968, pp. 2075–2091.

Cooke, H.J. Neural and humoral regulation of small intestinal electrolyte transport. Ch. 47. In: *Physiology of the Gastrointestinal Tract.* 2nd ed., L.R. Johnson, ed., New York: Raven Press, 1987, pp. 1307–1350.

Cooper, B.T., S.A. Douglas, L.A. Firth, J.H. Hannagan, and V.S. Chadwick. Erosive gastritis and gastrointestinal bleeding in a female runner. Prevention of the bleeding and healing of the gastritis with H2-receptor antagonists. *Gastroenterol.* 92(6):2019–2023, 1987.

Cooper, H., R. Levitan, J.S. Fordtran, and F.J. Ingelfinger. A method for studying absorption of water and solute from the human small intestine. *Gastroenterology* 50:1–7, 1966.

Costill, D.L. Sweating: Its compostion and effects on body fluids. In: *Annals of the New York Academy of Sciences. The Marathon: Physiological, Medical, Epidemiological, and Psychological Studies,* P. Milvey, ed., 1977, 301:160–174.

Crane, R.K. Hypothesis for mechanism of intestinal active transport of sugars. *Fed. Proc.* 21:891–895, 1962.

Cummins, A.J. Absorption of glucose and methionine from the human intestine: the influence of the glucose concentration in the blood and in the intestinal lumen. *J. Clin. Invest.* 31:928–937, 1952.

Curran, P.F. Coupling between transport processes in intestine. *Physiologist,* 11:3-23, 1968.
Curran, P.F. Na, Cl and water transport by rat ileum in vitro. *J. Gen. Physiol.* 43:1137-1148, 1960.
Curran, P.F. and J.R. McIntosh. A model system for biological water transport. *Nature* 4813:347-348, 1962.
Davis, J.M., D.R. Lamb, W.A. Burgess, and W.P. Bartoli. Accumulation of deuterium oxide in body fluids after ingestion of D_2O-labeled beverages. *J. App. Physiol.* 63:2060-2066, 1987.
Demigne, C., C. Remesy, F. Chartier, and J. LeFaivre. Effect of acetate or chloride anions on intestinal absorption of water and solutes in the calf. *Am. J. Vet. Res.* 42:1356-1359, 1981.
Dueno, M.I., J.C. Bai, W.C. Santangelo, and G.J. Krejs. Effect of somatostatin analog on water and electrolyte transport and transit time in the human small bowel. *Dig. Dis. Sci.* 32:1092-1096, 1987.
Ehrlein, H.J., M. Schemann, and M.L. Siegle. Motor patterns of the canine small intestine. *Dig. Dis. Sci.* 30:767, 1985.
Evans, D.F., G.E. Foster, and J.D. Hardcastle. Does exercise affect the migrating motor complex in man? In: *Gastrointestinal Motility,* C. Roman, ed., Lancaster, UK: MTP, 1984, p. 277-284.
Ewe, K. Effect of bisacodyl on intestinal electrolytes and water net transport and transit. *Digestion* 37:247-253, 1987.
Feldman, M. and J.V. Nixon. Effect on exercise on postprandial gastric secretion and emptying in humans. *J. Appl. Physiol.* 53:851-854, 1982.
Field, M. and I. McColl. Ion transport in rabbit ileal mucosa III. Effects of catecholamines. *Am. J. Physiol.* 225:852-857, 1973.
Fisher, R.L., L.F.McMahon, Jr., M.J. Ryan, et al. Gastrointestinal bleeding in competitive runners. *Dig. Dis. Sci.* 31(11):1226-1228, 1986.
Fogoros, R.N. Runner's trots. Gastrointestinal disturbance in runners. *JAMA* 243(17):1743-1744, 1980.
Fordtran, J.S. Stimulation of active and passive sodium absorption by sugars in the human jejunum, *J. Clin. Invest.* 55:728-737, 1975.
Fordtran, J.S., F.C. Rector, Jr., and N.W. Carter. The mechanisms of sodium absorption in the human small intestine. *J. Clin. Invest.* 47:884-900, 1968.
Fordtran, J.S. and B. Saltin. Gastric emptying and intestinal absorption during prolonged severe exercise. *J. Appl. Physiol.* 23:331-341, 1967.
Gardner, E., D.J. Gray, and R. O'Rahilly. In: *Anatomy,* Philadelphia: W.B. Saunders, 1967.
Gisolfi, C.V. Electrolyte supplementation. In: *The theory and Practice of Athletic Nutreition: Bridging the Gap,* Columbus, Ohio: Ross Laboratories, A.C. Grandjean and J. Storlie, eds., 1989, pp. 11-21.
Gisolfi, C.V., R.W. Summers, H.P. Schedl, T.L. Bleiler, and R.A. Oppliger. Human intestinal water absorption: Direct vs. indirect measurements. *Am. J. Physiol.* (In Press) 1990.
Gracey, M., V. Burke, and A. Oshin. Active intestinal transport of D-fructose. *Biochim. Biophys. Acta.* 226:397-406, 1972.
Granger, D.N., G. Rytilli, and J. McCord. Superoxide radicals in feline intestinal ischemia. *Gastroenterol.* 81:22-29, 1981.
Granger, D.N., M. Sennett, P. McEleanney, and A.E. Taylor. Effect of local arterial hypotension on cat intestine capillary permeability. *Gastroenterol.* 79:474-480, 1980.
Guenter, J.K. and J.S. Fordtran. Effect of VIP infusion on water and ion transport in the human jejunum. *Gastroenterol.* 78:722-727, 1980.
Gunther, R.D. and E.M. Wright. Na^+, Li^+, and Cl^- transport by brush border membranes from rabbit jejunum. *J. Membrane Biol.* 74:85-94, 1983.
Halvorsen, F.A., J. Lyng, and S. Ritland. Gastrointestinal bleeding in marathon runners. *Scan J. Gastroenterol.* 21(4):493-497, 1986.
Hartley, L.H., J.W. Mason, R.P. Hogan, L.G. Jones, T.A. Kotchen, E.H. Mougey, F.E. Wherry, L.L. Pennington, and P.T. Ricketts. Multiple hormonal responses to graded exercise in relation to physical training. *J. Appl. Physiol.* 33:602-606, 1972a.
Hartley, L.H., J.W. Mason, R.P. Hogan, L.G. Jones, T.A. Kotchen, E.H. Mougey, F.E. Wherry, L.L. Pennington, and P.T. Ricketts. Multiple hormonal responses to prolonged exercise in relation to physical training. *J. Appl. Physiol.* 33:607-610, 1972b.
Hellier, M.D., C. Thirumalai, and C.D. Holdsworth. The effect of amino acids and dipeptides on sodium and water absorption in man. *Gut* 14:41-45, 1973.
Hicks, T. and L.A. Turnberg. The influence of secretion on ion transport in the human jejunum. *Gut* 14:485-490, 1973.
Higuchi, S., G. Fukushi, T. Baba, D. Sasaki, and Y. Yoshida. New method of testing for carbohydrate absorption in man. Xylose and sucrose absorption; Effects of sucrase inhibition. *Dig. Dis. Sci.* 31:369-375, 1986.
Holdsworth, C.D. and A.M. Dawson. Absorption of fructose in man. *Proc. Soc. Exp. Biol. Med.* 118:142-145, 1965.
Holdworth, C.D. and A.M. Dawson. The absorption of monosaccharides in man. *Clin. Sci.* 27:371-379, 1964.
Hunt, J.N. and M.T. Knox. Regulation of gastric emptying. In: *Handbook of Physiology IV, Alimentary Canal.* Washington, D.C.: American Physiological Society, 1969, pp. 1917-1935.
Jones, B.J.M., A.K. Beavis, D. Edgerton, and D.B.A. Silk. Intestinal absorption of glucose polymers in man. *Gut* 21:A450, 1980.

Jones, B.J.M., B.E. Higgins, and D.B.A. Silk. Glucose absorption from maltotriose and glucose oligomers in the human jejunum. *Clin. Sci.* 72:409–414, 1987.
Keeffe, E.B.,D.K. Lowe, J.R. Goss, and R. Wayne. Gastrointestinal symptoms of marathon runners. *West J. Med.* 141:481–484, 1984.
Keeling, W.F. and B.J. Martin. Gastrointestinal transit during mild exercise. *J. Appl. Physiol.* 63:978–981, 1987.
Kenney, M.J., A. Flatt, R.W. Summers, C.K. Brown, and C.V. Gisolfi. Changes in jejunal myoelectrical activity during exercise in fed untrained dogs. *Am. J. Physiol.* 254:G741–G747, 1988.
Knochel, J.P., L.N. Dotin, and R.J. Hamburger. Pathophysiology of Intense Physical Conditioning in a Hot Climate. I. Mechanisms of Potassium Depletion. *J. Clin. Invest.* 51:242–255, 1972.
Konturek, S.J., J Tasler, and W. Obtulowicz. Effect of exercise on gastrointestinal secretions. *J. Appl. Physiol.* 34:324–328, 1973.
Lee, J.S. Luminal and plasma glucose concentrations on intestinal fluid absorption and lymph flow. *Am. J. Physiol.* 252:G568–G573, 1987.
Leiper, J.B. and R.J. Maughan. Effect of bicarbonate or base procursor on water and solute absorption from a glucose-electrolyte solution in the human jejunum. *Digestion* 41:39–45, 1988.
Leiper, J.B. and R.J. Maughan. Experimental models for the investigation of water and solute transport in man. Implications for oral rehydration solutions. *Drugs* (In Press), 1989.
Leiper, J.B. and R.J. Maughan. Improved reproducibility in measurement of jejunal absorption rates in vivo in man. *J. Physiol.* 380:11P, 1986.
Levens, N.R. Control of intestinal absorption by the renin-angiotensin system. *Am. J. Physiol.* 249:G3–G15, 1985.
Levins, N.R., M.J. Peach, and R.M. Carey. Interactions between angiotensin peptides and the sympathetic nervous system mediating intestinal sodium and water absorption in the rat. *J. Clin. Invest.* 67:1197–1207, 1981.
Levitt, M.D. Use of the constant perfusion technique in the nonsteady state. *Gastroenterol.* 73:1450–1453, 1977.
Lewis, L.D. and J.S. Fordtran. Effect of perfusion rate on absorption, surface area, unstirred water layer thickness, permeability, and intraluminal pressure in the rat ileum in vivo. *Gastroentero.* 68:1509–1516, 1975.
Lifshitz, F. and R.A. Wapnir. Oral hydration solutions: experimental optimization of water and sodium absorption. *J. Pediatr.* 106:383–389, 1984.
Lorber, S.H., Gastrointestinal Disorders and Exercise. Ch. 13. In: *Exercise Medicine: Physiological Principles and Clinical Application,* A.A. Bove & D.T. Lowenthall, eds., New York: Academic Press, 1983, pp. 279–290.
Macrae, A.R. and T.S. Neudoerffer. Support for the existence of an active transport mechanism of fructose in the rat. *Biochim. Biophys. Acta* 288:137–144, 1972.
Madara, J.L. and J.R. Pappenheimer. Structural basis for physiological regulation of paracellular pathways in intestinal epithelia. *Membrane Biol.* 100:149–164, 1987.
Malawer, S.J., M. Ewton, J.S. Fordtran, and F.J. Ingelfinger. Interrelation between jejunal absorption of sodium, glucose, and water in man. *Am. J. Clin. Invest.* 44:1072–1073, 1965.
Mathias, J.R., G.M. Carlson, A.J. DiMarino, G. Bertiger, H.E. Morton, and S. Cohen. Intestinal myoelectric activity in response to live *Vibrio cholerae* and colear enterotoxin. *J. Clin. Invest.* 58:91–96, 1976.
Mathias, J.R., J.L. Martin, T.W. Burns, G.M. Carlson, and R.P. Shields. Ricinoleic acid effects on the electrical activity of the small intestine in rabbits. *J. Clin. Invest.* 61:640–644, 1978.
McCabe, M.E., III, D.A. Peura, S.C. Kadakia, Z. Bocek, and L.F. Johnson. Gastrointestinal blood loss associated with running a marathon. *Dig. Dis. Sci.* 31(11):1229–1232, 1986.
McMahon, L.R., Jr., M.J. Ryan, and D. Larsons. Occult gastrointestinal blood loss in marathon runners. *Ann. Intern. Med.* 100(6):846–847, 1984.
Modigliani, R. and J.J. Bernier. Absorption of glucose, sodium, and water by the human jejunum studied by intestinal perfusion with a proximal occluding balloon and at variable flow rates. *Gut* 12:184–193, 1971.
Modigliani, R., J.C. Rambaud, and J.J. Bernier. The method of intraluminal perfusion of the human small intestine. *Digestion* 9:176–192, 1973.
Morris, A.I. and L.A. Turnberg. Influence of isoproterenol and propranolol on human intestinal transport in vivo. *Gastroenterol.* 81:1076- 1079, 1981.
Moses, F.M., T.G. Brewer, and D.A. Peura. Running-associated proximal hemorrhagic colitis. *Ann. Intern. Med.* 108:385–386, 1988.
Newton, C.R., P.B. McIntyre, J.E. Lennard-Jones, J.J. Gonvers, and D.M. Preston. Effect of different drinks on fluid and electrolyte losses from a jejunostomy. *J. Roy. Soc. Med.* 78:27–34, 1985.
Nielsen, B., G. Sjogaard, J. Ugelvig, B. Knudsen, and B. Dohlmann. Fluid balance in exercise dehydration and rehydration with different glucose-electrolyte drinks. *Europ. J. Appl. Physiol.* 55:318–325, 1986.
Norryd, C., H. Dencker, A. Lundenquist, T. Olin, and U. Tylen. Superior mesenteric blood flow during digestion in man. *Acta Chir. Scand.* 141:197–202, 1975.
Oddsson, E., J. Rask-Madsen, and E. Krag. Transmural ionic fluxes and electrical potential differences in the human jejunum during perfusion with a dihydroxy bile acid. *Scand.J. Gastroenterol.* 12:453–456, 1977.

Papaioannides, D., C. Giotis, N. Karagiannis, and C. Voudouris. Acute upper gastrointestinal hemorrhage in long-distance runners (letter). *Ann. Intern. Med.* 101:719, 1984.
Pappenheimer, J.R. Physiological regulation of transepithelial impedance in the intestinal mucosa of rats and hamsters. *J. Membrane Biol.* 100:137–148, 1987.
Pappenheimer, J.R. and K.Z. Reiss. Contribution of solvent drag through intercellular junctions to absorption of nutrients by the small intestine of the rat. *J. Membrane Biol.* 100:123–136, 1987.
Parks, D.A., G.B. Bulkley, D.N. Granger, S.R. Hamilton, and J.M. McCord Ischemic injury in the cat small intestine: role of superoxide radicals. *Gastroenterol.* 82:9–15, 1982.
Parsons, D.S. Methods for investigation of intestinal absorption, Ch. 64. In: *Handbook of Physiology—Alimentary Canal III*, C.F. Code (ed.), 1968, pp. 1177–1216.
Parsons, B.J., J.A. Poat, and P.A. Roberts. Studies of the mechanism of noradrenaline stimulation of fluid absorption by rat jejunum in vitro. *J. Physiol.* 355:427–439, 1984.
Patra, F.C., D. Mahalanabis, and K.N. Jalan. Stimulation of sodium and water absorption by sucrose in the rat small intestine. *Acta Paediatr. Scand.* 71:103–107, 1982a.
Patra, F.C., D. Mahalanabis, K. Jalan, A. Sen, and P. Banerjee. Is oral rice electrolyte solution superior to glucose electrolyte solution in infantile diarrhea? *Arch. Dis. Child.* 57:910–912, 1982b.
Persson, B.-E. and K.R. Spring. Gallbladder epithelial cell hydraulic water permeability and volume regulation. *J. Gen. Physiol.* 79:481–505, 1982.
Pinson, E.A. Water exchanges and barriers as studied by the use of hydrogen isotopes. *Physiol. Rev.* 21:123–134, 1952.
Pitts, R.F. *Physiology of the kidney and body fluids.* Chicago: Year Book Medical Publishers, 1963.
Porter, A.M. Do some marathon runners bleed into the gut? *Br. Med.J.* 287(6403):1427, 1983.
Powell, D.W. Intestinal water and electrolyte transport. Ch. 46. In: *Physiology of the Gastrointestinal Tract*, 2nd ed. L.R. Johnson, ed., New York: Raven Press, 1987, pp. 1267–1305.
Powell, D.W., H.M. Berschneider, L.D. Lawson, and H. Martens. Regulation of water and ion movement in intestine. In: *Microbial toxins and diarrhoeal disease.* Pitman: London (Ciba Foundation Symposium 112), 1985, pp. 14–33.
Quamar, M.I. and A.E. Read. Effect of exercise on mesenteric blood flow in man. *Gut* 28:583–587, 1987.
Reitemeier, R.J., C.F. Code, and A.L. Orvis. Comparison of rate of absorption of labeled sodium and water from upper small intestine of healthy human beings. *J. Appl. Physiol.* 10:256–260, 1957.
Riklis, E. and J. Quastel. Effects of cations on sugar absorption by isolated surviving guinea pig intestine. *Can. J. Biochem. Physiol.* 36:347–362, 1958.
Robertson, J.D., R.J. Maughan, and R.J.L. Davison. Faecal blood loss in response to exercise. *Br. Med. J.* 295:303–305, 1987.
Robinson, J.W.L., V. Mirmovitch, B. Winistorfer, and F. Saegesser. Response of the intestinal mucosa to ischemia. *Gut* 22:512–527, 1981.
Robinson, S. and A.H. Robinson. Chemical compounds of sweat. *Physiol. Rev.* 34:202–220, 1954.
Rolston, D.D.K., K.J. Moriarty, M.J.G. Farthing, M.J. Kelly, M.L. Clark, and A.M. Dawson. Acetate and citrate stimulate water and sodium absorption in the human jejunum. *Digestion* 34:101–104, 1986.
Rowell, L.B., J.R. Blackman, and R.A. Bruce. Indocyanine green clearance and estimated hepatic blood flow during mild exercise to maximal exercise in upright man. *J. Clin. Invest.* 43:1677–1690, 1964.
Rumessen, J.J. and E. Gudmand-Hoyer. Absorption capacity of fructose in healthy adults. Comparison with sucrose and its constituent monosaccharides. *Gut* 27:1161–1168, 1986.
Saltzman, D.A., F.C. Rector, Jr., and J.S. Fordtran. The role of intraluminal sodium in glucose absorption in vivo. *J. Clin. Invest.* 51:876–885, 1972.
Sandle, G.I., M.J. Keir, and C.O. Record. Inter-relationship between the absorption of hydrocortisone, sodium, water, and actively transported organic solutes in the human jejunum. *Eur. J. Clin. Pharmacol.* 23:177–182, 1982.
Saunders, D.R. and J.K. Sillery. Absorption of carbohydrate-electrolyte solutions in rat duodenojejunum. Implications for the composition of oral electrolyte solutions in man. *Dig. Dis. Sci.* 30:154–160, 1985.
Schaub, N., H.P. Spichtin, and G.A. Stalder. Ischamische kolitis als ursache einer darmblutung bei marathonlauf? *Schweiz Med. Wschr.* 115(13):454–457, 1985.
Schedl, H.P. and J.A. Clifton. Solute and water absorption by the human small intestine. *Nature* 199:1264–1267, 1963.
Schoch, D.R., A.L. Sullivan, R.J. Grand, and W.F. Eagan. Gastrointestinal bleeding in an adolescent runner. *J. Pediatr.* 111(2):302–304, 1987.
Scholer, J.F. and C.F. Code. Rate of absorption of water from stomach and small bowel of human beings. *Gastroenterol.* 27:565–577, 1954.
Schultz, S.G. and P.F. Curran. Coupled transport of sodium and organic solutes. *Physiol. Rev.* 50:637–718, 1970.
Schultz, S.G. and P.F. Curran. Intestinal absorption of sodium chloride and water, Ch. 66. In: *Handbook of Physiology—Alimentary Canal III*, 1964, pp. 1245–1275.
Scobie, B.A. Recurrent gut bleeding in five long-distance runners. *NZ Med. J.* 98(790):966, 1985.
Scott, L.D. and R.W. Summers. Correlation of contractions and transiet in rat small intestine. *Am. J. Physiol.* 230:132–137, 1976.

Selby, G., D. Frame, and E.R. Eichner. Effort-related gastrointestinal blood loss in young distance runners during a competitive season. (Abstract). *Med. Sci. Sports Exerc.* 20(2):S79, 1988.
Sforzo, G.A. Opioids and exercise: an update. *Sports Med.* 7:109-124, 1989.
Shoemaker, W.C. and W.F. Walker. *Fluid-Electrolyte Therapy in Acute Illness.* Chicago: Year Book Medical Publishers, 1974.
Sit, S.P., R. Nyhof, R. Gallavan, and C.C. Chou. Mechanisms of glucose-induced hyperaemia in the jejunum. *Proc. Soc. Exp. Biol. Med.* 163:273-277, 1980.
Sjovall, H., H. Abrahamsson, G. Westlander, R. Gillberg, S. Redfors, M. Jodal, and O. Lundgren. Intestinal fluid and electrolyte transport in man during reduced circulating blood volume. *Gut* 27:913-918, 1986.
Sjovall, H., S. Redfors, B. Biber, J. Martner, and O. Winso. Evidence for cardiac volume-receptor regulation of reline jejunal blood flow and fluid transport. *Am. J. Physiol.* 246:G401-G410, 1984.
Sjovall, H., S. Redfors, S. Eklund, D.A. Hellback, M. Jodal, and O. Lundgren. The effects of splanchnic nerve stimulation on blood flow distribution, villans tissue osmolality and fluid and electrolyte transport in the small intestine of the cat. *Acta Physiol. Scand.* 117:359-365, 1983.
Sjovall, H., S. Redfors, M. Jodal, and O. Lundgren. The effect of carotid occlusion on net fluid absorption in the small intestine of rats and cats. *Acta Physiol. Scand.* 115:447-453, 1982.
Slanden, G.E. Methods of studying intestinal absorption in man. In: *Intestinal Absorption in Man,* I. McColl & G.G.G. Sladen, eds. London: Academic Press, 1975, pp. 1-49.
Sladen, G.E. and A.M. Dawson. Interrelationships between the absorptions of glucose, sodium and water by the normal human jejunum. *Clin. Sci.* 36:119-131, 1969.
Sladen, G.E., and M.A. Dawson. Effect of bicaronate on sodium absorption by the human jejunum. *Nature* 218:267-268, 1968.
Smithson, K.W., D.B. Millar, L.R. Jacobs and G.M. Gray. Intestinal diffusion barrier: unstirred water layer or membrane surface mucous coat? *Science* 214:1241-1244, 1981.
Spiller, R.C., B.E. Higgins, P.G. Frost and D.B.A. Silk. Inhibition of jejunal water and electrolyte absorption by therapeutic doses of clindamycin in man. *Clin. Sci.* 67:117-120, 1984.
Spiller R.C., B.J.M. Jones, and D.B.A. Silk. Jejunal water and electrolyte absorption from two proprietary enteral feeds in man: importance of sodium content. *Gut* 38:681-687, 1978.
Spranger, K.J., T.L. Bleiler, and C.V. Gisolfi. The effect of exercise on intestinal absorption of water and carbohydrate-electrolyte solution. *J. Iowa Acad. Sci.* 96:A28, 1989.
Stevens, B.R., H.J. Ross, and E.M. Wright. Multiple transport pathways for neutral amino acids in rabbit jejunal brush border vesicles. *J. Mem. Biol.* 66:213-225, 1982.
Stewart, J.G., D.A. Ahlquist, D.B. McGill, D.M. Ilstrup, S. Schwartz, and R.A. Owen. Gastrointestinal blood loss and anemia in runners. *Ann. Intern. Med.* 100(6):843-845, 1984.
Sullivan, S.N. Exercise-related symptoms in triathletes. *Phys. Sportsmed.* 15(9):105-110, 1987.
Summers, R.W. and N.S. Dusdieker. Patterns of spike burst spread and flow in the canine small intestine. *Gastroenterol.* 81:742-750, 1981.
Thompson, P.D., E.J. Funk, R.A. Carleton, and W.Q. Sturner. Incidence of death during jogging in Rhode Island from 1975 through 1980. *JAMA* 247(18):2535-2538, 1980.
Turnberg, L.A., F.A. Bieberdorf, S.G. Morawski, and J.S. Fordtran. Interrelationships of chloride, bicarbonate, sodium, and hydrogen transport in the human ileum. *J. Clin. Invest.* 49:557-567, 1970a.
Turnberg, L.A., J.S. Fordtran, N.W. Carter, and F.C. Rector, Jr. Mechanisms of bicaronate absorption and its relationship to sodium transport in the human jejunum. *J. Clin. Invest.* 49:548-556, 1970b.
Vanatta, J.C. and M.J. Fogelman. *Moyer's Fluid Balance. A Clinical Manual.* Chicago: Year Book Medical Publishers, 1976.
Van Trappen, G., J. Janssens, and G. Coremans. Gastrointestinal motility disorders. *Dig. Dis. Sci.* 31:5S-25S, 1986.
Varro, V., G. Blaho, L. Csernay, I. Jung, and F. Szarvas. Effect of decreased local circulation on the absorptive capacity of a small intestine loop in the dog. *Am. J. Dig. Dis.* 10:170-177, 1965.
Welsh, M.J., P.L. Smith, M. Fromm, and R.A. Frizzell. Crypts are the site of intestinal fluid and electrolyte secretion. *Science* 218:1219-1221, 1982.
Wheeler, K.B. and J.G. Banwell. Intestinal water and electrolyte flux of glucose-polymer electrolyte solutions. *Med. Sci. Sports Exer.* 18:436-439, 1986.
Williams, J.H., M. Mager, and E.D. Jacobson. Relationship of mesenteric blood flow to intestinal absorption of carbohydrates. *J. Lab. Clin. Med.* 63:853-863, 1964.
Winne, D. Models of the relationship between drug absorption and intestinal blood flow. In: *Physiology of Intestinal Circulation.* A.P. Shepherd and D.N. Granger, eds. New York: Raven Press. 1984, p. 289.

DISCUSSION

SUMMERS: Nausea, vomiting, cramping pain, diarrhea, and gastrointestinal blood loss have all been reported after prolonged strenuous exercise. The minimal changes in absorption or secretion mentioned by Carl do not seem to explain any of these symptoms. It is possible that changes in GI motility could be playing a role; however, very few data are available with regard to motor activity and exercise. In our laboratory, Carl and I have reported some studies in dogs and we are beginning to study humans to look for abnormal patterns of motor activity that might contribute to diarrhea. Highly propulsive peristaltic waves might rapidy move intestinal contents through the gut, either in the small intestine or the colon, interfering with normal absorption. We have not found any of these patterns. Some subtle changes did occur, but we have found no evidence of marked changes in motor activity in the small intestine. We have not yet examined the colon. Changes in colonic absorption, secretion, or motility could be affected to cause diarrhea, but that remains to be proven. Another function affected by exercise is gastrointestinal blood flow. It is fairly well accepted that with severe exercise, GI blood flow may decrease to as low as 20% of control levels. The intestine seems to have a great deal of reserve capacity, and decreases in blood flow to that degree do not seem to dramatically affect the gastrointestinal absorption. At some point, however, reduced blood flow will affect the gastrointestinal absorption and will impair absorption of water, electrolytes, and nutrients. Eventually, lowered blood flow will not maintain mocosal viability, and ischemic necrosis will occur. That is the presumed mechanism of gastrointestinal blood loss that has been described in numerous cases of extreme exertion.

KACHADORIAN: With regard to the formation of blisters at the tight junction that you showed in electron micrographs, I should point out that a morphological event usually is caused by a reverse osmotic gradient across the epithelium. In this case, the causative agent for opening tight junctions probably would be glucose. I know of no data to support the possibility that this would be associated with water movement across the epithlia in the direction you suggest. In fact, based on experiments using in vitro preparations, I thought the reverse would hold. The mechanism for this was worked out in the early 1970s, and involves solute movement into the junction according to a transepithelial gradient. In turn, water is drawn from the serosal side of the epithelium into the junction, and blister formation occurs. In freeze fracture, a loss or disruption of junctional elements is seen. Associated with this, water movement occurs in a serosal to mucosal direction; in other words, into the lumen. This type of mechanism has been hypothesized as being important in controlling leakiness in kidney proximal tubule, which is morphologically similar to gut in some ways. In terms of mechanism, your view of solute-water movement across the epithelium through open tight junctions would be a novel phenomenon, which, I think, requires further study. The other consideration is that the area of the tight junction in the gut is more than 10^4 times less than the area of the cell membrane facing the lumen. Considering this, and regardless of permeability characteristics, paracellular fluid movement in the gut is less important than transcellular movement.

GISOLFI: What you're suggesting is that most of the water would be moving transcellularly from mucosal to the serosal side of the cell and that the paracellular pathway would allow movement in the opposite direction.

KACHADORIAN: That's my view on the matter. What I'm suggesting is that the interpretation that was given to the micrograph you showed may not be correct. This has to do with the issue of physiological mechanism, but not necessarily the rationale for including glucose in a fluid replacement solution. What I'm talking about is the mechanism by which fluid moves across the epithelium of the gut when fluid replacement solutions are given. I guess an extension of it is to say that too much glucose, in fact, may have an undesirable effect in terms of opening tight junctions and having fluid move into the lumen from the serosal side. In vitro studies to deal with this would seem desirable.

GISOLFI: Evidence to support the hypothesis of Pappenheimer comes from physiological and histological data. In one study, a 50–80 cm segment of rat intestine was perfused with solutions of inert solutes of varying molecular size and with 25 mM glucose. Ferrocyanide was added as an osmotically active solute to adjust the rate of fluid absorption and to measure the coefficient of osmotic flow. From measurements of osmotic flow and the clearance (steady-state transepithelial fluxes per unit concentration) rates of glucose and the inert solutes as a function of fluid absorption, estimates were made of paracellular fluid absorption, the rate of active glucose transport, the amount of glucose carried paracellularly by solvent drag or back diffusion, and glucose concentration in the absorbate. When luminal glucose concentration exceeded 10–20 mM (that required to saturate the active transport mechanism), glucose concentration in the basolateral absorbate was calculated to be 80 mM above that in luminal fluid. This concentration difference was able to account for the measured rate of fluid absorption. Thus, solvent drag through the paracellular pathway was calculated to be the primary avenue of glucose absorption under physiological concentrations of glucose (3–5%) in the luminal solution.

A second series of experiments was designed to determine if the paracellular pathway was under physiological control. Is the increase in clearance of luminal solutes the result of opening tight junctions, or can such clearances occur through junctions of fixed dimensions? This question was answered by measuring the impedance across isolated segments of rat or hamster intestine reperfused with salt solutions with and without nutrient (glucose, amino acids). The results showed that NA^+ coupled nutrient transport reduced transepithelial impedance 2- to 3-fold while increasing capacitance (membrane surface) and conductance (width of intercellular junctions and lateral sacs). Moreover, this reduction in impedance was reversibly dependent upon O_2 tension. It was not due to passive widening of tight junctions secondary to increased osmotic flow because adding 10 mM ferrocynamide to a luminal glucose solution, which prevents osmotic flow, failed to block the changes in resistance and capacitance induced by glucose. Evidence that this reduction in resistance was an active contractile process was illustrated in the electronmicrographs that I showed of tight junctions during perfusion of rat or hamster small intestine with solutions containing just electrolytes or electrolytes with glucose.

SCHEDL: In the small intestine, the studies showing dilatation of the lateral intracellular space are associated with absorption rather than secretion. It appears that one can open up another absorption pathway that can give a synergistic effect at higher glucose concentrations. Glucose absorption increases as glucose concentration is raised up to a certain level. Then there is a break in the curve at higher concentrations as absorption increases exponentially in the proximal small intestine. In the rat, this occurs in the range of 20 to 30 mM. But it's thought in the human to occur at higher concentrations. There may be a difference between the proximal and distal small intestine in this process.

GISOLFI: Sweat is hypotonic to plasma and contains approximately 45–50 mEq/L Na^+ in a fit individual. If sweat rate averages 1 L/h over the course of a triathalon (13 h), the total Na^+ loss would be about 600 mEq. This amount of Na^+ loss could result in hyponatremia. For shorter forms of competition, hyponatremia is usually not a concern because the majority of athletes do not replace all the fluid they lose in sweat. However, when all the fluid lost in sweat is replaced and water is the replacement beverage, hyponatremia can occur. The addition of sodium to a replacement beverage is to enhance carbohydrate absorption, improve palatability, and to promote fluid homeostasis. In two recent papers from our laboratory, the inclusion of electrolytes in a replacement beverage maintained plasma volume more effectively than ingesting plain water. This can be accomplished with approximately 10–20 mEq of salt. On the other hand, the World Health Organization recommends 90–100 mEq of salt in a replacement beverage to count diarrheal fluid loss. However, the Na^+ loss in diarrhea is 2–3 times the loss of sweat.

CONVERTINO: This discussion reflects back to the days when we were interested in calcium and sodium and their effects on thermoregulation. Based on some studies, I think there is an indication for eliminating sodium in drinks for exercise events of four hours or less duration. This may be leading to the point where we're recommending two different drinks for two different types of events. With regard to thermoregulation, do you see an advantage to limiting sodium in drinks? I used to include an experiment for my students in which we were able to demonstrate that if we increased sodium in a drink, we inhibited sweating and heat dissipation, and increased body temperature.

GISOLFI: That's a good point. There is a relationship between plasma sodium concentration and a rise in internal body temperature. Harrison showed that drinking a 1% saline solution (172 mEq) significantly increased core body temperature, but perfusing the intestine with a solution containing 50 mEq Na^+, twice the amount usually present in sport drinks, had no effect on plasma [Na^+] and therefore presumably no effect on body temperature. Thus, I would not be concerned about the amount of Na^+ in typical fluid replacement beverages.

CONVERTINO: I'm not sure there's evidence to suggest that the amount of sodium lost in sweat in an event lasting 2–4 h is so significant that we need to have sodium in the drink. There is little argument regarding a triathlon type of event that we probably need to be concerned with sodium replacement. That's really what I'm getting at; you've shown very convincing data that we don't need sodium to help with absorption of these substances.

GISOLFI: There is a possibility of developing hyponatremia in a 2–4 h event such as the marathon. If we assume a sweat rate of 1.5 L/h over a 3 h period and a sweat [Na^+] of 45 mEq, total sweat Na^+ loss is 203 mEq. If urinary Na^+ loss is 30 mEq, the total Na^+ loss would be 233 mEq. Such a loss is often accompanied by a rise in plasma [Na^+] because most athletes replace only 20% to 30% of the fluid lost in sweat. However, if the 4.5 L of sweat lost were replaced by plain water, plasma [Na^+] would fall to 130 mEq/L. This plasma [Na^+] would be considered borderline hyponatremia. If this athlete overhydrated, i.e., drank more than 4.5L, hyponatremia would surely occur.

CONVERTINO: I am aware of that. Are there data on palatability with different levels of sodium?

MURRAY: There certainly seems to be a tendency for a small amount of sodium to increase the palatability of the beverage, much like the small amount of sodium increases the palatability of the steak on your plate.

SUTTON: How often do we actually see diarrhea among athletes, and what impact does this actually have in terms of the study in fluid losses? Do you have any suggestions as to how one might go about minimizing that impact?

SUMMERS: "Runners Trots" are well known. Some authors have reported an incidence of diarrhea in marathoners as high as 30%. It may be more of a problem in the poorly trained individual or those who "overdo," but even world class athletes have had to divert to the bushes during a race. Some even have bloody diarrhea.

MURRAY: The research on sodium feeding and fluid homeostasis is a puzzlement because the results often don't match up with what you would theoretically expect sodium feeding to do. We discussed the positive influence of sodium on beverage palatability and also that a small amount of sodium might increase gastric emptying. The presence of sodium may also minimize urine production, thereby helping to conserve fluid and helping to maintain extracellular fluid volume. Perhaps a certain amount of sodium is also an impetus for thirst as Roger mentioned earlier. All such responses could be theoretically expected from sodium feedings.

5

Influence of Fluid Replacement Beverages on Body Fluid Homeostasis during Exercise and Recovery

ETHAN R. NADEL, PH.D.

GARY W. MACK, PH.D.

HIROSHI NOSE, M.D., PH.D.

INTRODUCTION

Water is the body's most abundant component, comprising about 65–70% of the body mass in an average adult. Water is the solvent in which numerous materials, organic and inorganic, are dissolved and thereby made available for transport from one site to another. A change in the water content of any of the body's fluid compartments will result in a redistribution of body water and an alteration of the solute concentration in all of the compartments.

Because dramatic changes in body water and solute concentrations can exert profound effects on cellular and organ system function, sophisticated mechanisms have evolved to regulate body fluid volume and composition so that these remain relatively constant despite sudden fluxes in water intake or loss. The regulatory mechanisms involve reflexes whose receptor elements within the vasculature, brain, and gut are sensitive to mechanical and chemical changes that occur during shifts in water and/or electrolyte content, and whose effector systems act to modify rates of fluid intake (e.g., thirst) and fluid output (e.g., the kidneys).

The details concerning the volume and distribution of the body fluids and the forces that cause the movement of fluids and solutes among the body compartments are covered in other chapters in this volume and in textbooks (Pitts, 1974; Ruch and Patton, 1974). They will not be delineated in any detail here. Total body water is determined by the quantity of solutes in the body. The distribution of water among the various body fluid compartments (intracellular, interstitial, plasma) is a function of the quantity of solutes in each compartment. Water moves passively along with the solutes as they are transported across boundaries between compartments. Water also moves down a total energy gradient, which includes that provided by the hydrostatic pressure head. Thus, major shifts of water from the plasma compartment to the interstitial fluid compartment take place, for example, just by changing from the supine to the upright posture (Hagan et al., 1978).

Water moves by passive diffusion and, more importantly, by bulk flow across the capillary endothelium through membrane slit-pores, fenestrations, or clefts. Osmotic and hydrostatic forces cause water to move between the intravascular and interstitial compartments (see Pappenheimer, 1953, for a complete review of the dynamics of capillary filtration and reabsorption); forces causing water to move between the interstitial and intracellular compartments are entirely osmotic.

Exercise is one condition that presents a potential threat to the maintenance of body fluid volume. During exercise, shifts in body water distribution can occur as a result of changes in muscle perfusion pressure that affect the filtration/reabsorption balance across the capillary endothelium, an increased capillary surface area for transfer, and also as a result of an increased rate of evaporation of water from the skin and pulmonary system.

The sweating rate is, in simplest analysis, a function of the total thermal load, which is the combined internal (related to the exercise intensity) and external (ambient temperature) load (Nadel, 1979). Water losses from the body can exceed 30 g/min (1.8 L/h) in heavy sweating conditions, and the water lost from the body is derived from all body fluid compartments, including the intravascular compartment.

During exercise, plasma water losses are partly compensated for by shifts in water from the other body fluid compartments, but there must be other compensatory adjustments to prevent a fall in the heart's ability to maintain an output appropriate to the requirements from muscle and skin. Progressive, uncompensated reductions in blood volume will result in a fall in the filling pressure of the heart (preload) and cardiac stroke volume and, eventually, in the heart's ability to maintain its output. Should these events occur during exercise, fuel and oxygen delivery to the contracting muscles may become compromised, as might heat delivery to the skin, the site of heat dissipation.

Among the body's compensations to progressive dehydration are a) an increase in cardiac frequency, which attenuates the fall in cardiac output; b) mobilization of water from the extravascular to the intravascular space (Nose et al., 1988a); and c) increases in splanchnic vascular resistance (Rowell et al., 1965) and forearm vascular resistance (Nadel et al., 1980) and a decrease in forearm venous capacitance (Fortney et al., 1983), all of which serve to shift the blood volume centrally and attenuate the fall in cardiac stroke volume. These compensations have the short-term benefit of providing for the maintenance of adequate oxygen and fuel delivery, but the longer term liabilities of progressively altering the intracellular environment and reducing the body's heat transfer ability. Thus, the optimal way to resist the ill effects of progressive dehydration during exercise would be to ingest water and electrolytes at the same rates as they are lost. The purpose of this chapter is to examine this premise.

BODY FLUID BALANCE DURING DEHYDRATION

In 1947, Adolph reported that water is not drawn equally from all the body compartments during dehydration. Rather, plasma water losses are 2.5 times greater (on a relative basis) than from the other compartments. The relatively greater plasma water loss may be due to the fact that the major ions lost in sweat are those from the extracellular space.

More recently, Senay (1979) reviewed the dehydration literature and concurred with the older view of Adolph (1947) that water was lost from the plasma compartment at a relatively greater rate than that from the other body fluid compartments during progressive dehydration. Costill (1977) ascribed the relatively greater plasma water loss to outward movement accompanying the ions lost in sweat, which are Na^+ and Cl^-, the major ions of the extracellular compartment. There would then be less mobilization of water from the intracellular compartment. Durkot et al. (1986) demonstrated that there was a greater water loss from the extracellular fluid compartment in rats than from the intracellular compartment during a 10% dehydration. Nose et al. (1985) suggested that water movement might be linked to the electrolyte losses from each compartment. However, selective dehydration of the extracellular compartment would presumably result in water movement from the intracellular compartment down its concentration gradient, and the effects of dehydration would eventually be distributed among the body fluid spaces.

Sweat is hypotonic with respect to the blood plasma, although the concentration of the different electrolytes in sweat varies widely: a) among individuals, b) at different rates of sweating, and c) according to the level of heat acclimatization and physical fitness (Costill, 1977). The concentrations of Na^+ and Cl^-, the major ions in sweat, average 40–60 and 30–45 mEq/L, respectively, whereas their concentrations in plasma average 140 and 105 mEq/L. It is well known that the sweat [Na^+] decreases during the process of heat acclimation (Costill and Sparks, 1973), but until recently there has been no experimental evidence demonstrating a relation between sweat [Na^+] and water mobilization from any of the body fluid compartments.

In 1988, Nose et al. (1988a) reported that at a given level of dehydration the [Na^+] in sweat determines the volume of fluid mobilized from the intracellular fluid compartment, which in turn determines the effective maintenance of the circulating blood volume. They followed the body fluid and electrolyte fluxes of 10 volunteers during 2 h of exercise-induced dehydration and 1 h of resting recovery without fluid intake. The average [Na^+] and [K^+] in sweat was 56.4 (range 30.6–105.7) and 9.6 (range 6.9–11.5) mEq/L, respectively.

Changes in the body fluid compartments following a mild dehydration of 2.3% of body water are shown in Figure 5-1. Changes in the intracellular fluid compartment after dehydration leveled off around -10 mL/kg body weight after 30 minutes of equilibration. Changes in the extracellular fluid compartment averaged -12.3 mL/kg body weight after equilibration had occurred. In the 30 min directly following the exercise period, there was a partial recovery of the plasma water deficit, at the expense of the interstitial fluid compartment. Plasma volume was reduced by 9.4% immediately following exercise, but this deficit was restored to -5.0% after 30 min of recovery and -5.6% after 60 min.

From relationships developed in their analyses of the water and electrolyte movements in the post dehydration period, Nose et al. (1988a) arrived at the following conclusions. The increase in plasma osmolality during dehydration is primarily a function of the loss of free water from the body ($r=0.78$, $p<0.01$), where free water loss is analogous to free water clearance in renal function studies. Secondly, the decrease in the intracellular fluid compartment was closely related to the increase in plasma osmolality ($r=0.74$, $p<0.02$), implying that water movement out of the cells followed the osmotic gradient. Thirdly, there is a strong inverse correlation between free water loss and the sweat [Na^+] over a wide range ($r=-0.97$, $p<0.01$). They concluded that the free water loss caused the increase in the plasma osmolality during dehydration, resulting in fluid mobilization from the intracellular fluid compartment to maintain the extracellular fluid volume. Finally, as shown in Figure 5-2, they noted that the decrease in plasma volume during dehydration was a function of the decrease in the extracellular fluid volume ($r=0.77$, $p<0.01$), which itself was related to the sweat [Na^+] ($r=0.80$, $p<0.01$), as shown in Figure 5-3. Thus, a more dilute sweat allows a greater conservation of the

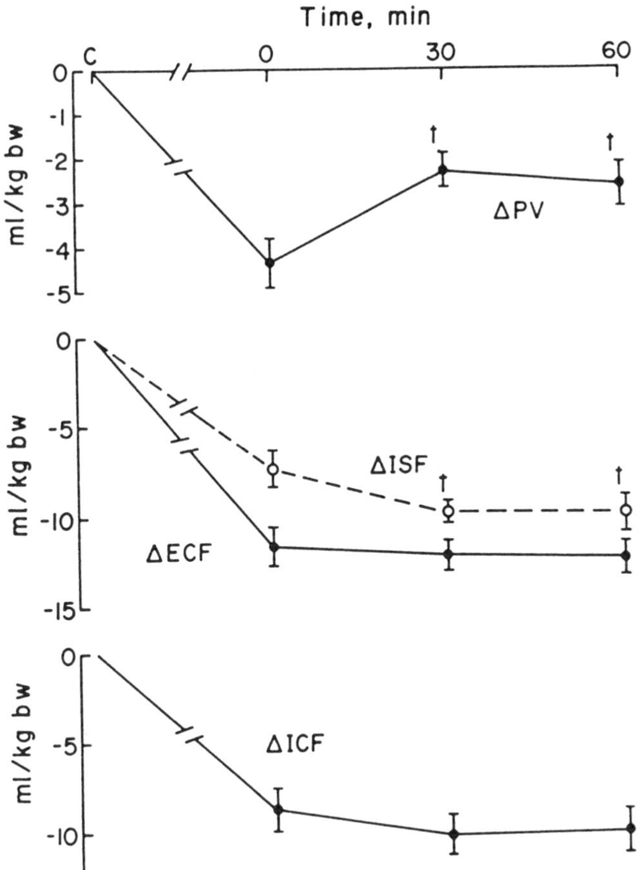

FIGURE 5-1. *Changes in the body fluid compartments from control values following 2 h dehydration exposures. ΔPV, ΔISF, ΔECF and ΔICF denote the plasma, interstitial, extracellular, and intracellular fluid compartment changes. All variables were significantly changed from control and the daggers indicate significant differences from the 0 min points. From Nose et al. (1988b), with permission from the American Physiological Society.*

plasma volume during dehydration, primarily due to the greater movement of water from the intracellular fluid compartment.

Once the phenomena governing the body fluid shifts during and following a period of dehydration are better understood, it becomes easier to predict the factors that affect the restoration of the body fluid compartments during rehydration.

BODY FLUID BALANCE DURING RECOVERY FROM DEHYDRATION

It is well established that humans have a prolonged period in which they are not capable of fully rehydrating after thermal- or exercise-

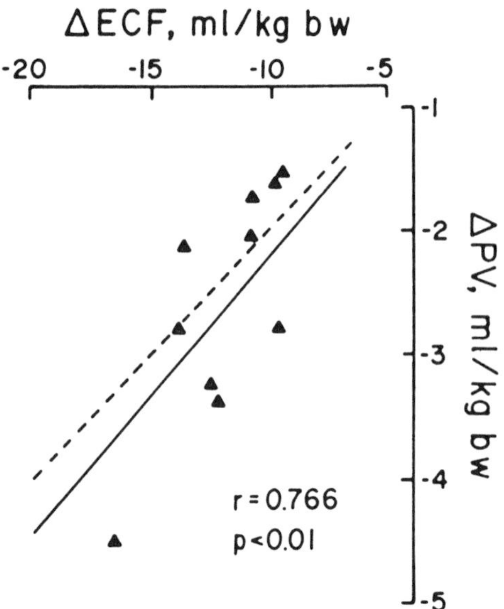

FIGURE 5-2. *Relation between the decreases in the ECF compartment and the plasma volume in different individuals following dehydration. The solid line is from the experimental data and the dashed line represents the theoretical relation. From Nose et al. (1988b), with permission from the American Physiological Society.*

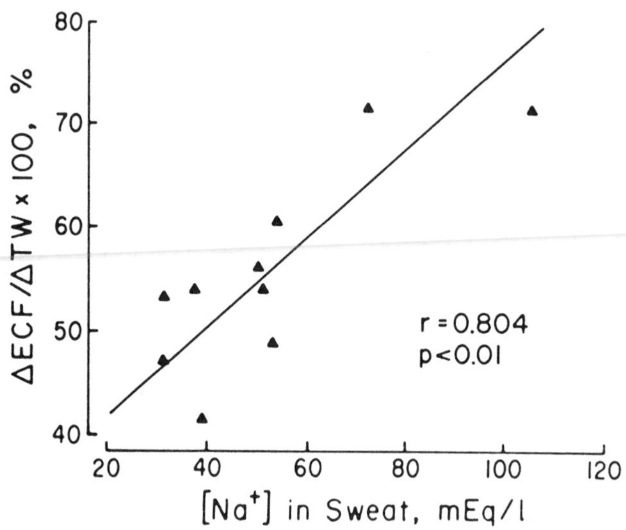

FIGURE 5-3. *Relation between sweat [Na$^+$] and the decrease in the extracellular fluid compartment in different subjects following dehydration. From Nose et al. (1988b), with permission from the American Physiological Society.*

induced dehydration. This phenomenon has been known for years as voluntary dehydration (Rothstein et al., 1947), but it is now customarily referred to as involuntary dehydration, precisely because the dehydrated individual has no volition to rehydrate. Greenleaf (1982) stated that two factors unique to humans contributed to this involuntary dehydration. These were: a) an excessive extracellular fluid loss due to the Na^+ lost with sweat, and b) the upright posture. Dill (1933) had, in fact, claimed many years ago that thirst was primarily related to the plasma Na^+ concentration, not the plasma volume. Rehydrating with water should dilute the plasma rapidly as the water is absorbed and therefore remove the drive for drinking.

Costill and Sparks (1973) reported that rehydration with a glucose/electrolyte solution resulted in a more rapid recovery of the plasma volume deficit than when the same subjects rehydrated with water. Morimoto et al. (1981) found that the degree of involuntary dehydration in humans was reduced when a glucose/electrolyte solution was ingested rather than water after thermal dehydration. However, both of these results are a bit difficult to interpret because the sweet taste of the glucose in the drinking solution may have influenced drinking behavior.

More recently, Nose et al. (1985, 1986) demonstrated a reduction in the absolute involuntary dehydration (a better rehydration) in rats when they were supplied with drinking water containing Na^+, which compensated in part for the Na^+ lost during dehydration. Their results argued for the involvement of osmotic factors affecting the ability to rehydrate and accounting for the phenomenon of involuntary dehydration.

Osmotic factors may not be all-important in the drive to rehydrate. Nose et al. (1986) also demonstrated, in rats, that a disproportionately high percentage of ingested water, about twice as much as would be expected assuming that ingested water is distributed proportionally among the body fluid compartments, is retained in the vascular compartment during rehydration. Thus, the high retention of ingested fluids in the vascular space might, along with the removal of the osmotic drive for drinking, act to diminish the volume-dependent drive for drinking despite the incomplete recovery of the total water deficit.

Nose et al. (1988b) recently reported the results of a study to assess the phenomenon of involuntary dehydration in humans. Their intent in this study was to examine the distribution and fate of water taken in during rehydration and thus to determine the mechanisms responsible for the high retention of ingested water within the vascular space. They studied six volunteers over 4 h of recovery from a whole body dehydration of 2.3%. During the first hour, no fluids were provided to allow the body fluid compartments to stabilize. During the following 3 h, the volunteers rehydrated in a thermoneutral environment with water ad libitum and capsules provided with each 100 mL of water ingested. Capsules contained either 0.2 g sucrose (placebo) or 0.45 g NaCl, so that rehydration in the experimental condition was with a 0.45% saline solution, without the salty taste.

Figure 5-4 illustrates the cumulative fluid intake, urine volume, and net fluid gain during the 3 h of rehydration with water and with 0.45% saline. Differences became apparent after 2 h of recovery, and these were magnified as time progressed. Taking urinary losses into account, the net fluid gain at 180 min was 12.1 +/- 1.6 mL/kg body weight in the water rehydration condition and 15.3 +/- 2.4 mL/kg in the saline recovery condition. In other words, the volunteers restored only 53% and 67% of the water lost, respectively, in the 3-h period of rehydration, despite the fact that they were able to drink as much as they wished.

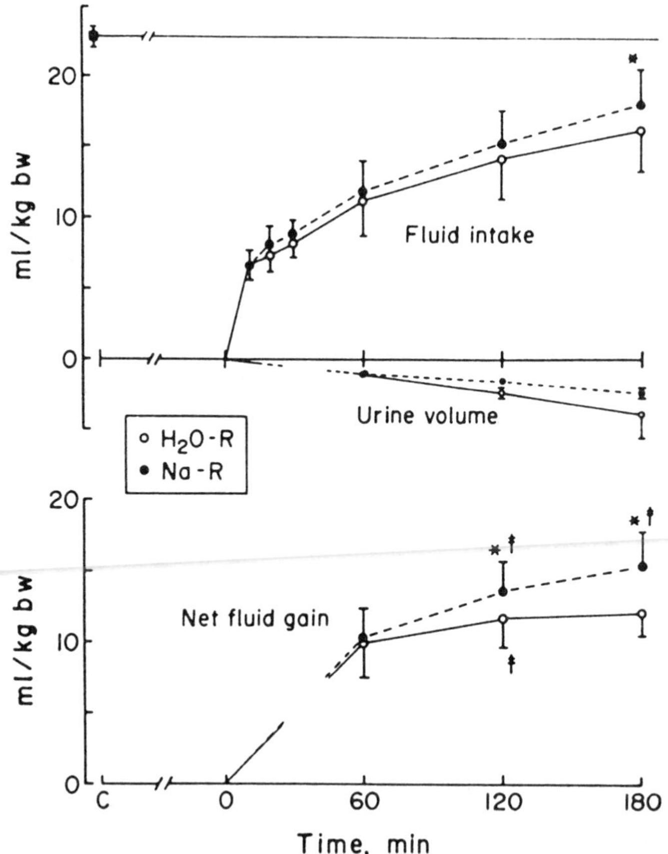

FIGURE 5-4. *Cumulative body fluid changes during 180 min of rehydration (from a dehydration of 2.3 mL/kg body weight dehydration) and water (H_2O-R) and water plus salt capsules resulting in a 0.45% Na^+ intake (Na-R). Asterisks denote differences between H_2O-R and Na-R and daggers denote differences from the 60-min point. From Nose et al. (1988a), with permission from the American Physiological Society.*

During the rehydration period, subjects restored plasma volume by 30 min in the saline recovery condition and by 120 min in the water recovery condition. Plasma [Na^+] was restored in the water recovery condition almost immediately upon drinking and plasma osmolality was restored 30 min after the onset of drinking. In the saline recovery condition, plasma [Na^+] and plasma osmolality remained elevated at 120 min.

Nose et al. (1988b) attempted to explain the reason for the involuntary dehydration from an analysis of the body fluid and electrolyte balance during recovery from dehydration, as shown in Figure 5-5. In this figure, the intersection of the x and y axes represents the point of origin, or the pre-dehydrated condition (control) and the solid line indicates the theoretical isotonic line, where $y = 0.15x$. The area above the isotonic line reflects hypertonic body fluids, and the area below the isotonic line reflects hypotonic body fluids. The two points on the left are those following dehydration, in which the body fluid balance was about −2.3 mL/kg body weight and the body cation balance was about −1.4 mEq/kg body weight (since sweat is hypotonic to plasma, relatively more water than cation is lost, and the body fluids become hypertonic).

In both recovery conditions, body fluid and electrolyte balance moved toward the isotonic line. When there was no cation in the rehydration drink (open points), the water deficit but not the cation deficit was restored, and recovery could occur in the lateral direction at best (in fact,

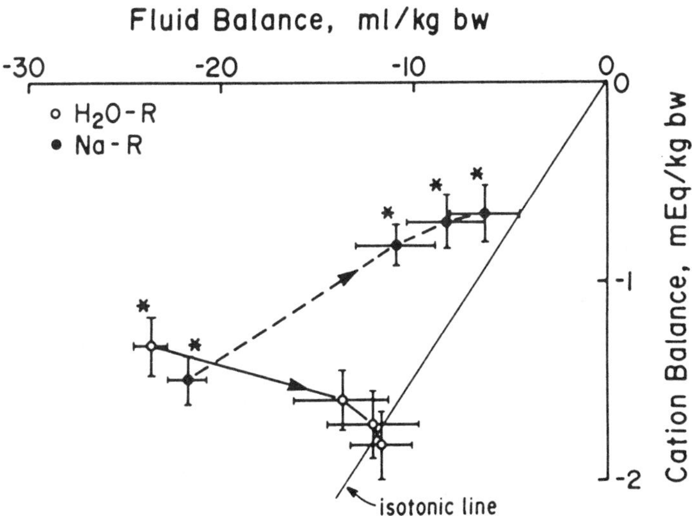

FIGURE 5-5. *Recoveries of body fluid cation status during rehydration as described in Figure 5-4. Asterisks denote points that differ from the isotonic line. From Nose et al. (1988a), with permission from the American Physiological Society.*

since there was some sweat loss, and therefore cation loss, in the rehydration period, recovery could not even proceed in the lateral direction). When cations were incorporated into the rehydration drink (filled points), both the body fluid deficit and the body cation deficit were restored, and recovery proceeded toward the point of origin. At 180 min of rehydration, the cation deficit was -1.8 mEq/kg body weight in the water recovery condition and -0.7 mEq/kg body weight (nearly all of which was made up of a K^+ deficit) in the saline recovery condition. Thus, the degree of involuntary dehydration after 180 min of recovery was determined primarily by the cation deficit, because the rate of fluid intake was attenuated and the rate of urine output was potentiated as the body fluid and electrolyte balance approached the isotonic line.

One further point from this study is worth emphasizing. At 180 min of rehydration the deficit in recovery of the intracellular fluid compartment was nearly the same in the two recovery conditions, reflecting the K^+ deficit. The authors calculated that around 80% of the water loss from the intracellular space was due to water movement following the outward flux of K^+. In the saline recovery condition, the subjects regained 95% of the Na^+ lost during rehydration and thus nearly all of the extracellular fluid space was restored by 180 min; therefore, the entire body fluid deficit was attributed to the intracellular fluid deficit. Because the recovery of the plasma volume was a function of the recovery of the extracellular fluid space ($r=0.87$, $p<0.01$), there was a better plasma volume restoration in the saline recovery condition. One can surmise that inclusion of some K^+ in the fluid replacement beverage might provide for an even better restoration of the body fluids lost during dehydration.

To summarize the message of this important study, when humans become fluid depleted and hypertonic due to dehydration, there is both an osmotic drive and a volume-dependent drive to drink. As fluid is absorbed from the gut after drinking begins, the plasma volume will be restored first due to the selective retention of ingested fluid in the vascular space, and the volume-dependent drive will be removed. If there is no cation in the fluid replacement drink, the plasma will be diluted as the fluid is absorbed, and the osmotic drive for drinking will be removed as well. As the fluid recovery approaches the isotonic line, increased formation of a dilute urine will occur to prevent the body fluids from becoming hypotonic. If cation is present in the fluid replacement beverage, the plasma osmolality will remain elevated during the rehydration period and the osmotic drive for drinking will therefore be retained. Drinking will persist as the subject approaches the isotonic line; because cations are being restored, the recovery point on the isotonic line will intersect closer to the origin, and the degree of involuntary dehydration will be accordingly less.

BODY FLUID BALANCE WITH FLUID INTAKE PRIOR TO EXERCISE

For reasons that should be apparent from the preceding section, it is difficult to overhydrate an individual in anticipation of the ill effects of impending dehydration. Taking in a large volume of water prior to an exercise bout will result in plasma volume expansion and plasma hypotonicity as the fluid is absorbed, followed by the rapid increase in the formation of dilute urine and a marked diuresis. It might be more reasonable to use saline instead of pure water to overhydrate an individual prior to exercise, although the taste of saline will not be tolerated by most people. Hypothetically, one would predict that saline intake would cause the body water and electrolyte balance to move up the isotonic line from the point of origin. This notion has yet to be tested in the laboratory, although the recent study of Candas et al. (1988) provided some insight into this question. They reported that prehydration with an isosmotic solution prevented the development of blood hyperosmolality that otherwise occurred during prolonged exercise in the heat without fluid replacement. Still, the best guesses concerning the effects of prehydration must be derived from the few studies that used this intervention to study its effects on the thermal and circulatory regulations during exercise.

In 1965, Moroff and Bass studied the effects of ingesting 2 L of water prior to a 90-min treadmill walk in the heat. They also gave water or saline to the subjects during the treadmill task. Despite the fourfold elevation in urine output during the pre-exercise and exercise periods, the subjects remained overhydrated throughout. When volume loaded, subjects maintained lower heart rates, higher sweating rates, and lower body core temperatures during exercise than when not, implying that the greater initial body water content conferred a certain resistance to the effects of dehydration. Others (Greenleaf and Brock, 1980; Greenleaf and Castle, 1971; Nielsen et al., 1971) employed simlar protocols to test the question of whether prehydration protects one against the effects of dehydration. Nielsen et al. (1971) found that subjects prehydrated with water had lower heart rates and body core temperatures during moderate exercise than when not pretreated. Prehydration with 2% saline had no effect on these variables, but when the subjects were dehydrated prior to exercise, they had higher heart rates and body core temperatures than when in the control condition.

Fortney et al. (1983) found that selective expansion of the plasma volume by 8% prior to exercise, by infusing an isotonic lactated Ringer solution contained 5% serum albumin, provided an increased cardiac stroke volume (from 100 to 111 mL/beat) and cardiac output (by 1.5 L/min from a mean of 16.1 L/min) during 30 min of exercise in the heat and an improved heat transfer capability, as demonstrated by a lower body core temperature. Thus, it appears that at least a part of the benefit of hyperhydration prior to exercise is the consequence on the circulation of an expansion of the vascular space.

BODY FLUID BALANCE WITH FLUID INTAKE DURING EXERCISE

Most studies involving fluid intake during exercise have been concerned with the replacement of the glucose primarily and have only been concerned with water replacement as a secondary notion (see Murray's review [1987] for a complete picture). For this reason, it has been difficult to separate the effects of the fuel replacement from the effects of the water and electrolyte replacement on the ability to resist fatigue during exercise. Since the physiological changes accompanying dehydration can limit exercise in certain conditions in which fuel availability is not an issue (e.g., moderately heavy exercise in the heat, where the optimal regulation of both arterial blood pressure and body temperature depends upon the maintenance of blood volume), it is of interest to examine the question of whether fluid and electrolyte intake during exercise can act to maintain the body water content and prevent the fatigue otherwise caused by a developing body fluid deficit. In the following discussion, the body fluid issues, but not the fuel issues will be explored.

Nearly half a century ago, Pitts et al. (1944) tested a group of men who exercised on a treadmill in a warm environment with or without fluid replacement. They found that heart rates and rectal temperatures were considerably elevated after 4 h when fluid was withheld as compared to when fluid was provided for the volunteers to drink ad libitum. Further, when water or a 0.2% NaCl solution or a 3.5% glucose solution was given at a rate equal to the evaporative rate, the heart rates were even lower than when water was provided ad lib, and rectal temperatures were marginally lower as well. This was among the earliest unequivocal demonstrations of the physiological changes that occur during progressive dehydration and an early indication that humans have an extremely poor sense of their body water status and do not recognize the characteristics of dehydration as it develops. Subsequently, it has been demonstrated repeatedly that dehydration results in an early onset of exhaustion and that an enforced regime of fluid intake will postpone this onset (Brown, 1947; Rothstein and Towbin, 1947) or provide an improved thermal and circulatory status (Candas et al., 1986; Costill et al., 1970; Francis, 1979).

In 1947 Rothstein et al. reported that replacement of the salt lost in sweat in the rehydration drink reduced the body weight deficit during dehydration by increasing the fluid intake and reducing the urinary output. Dill et al. (1973) confirmed this finding and demonstrated that plasma volume was expanded when salt was replaced with water every 7–8 min in small samples; plasma volume was contracted when no salt replacement occurred.

In their discussion of the efficacy of electrolyte replacement during prolonged exercise, Sherman and Lamb (1988) noted that there is scanty evidence to support this practice for individuals other than the small numbers of endurance athletes. They correctly recognized that the plasma electrolyte concentrations are elevated during prolonged exercise, and asked whether it would be advisable to provide electrolytes in such circumstances. They did not comment on the fact that athletes usually have acquired, through the adaptations of the sweat glands themselves, a relatively low sweat [Na^+] and thus may not require Na^+ replacement at the same rate as their less well trained counterpart. Further, they recognized the slight, but very real risk of hyponatremia in athletes who force great volumes of fluids low in electrolytes during endurance exercise (see Noakes et al., 1975). They concluded, however, that while fluid replacement during exercise (*N.B.* especially in the heat) appears to be beneficial insofar as the cardiovascular and thermoregulatory systems are concerned, the jury is still out on the value of electrolyte replacement.

In a recently completed study, Nose et al. (1989) simulated the ideal rate of fluid ingestion during exercise by infusing 8.75 mL/kg body weight of isotonic saline into subjects between 20 and 50 minutes of moderate exercise in a warm environment. By carefully selecting the infusion rate, they were able to return the plasma volume to the pre-exercise level by the end of the infusion period. Approximately half of the infused volume remained in the vascular space during the infusion period. Plasma volume expansion during exercise provided a lower heart rate, a higher forearm blood flow, and a lower body core temperature by the end of exercise when compared to the non-expanded condition, in which plasma volume was reduced by around 10%. Volume expansion promoted a better core-to-skin heat transfer by allowing the forearm blood flow to continue to rise, rather than to level off with increases in internal temperature (Figure 5-6). The total sweat produced during exercise was the same in the two conditions. Urine volume was 40% greater in the volume expanded condition, averaging 1.95 vs. 1.36 mL/kg body weight.

They concluded from this study that acute plasma volume expansion during exercise restores any decrease in preload that might occur in conditions of gradual volume depletion and thereby allows a lower heart rate and a progressive increase in peripheral blood flow with continuous body heating. Although they attempted to reproduce the effects caused by drinking, saline infusion was used specifically to avoid the variability resulting from differential rates of gastric emptying and absorption, and

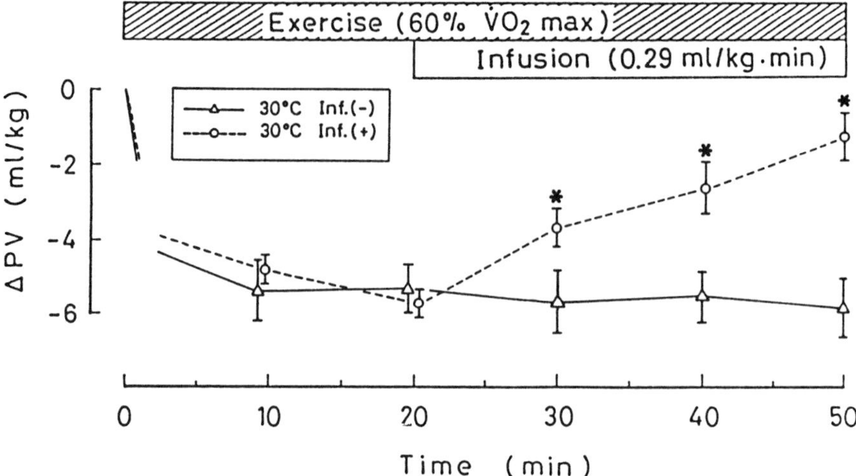

FIGURE 5-6a. *Changes in plasma volume with and without saline infusion during exercise. Asterisks denote differences between conditions. From Nose et al. (in press), with permission.*

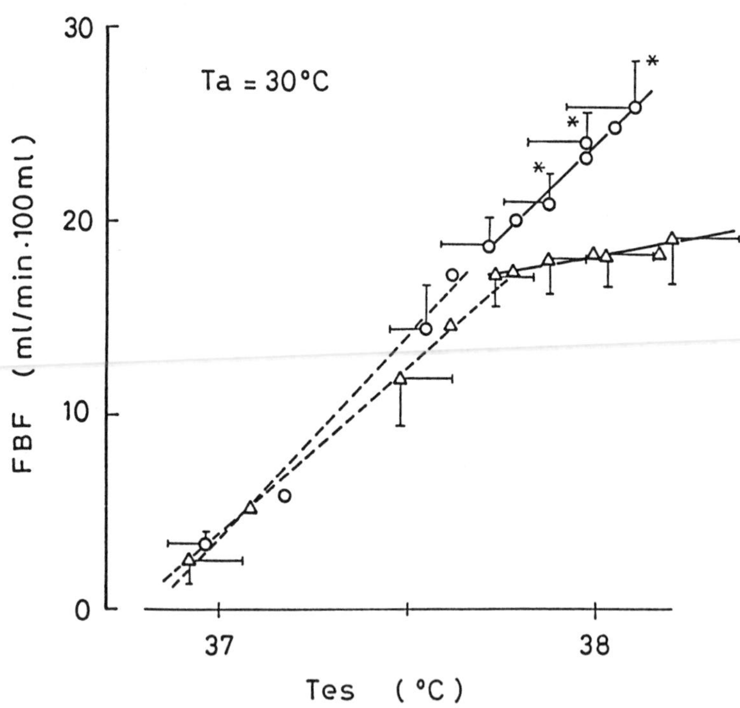

FIGURE 5-6b. *Forearm blood flow as a function of esophageal temperature during exercise in a 30°C environment with (△) and with (○) infusion. Modified from Nose et al. (in press), with permission.*

they were not able to claim that fluid replacement via drinking would have the same effect. Thus, we are left with the question about the ideal fluid replacement beverage that could be used during exercise.

SUMMARY

It is clear from the studies of Nose et al. (1988a,b) that the ideal fluid replacement beverage during recovery from dehydration should contain sufficient Na^+ to restore the amount lost in sweat. Because body water distribution is a function of solute distribution, and because Na^+ is the major cation in the extracellular fluid space, Na^+ replacement is necessary to restore the extracellular fluid volume lost. Because restoration of the plasma volume is a function of the restoration of the extracellular fluid space, a relatively high Na^+ content in the beverage is important.

A simple tank model illustrating the factors involved in the control of fluid intake and output during rehydration is shown in Figure 5-7. This simple model illustrates two inputs to the drinking controller, a volume input and a Na^+ input, and one input to the renal controller, a volume input. During progressive dehydration, blood volume is reduced and the float drops, thereby stimulating fluid intake through drinking and inhibiting fluid output via the renal system. The increases in blood [Na^+] during progressive dehydration stimulate fluid intake as well. During rehydration with water, the blood volume is restored first and the float rises, thereby inhibiting the drive for drinking and stimulating the drive for fluid output. Concurrently, the blood is diluted and [Na^+] decreases, re-

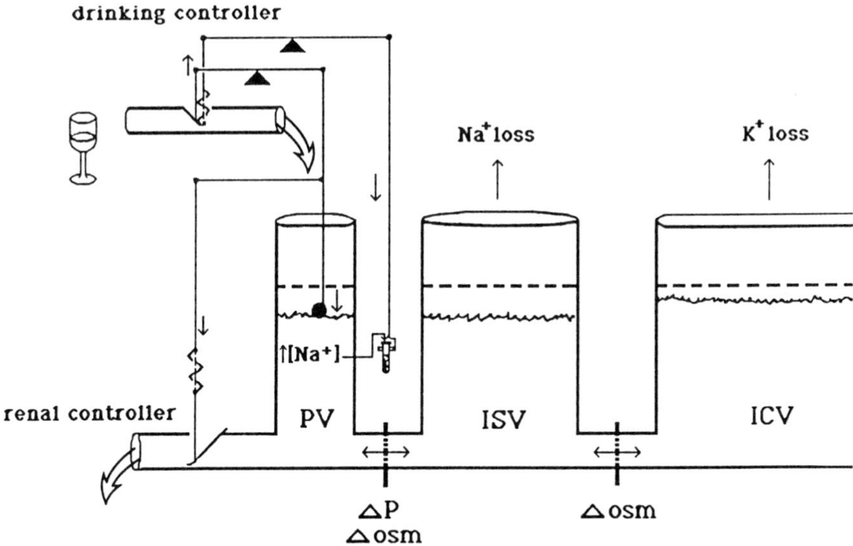

FIGURE 5-7. *A simple tank model illustrating the factors that affect the distribution of body water among the fluid compartments and the factors that influence the intake and output controllers.*

moving the osmotic drive for drinking. Gradually, as water is redistributed throughout the fluid compartments down its concentration gradient, the blood volume falls a bit and the drive for fluid intake increases, but not to the former level. If there is Na^+ in the fluid replacement beverage, it becomes distributed within the entire extracellular fluid space after it is absorbed, along with the water, and the plasma $[Na^+]$ remains somewhat elevated, thereby providing for a partial retention of the osmotic drive for drinking. Only with K^+ in the fluid replacement beverage can one expect to have a restoration of the intracellular fluid space.

If palatability were not an issue, the ideal fluid replacement beverage, insofar as the restoration of body fluid balance is concerned, might have a $[Na^+]$ between 40 and 60 mEq/L and a $[K^+]$ between 5 and 10 mEq/L, as these are the respective concentrations of these cations lost in sweat. Drinking a beverage with such concentrations of Na^+ and K^+ would maintain an elevated plasma osmolality and an osmotic drive for drinking.

Since palatability is most definitely an issue, and this concentration of Na^+ will have an unpleasantly strong taste, the drink designers must find a way to mask the salt taste to restore the lost cations. Otherwise, both the osmotic and volume-dependent drives for drinking will be removed as the dilute beverage is consumed and absorbed, and drinking will terminate before complete rehydration has occurred. It is important to add that the proper study to validate this claim has not been done. It is also important to add that many factors, still not well understood (see below), affect the ability to rehydrate.

A potentially important study is one that uses the design of the Nose et al. (1988b) paper, but provides the drink at various intervals and in various volumes in different experiments during exercise rather than during recovery. The $[Na^+]$ and $[K^+]$ should be varied in different experiments as well. Further, the initial levels of hydration should be varied in different experiments to verify the observation that this affects the ability to rehydrate adequately with a given drink (Candas et al., 1988). The exercise intensity, and therefore the required rate of energy dissipation, should also be varied in different experiments to learn how the rate of dehydration affects the ability to rehydrate. Once the data from such a study are available, our understanding of the dynamics of fluid movement during exercise will be advanced considerably. Until this study has been done, we are left to speculate based on the few studies that are available to us.

One other issue relevant to concerns about body fluid balance during exercise and recovery is whether the elderly are able to manage as well as the young. This issue is an important one since this country's population of elderly is growing at a rapid rate and the members of this population are increasingly active. There is preliminary evidence that the elderly demonstrate a reduced thirst during dehydration (Phillips et al., 1984), although the cause of the deficit is not at all clear. The elderly may also experience other deficits during dehydration and may not be capable of rehydrating as well as their younger counterparts, although it is not known whether such deficits are related to the aging process itself or the great inactivity and associated physiological changes within this population. Mechanistic studies of the physiological controls and regulations in the elderly will be an especially important research area in the next decade.

BIBLIOGRAPHY

Adolph, E.F. Blood changes in dehydration. In: *Physiology of Man in the Desert* (edited by E.F. Adolph et al.). Interscience, New York, 160-171, 1947.

Brown, A.H. Dehydration exhaustion. In: *Physiology of Man in the Desert* (edited by E.F. Adolph et al.). Interscience, New York, 208-225, 1947.

Candas, V., J.P. Libert, G. Brandenberger, J.C. Sagot, C. Amoros and J.M. Kahn. Hydration during exercise: effects on thermal and cardiovascular adjustments. *Eur. J. App. Physiol.* 55:113-122, 1986.

Candas, V., J.P. Libert, G. Brandenberger, J.C. Sagot, and J.M. Kahn. Thermal and circulatory responses during prolonged exercise at different levels of hydration. *J. Physiol. (Paris)* 83: 11-18, 1988.

Costill, D.L. Sweating: its composition and effects on body fluids. In: *The Marathon: Physiological, Medical, Epidemiological and Psychological Studies* (edited by P. Milvy). N.Y Acad. Sci., New York, 160-174, 1977.

Costill, D.L., W.F. Kammer and A. Fisher. Fluid ingestion during distance running. *Arch. Environ. Health* 21:520-525, 1970.

Costill, D.L. and K.E. Sparks. Rapid fluid replacement following thermal dehydration. *J. Appl. Physiol.* 34: 299-303, 1973.

Dill, D.B., A.V. Bock and H.T. Edward. Mechanism for dissipating heat in man and dog. *Am. J. Physiol.* 104: 36-43, 1933.

Dill, D.B., M.K. Yousef and J.D. Nelson. Responses of men and women to two-hour walks in desert heat. *J. App. Physiol.* 35:231-235, 1973.

Durkot, M.J., O. Martinez, D. Brooks-McQuade and R. Francesconi. Simultaneous determination of fluid shifts during thermal stress in a small-animal model. *J. Appl. Physiol*, 61:1031-1034, 1986.

Fortney, S.M., C.B. Wenger, J.R. Bove and E.R. Nadel. Effect of blood volume on forearm venous volume and cardiac stroke volume during exercise. *J. Appl. Physiol.* 55:884-890, 1983.

Francis, K.T. Effect of water and electrolyte replacement during exercise in the heat on biochemical indices of stress and performance. *Aviat. Space Environ. Med.* 50:115-119, 1979.

Greenleaf, J.E. Dehydration-induced drinking on humans. *Fed. Proc.* 41:2509-2514, 1982.

Greenleaf, J.E. and P.J. Brock. Na^+ and Ca^{++} ingestion: plasma volume-electrolyte distribution at rest and exercise. *J. Appl. Physiol*, 48:838-847, 1980.

Greenleaf, J.E. and B.L. Castle. Exercise temperature regulation in man during hypohydration and hyperhydration. *J. Appl. Physiol.* 30:847-853, 1971.

Hagan, R.D., F.J. Diaz and S.M. Horvath. Plasma volume changes with movement to supine and standing positions. *J. Appl. Physiol.* 45:414-418, 1978.

Locke, W., N.B. Talbot, H.S. Jones and J. Worcester. Studies on the combined use of measurements of sweat electrolyte composition and rate of sweating as an index of adrenocortical activity. *J. Clin. Invest.* 30:325-337, 1951.

Moroff, S.V. and D.E. Bass. Effects of overhydration on man's physiological responses to work in the heat. *J. Appl. Physiol.* 20:267-270, 1965.

Morimoto, T., K. Miki, H. Nose, S. Yamada, K. Hirakawa and C. Matsubara. Changes in body fluid and its composition during heavy sweating and effect of fluid and electrolyte replacement. *Jpn. J. Physiol.* 18:31-39, 1981.

Murray, R. The effects of consuming carbohydrate-electrolyte beverages on gastric emptying and fluid absorption during and following exercise. *Sports Med.* 4:322-351, 1987.

Nadel, E.R. Control of sweating rate while exercising in the heat. *Med. Sci. Sports Ex.* 11:31-35, 1979.

Nadel, E.R., S.M. Fortney and C.B. Wenger. Effect of hydration state on circulatory and thermal regulations. *J. Appl. Physiol.* 49:715-721, 1980.

Nielsen, B., G. Hansen, S.O. Jorgensen and E. Nielsen. Thermoregulation in exercisng man during dehydration and hyperhydration with water and saline. *Int. J. Biometeorol.* 15:195-200, 1971.

Noakes, T.D., N. Goodwin, B.L. Rayner, T. Branken and R.K.N. Taylor. Water intoxication: a possible complication during endurance exercise. *Med. Sci. Sports Ex.* 17:370-375, 1975.

Nose, H., G.W. Mack, X. Shi, K. Morimoto and E.R. Nadel. Effect of saline infusion during exercise on circulatory and thermal regulations. *J. Appl. Physiol.* in press.
Nose, H., G.W. Mack, X. Shi and E.R. Nadel. Role of osmolality and plasma volume during rehydration in humans. *J. Appl. Physiol.* 65:325–331, 1988.
Nose, H., G.W. Mack, X. Shi and E.R. Nadel. Shift in body fluid compartments after dehydration in man. *J. Appl. Physiol.* 65:318–324, 1988.
Nose, H., M. Morita, T. Yawata and T. Morimoto. Recovery of blood volume and osmolality after thermal dehydration in rats. *Am. J. Physiol.* 251:R492–R498, 1986.
Nose, H., T. Yawata and T. Morimoto. Osmotic factors in restitution from thermal dehydration in rats. *Am. J. Physiol.* 249:R166–R171, 1985.
Pappenheimer, J.R. Passage of molecules through capillary walls. *Physiol. Rev.* 33:387–423, 1953.
Phillips, P.A., B.J. Rolls, J.G. Ledingham, M.L. Forsling, J.J. Morton, M.J. Crowe, and L. Wollner. Reduced thirst after water deprivation in healthy elderly men. *New Engl. J. Med.* 311:753–759, 1984.
Pitts, R.F. *Physiology of the Kidney and Body Fluids*, 3rd Edition. Year Book, Chicago, 1974.
Pitts, G.C., R.E. Johnson and F.C. Consolazio. Work in the heat as affected by intake of water, salt and glucose. *Am. J. Physiol.* 142:253–259, 1944.
Rothstein, A., E.F. Adolph and J.H. Wills. Voluntary dehydration. In: *Physiology of Man in the Desert* (edited by E.F. Adolph et al.). Interscience, New York, 254–270, 1947.
Rothstein, A. and E.J. Towbin. Blood circulation and temperature of men dehydrating in the heat. In: *Physiology of Man in the Desert* (edited by E.F. Adolph et al.). Interscience, New York, 172–196, 1947.
Rowell, L.B., J.R. Blackmon, R.H. Martin, J.A. Mazzarella and R.A. Bruce. Hepatic clearances of indocyanine green in man under thermal and exercise stresses. *J. Appl. Physiol.* 20:384–394, 1965.
Ruch, T.C. and H.D. Patton. *Physiology and Biophysics*, 20th Edition. Saunders, Philadelphia, 1974.
Senay, L.C., Jr. Temperature regulation and hypohydration: a singular view. *J. Appl. Physiol.* 47:1–7, 1979.
Sherman, W.M. and D.R. Lamb. Nutrition and prolonged exercise. In: *Perspectives in Exercise Science and Sports Medicine. Volume 1. Prolonged Exercise* (edited by D.R. Lamb and R. Murray). Benchmark, Indianapolis, 213–280, 1988.

DISCUSSION

YOUSEF: The idea that saltiness of the sweat as related to the ability of an individual to rehydrate is well established. If we look at the change in the concentration of salt in the sweat with age, one finds that the elderly have a much saltier sweat. Thus many of the elderly who are participating in various long athletic events such as marathons and so on would seem to have a real problem. What would you recommend for these people?

NADEL: That's a good question. You pointed out in your recent letter to me that we should be concerned for the welfare of the elderly population. The direct answer is if these findings about the importance of sweat [Na^+] follow, we should expect the elderly with more concentrated sweat [Na^+] would suffer a greater loss of plasma volume during exercise and should be expected to perform less well relative to their younger counterparts, everything else being equal. The real question, as far as I'm concerned, is whether the changes in sweat sodium concentration are due to the aging process itself, and not to the increased inactivity that people generally experience as they become older. The necessary studies haven't been done. In the last ten years there have been a few studies, not only from your lab but also several other labs, which have concentrated on changes in physiological controls that occur with older people. Some of these changes are part of the aging process. For example, the changes in myocardial contractility documented by Lakatta. There may also be greater changes in plasma volume during exercise in older people, some of whom might be relatively dehydrated to begin with.

YOUSEF: Would you recommend addition of sodium to their drink?

NADEL: I think the jury is still out on this. Obviously, we are operating on two different levels here. Older people are told to have a sodium-free diet because high sodium in the diet is correlated with hypertension, so older people are being asked to avoid sodium. On the other hand, if people are sweating and losing sodium, it seems to me that they should increase their sodium intake. People in our discipline must be careful about determining whether sodium supplementation is important for older people. It may be important, for example, to the person who lives in Honolulu and is out on the tennis court.

YOUSEF: I think this is what I really wanted to say, because the recommendation to provide sodium in drinks should be qualified with age.

SUTTON: As a point of clarification, Ethan, in regard to Yousef's question, "Do we know how different the sweat sodium is in the elderly compared with younger persons?" Aging, per se, may be one factor, but if you take into account comparable levels of fitness, what influence does that actually have?

NADEL: I don't know the answer. I was going to suggest that Mo might know. Maybe instead of my guessing, Mo can tell us.

YOUSEF: It's very difficult to really have totally equal levels of fitness in young and old individuals. We have individuals who are above the age of 60 and have been in physical fitness programs for about 15 continuous years. These people do have a somewhat higher sodium in their sweat as compared to young individuals. The $\dot{V}O_2max$ of the two groups is not equal. It's very difficult to match $\dot{V}O_2max$ in young and old.

SUTTON: The only part I wanted to clarify was that in your presentation, you only compared sodium, and yet we heard yesterday about the importance of glucose in the salt contained drinks in terms of the absorption of sodium. Surely one of the important issues for experiments would be to test that combination.

NADEL: Yes. In fact, those studies have been done and Dave Costill with Sparks in 1973 and Taketeshi Morimoto have published several papers. There is a better rehydration drinking the glucose/electrolyte solution than when drinking water. The improved rehydration is similar to what we have found. The difference between those studies and ours is that it was not clear how the sweet taste of the glucose/electrolyte solution affected the drinking. In our study, we eliminated the sweet taste by eliminating carbohydrate from the solution and the salty taste by giving the salt in capsules. In this way, we allowed our subjects to drink ad lib and then studied the total fluid and electrolyte balance. As Ed Zambraski emphasized yesterday, we try to keep tabs on all of the electrolytes and water going into and out of the body. I'm not trying to diminish the importance of those studies, because obviously, when one is assessing drinking behavior, the taste is important. But, we tried to leave out the taste.

SCHEDL: I wondered, Ethan, if you could gain some other information from your data by considering the one subject who had the 105 milliequivalent sodium and chloride in the sweat, because I think he was almost two standard deviations from the median of the other cluster group. I wonder if he could have had some form of cystic fibrosis or maybe adrenogenital syndrome. Certainly he couldn't have been adrenally insufficient. But he might biochemically differ from the rest of the population.

NADEL: This fellow was at the top of the normal range. All of our people have to pass a very rigorous clinical examination to enter into the experimental protocol, so this fellow had no history of renal disease. Secondly, he was within the normal range. Granted, he was on the top end of the range, but Mo Yousef has in the past talked about how Dill and Hall had very different sweat sodium concentrations, and despite these differences, remained friends throughout their lives. I appreciate your point. One can learn a lot from studying outliers. I'd just like to come back to one earlier point, because I think it is important. The point about combining sodium and carbohydrates in solution is a good one. If we were to do this study again, it might be interesting and informative to add carbohydrate to the capsules so we could both eliminate the sweet taste and study rehydration with sodium and glucose.

HARVEY: I'd like to provide just a little clinical correlation to your last item on the hydration. With our elite cyclists, one of the things we found was that when they would cross the finish line after 4 or 6 h of cycling and literally fall off their bikes with heat illness or exhaustion, we found that by infusing 2–4 L of cold lactated Ringer's with glucose rapidly they would come around in 15–20 minutes. About the time you're hooking up the 2nd or 3rd liter, they're ready to leave the medical camp. Not only that, they get back on their bikes the next day and ride another 3 or 4 h. The results are so dramatic that our problem became, after a while, the team members coming in and feigning heat illness because they knew they could recover quicker with the IV. I think it would be interesting to extend your study by comparing oral hydration vs. IV hydration to repeated exercise bouts and see if we can't make people recover a lot quicker with a couple of liters of IV fluids rather than oral solution.

NADEL: I think that's a real good point. Obviously, when we're changing the body fluid compartments directly, by infusion, we're avoiding the delays that occur by gastric emptying and absorption.

KACHADORIAN: I want to return to some previous comments concerned with aging and the so-called "elderly." I think it is first of all important to separate conceptually aging from disease. Secondly, it's worth considering that the health of elderly represent different physiological categories and therefore it is unreasonable to group all people over a certain age, say 55 years, as a single homogenous group for the purpose of making dietary recommendations. If one is going to consider any kind of mineral replacement therapy for the "elderly," certain fundamental information appears necessary. First of all, who the elderly are needs to be defined and then in relation to this, the effect of the normal aging process with respect to dietary intake of minerals, calories, vitamins, etc. needs to be assessed. After this, one may then ask other questions about how adjustments for different kinds of activities and different kinds of environments should be made.

NADEL: I appreciate your raising this. Mo Yousef pointed out to me the 1974 paper by Phillips et al. in the *New England Journal of Medicine*. They showed that the elderly suffer some deficits in several organ systems. The question, of course, is separating the biological aging process from the increasing inactivity that most of our older population develops. Whether older people can change sweat sodium concentration the same way that younger people can by sweat gland training has not been studied as far as I know.

DAVIS: Ethan, my question is related specifically to the chapter and also to Sutton's comment. The title of your chapter is "Influence of Fluid Replacement Beverages on Body Fluid Homeostasis During Exercise and Recovery," and there is clearly an absence in the chapter of conventional fluid replacement beverages, the glucose/electrolyte beverages, and there are considerable recent papers on the issue of optimal fluid replacement beverages during exercise. Likewise, I think most of the stuff that is in here is on recovery. My question is, why was there a lack of information on conventional glucose/electrolyte replacement during exercise?

NADEL: You are right, Mark, and this comment was made to me by both of the reactors, Dave Lamb and Mo Yousef. In the rewrite of my chapter, I am including about half a dozen papers concerning fluid replacement during exercise. The chapter is titled "Body Fluid Homeostasis," and the problem is that most of the papers in the area have not been overly concerned with body fluid homeostasis, but rather with performance. So in trying to examine body fluid homeostasis, I'm still at a bit of a loss, because there haven't been a lot of good studies. I thought it best to leave the performance papers to Mike Sawka, and he covered them quite well.

GISOLFI: Do the elderly have a greater sodium concentration in their sweat compared with their younger counterparts? You directed this question to Yousef, but I did not hear the answer.

YOUSEF: My answer was: the only data that I'm aware of is the information that was collected on Dill, Hall, and Consolazio. In these three subjects, although the saltiness of their sweat was quite variable in their young age group, the concentration of salt increased with aging. I think the only reason for increased sweat saltiness in elderly may be associated with decreased adrenal cortical activity. Evidence to support this hypothesis comes from Dill who had asthma and was treated by an injection of a long-lasting adrenal cortical preparation. As soon as he received the injection, his sweat sodium concentration decreased immediately. At the end of three months postinjection, sweat sodium concentration increased significantly. This observation was repeated several times.

GISOLFI: Can a person prehydrate to prepare for a potentially dehydrating activity?

NADEL: That's a good question, Carl. I didn't include in my talk the questions about prehydration before exercise. Clearly prehydration is possible but difficult. The question is how to best prehydrate before an activity. Water and salt intake prior to activity may produce a natruresis and diuresis by influencing the volume receptors on the low pressure side of the heart. It's going to be fairly difficult to overhydrate significantly prior to exercise.

GISOLFI: In the past, people have tried to overhydrate just with water. Should we include electrolytes in a prehydration beverage?

NADEL: I think the jury is still out on that. Overhydration with water is obviously ill-advised because one will dilute the plasma, and inhibit antidiuretic hormone stimulation and there will be a large diuresis. It should be better to prehydrate with electrolytes. We should be able to prehydrate to a certain extent by moving up the isotonic line. In other words, ingest sodium at the proper concentration to maintain plasma isotonicity. But, this probably will stimulate a natriuresis and diuresis eventually.

COSTILL: Since a lot of your calculations on ion exchange and the effects of sodium loss depend upon the method you use to measure or estimate the losses, can you identify the difference between forearm or hand sweat and whole body losses? In most studies that compare the two methods, there is a remarkable difference between the ion losses from the forearm and the whole body (washdown technique).

NADEL: That is a valid criticism, Dave. We weren't using whole body washdowns. We were collecting sweat from arm bag samples. We changed the arm bag at frequent intervals to prevent sweat gland fatigue. We are using these to estimate whole body sodium concentrations in sweat.

SAWKA: I have a question and a comment. You say that with the sodium replacement in fluids that there was preferential expansion of plasma volume. As I look at your data, it seems that the expansion of plasma volume follows the expansion of the extracellular fluid volume, not necessarily plasma. Secondly, and more important to me, often you see dehydration, but not always a decrease in total circulating protein.

When you gave the individual the sodium and you reestablished interstitial volume as well as plasma volume, did you look at total circulating protein? Were proteins washing back into the vascular volume and did that help to maintain plasma volume?

NADEL: The plasma protein concentrations followed the red cell concentrations reasonably well, so without having made those calculations the way you are asking, my guess is that there were no dramatic changes in the total protein content.

SAWKA: Did the protein content stay constant?

NADEL: That's my guess.

SAWKA: Then you probably have sufficient changes in the total circulating protein mass.

NADEL: No, sorry. Plasma protein concentration increased with dehydration and then protein dilution occurred with water intake and so the total protein, my guess is, didn't change dramatically.

PHILLIPS: How quickly did the changes occur in recovery? It seems that they occurred almost immediately. If they occur immediately, that's too quick for the changes to be affected by absorption. Yesterday I mentioned that there is an oral pharyngeal reflex that occurs when you have water in the mouth, the blood pressure goes up. I'm wondering whether as soon as you have water in the mouth, maybe there is a neuroreflex that causes the change from one compartment to the other. It seems to me that your changes began awfully fast.

NADEL: The changes in the concentration of sodium and water in the plasma compartment were significant somewhere between 15–30 minutes after drinking water. Those were the most rapid changes. It seems to me that this is within the realm for gastric emptying and the absorption processes to occur. Nonetheless, I quite agree with your statement that there are other reflexes besides the volume and osmolality receptor inputs to the central nervous system. For example, these people drank a tremendous amount within the first 10–15 minutes and then the drinking rates decreased dramatically. If you plot drinking behavior as a function of plasma volume changes or the plasma osmolality changes, you will have a variable relationship; I think that is your point. The oropharyngeal reflex is important.

ZAMBRASKI: My question concerns the stimulus for the diuresis seen in your subjects when they received the oral infusions. By comparing the oral versus intravenous routes of administration, one can evaluate the possibility of an oropharyngeal reflex mediating this response. If that were the case, the diuresis should have been minimal, or greatly reduced, with the intravenous infusion.

NADEL: We did measure urine volumes following saline infusion during exercise. Urine volume during the infusion study was 40% and 70% greater than in the control, no infusion study in the 30°C and 22°C environments, respectively.

TIPTON: Ethan, you have the term homeostasis in your title. Consequently, I'd like to know when complete rehydration occurs after 3 L of fluid has been lost because of dehydration? Do you have any evidence on the intracellular and extracellular electrolyte concentrations after 3 h as I don't think your subjects had returned to baseline values in that time period?

NADEL: Three hours is certainly not enough time to rehydrate given the model that we used, with the rehydration drink containing 450 mg/100 mL of sodium. This wasn't enough to provide for restoration of the control state. Even with sodium in the rehydration drink, the people weren't able to restore the body water lost during the 3 h of recovery from dehydration. The question which remains is, "if they could restore the potassium that was lost, would they then restore the volume lost from the intracellular fluid compartments?" I don't know the answer to that question. The other important point is that without the sodium in the rehydration drink, the dilution of the blood that occurred as the water was absorbed removed the thirst drive completely. Simultaneously, and probably as important, is that blood dilution stimulates the kidneys to increase filtering and there follows a diuresis.

CONVERTINO: The time course and ability to replace body fluid losses may depend upon the manner in which the dehydration is brought about. In a heat/exercise acclimation study, we followed the 24 h recovery of body fluids in subjects after they had been exposed to exercising for 2 h at 50% of their maximal oxygen uptake in 42°C heat. At 24 h post-exercise, the subjects had completely recovered their plasma volume and body weight losses. In fact, there was a slight expansion of total body water of about 250 mL. These results suggest that rehydration can be rapid if induced by exercise and/or heat exposure. However, effective rehydration may be slower if dehydration is induced voluntarily. For instance, we observed that 4 days of voluntary dehydration and average loss of 8 kg body weight in wrestlers was not reversed by 3 days of voluntary rehydration. These results may raise the issue that effective rehydration may depend upon the stimulus of dehydration.

NADEL: I think much of the issue with rehydration concerns the solutes. The solute content in the body is going to determine the water content. If we're getting back the sodium lost in the sweat, then we can restore the compartment that is the sodium-containing compartment. This is the extracellular fluid compartment. We already know there is tremendous variability among us in our sweat sodium concentrations, and another variability induced by our level of training. Maybe the average sweat sodium is somewhere around 45–65 milliequivalents/L. The potassium concentration in sweat seems to range between 5–10 milliequivalents/L. Maybe we have to provide potassium in the rehydration drink to restore the volume lost from the intracellular compartment. Transiently, the intracellular fluid compartment can be shrunk to restore the extracellular fluid compartment, but eventually, it is the potassium content that determines the volume of the intracellular fluid compartment. I think 3 h is certainly too short for complete rehydration to occur, considering our model.

6

Hormonal Control of Blood Volume During and Following Exercise

CHARLES E. WADE, PH.D.

BEAU J. FREUND, PH.D.

INTRODUCTION

Blood volume is often decreased during heavy or prolonged exercise, particularly if dehydration occurs. The reduction in blood volume, predominantly due to changes in plasma volume, is initially the result of shifts among the various fluid compartments of the body. Thus, fluid may be translocated from one compartment to another without a net loss in total body fluids. Sweating during prolonged exercise eventually results in a net loss of body fluids predominantly due to sweating. Thus, blood volume is decreased during exercise due to the movement of fluid out of the vascular space as well as to the actual loss of fluids from the body via sweating. Following exercise, the loss of fluids is usually replaced within 24 h and with repeated daily exercise exposure, blood and plasma volume may be expanded.

The reduction of plasma volume during exercise and the subsequent rectification of this loss during recovery are mediated in part by hormonal mechanisms. In this chapter the following aspects will be considered: 1) endocrine responses to exercise, 2) fluid shifts during exercise, 3) fluid losses during exercise, 4) hormonal regulation of fluid alterations during exercise, 5) hormonally mediated rectification of the fluid losses following exercise, and 6) influence of hormones on the blood volume adaptations to exercise training.

ENDOCRINE RESPONSES TO EXERCISE

The intent of this chapter is to provide a summary of the responses of those hormones that may play a role in the regulation of blood volume during and following exercise. The hormones of interest are the sympatho-adrenal hormones, the renin-angiotensin system, aldosterone, vasopressin, cortisol, histamine, kinins, and prostaglandins (Share, 1974; Share & Claybaugh, 1972; Weitzman & Kleeman, 1980). There have been reviews of hormonal responses to exercise that provide a more comprehensive treatment than is possible here, e.g., Galbo (1983), Viru (1985), Wade et al. (1989), Bunt (1986), Francesconi (1988), and Sutton & Farrell (1988).

In response to exercise, the increase in the plasma concentrations of a hormone is usually interpreted as an increase in secretion of the hormone. However, other contributing factors may also be altered by exercise and should be considered as potential sources for the increase in the circulating levels of a hormone. For example, a decrease in plasma volume may account in part for an increase in hormone concentrations present in plasma because the quantity of hormone released by an endocrine organ would be distributed in a smaller volume. This explanation may apply if the hormones are distributed only in the vascular compartment. However, many hormones are of low molecular weight (less than 30,000) or can pass through cellular membranes, thereby permitting relatively free distribution outside of the vascular space (Renkin, 1985). Thus, plasma levels of such hormones are assumed to be indicative of hormone concentrations in extracellular fluid as well. Other hormones, however, are bound to plasma proteins; in these cases hormone concentrations in plasma may reflect changes in plasma volume during exercise. To calculate changes in total circulating content of those hormones limited to the vascular space, the effects of plasma volume changes may be quantified by using published equations (Harrison, 1985).

A decrease in the clearance or metabolism of a hormone may account in part for an increase in the plasma concentrations of the hormone during exercise. The concentration of a circulating hormone is a function of the rate at which the hormone is released from an endocrine organ and the rate at which it is cleared from the system. Though the clearance of hormones has not been well studied during exercise, it can be assumed that the rate of clearance is reduced because blood flow to organs such as the liver and kidneys, which are important in the metabolism and excretion of various hormones, is reduced (Rowell, 1974). Therefore, a decrease in the clearance of a hormone may account in part for an increase in plasma hormone levels during exercise.

During exercise, the actions of hormones are dependent upon interaction with a hormone "receptor." Alterations in access of the hormone to receptors may be affected by factors such as the redistribution of blood flow during exercise. A change in the number of the receptors for a specific hormone could also occur during exercise, thus affecting the activity of the hormones. Alteration in the number of receptors for hormones due to exercise has not yet been extensively investigated.

The volume of, distribution of, clearance of, and number of receptors for a hormone must be considered when interpreting the responses of the endocrine systems to exercise. In the present chapter, the absolute plasma concentrations and the above outlined contributing or confounding factors have been used in an attempt to explain the actions of the various hormones in the regulation of blood volume during and following exercise.

A. Sympatho-Adrenal System

Plasma catecholamines, i.e., norepinephrine and epinephrine, are derived from the adrenal medulla as well as the sympathetic nervous system and are collectively referred to as the sympatho-adrenal system. In response to exercise, both catecholamines are progressively increased as the intensity of the exercise is increased (Figure 6-1) (Bouissou et al., 1987; Svedenhag, 1985; Kotchen et al., 1971; Viru, 1985; Pluto et al., 1988; Galbo, 1983; Galbo et al., 1975; von Euler, 1974; Clutter et al., 1980). In response to maximal exercise, plasma norepinephrine levels are increased from 300–400 pg/mL at rest to 1,000–2,500 pg/mL (Kotchen et al., 1971; Viru, 1985; Galbo et al., 1975; Galbo, 1983). Plasma epinephrine concentrations increase from 30–80 pg/mL at rest to 400–700 pg/mL following maximal exercise (Kotchen et al., 1971; Viru, 1985; Galbo, 1983; Galbo et al., 1975). The duration of exercise also influences the response to catecholamines; submaximal exercise of long duration results in circu-

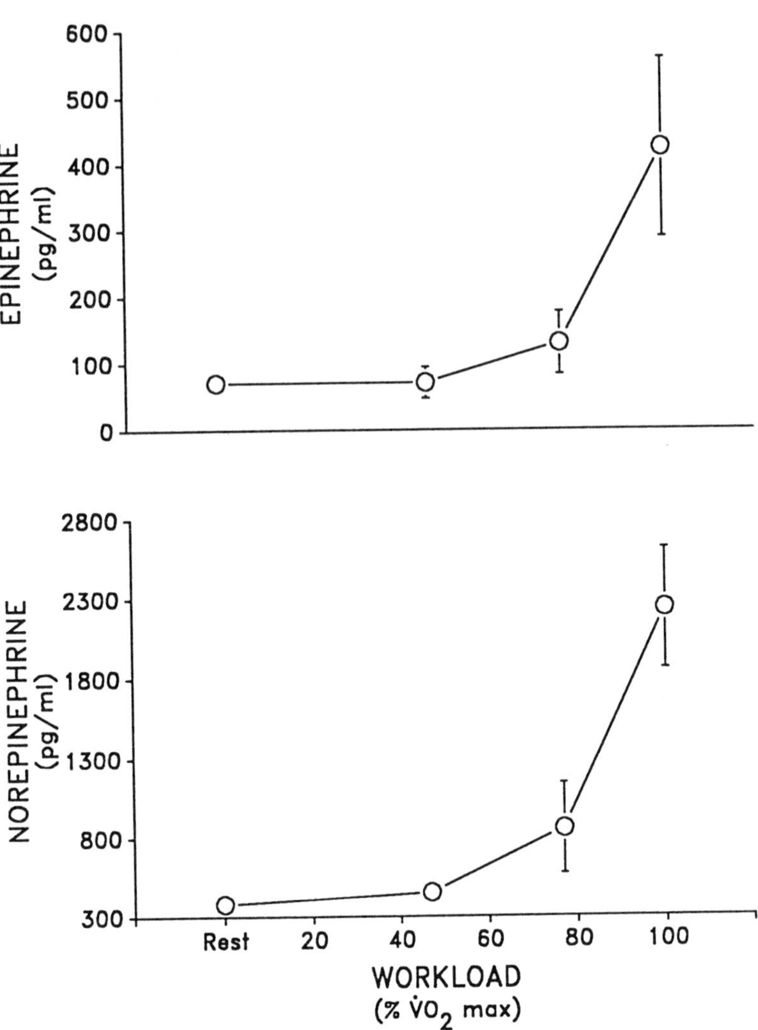

FIGURE 6-1. *Responses of plasma norepinephrine and epinephrine concentrations to graded exercise on a bicycle ergometer. (Redrawn from data of Galbo, 1983; Galbo et al., 1975.)*

lating catecholamine levels as great as those attained during brief, maximal exercise (Galbo et al., 1975). Catecholamines modulate the mobilization of metabolic substrates, cardiovascular responses, and the activity of other endocrine glands during exercise (Schnabel et al., 1984; Staessen et al., 1987; Svedenhag, 1985; Hespel et al., 1986; Manhem & Hoekfelt, 1981; Viru, 1985; Clutter et al., 1980). Blockade of cholinergic receptors, specifically beta receptors, results in a decrease in the plasma concentrations of glucose, free fatty acids, and lactate during the performance of exercise when compared to the unblocked state (Schnabel et al., 1984). Further, blockade leads to a decrease in heart rate at any given workload and may decrease blood pressure (Staessen et al., 1987; Hespel et al., 1986). Finally, the sympatho-adrenal system may influence the release of hormones. This is demonstrated by the reduced response of the renin-angiotensin system to standard exercise loads following beta blockage (Zambraski et al., 1984). Catecholamines thus have a multifaceted role in the regulation of responses to exercise.

B. Renin-Angiotensin System

Renin (an enzyme) is released from the juxtaglomerular apparatus of the kidneys and subsequently converts angiotensinogen to angiotensin I (Reid, 1984; Reid & Ganong, 1977). Angiotensin I is further converted to angiotension II (AII) in the lung by a converting enzyme. During exercise, this cascade is potentiated (Convertino et al., 1980a, 1981, 1983; Fagard et al., 1985a, 1985b; Geyssant et al., 1981; Freund et al., 1987a; Costill et al., 1976; Staessen et al., 1987; Adlercreutz et al., 1976; Kosunen & Pakarinen, 1976; Tanaka et al., 1986; Wade & Claybaugh, 1980; Wade et al., 1981, 1987; Castenfors, 1967a, 1967b, 1978). In response to maximal exercise, plasma renin activity (PRA) and angiotensin II levels both increased 5- to 10-fold (Fagard et al., 1985; Staessen et al., 1987; Tanaka et al., 1986). Plasma renin activity (PRA) is increased in response to workloads above a threshold corresponding to about 70% of $\dot{V}O_2max$ (Fig. 6-2) (Shvartz et al., 1981; Thomas & Etheridge, 1982; Wade & Claybaugh, 1980; Tanaka et al., 1986; Gleim et al., 1984).

Gleim and coworkers (1984) have correlated the increase in PRA with the attainment of the anaerobic threshold as determined by plasma lactate levels. The increase in PRA is correlated with the increase in angiotensin II during exercise (Staessen et al., 1987; Reid & Ganong, 1977), and it has been inferred that this increase in PRA is responsible for the increase in AII levels. This may not always be true because the responses have sometimes been dissociated. Fagard et al. (1985) have noted that in trained subjects, the response of PRA to exercise was not different from that in untrained controls, but the increase in AII was attenuated in the trained subjects. The reason for this disparity is not clear.

Several factors affect the response of the renin-angiotensin system to exercise (Wade & Claybaugh, 1980; Wade et al., 1987). The duration of the exercise may influence the response. Wade and Claybaugh (1980) noted that 20 min of exercise at 35% of maximum heart rate failed to alter PRA, whereas after 60 min an increase was reported. Convertino et al. (1980a, 1981) found that 2 h of cycle ergometry exercise at 65% of $\dot{V}O_2max$ increased PRA to 12 ng AI/mL x h compared to 7.5 hg AI/mL x h following 6 min at 90% $\dot{V}O_2max$.

The posture and type of exercise also influence the PRA response to exercise. Guezennec and co-workers (1986) found that maximal treadmill running increased PRA from 4.4 to 24.9 ng AI/mL x h, whereas max-

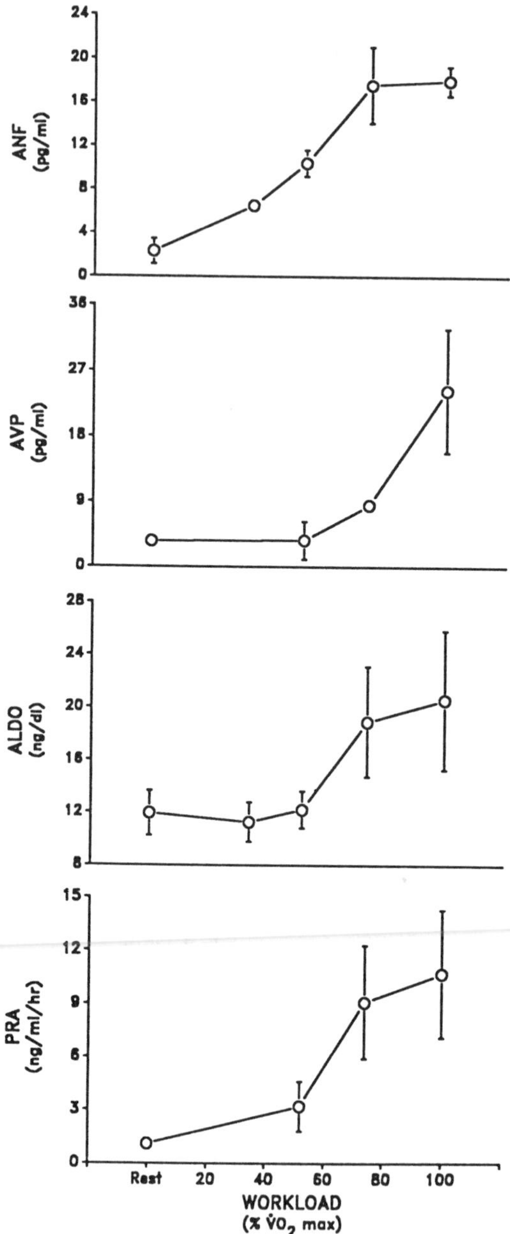

FIGURE 6-2. *Responses of plasma vasopressin, atrial natriuretic factor, aldosterone, and renin activity to graded exercise on a bicycle ergometer. (Redrawn from data of Tanaka et al., 1986.)*

imal swimming for a similar duration only resulted in an increase from 3.7 to 12.5 ng AI/mL x h.

The responsiveness of the renin-angiotensin system is regulated by the sympatho-adrenal system (Leenen et al., 1978; Bozovic & Castenfors, 1967; Manhem & Hoekfelt, 1981; Hespel et al., 1986; Zambraski et al., 1984) and is modulated by a variety of other factors. Activation of the renin-angiotensin system is consistently observed during and after exercise; it may function as an important modulator of the blood pressure response to exercise as well as a stimulus to the release of aldosterone during exercise (Wade et al., 1987; Reid & Ganong, 1977). Further, in animals angiotensin II has been shown to be a powerful stimulant of thirst (Adolph, 1967; Andersson, 1978; Denton, 1967; Reid, 1984; Stricker & Verbalis, 1988) and may have a function in the replacement of fluid losses following exercise.

C. Aldosterone

Plasma aldosterone concentrations are increased in response to exercise (Adlercreutz et al., 1976; Boudou et al., 1987; Brandenberger et al., 1986; Fagard et al., 1985b; Freund et al., 1987a; Geyssant et al., 1981; Costill et al., 1976; Kosunen & Pakarinen, 1976; Maher et al., 1975; Meehan, 1986; Melin et al., 1980; Tanaka et al., 1986; Staessen et al., 1987; Wade et al., 1987). Aldosterone is released from the adrenal cortex in response to increases in the circulating levels of angiotensin II, ACTH, and potassium or to a decrease in total body sodium (Reid & Ganong, 1977). In normal subjects, the increase in aldosterone in response to exercise mirrors that of renin and angiotensin II. Resting levels of aldosterone are highly variable and are dependent upon diurnal variation and sodium intake. Acute maximal exercise results in a two- to five-fold increase in plasma levels of aldosterone (Figure 6-2). The duration of exercise is a crucial factor in this response; submaximal exercise of long duration can elicit increases greater than those seen during brief maximal exercise. (Boudou et al., 1987; Wade et al., 1985; Fellman et al., 1988).

Of note is that the increase in plasma aldosterone during exercise persists for hours after exercise, unlike other hormones which return to resting concentration within 60 to 90 min after exercise (Wade et al., 1985; Costill et al., 1976). Exercise training typically does not affect plasma levels of aldosterone at rest (Freund et al., 1987a, 1988b; Geyssant et al., 1981; Melin et al., 1980). The response to exercise at similar relative workloads is likewise unaffected by training (Freund et al., 1987a; Geyssant et al., 1981; Melin et al., 1980). Interestingly, following prolonged heavy exercise by individuals unaccustomed to such demands, resting levels of aldosterone may be increased for at least 24 h (Wade et al., 1981, 1985).

The increase in circulating aldosterone levels during exercise may be important in the regulation of sodium reabsorption by the kidneys (Reid & Ganong, 1977; Morris, 1981) and possibly by the sweat glands (Kirby & Convertino, 1986; Collins, 1969; Reid & Ganong, 1977; Morris, 1981).

D. Vasopressin

The response of vasopressin to exercise has previously been reviewed by Wade (1984). The plasma levels of vasopressin are consistently reported to be elevated during exercise (Wade, 1984; Davies et al., 1981; Wade & Claybaugh, 1980; Tanaka et al., 1986; Wade et al., 1987; Convertino et al., 1980, 1981, 1983; Goetz et al., 1982). This increase in vasopressin release from the neurohypophysis appears to be mediated primarily by the increase in plasma osmolality accompanying exercise, though such factors as hydration status and posture of the subject can alter this relationship (Wade, 1984).

Vasopressin is released at workloads greater than 70% of $\dot{V}O_2max$, increasing progressively as exercise intensity increases (Fig. 6-2) (Wade, 1984; Convertino et al., 1981, 1983; Tanaka et al., 1986; Wade & Claybaugh, 1980). Vasopressin levels are increased from 1–2 pg/mL at rest to 8–20 pg/mL immediately following brief maximal exercise. The duration of exercise also affects plasma vasopressin levels; 60 min of exercise at 70% of maximal heart rate results in plasma vasopressin concentrations similar to those following maximal exercise of 20 min duration (Wade & Claybaugh, 1980).

Neither resting nor maximal exercise vasopressin concentrations are altered by physical training (Freund et al., 1987a; Convertino et al., 1981, 1983; Geyssant et al., 1981; Melin et al., 1980). Of interest is that the response of vasopressin is highly variable among subjects but is highly consistent within an individual (Maresh et al., 1985).

The increase in vasopressin in response to exercise may be important in the regulation of blood pressure, the handling of fluids by the kidneys and sweat glands, and the expansion of blood volume following exercise training (Legros et al., 1972; Baylis, 1987; Weitzman & Gleeman, 1980; Convertino et al., 1980a, 1980b; Schlein et al, 1971; Gibiniski et al., 1979; Fasciolo et al., 1969).

E. Atrial Natriuretic Peptide

The response of atrial natriuretic peptide to exercise has recently been reviewed by Freund et al. (1988c). Atrial natriuretic peptide (also referred to as atrial natriuretic factor, ANF) is increased in response to acute bouts of exercise (Freund et al., 1987a, 1988c; Somers et al., 1986; Petzl et al., 1987; Tanaka et al., 1986). Plasma levels of ANF are progressively increased during exercise in relation to exercise intensity (Figure 6-2). From resting values ranging from 10 to 45 pg/mL, ANF is increased to 70 to 90 pg/mL in response to the maximal exercise (Freund et al.,

1988a, 1988c; Tanaka et al., 1986). ANF is released from the atria in response to distention resulting from an increase in blood pressure or mechanical manipulations (Goetz, 1988). The initial increase in ANF during exercise is related to an increase in atrial volume or pressure (Freund et al., 1988c).

It has also been proposed that ANF is released during exercise as a response to increased heart rate (Somers et al., 1986; Saito et al., 1987). This role of tachycardia in regulating ANF during exercise is not clear but most likely reflects the direct relationship between an increase in heart rate and atrial pressure during acute exercise (Freund et al., 1988c; Thamsborg et al., 1987a, 1987b). Of note is the transitory characteristic of the increase in ANF during prolonged exercise. For instance, Freund et al., (1988a, 1988c) found an increase from baseline in ANF during the first 10 km of a marathon run, but not at the end of the race. Chan and co-workers (1988) reported the plasma concentrations of ANF to be decreased at the end of a marathon race. Thus, the duration of the exercise appears to play an important role in the response of ANF.

The actions of ANF during exercise are not yet clear. ANF may play a role in the diuresis and natriuresis that has been reported with low-intensity exercise (Freund et al., 1988c). In addition, ANF has powerful vasodilatory actions and may be important in modulating the blood pressure response to exercise (Freund et al., 1988c; Goetz, 1988). ANF also reduces plasma volume independently of renal effects (Weidmann et al., 1986) and hence may be involved in the translocation of fluid out of the vascular space during acute exercise. ANF may modulate the release of other hormones (Cuneo et al., 1986; Gaebelein & Senay, 1980; Samson, 1985), affect the satiation of thirst (Castenfors, 1967b; Januszewicz et al., 1986a, 1986b; Katsuura et al., 1986; Masotto & Negro-Vilar, 1985), and influence the secretion of fluid and electrolytes from sweat glands (Freund et al., 1988c).

F. Cortisol

The adrenal-cortical hormone, cortisol, is reported to be both increased and unchanged in response to exercise (Buono et al., 1987; Wade & Claybaugh, 1980; Wade et al., 1987; Luger et al., 1987; von Euler, 1974; Crandall & Gregg, 1986; Brandenberger et al., 1986). The variability in the reports concerning exercise is the result of a variety of factors such as diurnal variations, fitness levels of the subjects, and relationship of the exercise test to the last meal (Sutton & Farrell, 1988).

The increase in cortisol as a response to exercise is regulated by adrenocorticotropic hormone (ACTH) (Luger et al., 1987; Buono et al., 1987). However, ACTH levels may be increased during exercise in the absence of a change in plasma cortisol concentrations (Wade et al., 1987). This absence of an increase in cortisol may reflect a training-induced decrease in adrenal sensitivity to ACTH. For example, in response to exercise at 90% of $\dot{V}O_2max$ by trained and untrained subjects, similar increases in ACTH were observed, yet the cortisol response was attenuated in the trained subjects (Luger et al., 1987).

The duration of the exercise may also influence the response of cortisol. At submaximal workloads, Brandenberger et al. (1986) demonstrated that exercise of long duration increases cortisol.

The actions of elevated cortisol during exercise could be the modulation of cellular metabolism and gluconeogenesis as well as the alteration of cellular permeability (Bealer et al., 1985; Hartley et al., 1972; von Euler, 1974; Galbo, 1983).

G. Prostaglandins

Prostaglandins in the circulation are increased seven- to ten-fold following brief maximal exercise (Staessen et al., 1987; Demers et al., 1981; Fagard et al., 1985a; Kiyonaga et al., 1985; Nowak & Wennmalm, 1989). The increase is due to prostaglandin synthesis as shown by the fact that administration of indomethacin, a synthesis inhibitor, can inhibit the rise in prostaglandin levels during exercise (Staessen et al., 1987). The regulation of prostaglandins during exercise is unclear.

Prostaglandins modulate the release and actions of other hormones, have a direct action on the renal handling of sodium, and affect capillary permeability (Bealer et all, ; Dabney et al., 1988; Bolger et al., 1976, 1978; Crandall & Gregg, 1986). It is postulated that increases in prostaglandin concentrations during exercise result in similar actions.

H. Histamine

Histamine levels may be increased or unchanged during strenuous exercise (Morgan et al., 1983; Hartley et al., 1981; Barnes & Brown, 1981; Pavlik et al., 1978). Mast cells release histamine in response to a variety of stimuli, but the mechanism of release during exercise is unclear. There is a 50% increase in plasma histamine concentrations in normal subjects performing exercise on a bicycle ergometer at a heart rate of 146 b/min (Barnes & Brown, 1981). The renal excretion of histamine is also increased following heavy exercise.

Exercise training has not been shown to change the response of histamine to exercise, but training apparently suppresses cardiovascular responses to exogenously administered histamine (Morganroth et al., 1977). When both trained and untrained subjects were injected with histamine, the trained subjects experienced blunted increases in blood pressure and heart rate when compared to the untrained subjects. This suggests a change in receptor sensitivity.

An increase in histamine levels during exercise may affect the distribution of blood flow and permeability of capillaries (Bealer et al., 1985; Dabney et al., 1988).

I. Kinins

Kinins are increased in the circulation during exercise, at least in trained persons (Viru, 1985). The production of kinins from circulating globulins is mediated by a variety of proteolytic enzymes. As the kinins are short-lived, the changes are inferred from changes in the levels of the various kinases and kallikrein. The response of kinins to exercise may also be influenced by the training status of the subjects. The circulating levels of kinases tend to be reduced at rest in trained subjects and to be increased during exercise, whereas untrained subjects may exhibit a decrease during exercise (Viru, 1985).

Kinins are powerful vasoactive agents and seem to participate in the generation of the pain signal in response to tissue damage (Bealer et al., 1985). Bradykinin may play a role in the vasodilatation of local vascular beds and may modulate the actions of prostaglandins during exercise (Fossion et al., 1982). The significance of an increase in kinins during exercise has yet to be clarified; they may play a role in the redistribution of blood flow.

J. Effects of Exercise Training

Hormonal responses to exercise persist following training. As noted in Figures 6-1 and 6-2, the increase in the circulating concentrations of the various hormones is a function of the intensity of the exercise in relation to the subject's $\dot{V}O_2max$. Following exercise training, there is usually no alteration of hormone concentrations at rest or during maximal exercise (Convertino, 1983; Freund et al., 1987a, 1988; Galbo, 1983; Geyssant et al., 1981; Melin et al., 1980; Svedenhag, 1985). Further, there is no change with training in the hormonal response to the same relative intensity (% $\dot{V}O_2max$) of exercise (Convertino, 1983; Freund et al., 1987a; Svendenhag, 1985). However, at a given absolute workload (a lower % $\dot{V}O_2max$), the plasma concentration of a hormone is typically reduced following training. Most studies of the effects of training on hormonal responses are cross-sectional studies or involve exercise training of short duration with accompanying secondary factors; some of these factors may influence the responses of the hormones.

K. Summary

During exercise, increased concentrations of several hormones in the circulation suggest that they may contribute to the regulation of blood volume. Unfortunately, the role of these hormones in the modulation of blood volume during and following exercise must often be inferred. Investigations have focused on the responses of the specific hormones rather than on the actions of the hormones. Further, specific inhibitors of the synthesis or actions of a number of these hormones have not been available or have only recently been derived and have yet to be applied to the question of changes during exercise. In patients with various endocrine disorders, the study of exercise responses has been complicated because other endocrine systems are also compromised.

CHANGES IN BLOOD VOLUME DURING EXERCISE

The following discussion of the endocrine regulation of blood volume is often based upon inference from observations of hormone interactions in the resting state. These observations at rest may have little to do with exercise. An example of this complication might be the concomitant increase in aldosterone and ANF during exercise. Aldosterone is an antinatriuretic hormone, but ANF is natriuretic. The interaction of these hormones in the antinatriuresis associated with low-intensity exercise of short duration (10–30 min) has yet to be defined. The following discussion must be tempered in light of these limitations.

For the purpose of this discussion the responses of blood volume to exercise will be divided into four phases: 1) the acute shift at the onset of exercise; 2) the loss of fluids during exercise; 3) the rectification of fluid losses following exercise; and 4) fluid alterations caused by training. These phases represent unique changes in blood volume that may involve different endocrine systems.

A. Acute Shifts

There is usually a reduction in plasma volume caused by the redistribution of body fluids from the vascular space to the extravascular space within 5–10 min of the commencement of exercise. This movement of fluid out of the vascular compartment appears to be dependent on the intensity and type of exercise (Figure 6-3) (Sejersted et al., 1986; Fortney et al., 1981, 1983, 1984, 1988; Fortney & Vroman, 1985; Convertino et al., 1981, 1983; Miles et al., 1983; Senay et al., 1980; Wilkerson et al., 1977, 1982; Wade et al., 1987; Gaebelein & Senay, 1980, 1982; Wells et al., 1982). Harrison (1985, 1986) has emphasized the importance of experimental procedures, such as changes in posture, hydration status of the subjects, and methods of measurement in the evaluation of the acute changes in blood volume in response to exercise.

Bicycle ergometry at 100% $\dot{V}O_2max$ causes a 10–20% decrease in plasma volume (Bouissou et al., 1987; Convertino et al., 1981, 1983; Miles et al., 1983; Senay et al., 1980). This change corresponds to a 450–600 mL reduction in blood volume in a 70-kg man. Exercise of a short duration (0.5–3.0 min) at loads greater than 100% $\dot{V}O_2max$ decreases plasma volume by 10–11% (Green et al., 1984; Rotstein et al., 1982; Mohsenin & Gonzales, 1984). The rapid reduction of plasma volume in this and other studies emphasizes that the reduction is the result of fluid shifts rather than the actual loss of fluids from the body. The reduction in plasma volume induced by cycle ergometry is greater with

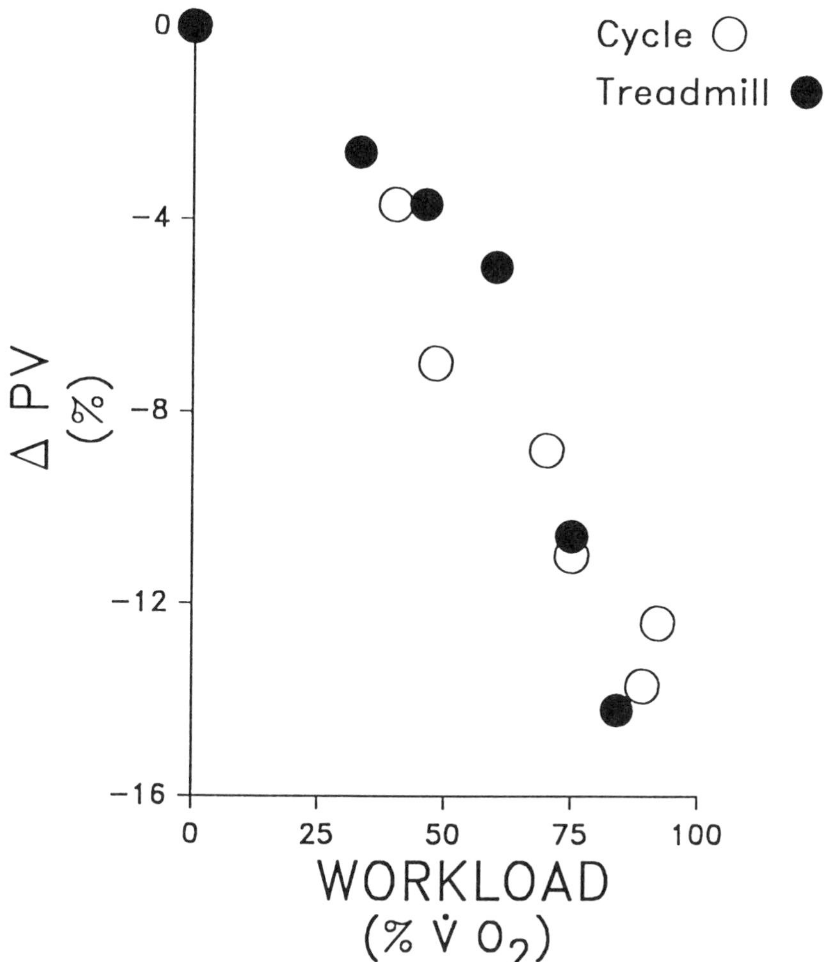

FIGURE 6-3. *Percent change of plasma volume in response to graded exercise (%VO_2max) performed on a bicycle ergometer or treadmill. (Redrawn from data of Wilkerson et al., 1977, 1982; Convertino et al., 1981, 1983.)*

greater loads (Pivarnik et al., 1985, 1988; Gaebelein & Senay, 1982; Miles et al., 1983; van Beaumont et al., 1981).

The change in plasma volume during maximal treadmill exercise is similar to the 10–20% decrease observed during cycle ergometer exercise (Galbo et al., 1975; Greenleaf et al., 1978; Wade & Claybaugh, 1980; Wilkerson et al., 1977, 1982). Harrison (1985) has suggested that this change was caused in many studies by subject movement from the seated position to standing. This comment is derived from the observation of Edwards and Harrison (1984) that subjects who stood unsupported and as motionless as possible for 20 min prior to prolonged running on the treadmill experienced no further decrease in plasma volume during exercise. Similar effects of postural changes on plasma volume were also documented earlier by Hagen et al. (1980). The absence of exercise-induced plasma volume changes in these studies and those of others may be attributed to prolonged motionless standing, which facilitates the movement of fluid into the extravascular space as a result of hydrostatic forces. Most studies demonstrate a decrease in plasma volume during treadmill exercise (Galbo et al., 1975; Greenleaf et al., 1978; Wade & Claybaugh, 1980; Wilkerson et al. 1977, 1982; Wade et al., 1987). The decrease in plasma volume during treadmill exercise is also a function of the intensity of exercise, i.e. greater reductions are observed at higher workloads (Wilkerson et al., 1977, 1982; Atherton et al., 1971; Wade & Claybaugh, 1980).

The similarity of the immediate decrease of 10–20% in plasma volume during maximal running or cycling exercise over short durations has suggested that there may be a limit to the hemoconcentration (Harrison, 1985). Maximal leg exercise with and without additional arm exercise results in a similar reduction in plasma volume (Wong et al., 1985). Miles and co-workers (1983) compared reductions in plasma volume during arm exercise with those during leg exercise and found arm exercise to result in a greater hemoconcentration at a given oxygen uptake. However, arm exercise caused a greater increase in mean arterial pressure than leg exercise at a given oxygen uptake. When differences in blood pressure responses were adjusted, the decreases in plasma volume were of the same magnitude (Figure 6-4). Exercise such as weight lifting, bench stepping, swimming, and canoeing also reduce plasma volume (Collins et al., 1986; Fulgraff et al., 1974; Knowlton et al., 1987; Gaebelein & Senay, 1982; Nielsen et al., 1984). The consistency of the decrease in plasma volume during various types of maximal exercise suggests that the response may be limited.

The acute shifts in plasma volume are assumed to be a function of the alteration in Starling forces (Starling, 1896; Sawka, 1988; Harrison, 1985; Mohsenin & Gonzalez, 1984; Bealer et al., 1985). These forces and their effects on the movement of fluid may be expressed as:

$$F=k[(P_c-P_i)-(O_c-O_i)]$$

where F= fluid flow rate

K= capillary filtration coefficient, which is a function of the permeability and surface area of the capillaries

P_c= capillary hydrostatic pressure

P_i= interstitial hydrostatic pressure

O_c= plasma colloid oncotic pressure

O_i= interstitial colloid oncotic pressure

Modulation of these forces presumably results in the shift of fluid among

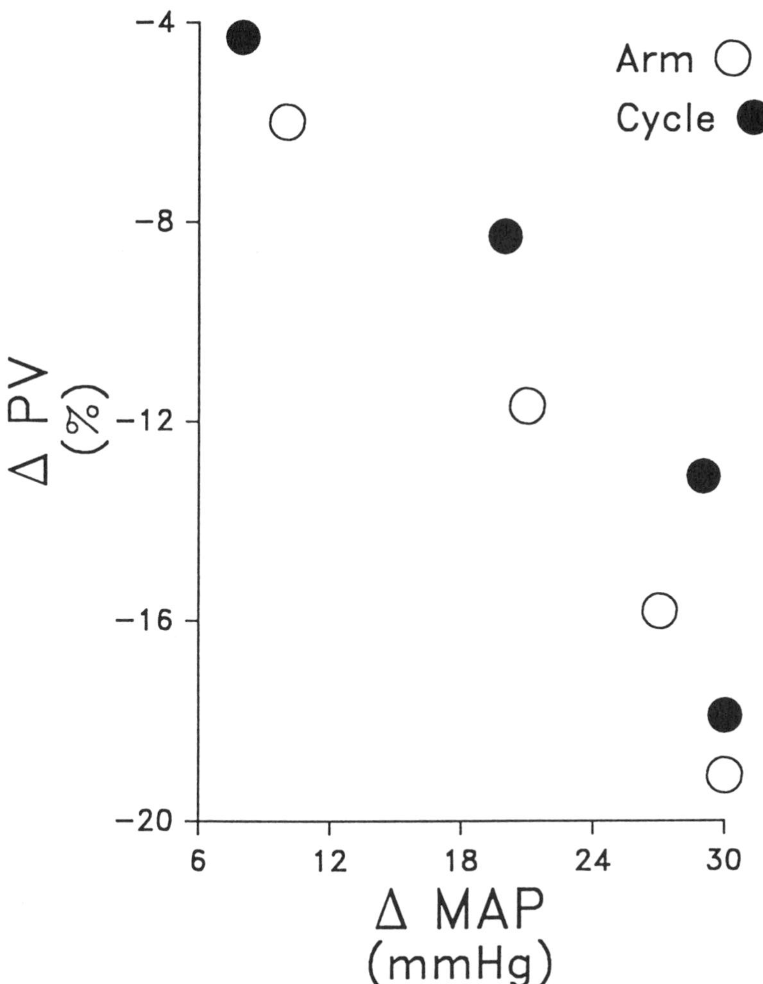

FIGURE 6-4. *Relationship of the percent change in plasma volume to the change in mean arterial pressure during arm cranking or leg ergometry. (Redrawn from data of Miles et al., 1983.)*

various compartments during exercise as well as during recovery. Changes in these forces may be due in part to hormonal effects (Bealer et al., 1985).

1. Capillary Hydrostatic Pressure. An increase in capillary hydrostatic pressure is suggested as the primary force in the efflux of fluid from the vascular space. Maximal exercise increases capillary hydrostatic pressure by 10 mmHg, with the increase proportional to the intensity of the exercise (Mohsenin & Gonzalez, 1984). Capillary hydrostatic pressure is a function of mean arterial pressure, venous pressure, precapillary resistance, and postcapillary resistance.

The mean arterial pressure is the primary factor modulating changes in capillary pressure. During maximal exercise, mean arterial pressure is increased by 10 to 22 mmHg, leading to an increase in capillary pressure (Wade et al, 1987; Wade & Claybaugh, 1980; Staessen et al., 1987; Hillman & Lundvall, 1981; Miles et al., 1983). As noted earlier, Miles et al. (1983) found the decrease in plasma volume to be related to the increase in blood pressure during arm or leg exercise (Figure 6-4). This increase in blood pressure is in part caused by the increase in circulating catecholamines and angiotensin II during exercise. The increase in circulating norepinephrine and epinephrine at the end of maximal exercise is sufficient to increase blood pressure (Hillman & Lundvall, 1981).

Following alpha adrenergic blockade, the blood pressure increase during maximal exercise was decreased by 10 mmHg (Staessen et al., 1987). Beta blockade decreased blood pressure by 12 mmHg during maximal exercise compared to a nonblockaded condition (Hespel et al., 1986).

Inhibition of the conversion of angiotensin I to angiotensin II also attenuated the increase in blood pressure during maximal exercise, but it failed to significantly alter the reduction in plasma volume (Wade et al., 1987).

The increase in vasopressin could also play a role in the increase in mean arterial blood pressure during exercise. However, the plasma concentrations of vasopressin necessary to increase blood pressure far exceed those reported during exercise (Wade, 1984; Weitzman & Kleeman, 1980; Share & Claybaugh, 1972). Vasopressin may indirectly affect blood pressure by potentiating the actions of catecholamines and angiotensin II.

Work by Staessen et al. (1987) showed that inhibition of prostaglandin synthesis increased mean arterial pressure by 5 mmHg during exercise. However, the change in blood volume during exercise was not altered following inhibition of prostaglandin synthesis.

Vasoactive hormones may change pre- and/or postcapillary resistance to redistribute blood flow and preferentially increase the capillary pressures in selective vascular beds. If these vascular beds have relatively great surface areas and permeabilities (capillary filtration coefficients), the vasoactive hormones might thereby facilitate the efflux of fluid from the vascular space. At the onset of exercise, the redistribution of blood flow away from the viscera to skeletal muscles may represent such a phenomenon (Rowell, 1974; Davidson et al., 1986; Aziz & Sommer, 1982; Lichtenstein et al., 1987). As circulating catecholamine levels rise, the surface area for filtration is increased in skeletal muscle but reduced in mesenteric tissues (McKeever et al., 1985; Lewis & Mellander, 1962; Rowell, 1974; Aziz & Sommer, 1982). The redistribution of blood flow is primarily due to constriction of the precapillary sphincters in tissues where flow is reduced and to dilation of precapillary sphincters in hyperemic tissues (Lewis & Mellander, 1962; Hillman & Lundvall 1981;

Haraldsson, 1985; Cotter et al., 1985; Thomson, 1984). The changes in precapillary resistance are modulated by vasoactive hormones. The net effect during exercise is an increase in capillary hydrostatic pressure and in the surface area for filtration.

2. Interstitial Hydrostatic Pressure. Immediately following short-duration supramaximal exercise, interstitial pressure is increased by 1.8 mmHg (Mohsenin & Gonzalez, 1984). Greater increases during muscle contraction can occur and may result in a value equal to that of capillary pressure (Mubarak & Hargens, 1981). The increase in interstitial pressure during or immediately following exercise is directly proportional to the workload (Mohsenin & Gonzalez, 1984). The efflux of fluid from the vascular space into the extravascular compartment and the contraction of the skeletal muscles during exercise appear to account for the increase in interstitital hydrostatic pressure (Thomson, 1984; Mohsenin & Gonzalez, 1984).

3. Oncotic Pressure. Oncotic pressures in the plasma and the interstitium may be modified by changes in muscle metabolism during exercise. Muscular activity produces metabolites that accumulate in the cell, thus favoring the movement of fluid into the cell (Sejersted et al, 1986; Costill et al., 1981; Felig et al., 1982). During exercise, the water content of active muscle cells increases (Sejersted et al., 1986; Costill et al., 1981; Felig et al., 1982). The movement of water into the cells increases the oncotic pressure in the interstitium due to the loss of fluids. This shift then favors movement of fluid from the vascular space to the interstitial space.

The metabolism in the muscle cells may be hormonally influenced, thereby altering the production of metabolites (von Euler, 1974; Clutter et al., 1980; Galbo, 1983; Viru, 1985). Catecholamines, for instance, stimulate glycogenolysis and thus promote the production of lactate (Viru, 1985). The mobilization of fats is also elicited by the increase in catecholamines during exercise (Clutter et al., 1980; Galbo, 1983). Schnabel et al. (1984) inhibited the metabolic action of catecholamines with beta blockade during exercise. Beta blockade reduced the exercise-induced elevation in lactate, glucose, free fatty acids, and glycerol (Schnabel et al., 1984). Reductions in plasma volume, however, were not significantly altered, being 13% in the control and 10% following beta blockade. The effects of the various hormonal systems on cell metabolism and the influence of these effects on the acute reduction of plasma volume during exercise are yet to be defined.

Plasma proteins may leave the vascular space and move into the interstitial space, resulting in a further increase in oncotic pressure (Cotter et al., 1985; Roztocil et al., 1983; Renkin, 1985). The rate of albumin escape from the capillaries is increased during exercise and is dependent upon the increase in blood pressure (Roztocil et al., 1983) and the exercise intensity (Pivarnik et al., 1985). Therefore, the movement of proteins out of the vascular space is facilitated by those hormones that increase blood pressure and shift blood flow during exercise.

As previously mentioned, the redistribution of blood flow during exercise to capillary beds having greater permeabilities can increase fluid loss from the vasculature. Further, the permeability of the capillary may be directly increased by the changes in hormones during exercise. Histamine, kinins, prostaglandins, and cortisol, all of which are increased during exercise, can increase capillary permeability (Bealer et al., 1985). Inhibition of prostaglandin synthesis, on the other hand, does not appear to affect the change in plasma volume induced by exercise (Pivarnik et al., 1985). However, these authors observed a decreased movement of proteins out of the vascular space during inhibition of prostaglandin synthesis. The authors suggested that factors other than prostaglandins influenced capillary permeability and that maintenance of proteins in the vascular space does not necessitate the retention of fluid. In light of this observation, it is interesting that catecholamines and vasopressin inhibit the efflux of proteins from the vasculature, primarily by inhibiting the actions of mediators of capillary permeability (Bealer et al., 1985). Although an efflux of proteins does occur during exercise, the factors modulating the movement of proteins appear to be primarily related to the increase in blood pressure.

Finally, circulating ANF is also increased during exercise. A recent report demonstrates that ANF is capable of inducing the movement of fluid from intravascular to extravascular compartments, presumably through alterations in capillary permeability and/or filtration pressure (Weidmann et al., 1986).

During exercise, the oncotic pressure of the plasma is increased despite the movement of proteins into the interstitial space. Plasma oncotic pressure may be increased by 5–6 mmHg during high power exercise of 3 min duration (Mohsenin & Gonzalez, 1984). This increase in plasma oncotic pressure is due in part to an increase in plasma protein concentration as the movement of fluid out of the vasculature exceeds that of proteins (Pivarnik et al., 1985, 1988; Convertino et al., 1980a, 1980b; Pivarnik & Senay, 1986). Thus, the increase in the plasma concentration of proteins occurs when the plasma protein content is decreased (Convertino et al., 1981; Mohsenin & Gonzalez, 1984; Wilkerson et al., 1982). However, the increase in protein concentration is greater than can be attributed to hemoconcentration alone (Pivarnik et al., 1988). Therefore, intravascular proteins are augmented by some yet to be determined means.

Proteins may be moved into the vascular space from the interstitium by an increase in lymph flow during exercise (Stebbins & Longhurst, 1985; Edwards & Harrison, 1984). This increase in lymph flow is primarily caused by the increase in the activity of the muscle pump. Lymph flow may also be increased by the greater interstitial pressure resulting from fluid efflux from plasma. Other factors that may increase lymph flow include kinins and histamine (Lindena et al., 1982).

The increase in plasma oncotic pressure during exercise is the net result of a loss of fluid into the extravascular space coupled with the movement of proteins into the vasulature. This maintenance of vascular oncotic pressure is essential in the defense of plasma volume during exercise and may account in part for the lower limit of the plasma volume decrease during exercise.

The rapid efflux of fluid from the intravascular to the extravascular space within the first few minutes of exercise is primarily the result of an increase in capillary hydrostatic pressure associated with the redistribution of blood flow and the increase in mean arterial pressure. The redistribution of blood flow and increase in blood pressure are mediated in part hormonally. Hormones also play a role in the increases in interstitial oncotic and hydrostatic pressures as well as the increase in plasma oncotic pressure. While all of the Starling forces are increased during exercise, the net effect is an increase in capillary hydrostatic pressure and surface area that favors the efflux of fluid out of the vascular space and results in a decrease in plasma volume.

B. Fluid Loss

During prolonged exercise, there is a continuing loss of total body fluids. In the absence of fluid ingestion, this loss is associated with a progressive reduction in total body water and body weight (Costill et al., 1981; Costill, 1984). The loss of total body water during long duration exercise varies from 900–1300 mL/h, depending on work intensity and environmental conditions (Myhre et al., 1982; Leiper et al., 1988; Boudou et al., 1987; Wade et al., 1981, 1985). Following exercise in the heat, the decrease in plasma volume has been reported to be as much as 37% (Adolph & associates, 1947). The loss of plasma volume *during the first minutes* of exercise has no relationship with the total decrease in body fluids during prolonged exercise (Convertino et al., 1980, 1981; Costill, 1984; Fortney et al., 1981; Pivarnik & Senay, 1986) (Figure 6-5). This finding suggests an unequal distribution of water loss from the various body fluid compartments as exercise progresses. Others have reported that the decrease in total body water during exercise is equally distributed among all compartments (Maughan et al., 1985; Sawka, 1988). Sawka (1988) found that during exercise in the heat, the decrease in plasma volume was correlated with the degree of total body water reduction. In the absence of fluid replacement during long-duration exercise, there is a continued loss of total body water that is typically accompanied by a reduction in blood volume.

1. Sweating. During exercise, there is a net loss of total body water due to sweating. Sweat rate during exercise of long duration typically

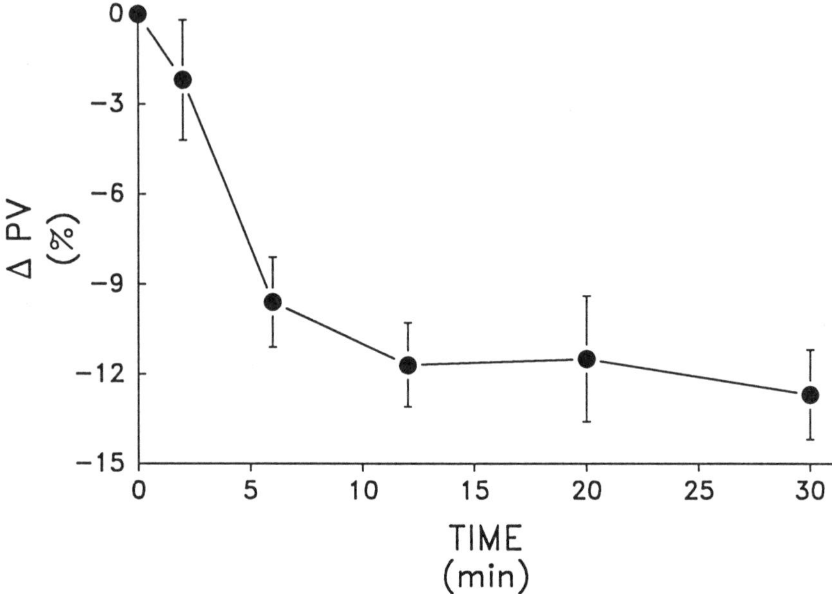

FIGURE 6-5. *The reduction in plasma volume during long duration bicycle ergometer exercise at 60–70% of maximum oxygen consumption in a warm environment (30°C, 40% humidity). Of note is the initial reduction of plasma volume followed by no significant change, although there was a progressive decrease in body fluids of more than 34 g/min. (Redrawn from data of Fortney et al., 1981.)*

ranges from 1.0–1.5 L/h (Buono & Sjoholm, 1988; Costill, 1984; Greenleaf & Sargent, 1965; Myhre et al., 1982; Edwards et al., 1983; Nadel, 1980). This rate may be increased in subjects who are adapted or acclimated to exercise or warm environments (Nadel et al., 1974; Kirby & Convertino, 1986; Convertino et al., 1980b; Buono & Sjoholm, 1988). The loss of fluid via sweat represents a 2–3% decrease in body water per hour in a 70-kg man. The sweat loss is probably derived equally from all body fluid compartments.

Electrolytes as well as water are lost via sweating. Though hypotonic in comparison to plasma, the concentration of solutes in the sweat results in a substantial loss of total body solutes. The concentration of sodium in sweat is 60 mEq/L, and a sweat rate of 1 L/h represents a 2% decrease in total body sodium (Wilkerson et al., 1982; Boling & Lipkind, 1963). Thus, the loss of fluid and electrolytes in sweat can represent a significant threat to the maintenance of fluid and electrolyte homeostatis if exercise continues for more than 3–4 h.

Sweating is initiated in response to increases in body heat stores and is the primary mechanism in the regulation of body temperature during exercise. Sweating is associated with a shift of blood flow to the skin, facilitating the movement of heat to the periphery. The shift in blood flow is modulated by the sympatho-adrenal system, vasopressin, and angiotensin II. These pressor hormones are increased in the circulation during exercise, but their role in the mobilization of heat to the periphery via redistribution of blood flow is not clear.

The sympatho-adrenal system may be involved in the regulation of sweating during exercise. Gordon et al. (1985) reported that although the rectal temperature response to exercise was not altered during beta adrenergic blockade, sweat production as measured by the decrease in body weight was increased. Similarly, Freund et al. (1987b) reported a greater body weight loss during prolonged exercise with beta blockade despite a reduction in forearm blood flow. Conversely, others have found no change (Allen et al., 1972) or a reduction (Mack et al., 1986; Davies et al., 1978) in sweat rate during exercise with beta blockade. Reasons for the discrepancies between studies are not clear. However, Freund et al. (1987b) suggest that the control of forearm blood flow (and presumably sweat rate) can be modified by baroreflexes. The evidence further suggests that perturbations of the blood pressure response to exercise, such as those produced by beta blockade, may affect thermoregulatory responses as well. By modulating blood pressure and flow, the sympatho-adrenal system may thus be involved indirectly in the regulation of sweating during exercise.

Vasopressin has been suggested to modulate sweat rate and composition. Fasciolo et al. (1969) found that subcutaneous injection of vasopressin decreased the rate of sweating induced by local heating of the skin surface and reduced the solute concentration of the sweat as well. The authors failed to account for possible effects of vasopressin on peripheral blood flow in their observation. A relationship between circulating levels of vasopressin and sweat rate or the concentration of solute has not been demonstrated during exercise. Further, in trained subjects at a given relative workload, the rate of sweating is increased, but the concentration of solutes decreased. Therefore, the increase in vasopressin during exercise does not appear to play a role in the regulation of the secretion or composition of sweat.

Aldosterone is associated with the reabsorption of sodium in the kidneys, and a similar function has been postulated for the sweat gland. Injection of aldosterone decreases the sodium concentration of sweat (Collins, 1969). However, Kirby and Convertino (1986) reported that the concentration of sodium in sweat was increased following the daily performance of submaximal bicycle ergometry in a hot environment that increased plasma aldosterone levels. Further, Wade et al. (1981, 1985) found that plasma aldosterone was increased at rest following heavy daily exercise. This increase resulted in higher aldosterone concentrations in blood during subsequent exercise, yet the decrease in body weight (presumably due to sweating) was not altered. Accordingly, it appears that the increase in plasma aldosterone during exercise does not usually affect sweat rate or sodium content.

The effect of ANF on the sweat gland has yet to be investigated. The possibility of such an effect is of interest because the response of ANF to exercise is transitory and appears to be related to the shifting of blood to the peripheral circulation, thereby facilitating the loss of heat. Freund et al. (1988c) has proposed that the transitory response of ANF during prolonged exercise such as a marathon is related to a decrease in atrial pressure associated with a reduction in venous return. Chan and coworkers (1988) found that plasma ANF was reduced at the end of a marathon race. This eventual reduction in ANF during prolonged exercise may facilitate the conservation of sodium at the sweat gland. This hypothesis has yet to be investigated.

2. Renal Function. During strenuous exercise, the loss of fluid and electrolytes via the kidneys is significantly reduced. (See the chapter in this volume by Zambraski.) At rest, urine flow rate ranges from 60 to 90 mL/h, whereas during moderate to heavy exercise, this rate is reduced by 50% (Dressendorfer et al., 1983; Refsum & Stromme, 1975, 1977; Wade & Claybaugh, 1980; Wade et al., 1985, 1987; Zambraski et al., 1982; Poortmans, 1977, 1984). The reduction in urine flow rate is accompanied by a decrease in the excretion of solutes (Wade & Claybaugh, 1980; Refsum & Stromme, 1975, 1977; Dressendorfer et al., 1983; Wade et al., 1985, 1987). Consequently, there is a net renal conservation of fluid and electrolytes during exercise.

The decrease in urine flow rate is due in part to a decrease in renal blood flow. Castenfors et al. (1967b, 1978) found the decrease in renal blood flow to be inversely related to the intensity of the exercise in subjects performing bicycle ergometry in the supine posture. The sympathoadrenal system is crucial to this decrease in renal blood flow (Castenfors, 1967b; Baer & McGiff, 1980). Catecholamines constrict afferent glomerular arterioles, yielding a decreased delivery of blood to the glomeruli. Of note is the increase in the filtration fraction, the ratio of glomerular filtration rate (GFR) to renal plasma flow (RPF). Because RPF is decreased during exercise, the increase in the filtration fraction is indicative of a constriction of efferent arterioles. This constriction of the efferent arterioles may be mediated in part by the increase in angiotension II during exercise (Baer & McGiff, 1980). The resulting net decrease in GFR accounts, in part, for the reduction in urine flow rate during moderate- to high-intensity or prolonged exercise.

The reduction in urine flow rate is also purported to be the result of the increase in vasopressin during exercise (Poortmans, 1977; 1984). The increase in vasopressin is expected to increase the reabsorption of water in the collecting tubule of the nephron, thereby yielding a concentrated urine (Weitzman & Kleeman, 1980; Share & Claybaugh, 1972). However, ability of the kidneys to produce a concentrated urine during exercise appears to be impaired, thereby refuting any major effect of vasopressin (Figure 6-6) (Wade & Claybaugh, 1980; Wade et al., 1989). In fact, the clearance of free water is increased (although still negative) during exercise (Wade & Claybaugh, 1980; Zambraski et al., 1982; Refsum & Stromme, 1975, 1977).

The inability of vasopressin to elicit an increase in tubular water reabsorption during exercise conceivably could be caused partly by the blockade of its actions by prostaglandins. However, Zambraski et al. (1982), who assessed the role of prostaglandins in the increase of free water clearance during exercise, found that inhibition of prostaglandin synthesis did not affect the increase in free water clearance during exercise in either euhydrated or hypehydrated subjects. The action of vasopressin in the conservation of fluids by the kidneys during acute exercise is thus questionable.

An increase in the reabsorption of solutes during exercise appears to account in part for the decrease in urine flow rate during exercise. The percent of the excreted filtered load is reduced during exercise for most solutes (Wade & Claybaugh, 1980; Dressendorfer et al., 1983; Poortmans, 1977, 1984). This increase in reabsorption of solutes is accompanied by passive reabsorption of water that conserves both water and electrolytes.

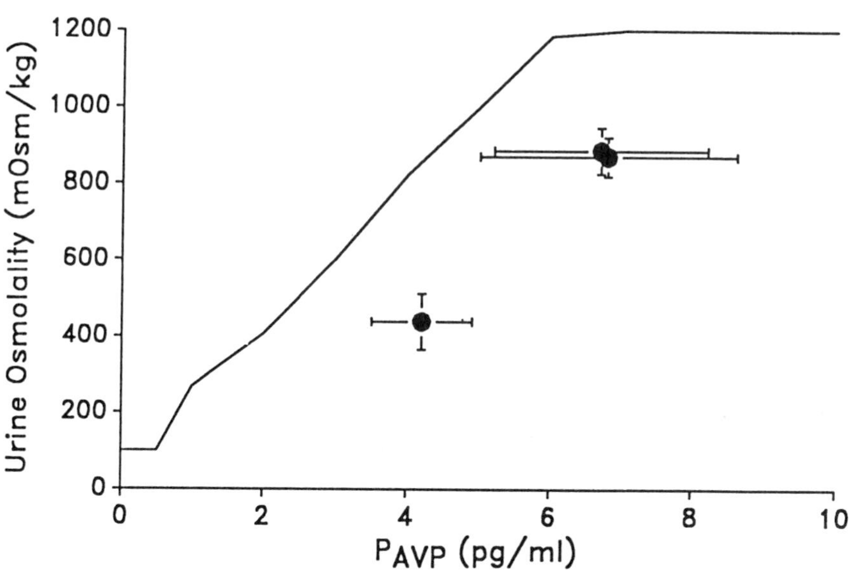

FIGURE 6-6. *The relationship of plasma vasopressin to the concentration of the urine (urine osmolality) in normal subjects at rest (solid line) compared to observations during maximal treadmill exercise at different states of hydration (Wade & Claybaugh, 1980). At a given plasma vasopressin level during exercise, the urine osmolality is decreased compared to that observed at rest, indicating a decreased renal concentrating ability.*

The increase in plasma aldosterone is associated with a decrease in the renal excretion of sodium during exercise (Figure 6-7). Aldosterone modulates the reabsorption of sodium in the distal tubule of the nephron (Reid & Ganong, 1977; Morris, 1981). At rest, an increased reabsorption of sodium in the distal tubule is associated with the secretion of potassium. This had led to the suggestion that increased circulating aldosterone during exercise could lead to hypokalemia (Knochel et al., 1972). However, no such hypokalemia occurs (Wade et al., 1981, 1985), possibly because sodium is exchanged for other cations, such as hydrogen, which mainten electroneutrality. In any event, there is a net reabsorption of sodium during exercise that is mediated in part by the increase in aldosterone.

The role of ANF in handling of solutes, primarily sodium, during exercise, is not well defined (Freund et al., 1988c). As noted earlier, ANF is increased at low work intensities prior to the increase in aldosterone

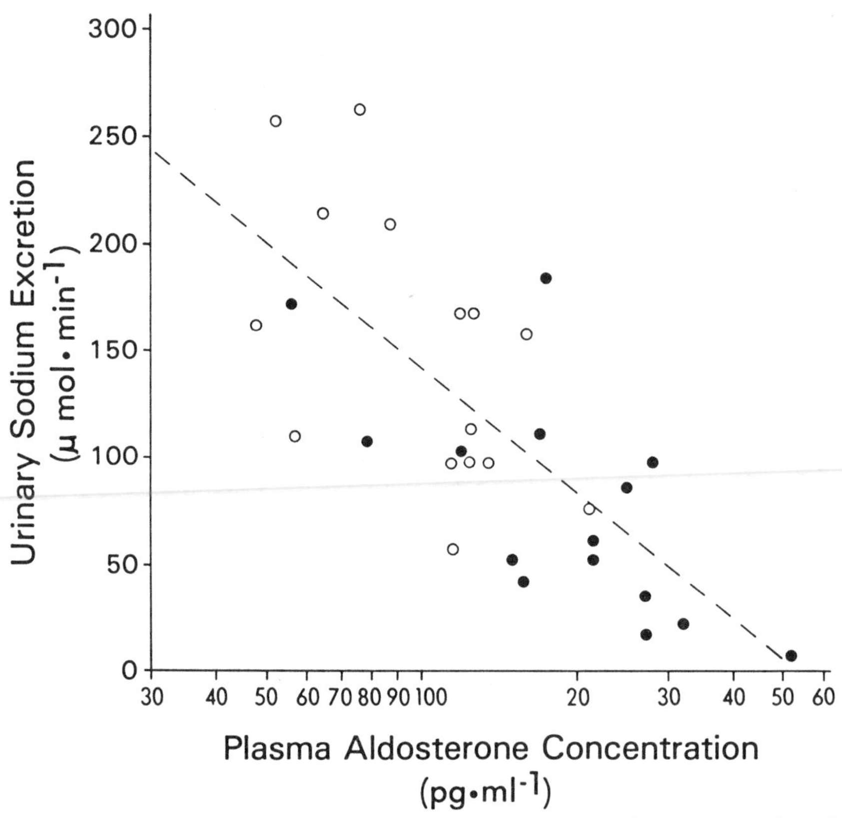

FIGURE 6-7. *The relationship of plasma aldosterone concentration to urinary sodium excretion on a day with 2 h of exercise (closed circles) and following 2 days of rest (open circles). (Reprinted from Wade et al., 1985.)*

(Tanaka et al., 1986; Freund et al., 1987a). The increase in ANF may account for the transient increase in urine flow rate and sodium excretion observed at workloads less than 40% of $\dot{V}O_2max$ (Virvidakis et al., 1986; Kachadorian & Johnson, 1970, 1971). Thus, the natriuresis and diuresis at low-intensity exercise could be due in part to the increase in ANF, which occurs prior to the rise in circulating aldosterone and vasopressin (Freund et al., 1988c).

Prostaglandins are suggested to have a direct effect on the renal handling of sodium as well as to modulate the action of other hormones (Bolger et al., 1976, 1978; Berl et al., 1977). However, blockade of the synthesis of prostaglandins did not alter the renal handling of water or solutes during exercise (Staessen et al., 1987; Zambraski et al., 1982). Johnson and Barger (1981) suggested that the exercise-induced increase in plasma epinephrine may also directly affect renal sodium conservation.

The conservation of water and solutes by the kidneys is increased during exercise and is modulated by a variety of endocrine systems. However, the renal conservation of water and solutes does not equal the loss incurred via sweating. Thus, there is a net loss of water and solutes during exercise; therefore, fluid ingestion is required to restore fluid balance.

C. Replacement of Fluids

Subjects lose body water during exercise even if fluids are available for ingestion (Maron et al., 1977; Wade et al., 1981, 1985, 1989; Myhre et al., 1982; Leiper et al., 1988; Boudou et al., 1987). This voluntary dehydration represents a change in the regulation of thirst as one exercises (Wade et al., 1989; Greenleaf & Sargent, 1965). Thirst is the motivation to seek water and is a subjective sensation which can only be defined in man. In the study of animals, the ingestion of fluids to satiation is assumed to be reflective of thirst. Thus, during exercise in human beings with and without access to fluid replacement, a loss is incurred that must be replaced following exercise. For example, daily running for 2 h (Wade & Claybaugh, 1980; Wade et al., 1985) or walking for 7 h (Leiper et al., 1988), caused a loss of fluids during exercise even with drinking water available. This fluid loss was replaced within 24 h of the onset of exercise. Urine flow rate also returned to normal by this time. The rectification of fluid losses incurred during exercise appears to be the result of thirst and the conservation of water by the kidneys.

The role of thirst in the replacement of fluid losses following exercise has not been well studied. The time necessary to replace fluid losses appears to be a function of the type of fluids ingested. Nose et al. (1988a, 1988b, 1988c) reported that 68% of the fluid losses induced during submaximal exercise in the heat was replaced within 3 h when water was provided. If the subjects were given an isotonic salt solution, 82% of the fluid loss was replaced within the same period. The difference in the degree of rehydration between the two solutions appeared to be related to changes in the renin-angiotensin system. The suppression of plasma renin activity and aldosterone release following water ingestion was associated with an inhibition of thirst. A decrease in renin activity and aldosterone after water ingestion is accompanied by a decrease in angiotensin II, a powerful dipsogen (Stricker & Verbalis, 1988). Nose et al. (1988a, 1988b, 1988c) concluded that the ingestion of water attenuated both the osmotic and volume stimuli of thirst, whereas the isotonic solution did not significantly alter the osmotic stimuli. A role for the renin-angiotensin system in the regulation of thirst following exercise could also be postulated.

Other hormones whose release is stimulated by exercise may play a role in the regulation of thirst. Vasopressin stimulates thirst in animals, but its action is of short duration (Adolph, 1967). It is possible that ANF may have antidipsogenic actions and thus influence voluntary dehydration during exercise (Castenfors, 1967b; Januszewicz et al., 1986a, 1986b; Katsuura et al., 1986; Masotto & Negro-Vilar, 1985). The roles of vasopressin and ANF in the modulation of thirst during and following exercise have yet to be clarified.

While the performance of exercise induces an increase in a variety of hormones, the act of drinking itself results in a rapid suppression of circulating hormone concentrations, with the exception of aldosterone (Geelen et al., 1984; Thrasher et al., 1981, 1984; Freund et al., 1988b). The role of the oral pharyngeal reflex in the modulation of thirst is not clear (Thrasher et al., 1981). Of note is the increase in urine flow rate that precedes the expansion of plasma volume by 30 min when an isotonic solution is ingested following exercise (Morgan et al., 1982). The suppression of various hormones by the act of drinking may initiate an increase in renal excretion that facilitates the elimination of metabolic waste.

Following exercise, renal function may remain suppressed and thereby aid the restoration of fluid balance. Urine flow rate is decreased for up to 3 h following exercise (Costill et al., 1976; Wade & Claybaugh, 1980). Of note is that during this period, GFR is normal, indicating that the decrease was predominantly caused by changes in the tubular handling of water and solutes (Wade & Claybaugh, 1980). Following exercise, free water clearance is decreased, possibly due to the action of vasopressin. However, vasopressin concentrations are returned to control values within 1 h after exercise, even in the absence of drinking. Thus, the influence of vasopressin on the decrease in free water clearance is not clear.

The excretion of solutes, including sodium, continues to be reduced following exercise, even after rehydration (Wade et al., 1985), and appears to reflect the continued elevation in plasma aldosterone concentration. Alteration of renal function thus participates in the rectification of fluid and electrolyte homeostasis following exercise.

D. Exercise Training

Endurance exercise training is generally associated with an expansion of blood volume (McKeever et al., 1985; Green et al., 1984, 1987; Convertino, 1983; Convertino et al., 1980a, 1980b; Mackintosh et al., 1983; Schmidt et al., 1988). Convertino (1983) and Convertino et al. (1980a, 1980b), in studies of subjects undertaking eight consecutive days of training in a warm environment, found blood volume to be increased by 427 mL or 12%. In a group of subjects in whom body temperature was increased passively by heat exposure to a similar degree as that observed in exercising subjects, blood volume was expanded by 177 mL or 5%. The authors (Convertino et al., 1980b) concluded that 40% of the expansion of blood volume during exercise training was the result of thermal factors and 60% was caused by other factors. The greater increases during exercise compared to heat exposure in plasma osmolality and vasopressin and a five-fold increase in plasma proteins at rest were suggested as factors contributing to plasma volume expansion. Of note in this study was that the subjects exposed to passive heating showed an 11% daily decrease in plasma volume, compared to an 8% reduction observed during exercise. The greater decrease in plasma volume during heat exposure alone suggests that exercise-induced large increases in plasma hormone levels may help defend plasma volume.

The defense of plasma volume is of interest because differences between endurance-trained subjects and controls have been observed in the recovery of plasma volume following acute exercise (Freund et al., 1987a) and during immersion in water (Boening et al., 1972; Claybaugh et al., 1986). Claybaugh et al., (1986) reported that trained subjects did not decrease urinary vasopressin or increase urine flow rate during immersion to the same degree as untrained subjects. Freund et al. (1987a) found that, although the decrease in plasma volume during maximal treadmill exercise was similar in trained and untrained subjects, 1 h following exercise the plasma volume of the trained subjects was expanded compared to pre-exercise volume, whereas the untrained subjects did not exhibit this acute hypervolemia. There was no difference between these groups during exercise or recovery in the plasma levels of vasopressin, renin activity, ANF or aldosterone. During the recovery period, the trained subjects had a greater plasma protein concentration that accompanied an expansion of plasma volume. Thus, it appears that trained subjects may increase the movement of proteins from the extravascular to the intravascular space following exercise and thereby better defend plasma volume (O'Toole et al., 1983).

The increase in plasma volume during training is associated with a chronic increase in plasma albumin content (Green et al., 1984; Convertino et al., 1980a, 1980b). This increase was observed 24 h after exercise in the absence of increases in vasopressin or plasma renin activity (Convertino et al., 1980a, 1980b). The return of these hormones to control (pre-training) values is paradoxical and may represent a resetting of the pressure systems regulating these hormones. Following training, blood volume is expanded, which should result in a decrease in the plasma levels of vasopressin and PRA.

A similar observation is the increase in plasma volume in trained subjects following maximal exercise when vasopressin and PRA values had returned to control values (Freund et al., 1987a). Acute expansion of blood volume is normally associated with a decrease in vasopressin and PRA, resulting in a diuresis and rectification of volume (Weitzman & Kleeman, 1980; Share, 1974; Share & Claybaugh, 1972). Even though these hormones were not decreased following training during the performance of maximal exercise in trained subjects, vasopressin and the renin-angiotensin system appear to play a permissive role in the expansion of blood volume following training.

The mechanism by which plasma protein content is increased, thereby facilitating the training-induced expansion of blood volume is not clear but may be associated with alterations in protein synthesis or distribution. Convertino et al. (1980a) suggested that protein synthesis was increased following training in the heat because extravascular water as well as plasma volume were expanded. The similar expansion of these compartments suggests an increase in total body protein content.

The movement of protein among fluid compartments may be altered by exercise training. As noted earlier, the efflux of proteins from the vascular to the extravascular space is dependent upon blood pressure. Exercise training sometimes decreases blood pressure, perhaps by reducing resting catecholamine levels (Greenleaf et al., 1981; Svedenhag, 1985; von Euler, 1974). The reduction in blood pressure during training may thus account for the retention of proteins in the vascular space.

Exercise training also decreases concentrations of circulating kinins and prostaglandins (Viru, 1985). The decrease in these hormones may influence the movement of fluids and plasma proteins in trained subjects.

SUMMARY

Exercise results in rapid fluid shifts among the various body compartments followed by the loss of fluids in sweat. The net effect is a decrease in blood volume that can affect the ability to perform work and maintain body temperature. The shift of fluids and rectification of the fluid loss during exercise may be modulated in part by hormonal systems that are activated during exercise. Following exercise, the fluids that were lost are replaced predominantly by fluid ingestion, which may be affected by a variety of hormonal systems. Finally, daily exercise training results in an increase in blood volume that may be influenced by various hormonal systems activated during exercise. The exact role of endocrine systems in the regulation of blood volume during and following exercise has yet to be elucidated and offers interesting areas of research for the future.

ACKNOWLEDGMENTS

The authors thank Mrs. Susan Siefert and Mrs. Marjorie Hunt for their assistance in the preparation of this manuscript.

The opinions and assertions contained herein are the private views of the authors and are not to be construed as official or as reflecting the views of the Department of the Army or the Department of Defense.

BIBLIOGRAPHY

Adlercreutz, H., M. Haerkoenen, K. Kuoppasalmi, K. Kosunen, H. Naeveri & S. Rehunen. Physical activity and hormones. *Adv. Cardiol.*, 1976, 18, 144–157.

Adolph, E.F. Regulation of water intake in relation to body water content. In *Handbook of Physiology: Alimentary Canal. Food and Water Intake.* Washington, DC: American Physiology Society, 1967. 163–172.

Adolph, E.F., & Associates, *Physiology of Man in the Desert.* New York: Interscience, 1947.

Allen, J.A., D.J. Jenkinson, & I.C. Roddie. The effect of beta-adrenoceptor blockade on human sweating. *Brit. J. Pharmacol.*, 1972, 47, 487–497.

Andersson, B. Regulation of water intake. *Am. Physiol. Soc.*, 1978, 58, 582–603.

Atherton, J.C., J.A. Evans, R. Green & S. Thomas. Influence of variations in hydration and in solute excretion on the effects of lysine-vasopressin infusion on urinary and renal tissue composition in the conscious rat. *J. Physiol.*, 1971, 213, 311–327.

Aziz, O. & E. Sommer. Transvascular fluid shifts accompanying short bodily activity in the alert rat and their relation to arterial pressure. *Basic Res. Cardiol.*, 1982, 77, 431–448.

Baer, P.G. & J.C. McGiff. Hormonal systems and renal hemodynamics. *Ann. Rev. Physiol.*, 1980, 42, 589–601.

Barnes, P.J. & M.J. Brown. Venous plasma histamine in exercise-and hyperventilation-induced asthma in man. *Clin. Science*, 1981, 61, 159–162.

Baylis, P.H. Osmoregulation and control of vasopressin secretion in healthy humans. *Am. J. Physiol.*, 1987, 253, R671–R678.

Bealer, S.L., F.J. Haddy, J.N. Diana, G.J. Grega, R.D. Manning, Jr., J.C. Rose & D.S. Gann. Neuroendocrine mechanisms of plasma volume regulation. *Fed. Proceed.*, 1985, 45, 2455–2463.

Berl, T., A. Raz, H. Wald, J. Horowitz & W. Czaczkes. Prostaglandin synthesis inhibition and the action of vasopressin: studies in man and rat. *Am. J. Physiol.*, 1977, 232(6), F529–F537.

Boening, D., H.-V. Ulmer, U. Meier, W. Skipka & J. Stegemann. Effects of a multi-hour immersion on trained and untrained subjects: I. renal function and plasma volume. *Aerospace Med.*, 1972, 43(3), 300–305.

Bolger, P.M., G.M. Eisner, P.W. Ramwell & L.M. Slotkoff. Effect of prostaglandin synthesis on renal function and renin in the dog. *Nature*, 1976, 259, 244–245.

Bolger, P.M., G.M. Eisner, P.W. Ramwell, L.M. Slotkoff & E.J. Corey. Renal actions of prostacyclin. *Nature*, 1978, 271, 467–469.

Boling, E.A. & J.B. Lipkind. Body composition and serum electrolyte concentrations. *J. Ap. Physiol.*, 1963, 18(5), 943–949.

Boudou, P., J. Fiet, C. Laureaux, M.C. Patricot, C.Y. Guezennec, M.J. Foglietti, J.M. Villette, F. Friemel & J.C. Haag. Variations of a few plasmas and urinary components in marathon runners. *Annales de Bioligie Clinique*, 1987, 45, 37–45.

Bouissou, P., G. Peronnet, G. Brisson, R. Helie & M. Ledoux. Fluid-electrolyte shift and renin-aldosterone responses to exercise under hypoxia. *Horm. and Metab. Res.*, 1987, 19, 331–334.

Bozovic, L. & J. Castenfors. Effect of dihydralazine on plasma renin activity and renal function during supine exercise in normal subjects. *Acta Physiol. Scand.*, 1967, 70, 281–289.

Brandenberger, G., V. Candas, M. Follenius, J.P. Libert & J.M. Kahn. Vascular fluid shifts and endocrine responses to exercise in the heat. *Europ. Ap. Physiol.*, 1986, 55, 123–129.

Bunt, J.C. Hormonal alterations due to exercise. *Sports Med.*, 1986, 30, 331–345.

Buono, M.J. & N.T. Sjoholm. Effect of physical training on peripheral sweat production. *J. Ap. Physiol.*, 1988, 65(2), 811–814.

Buono, M.J., J.E. Yeager & A.A. Sucec. Effect of aerobic training on the plasma ACTH response to exercise. *J. Ap. Physiol.*, 1987, 63, 2499-2501.

Castenfors, J. Effect of ethacrynic acid on plasma renin activity during supine exercise in normal subjects. *Acta Physiol. Scand.*, 1967a, 70, 215-220.

Castenfors, J. Renal function during exercise. *Acta Physiol.* Scand., 1967b, 70(suppl. 293), 1-44.

Castenfors, J. Renal function during prolonged exercise. *Ann. New York Acad. Sciences*, 1978, 301, 151-159.

Chan, K., A. Pipe & A.J. DeBold. Atrial natriuretic hormone in marathon running. *Med. Science in Sports*, 1988, 20(2), S39-S39. (Abstract)

Claybaugh, J.R., D.R. Pendergast, J.E. Davis, C. Akiba, M. Pazik & S.K. Hong. Fluid conservation in athletes: responses to water intake, supine posture, and immersion. *J. Ap. Physiol.*, 1986, 61, 7-15.

Clutter, W.E., D.M. Bier, S.D. Shah & P.E. Cryer. Epinephrine Plasma Metabolic Clearance Rates and Physiologic Thresholds for Metabolic and Hemodynamic Actions in Man. *J. Clin. Invest.*, 1980, 66, 94-101.

Collins, K.J. Action of exogenous aldosterone on the secretion and composition of drug-induced sweat. *Clin. Science*, 1969, 30, 207-213.

Collins, M.A., D.W. Hill, K.J. Cureton & J.J. DeMello. Plasma volume change during heavy-resistance weight lifting. *Europ. J. Ap. Physiol.*, 1986, 55, 44-48.

Convertino, V.A. Heart rate and sweat rate responses associated with exercise-induced hypervolemia. *Med. Science in Sports and Exercise*, 1983, 15, 77-82.

Convertino, V.A., P.J. Brock, L.C. Keil, E.M. Bernauer & J.E. Greenleaf. Exercise training-induced hypervolemia: role of plasma albumin, renin, and vasopressin. *J. Ap. Physiol.*, 1980a, 48, 665-669.

Convertino, V.A., J.E. Greenleaf & E.M. Bernauer. Role of thermal and exercise factors in the mechanism of hypervolemia. *J. Ap. Physiol.* 1980b, 48, 657-664.

Convertino, V.A., L.C. Keil & E.M. Bernauer. Plasma volume, osmolality, vasopressin, and renin activity during graded exercise in man. *J. Ap. Physiol.*, 1981, 50, 123-128.

Convertino, V.A., L.C. Keil & J.E. Greenleaf. Plasma volume, renin and vasopressin responses to graded exercise after training. *J. Ap. Physiol.*, 1983, 54, 508-514.

Costill, D.L. Water and electrolyte requirements during exercise. *Clinics Sports Med.*, 1984, 3, 639-648.

Costill, D.L., G. Branam, W. Fink & R. Nelson. Exercise induced sodium conservation: changes in plasma renin and aldosterone. *Med. Science in Sports*, 1976, 8, 209-213.

Costill, D.L., R. Cote, W.J. Fink & P. Van Handel. Muscle water and electrolyte distribution during prolonged exercise. *Int. J. Sports Med.*, 1981, 2. No. 3, 130-134.

Cotter, T.P.., E.M. Gebruers & W.J. Hall. The time course of plasma expansion and diuresis in man following drinking of isotonic salt solution. *Abstract-Royal Acad. Med. Ireland*, 1985, 125.

Crandall, M.E. & C.M. Gregg. In vitro evidence for an inhibitory effect of atrial natriuretic peptide on vasopressin release. *Neuroendocrin.*, 1986, 44, 439-445.

Cuneo, R.C., E.A. Espiner, M.G. Nicholls, T.G. Yandle, S.L. Joyce & N.L. Gilchrist. Renal, hemodynamic, and hormonal responses to atrial natriuretic peptide infusions in normal man, and effect of sodium intake. *J. Clin. Endocrin.*, 1986, 63, 946-953.

Dabney, J.M., M.J. Buehn & D.E. Dobbins. Constriction of lymphatics by catecholamines, carotid occlusion, or hemorrhage. *Am. J. Physiol.*, 1988, 255, H514-H524.

Davidson, R.J.L., J.D. Robertson & R.J. Maughan. Haematological changes due to triathlon competition. *Brit. J. Sports Med.*, 1986, 20 (4), 159-161.

Davies, C.T.M., J.R. Brotherhood & E. ZeidiFard. Effects of atropine and beta-blockade on temperature and performance during prolonged exercise. *Europ. J. Ap. Physiol.*, 1978, 58, 223-232.

Davies, J.A., M.H. Harrison, L.A. Cochrane, R.J. Edwards & T.M. Gibson. Effect of saline loading during heat acclimatization on adrenocortical hormone levels. *J. Ap. Physiol.*, 1981, 50, 605-612.

Demers, L.M., T.S. Harrison, D.R. Halbert & R.J. Santen. Effect of prolonged exercise on plasma prostaglandin levels. *Prostaglandins and Med.*, 1981, 6, 413-418.

Denton, D.A. Salt appetite. In *Handbook of Physiology: Alimentary Canal. Food and Water Intake.* Washington, DC: American Physiology Society, 1967. 433-459.

Dressendorfer, R.H., C.E. Wade & J.H. Scaff. Renal function during short-term and prolonged strenuous exercise in coronary heart disease patients. *J. Card. Rehab.*, 1983, 3, 575-582.

Edwards, R.J. & M.H. Harrison, Intravascular volume and protein responses to running exercise. *Medi. Science Sports Exer.*, 1984, 16, No.3, 247-255.

Edwards, R.J., M.H. Harrison, L.A. Cochrane & F. Mills. J. Blood volume and protein responses to skin cooling and warming during cycling exercise. *Europ. J. Ap. Physiol.*, 1983, 50, 195-206.

Fagard, R., R. Grauwels, D. Groeseneken, P. Lijnen, J. Staessen, L. Vanhees & A. Amery. Plasma levels of renin, angiotensin II, and 6-ketoprostaglandin Fla in endurance athletes. *J. Ap. Physiol.*, 1985a, 59, 947-952.

Fagard, R., P. Lijnen & A. Amery. Effects of angiotensin II on arterial pressure, renin and aldosterone during exercise. *Europ. J. Ap. Physiol.*, 1985b, 54, 254-261.

Fasciolo, J.C., G.L. Totel & R.E. Johnson. Antidiuretic hormone and human eccrine sweating. *J. Ap. Physiol.*, 1969, 27, 303-307.

Felig, P., C. Johnson, M. Levitt, J. Cunningham, F. Keefe & B. Boglioli. Hypernatremia induced by maximal exercise. *J.A.M.A.*, 1982, 248, No. 10, 1209-1211.

Fellman, N., M. Sagnol, M. Bedu, G. Falgairette, E.V. Praagh, G. Gaillard, P. Jouanel & J. Coudert. Enzymatic and hormonal responses following a 24 h endurance run and a 10 h triathlon race. *Europ. J. Ap. Physiol.*, 1988, 57, 545–553.

Fortney, S.M. & N.B. Vroman. Exercise, performance and temperature control: temperature regulation during exercise and implications for sports performance and training. *Sports Med.*, 1985, 2, 8–20.

Fortney, S.M., N.B. Vroman, W.S. Beckett, S. Permutt & N.D. LaFrance. Effect of exercise hemoconcentration and hyperosmolality on exercise responses. *J. App. Physiol.*, 1988, 65(2), 519–524.

Fortney, S.M., C.B. Wenger, J.R. Bove & E.R. Nadel. Effect of blood volume on sweating rate and body fluids in exercising humans. *J. Ap. Physiol.*, 1981, 51(6), 1594–1600.

Fortney, S.M., C.B. Wenger, J.R. Bove, & Nadel. Effect of blood volume on forearm venous and cardiac stroke volume during exercise. *J. Ap. Physiol.*, 1983, 55(3), 884–890.

Fortney, S.M., C.B. Wenger, J.R. Bove & E.R. Nadel. Effect of hyperosmolality on control of blood flow and sweating. *J. Ap. Physiol.*, 1984, 57(6), 1688–1695.

Fossion, A., F. Brauers, J. Juchmes & G. Camus. Modifications du volume plasmatique lors d'exercices d'intensite submaximale et de duree breve. *Comptes Rendus des Seances de la Societe de Biologie et de Ses Filiales*, 1982, 176, 95–98.

Francesconi, R.P. Endocrinological responses in stressful environments. *Exer. Sports Science Rev.*, 1988, 16, 255–284.

Freund, B., G. Hashiro, M. Buono, J. Claybaugh & S. Chrisney. Endocrine and electrolyte responses during and following a marathon in young versus middle-aged runners. *Med. Science Sports*, 1988a, 20(2), (Abstract)

Freund, B.J., J.R., Claybaugh, M.S. Dice & G.M. Hashiro. Hormonal and vascular fluid responses to maximal exercise in trained and untrained males. *J. Ap. Physiol.*, 1987a, 63, 669–675.

Freund, B.J., J.R. Claybaugh, G.M. Hashiro & M.S. Dice. Hormonal and renal responses to water drinking in moderately trained and untrained humans. *Am. J. Physiol.*, 1988b, 254, R417–R423.

Freund, B.J., M.J. Joyner, S.M. Jilka, J. Kalis, J.M. Nittolo, J.H. Taylor, H. Peters, G. Feese & J.H. Wilmore. Thermoregulation during prolonged exercise in heat: alterations with beta-adrenergic blockade. *J. Ap. Physiol.*, 1987b, 63(3), 930–936.

Freund, B.J., C.E. Wade & J.R. Claybaugh. Effects of exercise on atrial natriuretic factor: implications to fluid homeostasis. *Sports Med.*, 1988c, 6, 364–376.

Fulgraff, G., G. Brandenbusch & K. Heintze. Dose response relation of the renal effects of PGA1, PGE2, and PGF alpha in dogs. *Prostaglandins*, 1974, 8, 21–30.

Gaebelein, C.J. & L.C. Senay, Jr. Influence of exercise type, hydration, and heat on plasma volume shifts in men. *J. Ap. Physiol.*, 1980, 49(1), 119–123.

Gaebelein, C.J. & L.C. Senay, Jr. Vascular volume changes during cycling and stepping in women at two hydration levels. *Europ. J. Ap. Physiol.*, 1982, 48, 1–10.

Galbo, H. *Hormonal and Metabolic Adaptation to Exercise*. New York: Thieme-Stratton, Inc., 1983.

Galbo, H., J.J. Holst & N.J. Christensen. Glucagon and plasma catecholamine responses to graded and prolonged exercise in man. *J. App. Physiol.*, 1975, 38, 70–75.

Geelen, G., L.C. Keil, S.E. Kravik, C.E. Wade, T.N. Thrasher, P.R. Barnes, G. Pyka, C. Nesvig & J.E. Greenleaf. Inhibition of plasma vasopressin after drinking in dehydrated humans. *Am. J. Physiol.*, 1984, 247, R968–R971.

Geyssant, A., G. Geelen & C.H. Denis. Plasma vasopressin, renin activity, and aldosterone: Effect of exercise training. *Europ. J. Ap. Physiol.*, 1981, 46, 21–30.

Gibiniski, K., S. Kozbowski, J. Chwelbinska-Moneta, L. Giec, J. Zmudzinski & A. Markiewicz. ADH and thermal sweating. *Europ. J. Ap. Physiol.*, 1979, 42, 1-13.

Gleim, G.W., P.M. Zabetakis, E.E. DePasquale, M.F. Michelis & J.A. Nicholas. Plasma osmolality, volume, and renin activity at the "anaerobic threshold." *J. Ap. Physiol.*, 1984, 56, 57–63.

Goetz, K.L. Physiology and pathophysiology of atrial peptides. *Am. J. Physiol.*, 1988, 254, E1–E15. (Abstract)

Goetz, K.L., C.M. Maresh & B.C. Wang. Plasma vasopressin and plasma renin response to maximal treadmill exercise in physically-active college women. *Fed. Proceed.*, 1982, 1, 1677–1677.

Gordon, N.F., P.E. Kruger, J.P. Van Rensburg, A. Van Der Linde, A.J. Kielblock & J.F. Cilliers. Effect of beta-adrenoceptor blockade on thermoregulation during prolonged exercise. *J. Ap. Physiol.*, 1985, 58(3), 899–906.

Green, H.J., L.L. Jones, R.L. Hughson, D.C. Painter & B.W. Farrance. Training-induced hypervolemia: lack of an effect on oxygen utilization during exercise. *Med. Science Sports Exer.*, 1987, 19(3), 202–206.

Green, H.J., J.A. Thomson, M.E. Ball, R.L. Hughson, M.E. Houston & M.T. Sharratt. Alterations in blood volume following short-term supramaximal exercise. *J. Ap. Physiol.*, 1984, 56(1), 145–149.

Greenleaf, J.E., E.M. Bernauer, W.C. Adams & L. Juhos. Fluid-electrolyte shifts and VO_2max in man at simulated altitude (2,287 m). *J. Ap. Physiol.*, 1978, 44(5), 652–658.

Greenleaf, J.E. & F. Sargent, II. Voluntary dehydration in man. *J. Ap. Physiol.*, 1965, 20(4), 719–724.

Greenleaf, J.E., D. Sciaraffa, L.C. Shvartz, L.C. Keil & P.J. Brock. Exercise training hypotension: implications for plasma volume, renin, and vasopressin. *J. Ap. Physiol.*, 1981, 51(2), 298–305.

Guezennec, C.Y., G. Defer, G. Cazorla, C. Sabathier & F. Lhoste. Plasma renin activity, aldosterone and catecholamine levels when swimming and running. *Europ. J. Ap. Physiol.*, 1986, 54, 632–637.

Hagan, R.D., F.J. Diez, R.G. McMurray & S.M. Horvath. Plasma volume changes related to posture and exercise. *Proceed. Soc. Experimental Biol. Med.*, 1980, 165, 155–160.

Haroldsson, B. Effects of noradrenaline on the transcapillary passage of albumin, fluid and CrEDTA in the perfused rat hindlimb. *Acta Physiol. Scand.*, 1985, 125, 561–571.

Harrison, M.H. Effects of thermal stress and exercise on blood volume in humans. *Physiol. Rev.*, 1985, 65, No.1, 149–209.

Harrison, M.H. Heat and exercise effects on blood volume. *Sports Medi.*, 1986, 3, 214–223.

Hartley, J.P.R., T.J. Charles, R.D.H. Monie, A. Seaton, W.H. Taylor, A. Westwood & J.D. Williams. Arterial plasma histamine after exercise in normal individuals and in patients with exercise-induced asthma. *Clin. Science*, 1981, 61, 151–157.

Hartley, L.H., J.W. Mason, R.P. Hogan, L.G. Jones, T.A. Kotchen, E.H. Mougey, F.E. Wherry, L.L. Pennington & P.T. Ricketts. Multiple hormonal responses to graded exercise in relation to physical training. *J. Ap. Physiol.*, 1972, 33, No. 5, 602–606.

Hespel, P., P. Lijnen, L. Vanhees, R. Fagard & A. Amery. Beta-adrenoceptors and the regulation of blood pressure and plasma renin during exercise. *J. Ap. Physiol.*, 1986, 60, 108–113.

Hillman, J. & S. Lundvall. Further studies on beta-adrenergic control of transcapillary fluid absorption from skeletal muscle to blood during hemorrhage. *Acta Physiol. Scand.*, 1981, 112, 281–286.

Januszewicz, P., J. Gutkowska, G. Thibault, R. Garcia, C. Mercure, F. Jolicoeur, J. Genest & M. Cantin. Dehydration-induced changes in the secretion of atrial natriuretic factor in brattleboro rats: effect of water-drinking. *Neuroscience Letters*, 1986a, 67, 203–207.

Januszewicz, P., G. Thibault, J. Gutkowska, R. Garcia, C. Mercure, F. Jolicoeur, J. Genest & M. Cantin. Atrial natriuretic factor and vasopressin during dehydration and rehydration in rats. *Am. J. Physiol.*, 1986b, 251, E497–E501.

Johnson, M.D. & A.C. Barger. Circulating catecholamines in control of renal electrolyte and water excretion. *Am. J. Physiol.*, 1981, 240, F192–F199.

Kachadorian, W.A. & R.E. Johnson. Renal responses to various rates of exercise. *J. Ap. Physiol.*, 1970, 28, 748–752.

Kachadorian, W.A. & R.E. Johnson. The effect of exercise on some clinical measures of renal function. *Am. Heart J.*, 1971, 82, 278–280.

Katsuura, G., M. Nakamura, K. Inouye, M. Kono, K. Nakao & H. Imura. Regulatory role of atrial natriuretic polypeptide in water drinking in rats. *Europ. J. Pharmacol.*, 1986, 121, 285–287.

Kirby, C.R. & V.A. Convertino. Plasma aldosterone and sweat sodium concentrations after exercise and heat acclimation. *J. Ap. Physiol.*, 1986, 61, 967–970.

Kiyonaga, A., K. Arakawa, H. Tanaka & M. Shindo. Blood pressure and hormonal responses to aerobic exercise. *Hypertension*, 1985, 7, 125–131.

Knochel, J., L. Dotin & R. Hamburger. Pathophysiology of intense physical conditioning in a hot climate. I. mechanisms of potassium depletion. *J. Clin. Invest.*, 1972, 51, 242–255.

Knowlton, R.G., R.K. Hetzler, L.A. Kaminsky & J.J. Morrison. Plasma volume changes and cardiovascular responses associated with weight lifting. *Med. Science Sports Exer.*, 1987, 19(5), 464–468.

Kosunen, K. & A. Pakarinen. Plasma renin, angiotensin II, and plasma and urinary aldosterone in running exercise. *J. Ap. Physiol.*, 1976, 41, 26–29.

Kotchen, T.A., L.H. Hartley, T.W. Rice, E.H. Mougey, L.G. Jones & J.W. Mason. Renin, norepinephrine, and epinephrine responses to graded exercise. *J. Ap. Physiol.*, 1971, 31(2), 178–184.

Leenen, F.H., P. Boer & G.G. Geyskes. Sodium intake and the effects of isoproterenol and exercise on plasma renin in man. *J. Ap. Physiol.*, 1978, 45, 870–874.

Legros, J., J. Juchmes & H.V. Caunenreck. Influence de l'exercise musculaire sur le laux plasmatique de la neurophysine chez l'Homme. *Societie de le Biologie de Strasbourg*, 1972, 28, 1391–1398.

Leiper, J.B., K. McCormick, J.D. Robertson, P.H. Whiting & R.J. Maughan. Fluid homoeostasis during prolonged low-intensity walking on consecutive days. *Clin. Science*, 1988, 75, 63–70.

Lewis, D.H. & S. Mellander. Competitive effects of sympathetic control and tissue metabolites on resistance and capacitance vessels and capillary filtration in skeletal muscle. *Acta Physiol. Scand.*, 1962, 56, 162–188.

Lichtenstein, S.V., H. El-Dalati, A. Panos, T.W. Rice & T.A. Salerno. Systemic vascular effects of epinephrine adminstration in man. *J. Surg. Res.*, 1987, 42, 166–178.

Lindena, J., W. Kupper & I. Trautschold. Effect of transient hypoxia in skeletal muscle on enzyme activities in lymph and plasma. *J. Clin. Chem. Clin. Biochem.*, 1982, 20, 95–102.

Luger, A., A. Deuster, S. Kyle, W.T. Gallucci, L.C. Montgomery, P.W. Gold, D.L. Loriaux & G.P. Chrousos. Acute hypothalamic-pituitary-adrenal responses to the stress of treadmill exercise. *New Engl. J. Med.*, 1987, 316, 1309–1315.

Mack, G.W., L.M. Shannon, & E.R. Nadel. Influence of beta-adrenergic blockade on the control of sweating in humans. *J. Ap. Physiol.*, 1986, 61(5), 1701–1705.

Mackintosh, I.C., I.C. Dormehl, A.L. van Gelder & M. du Plessis. Blood volume, heart rate, and left ventricular ejection fraction changes in dogs before and after exercise during endurance training. *Am. J. Vet. Res.*, 1983, 44(10), 1960–1962.

Maher, J.T., L.G. Jones, H. Hartley, G.H. Williams & L.I. Rose. Aldosterone dynamics during graded exercise at sea level and high altitude. *J. Ap. Physiol.*, 1975, 39, 18–22.

Manhem, P. & B. Hoekfelt. Prolonged clonidine treatment: catecholamines, renin activity and aldosterone following exercise in hypertensives. *Acta Med. Scand.*, 1981, 209, 253–260.
Maresh, C.M., B.C. Wang & K.L. Goetz. Plasma vasopressin, renin activity, and aldosterone responses to maximal exercise in active college females. *Europ. J. Ap. Physiol.*, 1985, 54, 398–403.
Maron, M.B., S.M. Horvath & J.E. Wilkerson. Blood biochemical alterations during recovery from competitive marathon running. *Europ. J. Ap. Physiol.* 1977, 36, 231–238.
Masotto, C. & A. Negro-Vilar. Inhibition of spontaneous or angiotensin II-stimulated water intake by atrial natriuretic factor. *Brain Res. Bul.*, 1985, 15, 523–526.
Maughan, R.J., P.H. Whiting & R.J.L. Davidson. Estimation of plasma volume changes during marathon running. *Brit. J. Sports Med.*, 1985, 19(3), 138–141.
McKeever, K.H., W.A. Schurg & V.A. Convertino. Exercise training-induced hypervolemia in greyhounds: role of water intake and renal mechanisms. *Am. J. Physiol.*, 1985, 248, R422–R425.
Meehan, R.T. Renin, aldosterone, and vasopressin responses to hypoxia during 6 hours of mild exercise. *Aviat. Space Environ. Med.*, 1986, 57, 960–965.
Melin, B., J.P. Eclache & G. Geelen. Plasma AVP, neurophysin, renin activity, and aldosterone during submaximal exercise performed until exhaustion in trained and untrained men. *Europ. J. Ap. Physiol.*, 1980, 44, 141–151.
Miles, D.S., M.N. Sawka, R.M. Glaser & J.S. Petrofsky. Plasma volume shifts during progressive arm and leg exercise. *J. Ap. Physiol.*, 1983, 54(2), 491–495.
Mohsenin, V. & R.R. Gonzalez. Tissue pressure and plasma oncotic pressure during exercise. *J. Ap. Physiol.*, 1984, 56(1), 102–108.
Morgan, D.J.R., I. Moodley, M.J. Phillips & R.J. Davies. Plasma histamine in asthmatic and control subjects following exercise: influence of circulating basophils and different assay techniques. *Thorax*, 1983, 38, 771–777.
Morgan, D.J.R., M.J. Phillips, I. Moodley, E.V. Elliott & R.J. Davies. Histamine, neutrophil chemotactic factor and circulating basophil levels following exercise in asthmatic and control subjects. *Clin. Allergy*, 1982, 12, 29–37.
Morganroth, M.L., E.W. Young & H.V. Sparks. Protaglandin and histaminergic mediation of prolonged vasodilation after exercise. *Am. J. Physiol.*, 1977, 233(1), H27–H33.
Morris, D.J. The metabolism and mechanism of action of aldosterone. *Endocrine Rev.*, 1981, 234–247.
Mubarak, S.J. & A.R. Hargens. Clinical use of the wick-catheter technique. In *Tissue fluid pressure and composition*. A.R. Hargens, ed. Baltimore: Williams and Wilkins, 1981. 261–268.
Myhre, L.G., G.H. Hartung & D.M. Tucker. Plasma volume and blood metabolites in middle-aged runners during a warm-weather marathon. *Europ. J. Ap. Physiol.*, 1982, 48, 227–240.
Nadel, E.R. Circulatory and thermal regulations during exercise. *Fed. Proceed.*, 1980, 39, 1491–1497.
Nadel, E.R., K.B. Pandolf, M.R. Roberts & J.A. Stolwijk. Mechanism of thermal acclimatization to exercise and heat. *J. Ap. Physiol.*, 1974, 37, 515–520.
Neilsen, B., G. Sjogaard & F. Bonde-Petersen. Cardiovascular, hormonal and body fluid changes during prolonged exercise. *Europ. J. Ap. Physiol.*, 1984, 53, 63–70.
Nose, H., G.W. Mack, X. Shi & E.R. Nadel. Role of osmolality and plasma volume during rehydration in humans. *J. Ap. Physiol.*, 1988a, 65, (1), 325–331.
Nose, H., G.W. Mack, X. Shi & E.R. Nadel. Involvement of sodium retention hormones during rehydration in humans. *J. Ap. Physiol.*, 1988b, 65(1), 332–336.
Nose, H., G.W. Mack, X. Shi & E.R. Nadel. Shift in body fluid compartments after dehydration in humans. *J. Ap. Physiol.*, 1988c, 65(1), 318–324.
Nowak, J. & A. Wennmalm. A study on the role of endogenous prostaglandins in the role of exercise-induced and post occlusive hyperemia in human limbs. *Acta Physiol.* Scand., 1989, 106, 365–369.
O'Toole, M.L., A.M. Paolone, R.E. Ramsey & G. Irion. The effects of heat acclimation on plasma volume and plasma protein of females. *Internat. J. Sports Med.*, 1983, 4(1), 40–44.
Pavlik, G., A. Hegyi & R. Frenkl. Histamine reactions in blood pressure and heart rate in trained and untrained albino rats. *Agents and Actions*, 1978, 8(4), 404–405.
Petzl, D.H., E. Hartter, W. Osterode, H. Boehm & W. Woloszczuk. Atrial natriuretic peptide release due to physical exercise in healthy persons and in cardiac patients. *Klin Wochenschr*, 1987, 65, 194–196.
Pivarnik, J., T. Kayrouz & L.C. Senay, Jr. Plasma volume and protein content in progressive exercise: influence of cyclooxygenase inhibitors. *Med. Science Sports Exer.*, 1985, 17(1), 153–157.
Pivarnik, J.M., S.J. Montain, J.E. Graves & M.L. Pollock. Alterations in plasma volume, electrolytes and protein during incremental exercise at different pedal speeds. *Europ. J. Ap. Physiol.*, 1988, 57, 103–109.
Pivarnik, J.M. & L.C. Senay, Jr. Effects of exercise detraining and deacclimation to heat on plasma volume dynamics. *Europ. J. Ap. Physiol.*, 1986, 55, 222–228.
Pluto, R., S.A. Cruze, M. Weiss, T. Holtz, P. Mandel & H. Weicker. Cardiocirculatory, hormonal, and metabolic reactions to various forms of ergometric tests. *Internat. J. Sports Med.*, 1988, 9, S79–S88.
Poortmans, J.R. Exercise and renal function. *Exer. Sports Science Rev.*, 1977, 5, 255–294.
Poortmans, J.R. Exercise and renal function. *Sports Med.*, 1984, 1, 125–153.
Refsum, H.E. & S.B. Stromme. Relationship between urine flow, glomerular filtration, and urine solute concentrations during prolonged heavy exercise. *Scand. J. Clin. Lab. Invest.*, 1975, 35, 775–780.

Refsum, H.E. & S.B. Stromme. Renal osmol clearance during prolonged heavy exercise. *Scand. J. Clin. Lab. Invest.*, 1977, 38, 19–22.

Reid, I.A. Actions of angiotensin II on the brain: mechanisms and physiologic role. *Am. J. Physiol.*, 1984, 246, F533–F543.

Reid, I.A. & W.F. Ganong. Control of aldosterone secretion. In *Hypertension: Pathophysiology and Treatment*, J. Genest, E. Koiw, & O. Kuchel, eds. New York: McGraw-Hill, 1977. 265–292.

Renkin, E.M. Capillary transport of macromolecules: pores and other endothelial pathways. *J. Ap. Physiol.*, 1985, 58, 315–325.

Rotstein, A., O. Bar-Or & R. Dlin. Hemoglobin, hematocrit, and calculated plasma volume changes induced by a short, supramaximal task. *Internat. J. Sports Med.*, 1982, 3(4), 230–233.

Rowell, L.B. Human cardiovascular adjustments to exercise and thermal stress. *Physiol. Rev.*, 1974, 54, 75–159.

Roztocil, K., I. Prerovsky, R. Jandova, J. Widimsky & I. Oliva. Transcapillary escape rate of albumin in juvenile hypertension. *Clin. Physiol.*, 1983, 3, 289–295.

Saito, Y., K. Nakao, A. Sugawara, K. Nishimura, M. Sakamoto, N. Morii, T. Yamada, H. Itoh, & S. Shiono, et al. Atrial natriuretic polypeptide during exercise in healthy man. *Acta Endocrin. (Copenhagen)*, 1987, 116, 59–65.

Samson, W.K. Dehydration-induced alterations in rat brain vasopressin and atrial natriuretic factor immunoreactivity. *Endocrin.*, 1985, 117, 1279–1281.

Sawka, M.N. Body fluid responses and hypohydration during exercise heat stress. In *Human performance physiology and environmental medicine at terrestrial extremes*, K.B. Pandolf, M.N. Sawka & R.R. Gonzalez. eds., Indianapolis: Benchmark Press, 1988. 227–266.

Schlein, E.M., G.R. Spooner, C. Day, M. Pickering & R. Cade. Extrarenal water loss and antidiuretic hormone. *J. App. Physiol.*, 1971, 31(4), 569–572.

Schmidt, W., N. Maassen, F. Trost & D. Boning. Training induced effects on blood volume, erythrocyte turnover and haemoglobin oxygen binding properties. *Europ. J. Ap. Physiol.*, 1988, 57, 490–498.

Schnabel, A., W. Kindermann, V. Steinkraus, O. Salas-Fraire & G. Biro. Metabolic and hormonal responses to exhaustive supramaximal running with and without beta-adrenergic blockade. *Europ. J. Ap. Physiol.*, 1984, 52, 214–218.

Sejersted, O.M., N.K. Vollested & J.I. Medbo. Muscle fluid and electrolyte balance during and following exercise. *Acta Physiol. Scand.*, 1986, 128(Supp 1556), 119–127.

Senay, L.C., G. Rogers & P. Jooste. Changes in blood plasma during progressive treadmill and cycle exercise. *J. App. Physiol.*, 1980, 49, 59–65.

Share, L. Blood pressure, blood volume, and the release of vasopressin. In *Handbook of Physiology*, E. Knobil & W. Sawyer, eds. Washington, D.C.: American Physiological Society, 1974. 243–252.

Share, L. & J. Claybaugh. Regulation of body fluids. *Ann. Rev. Physiol.*, 1972, 34, 235–260.

Shvartz, E., V.A. Convertino, L.C. Keil & R.F. Haines. Orthostatic fluid-electrolyte and endocrine responses in fainters and nonfainters. *J. Ap. Physiol.*, 1981, 51(6), 1404–1410.

Somers, V.K., J.V. Anderson, J. Conway, P. Sleight & S.R. Bloom. Atrial natriuretic peptide is released by dynamic exercise in man. *Hormonal Metab. Res.*, 1986, 18, 871–872.

Staessen, J., R. Fagard, P. Hespel, P. Lijnen, L. Vanhees & A. Amery. Plasma renin system during exercise in normal men. *J. Ap. Physiol.*, 1987, 63, 188–194.

Starling, E.H. On the absorption of fluids from the connective tissue spaces. *J. Physiol.*, 1896, 19, 312–326.

Stebbins, C.L. & J.C. Longhurst. Bradykinin-induced chemoreflexes from skeletal muscle: implications for the exercise reflex. *J. Ap. Physiol.*, 59(1), 56–63.

Stricker, E.M. & J.G. Verbalis. Hormones and behavior: the biology of thirst and sodium appetite. *Am. Scientist*, 1988, 76, 261–267.

Sutton, J.R. & P. Farrell. Endocrine responses to prolonged exercise. *Perspectives in Exercise Science and Sports Medicine*, R. Murray & D. Lamb, eds. Indianapolis: Benchmark Press, 1988, 1, 153–212.

Svedenhag, J. The sympatho-adrenal system in physical conditioning. *Acta Physiol. Scand.*, 1985, 125 (Suppl. 543), 3–73.

Tanaka, H., M. Shindo, J. Gutkowska, A. Kinoshita, H. Urata, M. Ikeda & K. Arakawa. Effect of acute exercise on plasma immunoreactive-atrial natriuretic factor. *Life Sciences*, 1986, 39, 1685–1693.

Thamsborg, G., T. Storm, N. Keller, R. Sykulski & J. Larsen. Changes in plasma atrial natriuretic peptide during exercise in healthy volunteers. *Acta Med. Scand.*, 1987a, 221, 441–444.

Thamsborg, G., R. Sykulski, J. Larsen, T. Storm & N. Keller. Effect of betal-adrenoreceptor blockade on plasma levels of atrial natriuretic peptide during exercise in normal man. *Clin. Physiol.*, 1987b, 7, 313–318.

Thomas, T.R. & G.L. Etheridge. The effect of acute exercise on body density, body volume, and plasma volume. *Canad. J. Ap. Sport Science*, 1982, 7:4, 258–262.

Thomson, I.R., Cardiovascular physiology: venous return. *Canad. Anaesthetists Soc. J.*, 1984, 31:3, S31–S37.

Thrasher, T.N., J.F. Nistal-Herrera, L.C. Keil & D.J. Ramsay. Satiety and inhibition of vasopressin secretion after drinking in dehydrated dogs. *Am. J. Physiol.*, 1981, 240, E394–E401.

Thrasher, T.N., C.E. Wade, L.C. Keil & D.J. Ramsay. Sodium balance and aldosterone during dehydration and rehydration in the dog. *Am. J. Physiol.*, 1984, 247, R76–R83.

Van Beaumont, W., S. Underkofler & S. Van Beaumont. Erythorocyte volume, plasma volume, and acid-base changes in exercise and heat dehydration. *J. Ap. Physiol.*, 1981, 50(6), 1255–1262.

Viru, A., *Hormones in muscular activity*. Boca Raton: CRC Press, 1985.
Virvidakis, C., A. Loukas, D.M. Symvoulidou & T. Mountokalakis. Renal responses to bicycle exercise in trained athletes: influence of exercise intensity. *Internat. J. Sports Med.*, 1986, 7, 86–88.
von Euler, U.S. Sympatho-adrenal activity in physical exercise. *Med. Science Sports*, 1974, 6, 165–173.
Wade, C.E. Response, regulation, and actions of vasopressin during exercise: a review. *Med. Science Sports Exer.*, 1984, 16, 506–511.
Wade, C.E. & J. Claybaugh. Plasma renin activity, vasopressin concentration, and urinary excretory responses to exercise in men. *J. Ap. Physiol.*, 1980, 49, 930–936.
Wade, C.E., R.H. Dressendorfer, J.C. O'Brien & C. Claybaugh. Renal function, aldosterone, and vasopressin excretion following repeated long distance running. *J. Ap. Physiol.*, 1981, 50, 709–712.
Wade, C.E., B.J. Freund & J.R. Claybaugh. Fluid and electrolyte homeostasis during and following exercise: hormonal and non-hormonal factors. In *Hormonal regulation of fluids and electrolytes: environmental effects*, J.R. Claybaugh & C.E. Wade, eds. New York: Plenus Publishing Co., 1989. 1–46.
Wade, C.E., L.C. Hill, M.M. Hunt & R.H. Dressendorfer. Plasma aldosterone and renal function in runners during a 20-day road race. *Europ. J. Ap. Physiol.*, 1985, 54, 456–460.
Wade, C.E., S.R. Ramee, M.M. Hunt & C.J. White. Hormonal and renal responses to converting enzyme inhibition during maximal exercise. *J. Ap. Physiol.*, 1987, 63, 1796–1800.
Weidmann, P., L. Hasler, M.P. Gnadinger, R.E. Lang, D.E. Uehlinger, S. Shaw, W. Rascher & F.C. Reubi. Blood levels and renal effects of atrial natriuretic peptide in normal man. *J. Clin. Invest.*, 1986, 77, 734–742.
Weitzman, R. & C.R. Kleeman. Water metabolism and neurohypophyseal hormones. In *Clinical Disorders of Fluid and Electrolyte Metabolism*, M.H. Maxwell & C.R. Kleeman, eds. New York: McGraw-Hill, 1980. 531–645.
Wells, C.L., J.R. Stern & L.H. Hecht. Hematological changes following a marathon race in male and female runners. *Europ. J. Ap. Physiol.*, 1982, 48, 41–49.
Wilkerson, J., B. Gutin & S.M. Horvath. Exercise-induced changes in blood, red cell, and plasma volumes in man. *Med. Science Sports*, 1977, 9, 155–158.
Wilkerson, J.E., S.M. Horvath, B. Gutin, S. Molnar & F.J. Diaz. Plasma electrolyte content and concentration during treadmill exercise in humans. *J. Ap. Physiol.*, 1982, 53, 1529–1539.
Wong, N., J.E. SIlver, W. Greenawalt, S.E. Kravik, G. Geelen, P.R. Barnes & J.E. Greenleaf. Effect of hand-arm exercise on venous blood constituents during leg exercise. *Internat. J. Sports Med.*, 1985, 6(2), 86–89.
Zambraski, E., T. Rofrano & C. Ciccone. Effects of aspirin treatment on kidney function in exercising man. *Med. Science Sports Exer.*, 1982, 14, 419–423.
Zambraski, E.J., M.S. Tucker, C.S. Lakas, S.M. Grassl & C.G. Scanes. Mechanism of renin release in exercising dog. *Am. J. Physiol.*, 1984, 246, E71–E76.

DISCUSSION

CONVERTINO: We lack mechanistic studies of endocrine responses to exercise. We have continued to do descriptive studies, and we've tried to guess what might be going on. I'd like to mention a study that was just reported at the American College of Sports Medicine meeting by Maurie Luetkemeier. He used a drug, spironolactone, which inhibits aldosterone effects, and found in the first few days of exercise training that inhibiting aldosterone attenuated the increase in plasma volume. This is the type of study that needs to be done so that we can begin to determine if, in fact, aldosterone is an important contributing factor to the control of homeostatic control of plasma volume.

It is intriguing to me that some of these hormones exhibit vascular as well as renal affects that tend to work toward the maintenance of venous pressure and an adequate volume in the vascular space. That can be done in two ways: one is by expanding volume or trying to replace volume during exercise, and the other is to contract vascular space. I think it is interesting that many of these hormones can operate in both ways to defend plasma volume and venous pressure. Thus, hormone systems have developed a redundancy, i.e., a backup. It's difficult for me to see how we can at any time suggest that a particular hormone such as vasopressin does not have a potential role, even if it may not be acting under certain exercise conditions. Even though we may not find a significant reduction or even see an increase in free water clearance, vasopressin is still there, and under another situation, may work to our advantage if the aldosterone system, for some reason, is not adequate.

WADE: First, I agree with Vic that hormone research has been pointed toward descriptive studies and not toward a mechanistic approach. Secondly, the work of Maurie Luetkemeier was the right approach. Unfortunately, they did not show a full effect on aldosterone because a change in plasma sodium or sodium balance was not observed, suggesting that there was still adequate aldosterone available. Thirdly, as I alluded to, there is a mixed redundancy in hormonal systems. You may block or eliminate one set of hormones or one input to a hormone, and you often get another response. An example of this is the modulation of vasopressin by its two primary regulators, i.e., volume and osmolality. If you eliminate the input of one, the sensitivity of the other seems to increase in time. So there is, from the point of view of the regulation of a single hormone, a lot of redundancy.

Of interest about ANP is that ANP is only increased acutely in exercise. As you continue to exercise, the ANP levels come back down. ANP levels are increased prior to the rise in aldosterone, suggesting that they may be associated with the natriuresis that Kachadorian showed during low-intensity walking in some of his early work.

TIPTON: Does circulating ANP change at all with dehydration?

CONVERTINO: With dehydration, there is a decrease in ANP. That is just out of our laboratory. Charlie Wade, you've mentioned that there are data to suggest that during low-intensity exercise there is a natriuresis which is coincident with the increase in ANP; with high-intensity exercise, we find just the opposite effect, i.e., a reduced clearance of sodium, yet higher levels of ANP. We certainly would argue against a significant role of ANP in any exercise-induced natriuresis.

DAVIS: In one of your studies, you showed that aldosterone was maintained at a low level, despite an increase in plasma renin activity. What does that mean?

WADE: We blocked the renin-angiotensin system and were still able to elicit the rise in plasma aldosterone. During exercise, there appears to be a greater sensitivity of aldosterone to other modulators of its regulation. There are four components that can affect aldosterone secretion: sodium, potassium, ACTH, and the renin-angiotensin system. The major point appears to be that during exercise, the sodium drive or ACTH drive can override or overcome the blockade of the renin-angiotensin system. There are other conditions where one can observe dissociation of the renin-angiotensin system and aldosterone, not only in these types of studies, but also in clinical studies.

DAVIS: But what is keeping aldosterone down when you have high renin activity?

WADE: That may be related to the plasma sodium levels. We showed an inverse relationship between plasma sodium and plasma aldosterone, even though PRA was not changed. So as you drop the plasma sodium level, you increase the aldosterone.

PHILLIPS: Are trained athletes able to use the hormones differently than nonathletes? Are the hormones relevant to exercise?

WADE: The circulating hormone concentrations are often the same, but due to receptor changes, athletes are probably able to use the hormones differently.

CONVERTINO: As an example of this, in our heat acclimation study, we found resting levels of aldosterone were not altered, but the 24-h sodium clearance was significantly reduced. This suggests that there may be a training-induced increase in the receptor sensitivity or number of receptors available. Thus, it looks like the athletes use the hormones differently. They have the same circulating hormone content, but athletes might be able to use it differently.

YOUSEF: I am intrigued by the fact that at a lower workload of 50% $\dot{V}O_2max$, you don't have a change in the hormones. Does this mean that hormones don't play a role if the workload is 50% $\dot{V}O_2max$ or lower?

WADE: That is true if it is a brief work bout. Duration plays a major affect. If work at 35% of $\dot{V}O_2max$ is continued for over 30–60 min, then the hormones start increasing. Some of our early work demonstrates that.

SUTTON: I remain to be convinced that we've got any concrete evidence that the hormonal changes that we've been mentioning really have any importance at all in plasma volume expansion. Can you defend that hypothesis forcefully?

WADE: We can argue that one back and forth; Vic Convertino is on one side of the fence and I'm on the other. I don't believe that there is a hormonal role in the plasma volume expansion; I believe it has to do with protein flux. Whether or not hormones play a role in that is different. Vic has suggested that there may be a role for hormones in the conservation of fluids. All I'm saying is that with long-term, repeated exercise and in training states where we don't get any expansion of plasma volume, there are problems that can be corrected, such as hyponatremia. The role of hormones in the plasma volume expansion with heavy training has yet to be elucidated, I agree.

I think that there is an important heat component involved in the expansion of plasma volume. How it is mediated, I'm not sure. When we've done long-term training studies with moderate exercise in neutral environments, we've yet to see an expansion of plasma volume. But both Vic Convertino and Mike Sawka have been able to acutely expand plasma volume with training in the heat. Whether or not it is hormonally mediated is still a question.

SAWKA: I think you're correct; there is a heat component. There are several mechanisms involved. First, if you look at the effects of heat acclimation on resting plasma volume, you see an expansion of plasma volume within the first few days of acclimation that returns to baseline by the 8th to 10th day. Second, if the heat-acclimated individual initiates upright exercise in the heat, he will expand his plasma volume. I think there are at least two possible mechanisms occurring. One is that the combination of acute exercise and heat exposure may decrease hepatic blood flow and cause an increase in plasma protein synthesis early in heat acclimation. Then, later in acclimation, extracellular fluid may be further expanded by hormonal adaptations. The net effect is that the extra plasma proteins retain the additional extracellular fluid in the vascular space. With additional heat acclimation, the exercise-heat stress causes smaller reductions in hepatic flow so there is no additional stimulus for further enhanced production of plasma proteins. The second mechanism is one which Senay proposed for many years, that is, the intravascular protein mass is only a reflection of an equilibrium between the extravascular and intravascular protein mass. He has suggested that albumin and globulins may be sequestered in the cutaneous interstitial spaces. With heat stress, these proteins are washed into the intravascular space where they exert oncotic pressure to expand plasma volume. Thus, there may be two separate reasons for plasma volume expansion with heat acclimation: 1) an expansion of extracellular fluid volume, and 2) the accumulation of proteins in the plasma that hold fluid in the vascular space by oncotic pressure. The mechanisms underlying these adaptations are probably very complex and will be controversial for many years.

CONVERTINO: We find a net increase in total body water, not just in the plasma, that either is caused by increasing fluid intake with the same fluid output or by maintaining the same intake with greater retention. We find that fluid intake replaces the loss through sweat and respiration during the exercise/heat exposures and that there is also a net retention of salt and water by the kidneys during recovery. It seems reasonable to hypothesize that this salt and water retention is hormonally regulated. I think that Senay's argument is an appropriate one for events during exercise, when there is not a better way of rapidly replacing or defending plasma volume. During recovery, I think the hormones may come into play.

WADE: Vic, in your trained individuals, there was an elevation in plasma aldosterone levels. In our training studies we don't see a change in resting aldosterone.

CONVERTINO: We don't see a change in resting aldosterone, but we see it during the exercise bout. But we think there is an increase in renal sensitivity to aldosterone. We see a 50% reduction in sodium clearance with the same resting aldosterone levels.

WADE: One of the problems in interpreting changes in circulating aldosterone is that an exercise-induced increase in aldosterone may have effects on sodium conservation for up to 8 h, i.e., long after circulating concentrations of aldosterone have returned to resting baseline values. Thus, even though Vic sees an acute aldosterone elevation that subsequently returns to normal, there still may be a lingering conservation of sodium that leads to an expanded plasma volume.

7

Renal Regulation of Fluid Homeostasis During Exercise

EDWARD J. ZAMBRASKI, PH.D.

INTRODUCTION

The appropriateness of including a chapter on the renal regulation of body fluid homeostasis during exercise is obvious. When one thinks of body fluid balance, or imbalance, the organs that first come to mind should be the kidneys.

This chapter will delineate the essential role and importance of the kidneys in body fluid balance during and after exercise. Unfortunately, the specific reasons why the kidneys are so important in this regard are, for the most part, misunderstood. As will be shown, there are two major misconceptions about the kidneys or renal function. The first deals with the kidneys' role in the conservation of water and sodium. During exercise the renal response is a decrease in the excretion of water and sodium. Quantatively the magnitude and importance of this response is significantly overestimated. The second fallacy is that with exercise, even in a hypohydrated state, a large amount of blood is shunted away from the kidneys to allow for increased muscle and/or cutaneous blood flow.

The kidneys are important during and especially after exercise in the overall control of body fluid balance, but their major role and significance, especially during exercise, transcends a simple reduction of water and sodium excretion, or a redistribution of renal blood flow. The purpose of this chapter is to define the changes in kidney function during exercise in relation to body fluid homeostasis and to the extent possible, to delineate the mechanisms responsible for these changes. A major emphasis is placed on how changes in renal function mediate non-renal compensatory responses to body fluid deficits associated with exercise.

Because a major focus of this book is on performance, this chapter will emphasize renal function in humans. Studies from animal models will only be referred to when necessary to illustrate possible mechanisms of control. Also, similarities and dissimilarities between humans and specific animal models with regard to renal function and body fluid homeostasis will be pointed out. Lastly, several excellent reviews on the topic of renal function and exercise have been written (Castenfors, 1977; Poortmans, 1984). To emphasize the role of the kidneys in body fluid homeostasis, studies dealing with the kidneys and exercise that do not directly relate to body fluid balance will not be discussed.

REVIEW OF RENAL PHYSIOLOGY

The primary role of the kidneys is to filter plasma to remove various metabolic wastes. The structure of the kidneys, or that of their functional unit, the nephron, is unique in terms of the anatomy that allows for extensive interaction between the systemic circulation or circulatory compartment, and the renal tubule or excretory compartment.

The processes occurring in the kidneys, that are essentially interactions or movements of water/solute between the circulatory and renal tubule compartments, are glomerular filtration, tubular reabsorption, and tubular secretion. Glomerular filtration is the movement of water and solute from the circulation into the renal tubule at the glomerular capillary. Reabsorption is the movement of filtered water/solute from the renal tubular lumen, through the tubular cells, back into the peritubular capillaries, or the circulation. Secretion is the active transport of solute, but not water, from the peritubular capillaries into the renal tubular lumen. The excretion of water and solute is the net effect of glomerular filtration versus renal tubular reabsorption with renal tubular secretion influencing only selective solutes.

The kidneys, which comprise only 0.4% of body weight, receive 20–25% of the cardiac output at rest, or more blood flow than any other organ. The majority (90%) of this renal blood flow (RBF) perfuses the renal cortex, with only 10% or less distributed to the renal medulla. Within the cortex there is also a heterogenous flow pattern with the outer cortex receiving a greater fraction of flow as compared to the inner cortex.

Because only plasma is filtered by the glomerular capillaries, total renal plasma flow (RPF) is approximately 650 ml/min. The amount of plasma filtered per unit time, or glomerular filtration rate (GFR), is approximately 120 ml/min. Therefore, of the total RPF, which could potentially all be filtered, only 120/650 or 15–20% normally passes into the renal tubule. This fraction, GFR/RPF, is termed the filtration fraction (FF). By alterations in either RPF or GFR, or disproportionate changes in both parameters, FF can be altered.

It is important to note that in man we do not have the capacity to measure instantaneous RPF or GFR. These parameters are measured using the urinary clearance of substances such as para-aminohippurate (PAH) for RPF and inulin for GFR. Both PAH and inulin are compounds that must be infused. Endogenous creatinine clearance may be used in humans to estimate GFR; however, its accuracy is limited because some creatinine is secreted, which causes GFR to be overestimated. Also, confounding non-steady state changes in plasma creatinine concentration may occur. When urinary clearance techniques are utilized to measure RPF/GFR in humans, especially during exercise, there is a major limitation because this is a time-integrated measure; urine must be collected for at least 15–20 minutes to obtain an adequate volume. These measures will only indicate the average GFR or RPF over the entire urine collection period. To be accurate, steady-state conditions should exist. Nonetheless, urinary clearance measurements of RPF and GRF in humans during and after exercise have provided much valuable information. In animal models, the use of surgically implanted doppler or electromagnetic flow probes on the renal artery have enabled the instantaneous and continuous measurement of RBF during exercise. However, GFR for the most part must still be measured using the urinary clearance of inulin.

GFR is of primary importance in determining the renal handling of water and sodium because only through GFR can water and sodium gain access to the renal tubular lumen for potential excretion. If GFR is decreased, this reduction in the filtered load is an effective mechanism to decrease the excretion of water and electrolytes.

The forces governing glomerular filtration are similar to those at any capillary, namely the existing hydrostatic and oncotic pressure gradients. In the glomerular capillaries, there is always a net driving force causing filtration. This force acts on the plasma to filter water and various small solutes such as electrolytes, glucose, and amino acids. The filtration of larger molecules (>40Å), such as various plasma proteins, does not normally occur due to the glomerular capillary membrane's molecular size and charge selectivity. The actual amount of filtration also depends upon the K_f or glomeruler capillary ultrafiltration coefficient. In the kidneys, the K_f is an extremely dynamic variable. As will be discussed, it may be dramatically changed (usually reduced) by various hormonal and/or neural stimuli.

With a normal GFR of 120 ml/min, approximately 170 liters of plasma ultrafiltrate are translocated into the renal tubular lumen in 24 hours. Because we only excrete approximately 1.5 liters of urine (1.0 ml/min) during the same time period, the renal tubule is reabsorbing 99% of the filtered load of fluid (i.e. water) back into the circulation. Beyond adjustments of the filtered load (i.e. changes in GFR) it is the control of renal tubular reabsorption of water that determines urine output.

As discussed in Chapter 1, the maintenance of total body fluid homeostasis is accomplished by the tight regulation of total body sodium. Through changes in the renal handling of sodium the kidney precisely regulates body water and sodium. Because of the importance of being able to control or adjust urinary sodium excretion, there are multiple mechanisms that may influence renal tubular sodium reabsorption. Intrarenal control factors include local secretion of renin, angiotensin II, prostaglandins (PG), and dopamine; changes in FF; glomerulotubular balance; and possible intrarenal feedback systems involving the macula densa and juxtaglomerular apparatus. To quantitate the relative contribution of each of these intrarenal control systems to the renal handling of sodium in the exercise condition has been largely impossible.

Some of the extrarenal factors capable of altering renal tubular sodium reabsorption are: renal perfusion pressure; renal sympathetic nerve activity; and various hormonal substances such as norepinephrine (NE), epinephrine, aldosterone, antidiurectic hormone (ADH), atrial natriuretic peptide (ANP), and insulin. Because renal tubular chloride reabsorption is tightly linked to sodium reabsorption, factors that increase or decrease urinary sodium excretion usually modify urinary chloride excretion in a similar manner. In addition, active renal tubular reabsorption of chloride, as the primary ion, does occur. The regulation of urinary potassium excretion is accomplished by altering tubular reabsorption and tubular secretion. In the distal segments of the nephron, an aldosterone-induced increase in tubular sodium reabsorption increases tubular potassium and hydrogen ion secretion. Consequently, a beneficial renal conservation of sodium may be at the expense of increased renal potassium loss.

The renal handling of water is accomplished by two distinctly different mechanisms. The majority of all water reabsorbed by the kidney (80–85%) is accomplished by isotonic reabsorption. This process involves water reabsorption from the proximal tubule as a consequence of an osmotic pressure gradient created by the active tubular reabsorption of solutes, which for the most part are sodium and chloride. Because the concentration of sodium in the fluid reabsorbed is the same as that in the tubular luminal fluid and in the peritubular capillary blood, neither the sodium concentration in the tubular lumen or peritubular capillary is changed, hence reabsorption is isotonic. There are two major implications of this process. The first is that any factor that causes an increase in renal tubular sodium reabsorption will, via isotonic reabsorption, increase renal tubular water reabsorption. Because the majority of filtered sodium is reabsorbed by the end of the renal proximal tubule, most of the water will be returned to the circulation before the loop of Henle.

An example of increasing renal tubular sodium reabsorption to decrease urinary water excretion in the distal segments of the nephron is seen with aldosterone. The short-term effects of aldosterone on the urinary excretion of sodium/water are largely overestimated. At any point in time, aldosterone is only responsible for approximately 2% of renal tubular sodium reabsorption. However, the importance of aldosterone in long-term control should not be de-emphasized. Because huge amounts of water (170 liters) and sodium (24,000 mEq) are filtered each day, an aldosterone-mediated 1–2% change in renal tubular reabsorption of these large amounts can have a profound cumulative effect on body fluid/sodium homeostasis.

The second major implication of isotonic reabsorption is that it only enables one to produce a renal tubular luminal fluid that is isosmotic to plasma (285–300 mosm/kg). Isotonic reabsorption does not enable the tubular reabsorption of more water, in relation to solute, to form a concentrated or hyperosmotic fluid, relative to plasma. The ability to concentrate the final urine is due to the action of ADH or vasopressin in more distal segments of the nephron. By increasing the water permeability of the collecting duct, the extremely hyperosmotic medullary interstitium enables the abstraction of water from the tubular lumen to create a concentrated urine with an osmolality as high as 1200 mosm/kg (i.e. four times as concentrated as plasma). If tonicity of the medullary interstitium declines, the ability of ADH to form a hypertonic urine is limited. The factors responsible for regulating plasma ADH concentration during exercise have been discussed in Chapter 6. Without ADH, daily urine output would be 15–20 liters, as compared to a normal 1.5 liters/day. With 175 liters of water being filtered, this means that ADH is only mediating about 8–10% of total tubular reabsorption of water. As with aldosterone, the acute affects of ADH may be small, but the cumulative long-term effects on total body water and osmolality are of major significance.

In relation to isosmotic versus hyperosmotic reabsorption of water, it is necessary to define the concept of free water clearance (C_{H2O}). Because the kidneys are responsible for excreting various solutes, such as urea, fixed acids, etc., the excretion of any given solute load requires accompanying amount of water. For whatever given amount of solute that must be eliminated, if one excretes just enough water to excrete that load isosmotically to plasma (ie. osmolality 300 mosm/kg) then the C_{H2O} is zero. This means that no "pure water" over and above the amount needed to excrete this load isosmotically is added to the urine. If additional water is excreted, as in the case of a hypo-osmotic or dilute urine, C_{H2O} is positive. Because urine is normally concentrated by the action of ADH, C_{H2O} is usually negative and "free water" is returned to the plasma. With exercise and/or fluid deficits and concomitant increases in plasma ADH concentrations, the appropriate or expected response would be to further decrease C_{H2O}, or to make it more negative. This does not necessarily occur during exercise (see below).

ACUTE RESPONSE OF THE KIDNEYS TO EXERCISE

Deficits in total body water and sodium may result from intense and/or prolonged exercise. To understand and separate the renal responses to the stress of exercise, versus fluid and electrolyte loss, it is helpful to first evaluate the acute responses of the kidneys to an exercise stress alone. Fortunately, the renal responses with these two different perturbations are very similar, suggesting the existence of common control mechanisms.

A. Renal Hemodynamic Changes

Renal blood flow: Numerous studies in humans, using the urinary clearance of PAH, have demonstrated that RPF is decreased with heavy exercise (Castenfors, 1967; Chapman et al., 1948; Grimby, 1965; Radigan & Robinson, 1949; White & Rolf, 1948). In 1948, Chapman et al. reported decreases of 15, 27, and 35% in PAH clearance in men exercised at 3 different progressively increasing workloads. In the same year, White and Rolf (1948) ran 6 subjects at 6–7 mph, and PAH clearance decreased on the average by 57%. Baseline PAH clearance was approximately 700 ml/min. Radigan and Robinson (1949) also reported PAH clearance decreased from 695 to 422 ml/min, or a 43% decline in normal exercising subjects. Grimby (1965), using various workloads, reported reductions of PAH clearance averaging around 30%, with the largest recorded decreases being in the range of 40–55%. Lastly, Castenfors (1967) reported decreases in PAH clearance from 700 to 400 ml/min with strenuous exercise. These studies clearly demonstrate that RPF is significantly decreased with heavy exercise; the largest decrements appear to be in the 50–60% range.

Using various animal models, investigators have evaluated the RBF responses to exercise to see if similar changes occur and to elucidate the mechanism responsible for the renal vasoconstriction. In the exercising normal dog, the majority of studies have shown that RBF is not significantly decreased (Delgado et al., 1975; Musch et al., 1987). Interestingly enough, if dogs are made anemic, splenectomized, or manipulated to induce congestive heart failure, a significant decline in RBF is observed with exercise (Vatner et al, 1972; Vatner et al., 1971). In contrast to dogs, Hohimer and colleagues (1979, 1983) reported 16–19% decreases in RBF during acute exercise in the baboon. In a very elegant study they evaluated the effects of renal denervation on this response by measuring RBF bilaterally with unilateral renal denervation. During a 4-min exercise test, RBF to the innervated kidney decreased below the resting level, whereas RBF initially rose and then gradually decreased in the denervated kidney but only to the resting level. In Yucatan miniature swine, Sanders et al. (1976) have also shown that RBF is significantly decreased during treadmill exercise.

These results suggest that the decline in RBF during exercise is mediated by an increase in renal sympathetic nerve activity. Responses in primates and miniature swine resemble the responses observed in man. The normal dog is an inappropriate model to evaluate renal hemodynamic changes during exercise, presumably due to a powerful RBF autoregulatory mechanism that predominates over any alterations in renal sympathetic activity. In man, indirect evidence suggests that increased plasma angiotensin II concentration is not responsible for the renal vasoconstriction during exercise. Castenfors (1967) used ethacrynic acid administration to elevate renin-angiotensin system activity, but could not alter the normal decline in PAH clearance with exercise. Very recently Wade et al. (1987) used angiotensin I converting enzyme inhibitors to block the formation of angiotensin II in exercising men. PAH clearance was not measured, but the failure of the converting enzyme inhibitor to alter the normal decrement in GFR, urinary flow rate, and sodium excretion suggests that the renal vasoconstriction during exercise is not due to angiotensin II.

Because of technical difficulties, the measurement of the intrarenal distribution of RBF during exercise has not been made in man. In the dog and miniature pig there is no redistribution of RBF within the kidney during exercise (Delgado et al., 1975; Sanders et al., 1976).

Glomerular filtration rate: Significant changes in GFR have been observed during exercise. Some of the early studies using relatively light exercise (Kattus et al., 1949), and experiments in which subjects were excessively hydrated prior to testing (Castenfors, 1967), have reported no changes in GFR. An evaluation of the GFR response to 3 different exercise workloads was made by Kachadorian and Johnson (1970). They found that GFR was either increased or unchanged at light-moderate exercise and significantly decreased only at heavy exercise. Another study by Grimby (1965) reported decreases in GFR of 6–10% with light-moderate exercise, while with heavy exercise GFR declined 30–50%. Radigan and Robinson (1949) reported no change in GFR with exercise, while White and Rolf (1948) observed an average decrement in GFR of 53% during exhaustive exercise. To date, very few animal studies have systematically evaluated the changes in GFR during exercise or in particular, possible increases in GFR seen in some studies with light exercise. In man, decrements in GFR during exercise, when they occur, are probably the result of increased renal sympathetic nerve activity.

Filtration fraction: The renal hemodynamic results discussed thus far, indicating a significant fall in RPF with less dramatic changes in GFR support the consensus view that filtration fraction (FF) is increased with acute exercise (Castenfors, 1967; Castenfors, 1977; Grimby, 1965; Radigan & Robinson, 1949; White & Rolf, 1948). This is illustrated in Figure 7-1. In the exercise situation with profound renal vasoconstriction causing decreases in RBF without changes in GFR, there are two possible explanations for this increased FF. One possibility is a relatively greater constriction of the efferent glomerular arteriole as compared to the afferent glomerular arteriole. This would maintain glomerular capillary hydrostatic pressure and preserve GFR, despite a fall in RPF. The existence of differential responses of the afferent versus efferent arterioles to circulating catecholamines or neuronally released norepinephrine has not been supported in the literature. Another attractive hypothesis is that during exercise, locally formed (i.e. intrarenal) angiotensin II, which may preferentially cause efferent arteriolar constriction, is responsible for increasing FF. This is difficult to prove in the exercising condition. In fact, assuming that captopril treatment blocks the synthesis of angiotensin II at the efferent arterioles, the data of Wade et al. (1987) showing that captopril did not alter the GFR response to exercise, argue against this possibility. Unfortunately, they did not measure RPF in their study so changes in FF with captopril could not be evaluated.

The other possibility to explain the increase in FF during exercise is an increase in glomerular capillary K_f. An increase in glomerular capillary K_f at times when afferent arteriolar constriction is decreasing glomerular capillary hydrostatic pressure, would assist in maintaining GFR. Numerous hormones and autocoids, such as ADH, PG, and angiotensin II, which are probably released during exercise, conceivably could alter K_f (Dunn, 1984). Unfortunately, it is not feasible to directly test this possibility by measuring K_f in an exercise setting.

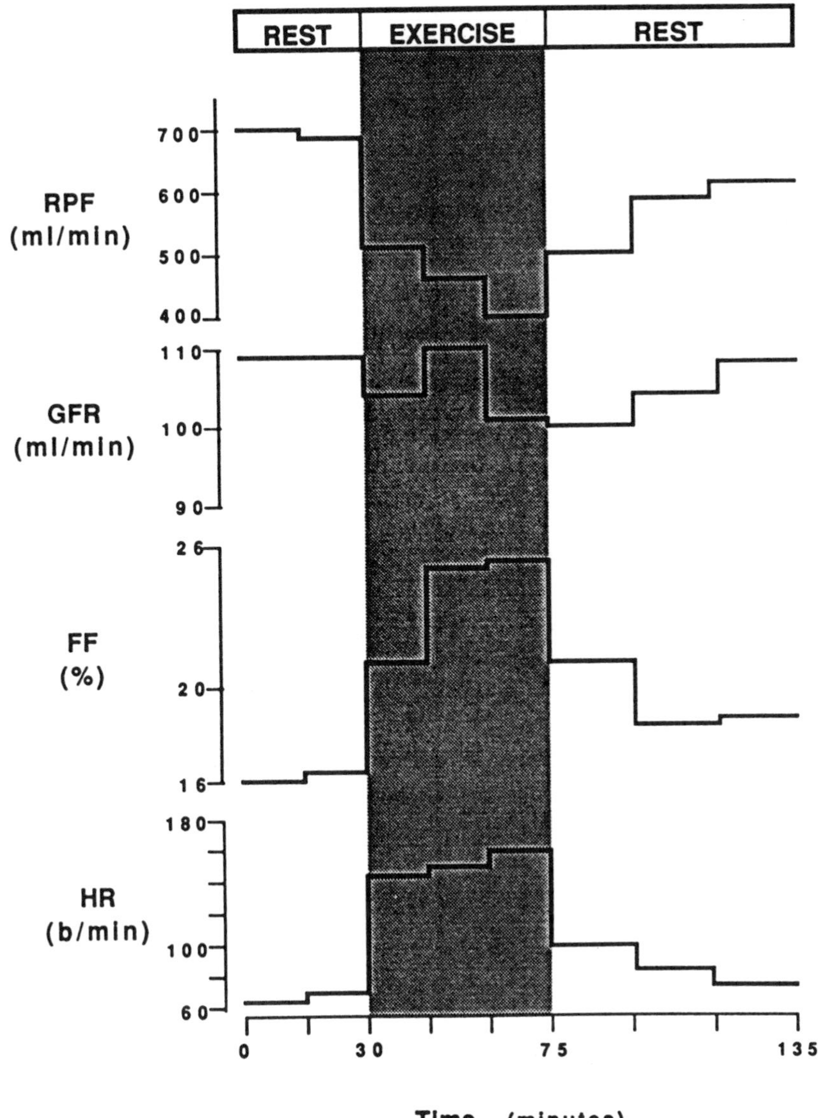

FIGURE 7-1. *The effects of acute moderate-heavy exercise in 14 men on renal plasma flow (RPF), glomerular filtration rate (GFR), filtration fraction (FF), and heart rate (HR) are shown. Values for RPF and GFR have been normalized for body size (1.73m²). This figure has been constructed from published data (Castentors, 1977).*

Importance of the Decrease in Renal Blood Flow During Exercise: It has become ingrained in our teaching, and our minds, that the shunting or diversion of blood away from the kidneys to metabolically active tissue (i.e. skeletal muscle) is an important and necessary cardiovascular adjustment to acute exercise. Diagrams, such as that in the text by Astrand

and Rodahl (1986), showing that the fraction of the cardiac output going to the kidneys decreases from 20 to 2–4%, reinforce the belief that this response is of major importance.

During the most intense exercise, the amount of blood flow actually diverted from the kidneys for use as cardiac output to non-renal areas is small. As discussed earlier, measured absolute RBF may decrease from 700 to 400 ml/min during exercise which is a reduction of some 300 ml/min. During heavy exercise when cardiac output may be 20–25 l/min, gaining 300 ml/min of blood flow from the kidneys is a very small contribution (<2%). This fact was pointed out by Rowell (1974) years ago. Rowell (1974) also indicated that such a redistribution of blood flow would only be of consequence to someone who had a severely limited cardiac output, such as a patient with cardiac failure. It should be emphasized that a 30–40% reduction in absolute RBF is clearly a significant event for the kidneys. The impact that this reduction in RBF has on renal function is largely unknown.

Despite the fact that the absolute amount of blood flow redistributed is limited, renal vasoconstriction, which increases renal vascular resistance during exercise, is extremely important. Because the kidneys generally receive a large amount of blood flow (fraction of cardiac output), they potentially comprise a large fraction of total peripheral resistance. During exercise, with metabolic and neurally mediated dilation of skeletal muscle blood vessels, the increase in renal vascular resistance is essential in maintaining the increased systemic arterial pressure needed to perfuse active skeletal muscle.

B. Changes in Excretory Function with Exercise

Urinary Flow Rate: It is well accepted that moderate to heavy exercise reduces urinary flow rate. It is difficult to quantify the magnitude of this exercise-induced antidiuresis from the literature because of differences in control urine flow rates, often due to the pre-exercise hydration of subjects. Normal resting urine flow rates range from 0.8 to 1.5 ml/min. Using non-hydrated subjects, urine volume declines of 22%, 48%, 14%, and 37% in studies by Wade et al., (1980), White and Rolf (1948), Wade et al. (1987), and Kachadorian and Johnson (1970), respectively, have been reported. In excessively hydrated subjects performing heavy exercise, urinary flow rate was not significantly altered in a study by Grimby (1965) and decreased 56% in a report by Castenfors (1967). In field studies, the effects of prolonged exercise on urinary flow rate have been reported. Castenfors (1967) reported that urinary flow rate decreased from 0.73 to 0.50 ml/min after an 85-km cross-country ski race. After a 29-km average daily run, as part of a 20-day road race, Wade et al. (1985) reported that urinary flow rate decreased from 1.2 to 0.8 ml/min.

These studies indicate that during acute moderate exercise or strenuous prolonged exercise a decrease in urinary flow rate usually occurs.

An important point is that with "normal" pre-exercise urine flow rates, the actual amount of water retained due to decreased urinary excretion is relatively small, ranging from 0.2 to perhaps 0.75 ml/min. As indicated earlier, because we are normally in a state of negative C_{H2O} (i.e. hyperosmotic concentrated urine) urine flow rate at rest is low. Consequently, the amount of water that can be conserved due to a reduction in urinary flow rate is quite small.

Urinary Sodium Excretion: Several studies have examined the effects of acute exercise on urinary sodium excretion. Using various workloads, Aurell et al. (1967) indicated that urinary sodium excretion increased or showed variable changes at light to moderate workloads, but was dramatically reduced at heavier (>450 kpm/min) work-loads. The decrease in urinary sodium excretion was greater than what could be accounted for by a decrease in filtered sodium load (i.e. decreased GFR), suggesting increased renal tubular sodium reabsorption. Castenfors (1967) also reported significant decreases in urinary sodium excretion in hydrated subjects prior to testing. This exercise test did not decrease GFR, but did increase FF. The decrease in sodium excretion was attributed to increased renal tubular sodium reabsorption. Lastly, Raisz et al. (1959) reported large decreases in urinary sodium excretion during acute exercise, along with significant decreases in GFR; estimates of renal tubular sodium reabsorption were not made.

Increased urinary sodium excretion has been reported in some studies evaluating the effects of light exercise (Kachadorian & Johnson, 1970). The mechanism responsible for this is unclear. Possibilities might include the effects of increased atrial natriuretic peptide (discussed later in the chapter). Increased renal perfusion pressure could increase sodium excretion during light exercise, due to the lack of several antinatriuretic influences (i.e., endocrine, neural) that may not be fully activated until exercise of moderate-heavy intensity is reached.

Various studies have also evaluated the effects of prolonged exercise on urinary sodium excretion. Castenfors (1967) found that urinary sodium excretion declined by 43% after an 85-km cross-country ski race, even when normalized for changes in GFR. Urinary potassium excretion increased. In 1981, Wade and associates (1981) examined how a 20-day road race with the subjects running 28 km/day affected the excretion of electrolytes. By 12 hours post-race, urinary sodium excretion was generally reduced, but urinary flow rate did not fall. Renal retention of sodium appeared to continue for up to 20 hours of recovery. By retaining sodium, these subjects were able to replace average daily body weight losses of 2.0–2.5 kg. In a subsequent study of the same prolonged race, Wade et al. (1985) confirmed the prolonged decrease in urinary sodium excretion and reported a significant inverse relationship between urinary sodium excretion and plasma aldosterone concentration (r^2=0.73). This prolonged elevation in plasma aldosterone concentration with these intense daily exercise periods has also been reported by Kosunen et al. (1980). These studies demonstrate a consistent anti-natriuretic effect of acute exercise with continued sodium retention over longer periods of time with intense intermittent work. Changes in urinary potassium excretion, which may increase after acute heavy exercise, are much less consistent.

During acute exercise, several factors could be responsible for the increase in renal tubular sodium (and chloride) reabsorption. These would include increased renal sympathetic nerve activity, increased FF, increased plasma angiotensin II concentration, increased plasma aldosterone concentration, and increased plasma ADH concentration. The antinatriuresis observed during acute exercise has been correlated with increased plasma aldosterone concentration (Poortmans, 1984). However, as noted by Castenfors (1967), the time course for the increase in renal tubular sodium reabsorption is very rapid, well before the 30–45 minute minimal time period required for plasma aldosterone concentration to increase and exert its effect. In the study by Wade et al. (1987), the failure of an angiotensin I-converting enzyme inhibitor to influence the exercise effect on urinary sodium excretion suggests that angiotensin II is not mediating the antinatriuresis. A confounding factor in that study was that a significant increase in renal tubular sodium reabsorption was not observed in the subjects during the control runs.

Data from animal models may illustrate the mechanism(s) responsible for the decrease in urinary sodium excretion with acute exercise. During acute exercise in the dog, urinary sodium excretion has been reported to remain unchanged (Carlin et al., 1950), or even increase (Grignolo et al., 1981). A study by Sadowski et al. (1981) evaluated the excretory response to exercise in dogs with unilateral denervation. The results, which showed that exercise caused a greater renal vasoconstriction and antinatriuretic effect in the denervated compared to the innervated kidneys, were not predicted and may have been due to a denervation-induced renal vascular and tubular hypersensitivity to circulating catecholamines (i.e., norepinephrine). These studies demonstrate that, in the dog, inconsistent changes in urinary sodium excretion during exercise have been reported.

In the last decade it has been documented that renal sympathetic (adrenergic) nerves have the capacity to directly increase renal tubular sodium reabsorption. Various aspects of this direct neurogenic control over renal tubular sodium reabsorption have been recently reviewed (DiBona, 1978; DiBona, 1982). Miniature swine appear to have large increases in renal sympathetic nerve activity that results in significant renal vasoconstriction during exercise. The data for six animals is shown in Figure 7-2 (unpublished results). In all animals, there was a pronounced decrease in urinary sodium excretion during acute exercise. This decrease in urinary sodium excretion could not be attributed to changes in

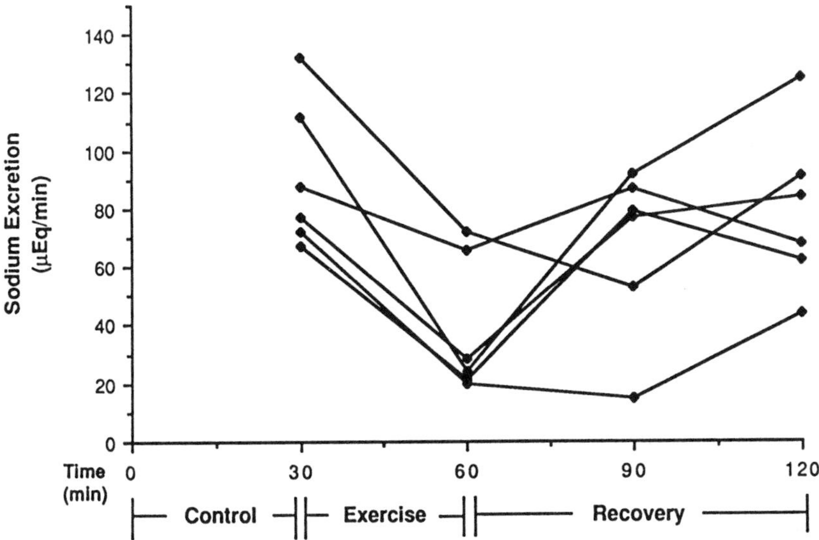

FIGURE 7-2. *The effects of 30 min of treadmill exercise, at 80% of maximal heart rate, on sodium excretion in 6 Yucatan miniature swine. The time course for the antinatriuresis suggests a neurally mediated event.*

filtered load because there were no significant changes in GFR. Within the first 30 minutes of recovery, the majority of the animals had increased urinary sodium excretion back to control levels with all of the animals re-achieving baseline urinary sodium excretion by 60 minutes of recovery. The time course for the onset/recovery of this antinatriuretic effect suggests a neural mechanism compared to a slower, longer lasting hormone effect (e.g., aldosterone). Also, three of the six animals in Figure 7-2 were receiving chronic mineralocorticoid treatment (DOCA) to suppress their renin-angiotensin systems. The demonstrated antinatriuretic effect in these three renin-suppressed animals, which is indistinguishable from the three normals, indicates that this antinatriuresis is not mediated by angiotensin II. In these animals, exercise also reduced urinary flow rate by approximately 70%. At 60 minutes post-exercise, even though urinary sodium excretion had recovered, urinary flow rate was still significantly decreased. As yet, we have not evaluated the effects of renal denervation in the miniature swine to conclusively implicate a neurogenic control over urinary sodium excretion during acute exercise.

KIDNEY AS AN ENDOCRINE ORGAN DURING EXERCISE

A. Renin—Angiotensin

It has been well documented that acute or prolonged exercise causes an increase in the renal synthesis and release of renin (Convertino et al.,

1981; Convertino et al., 1983; Hesse et al., 1978; Koch et al., 1980; Wade & Claybaugh, 1980). This is usually expressed as an increase in plasma renin activity (PRA). During exercise, measured circulating PRA is significantly less than what can be detected in the renal venous effluent (Hesse et al., 1978). Pro-renin, or inactive renin, decreases during exercise (Fujita et al., 1982). Several early studies in man have correlated the increment in PRA with increased exercise intensity and/or an increase in sympathetic drive (Convertino et al., 1981, Fujita et al., 1982; Hesse et al., 1978; Wade & Claybaugh, 1980). Decreased renal perfusion pressure, increased prostaglandins, increased sympathetic activity, and intrarenal mechanisms involving glomerular-tubular feedback and changes in renal hemodynamics, such as a decline in RPF as seen with exercise, may also evoke renal renin release (Stella & Zanchetti, 1987).

One of the first studies to suggest a direct sympathetic control of renin release during exercise was by Zambraski et al. (1984) in the exercising dog. The dog model was chosen because renal hemodynamic changes during exercise are minimal in this species. In that study, interruption of renal sympathetic nerve activity using guanethidine or administration of a beta-l adrenergic receptor antagonist (metoprolol) completely abolished the exercise-induced increase in renin release. These data implicated a sympathetic neural beta-l adrenoceptor mediated effect. Prostaglandin inhibition did not alter the response, indicating that the exercise renin response was prostaglandin-independent.

Numerous subsequent studies in humans have shown that either non-selective beta adrenoceptor-blockade or selective beta-l adrenoceptor blockade attenuates the renin response to exercise (Hansson et al., 1977; Hansson & Hokfelt, 1975; Lammintausta et al., 1979; Winer et al., 1979). Although epinephrine can increase renin release, it is probably not involved in the exercise response because guanethidine leaves the response to epinephrine intact; however guanethidine abolishes the increase in PRA (Zambraski et al., 1984). Also, Guezennec et al. (1986) compared the PRA response to swimming versus running and observed a blunted PRA with swimming even though plasma epinephrine was higher after swimming.

The release of renin during exercise appears to be limited by an angiotensin II-mediated negative feedback loop. If this loop is pharmacologically interrupted, the PRA response to exercise is increased (Fagard et al., 1985). Sodium deprivation or hypohydration, which increases basal PRA, does not change the PRA response to exercise (Francesconi et al., 1985; Leenen et al., 1978). For reasons that are unclear, the PRA response to exercise is blunted in hypertensives and also in their normotensive offspring (Fasola et al., 1968; Fasola et al., 1966).

An increase in renin will generate angiotensin II. A major effect of angiotensin II is the stimulation of aldosterone release. Although there are parallel increases in renin-angiotensin and aldosterone during exercise (Convertino et al., 1981), several recent studies dissociate the two factors (Hohimer et al., 1983; Lijnen et al., 1979; Melin et al., 1980; Staessen et al., 1987), suggesting that the increase in aldosterone may not be totally renin-dependent. The most recent of these studies by Wade et al. (1987) found that, in man, captopril treatment had no affect on the exercise-stimulated aldosterone response. There is an increased awareness that the sympathetic nervous system may affect not only adrenal medullary function, but also adrenal cortical steroid synthesis (Rauch & Campbell, 1988). The possibility that the exercise-induced increase in aldosterone is neurogenically mediated remains to be determined.

Data are available indicating that the increase in plasma angiotensin II concentration with heavy exercise contributes to the increase in systemic arterial pressure. This conclusion derives from studies in which either angiotensin II receptor blockade or converting enzyme inhibition attenuated the arterial pressure rise during exercise (Fagard et al., 1977; Fagard et al., 1978; Wade et al., 1987).

Angiotensin II may have a stimulating effect on the autonomic nervous system to increase sympathetic outflow. In normal man, interruption of the renin-angiotensin system has equivocal effects on the increase in plasma catecholamine concentrations observed during exercise. However, McGrath and Arnolda (1986) have recently shown that in patients with cardiac failure, converting enzyme inhibition markedly reduces the increment in plasma norepinephrine concentration during exercise.

The potential intrarenal effects of angiotensin II are numerous. Angiotensin II can cause glomerular arteriolar constriction, decrease K_f, increase renal prostaglandin synthesis, increase renal tubular sodium reabsorption, and facilitate the release of neurotransmitters from adrenergic nerve terminals. It is extremely difficult to differentiate between the systemic effects (i.e. increased arterial pressure, change in sympathetic activity) and the potential intrarenal effects of angiotensin II during exercise stress.

B. Norepineprhine

Circulating plasma norepinephrine (NE) is believed to be the result of NE spillover from sympathetic nerve endings. The resultant plasma concentration of NE is a function of the amount of NE released into the circulation from various circulatory beds. The amount of NE release from a particular region will depend upon the degree to which that tissue is sympathetically innervated, as well as the relative sympathetic activity.

To quantify the degree to which various organs and circulating beds contribute to the increase in plasma NE concentration, Esler and associates (1988) performed a series of studies measuring local sites of NE spillover. In man, they have estimated that at rest, the kidneys contribute approximately 25% of the total NE spillover into plasma. In contrast, by their estimates, the adrenal gland and skeletal muscle contribute only 2 and 20%, respectively. Therefore, at rest, the kidneys may be the greatest contributors to circulating NE. These measurements have not been made in exercising man.

In the exercising dog, Peronnet et al. (1988) have recently suggested that the skeletal muscle contributes the greatest amount of NE to the circulation. Since NE release is proportional to the amount of local sympathetic innervation and tone, how applicable the results in the dog are to man is questionable. As discussed, in the dog the amount of sympathetic adrenergic activity to the kidneys during exercise is minimal. On a relative scale, as compared to skeletal muscle, one would envision a much greater increase in sympathetic adrenergic activity directed to the kidneys during exercise. This being the case, the kidneys would be the major source of circulating NE during exercise. By releasing NE into the plasma, the kidneys would be indirectly influencing many systemic circulatory and metabolic events.

C. Prostaglandins

The kidneys have a large capacity to synthesize prostaglandins (PG). The major PG in the kidneys appear to be PGE_2 and PGI_2. In the kidneys, PGs are generally thought to be vasodilators, natriuretic, and stimulators of renin release (Dunn, 1984). They also increase K_f by attenuating the effects of angiotensin II and ADH and inhibiting the actions of ADH on the collecting duct. PGs are not true hormones; they are better described as autocoids or substances that are produced and have a very local influence.

The question of whether exercise causes an increase in renal PG synthesis has been difficult to answer. Reported increases in peripheral venous plasma PG during exercise (Demers et al., 1981) do not necessarily represent increases in renal PG synthesis. Nowak and Wennmalm (1978) did report increases in renal venous PG concentrations in exercising man. The same group reported an increase in the urinary excretion of the PGI_2 metabolite after leg exercise (Wennmalm et al., 1988). The urinary excretion of PG in the female is believed to reflect renal PG synthesis. A study of treadmill exercised females reported extremely variable increases in urinary PGE_2 and $PGF_{2\alpha}$ excretion (Zambraski et al., 1986). The administration of indomethacin, a known renal PG synthesis inhibitor, abolished the increases in urinary PG excretion observed during exercise with placebo treatment. Indomethacin did not alter the normal exercise responses of GFR, urinary flow rate, or sodium excretion (Zambraski et al., 1986). During exercise, various stimuli such as increased sympathetic activity, catecholamines, ADH, and angiotensin II are present. Despite the fact that these factors are known to increase renal PG synthesis, the role that PGs play in determining kidney function during exercise has not been defined.

KIDNEY AS AN ENDOCRINE TARGET ORGAN DURING EXERCISE

The renal response, in terms of body fluid homeostasis, may be largely controlled by intra- and extrarenal hormonal stimuli. The actions of various intrarenal hormones, such as renin and PG, have already been discussed. The effects that ADH have on the kidney have been reviewed in Chapter 6. One additional extrarenal hormone which should be discussed is atrial natriuretic peptide (ANP).

In 1981, DeBold and colleagues reported that the administration of extracts of rat atria had a diuretic and natriuretic effect (Goetz, 1988). In less than three years, a 28 amino-acid peptide was isolated, characterized, and is now referred to as atrial natriuretic peptide (ANP). This endogenous peptide has raised considerable interest because it has the unique properties of being a vasodilator and its hypotensive effects are associated with a natriuresis and diuresis. Early work suggested that the major effect of ANP on the kidney was an increase in GFR with little if any influence on renal tubular solute and water reabsorption. More recent studies clearly establish that ANP can cause a significant increase in sodium and water excretion without any change in GFR (i.e., a direct effect to decrease renal tubular sodium and water reabsorption) (Banks, 1988).

ANP is postulated to be a major hormone regulating body fluid volume. With an absolute increase in intravascular volume or a redistribution of intravascular volume towards the central cardiopulmonary circulation, as observed with water immersion, an increase in atrial volume or stretch releases ANP from the cardiac atria. Increased ANP would evoke a natriuretic/diuretic response to normalize intravascular volume. It is clear that ANP's role has extended beyond its function of regulating body fluid homeostasis. ANP affects various other hormones, (i.e., suppression of renin, angiotensin, and aldosterone) and also interacts with the autonomic nervous system (Goetz, 1988; Shenker, 1988).

Interest in ANP and exercise was stimulated by studies showing an increase in plasma ANP concentration during acute exercise as well as after running a marathon (Lijnen, et al., 1987). The effects of ANP on the kidneys during exercise are probably negligible. First, ANP's renal actions would be to cause an increase in GFR, a diuresis, and a natriuresis. As previously described, during exercise at workloads where ANP is significantly elevated, the renal responses are in the opposite direction.

A major issue with ANP is that its natriuretic properties, which are profound in a normal animal or man, are significantly blunted or absent in situations where various other antinatriuretic stimuli cause increased renal tubular sodium reabsorption (Freeman et al., 1985; Koepke & DiBona, 1987). In various disease states, the vasoconstrictor and antinatriuretic properties of circulating catecholamines, angiotensin II, aldosterone, and ADH appear to oppose and often negate the renal effects of ANP. These same factors, which are stimulated during exercise, are probably offsetting ANP's influence on renal function. Thus, ANP may play a more important role in the control of renal function during the post-exercise or recovery period (see below).

INAPPROPRIATE RESPONSES OF THE KIDNEY TO EXERCISE AND THE STRESS OF FLUID IMBALANCE

Thus far, the changes described in renal function during exercise have been favorable. Some RBF is redistributed making a small contribution to CO, and very limited amounts of water and sodium are conserved. There are, however, several responses of the kidney that are inappropriate, or deleterious, when one is attempting to maintain body fluid homeostasis during exercise and/or fluid imbalance.

A. Increases in Free Water Clearance With Exercise

With acute exercise it would be predicted that C_{H2O} should decrease as a consequence of increased plasma ADH concentration and renal tubular water reabsorption. Throughout the literature, however, there are studies showing that exercise may actually be associated with an increase in C_{H2O}. Early reports by Raisz et al. (1959), Castenfors et al. (1967), and Refsum et al. (1975) show impaired renal concentrating capacity during exercise, indicated by an increase in C_{H2O}. This response is not always seen. Studying different workloads, Kachadorian and Johnson (1970) reported either increases or no change in C_{H2O}. Over all workloads studied, Grimby (1965) noted a large variability between subjects in C_{H2O}.

An increase in C_{H2O} is unexpected because several studies have documented a concurrent increase in plasma ADH concentration during the exercise bout (Convertino et al., 1981; Melin et al., 1980; Wade & Claybaugh, 1980). Exogenous ADH does not appear to alter the impaired renal concentrating capacity associated with exercise (Raisz et al., 1959). Wade and Claybaugh (1980) suggested that the increase in C_{H2O} could be due to an inhibitory effect of increased renal PG on the hydro-osmotic affects of ADH. This possibility was tested by Zambraski and associates. In exercising males and females, administration of either aspirin (1982) or indomethacin (1986) did not alter the changes in C_{H2O} observed during exercise, suggesting that PG are not involved. This paradoxical increase in C_{H2O} in the presence of elevated plasma ADH concentration could be explained if there was a redistribution of RBF towards the medulla in exercising human subjects. This would tend to decrease the osmolality of the medullary interstitium, limiting the ability to concentrate urine even in the presence of elevated plasma ADH concentration (i.e. medullary washout). However, this redistribution of RBF during exercise has not been seen in either the dog (Delgado et al., 1975) or miniature pig (Sanders et al., 1976).

A diuretic response has also been reported in swimmers (Guezennec et al., 1986; Nielsen et al., 1984). This effect could be explained by a central cardiopulmonary redistribution of intravascular volume as observed with water immersion (Norsk & Epstein, 1988). Predictable decreases in renal sympathetic nerve activity, plasma concentrations of ADH, aldosterone, and renin, or increases in ANP would contribute to an increase in urine flow rate.

One other deleterious response of the kidney is an increase in urinary sodium excretion, which is sometimes observed in dehydrated subjects. Although studied more in a clinical situation, a natriuresis in a water deprived state may be due to a normal renal response to suppressed levels of aldosterone (Merrill et al., 1986).

B. Hyponatremia—Water Intoxication

There are reports in the literature of hyponatremia during long distance running (Nelson et al., 1988; Noakes et al., 1985). In an Ironman Triathalon, of 64 subjects studied, 27% were found to be hyponatremic (Nelson et al., 1988). This condition results from a combination of excess sodium loss, via sweating, and the failure to excrete the large amounts of hypotonic fluid that have been ingested. In many of these hyponatremic individuals, the ingestion of 6–20 liters of water during the course of the race has been noted (Nelson et al., 1988). Even though this amount of fluid ingestion would be predicted to decrease plasma ADH concentration and possibly increase plasma ANP concentration to increase urinary flow rate and C_{H2O}, this response is not observed.

With prolonged exercise, especially when coupled with heat stress/dehydration, the factors causing fluid retention appear to predominate and prevent the sometimes necessary excretion of increased volumes of hypotonic urine. This is demonstrated by the study of Poortmans in Figure 7-3 (1984). In hyperhydrated men, pre-exercise urine flow rates as high as 12 ml/min were reduced to 1-2 ml/min by exhaustive exercise, even though the subjects continued to drink 200 ml of water every 20 minutes. The failure of the kidney to increase C_{H2O} to prevent hyponatremia is probably not a result of an abnormality in renal function but more of an imbalance in the extrarenal factors controlling renal water excretion.

C. Attenuation of Rapid Rehydration

The importance of fluid replacement has been discussed in Chapter 5. Failure to retain adequate sodium during attempts to rehydrate is believed to be an important component in causing involuntary dehydration (Nose et al., 1988). An increase in urinary sodium excretion at a time when one is consuming fluid to restore extracellular fluid volume is un-

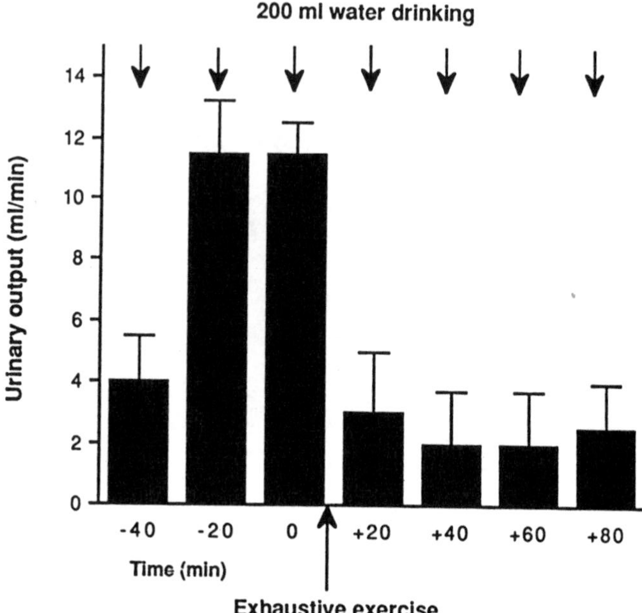

FIGURE 7-3. *The inhibitory effect of exhaustive exercise on the production of urine in excessively hydrated human subjects is shown. Despite high pre-exercise urine flow rates and the continued consumption of water, exercise prevented the excretion of a hypotonic urine. This figure has been adapted from Poortmans (1984).*

desirable. The mechanism causing this natriuresis during rehydration is not known. In addition to decreases in PRA and plasma aldosterone concentration observed with rapid rehydration (Nose et al., 1988), decreases in plasma ADH concentration have also been reported (Blair-West et al., 1985; Freund et al., 1988; Geelen et al., 1984). A decrease in plasma ADH concentration would cause an increase in C_{H2O}.

In studies evaluating the rehydration process, data suggest that ANP may influence the renal response. In dehydrated rats, significantly decreased basal plasma concentrations of ANP were dramatically increased in minutes after allowing the animals to drink (Januszewicz et al., 1986). Furthermore, in the dehydrated rat, glomerular ANP receptors appear to be increased (Gauguelin et al., 1988). This would potentially exaggerate a diuretic/natriuretic response to rapidly changing plasma ANP concentrations during attempted rehydration. In humans, studies using normally hydrated subjects have failed to show any changes in plasma ANP concentration (Freund et al., 1988) with fluid consumption; a key factor, however, may be the prerequisite of dehydration.

Studies on fluid replacement and the chemical composition of the fluid consumed have been focused on gastric emptying and intestinal absorption. The problem is not only to assure that the solution is absorbed, but also to prevent it from being excreted. Studies performed in animal models suggest that chemical composition (i.e. sodium concentration) may differentially influence the reactive renal excretory response (Okuno et al., 1988). If possible, the choice of a rehydration fluid should also weigh the renal response, i.e., a fluid that eliminates or evokes the smallest possible diuretic/natriuretic response.

EFFECTS OF DEHYDRATION/ENVIRONMENTAL STRESS ON THE RENAL RESPONSE TO EXERCISE

The effects of dehydration on systemic function have been described in Chapter 1. Figure 7-4 illustrates the various factors previously discussed that conserve sodium and water during exercise. As shown, dehydration, sodium deficits, and/or heat stress initiate many of the same control mechanisms. Exercise, plus the combination of one or more of these stresses, influence the kidneys in an additive manner. For example, Radigan and Robinson (1949) evaluated the effects of exercise on RPF and GFR in men exposed to a cool versus hot environment. At rest, heat exposure reduced RPF and GFR 39% to 22%, respectively. The combined effects of exercise and heat caused a reduction of RPF that was 20% greater than the effect of exercise alone. The additive effects of exercise

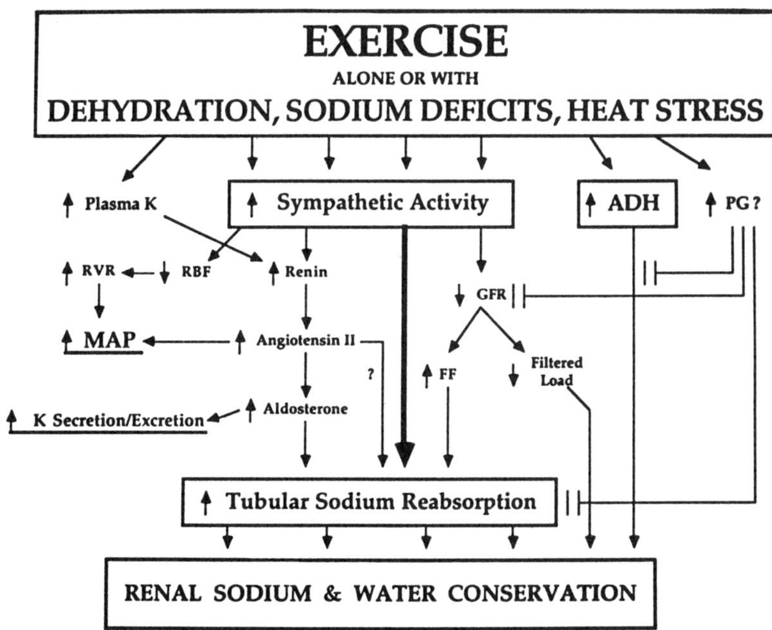

FIGURE 7-4. *A scheme illustrating all of the control factors influencing renal function with exercise alone or in conjunction with dehydration, sodium deficits, and/or heat stress. All of these pathways, which assist in the renal conservation of sodium and water, are discussed in the text.*

and heat also reduced GFR by 29% more than the change observed with exercise alone. In a follow-up study, the same investigators evaluated the combined stresses of exercise, heat, and dehydration (Smith et al., 1952). Again, the decreases in RPF and GFR were significantly greater than the combined stresses of exercise, dehydration, and heat compared to the effects of the exercise alone.

The degree to which dehydration and/or heat stress alters extrarenal control factors, such as aldosterone, PRA, or sympathetic nerve activity, predicts the changes observed in the renal handling of sodium and water. To date, there is little support for a direct intrarenal effect of dehydration. However, studies must begin to evaluate the sensitivity of the kidneys, and different parts of the nephron, to the various stimuli associated with a dehydrated state. The importance of this "next step" has been demonstrated by Steiner and Phillips (1988) who have recently reported that in the rat, ADH V_2 receptors are down regulated by dehydration, possibly in response to increased plasma ADH concentration. The effects of dehydration and training on various renal receptors (adrenergic, angiotensin II, PG) should be investigated.

EFFECTS OF TRAINING ON THE RENAL RESPONSE TO EXERCISE AND FLUID IMBALANCE

Changes in renal function with training will largely reflect changes in extrarenal factors that influence renal handling of sodium and water. The changes with training in various hormones, such as renin-angiotensin, aldosterone, ADH, or circulating catecholamines have been described in Chapter 6. Resultant alterations in renal function, as a consequence of a change in hormonal control with training are predictable. Although the quantitative importance has not been assessed, the most dramatic change within the kidneys after exercise training may be due to a decrease in the response of peripheral sympathetic nerve activity to any given workload, as measured by circulating plasma NE concentration (Peronnet et al., 1981). Because renal sympathetic nerve activity may produce renal vasoconstriction (i.e. decreased RPF and GFR), increased renin release, and renal tubular sodium reabsorption, a reduced peripheral sympathoexcitatory response at a given absolute workload could potentially alter all of these parameters. In normal individuals at rest, changes in these neurohumoral systems do not seem to occur with training.

With training, changes within the kidneys that could influence the renal handling of sodium have not been described. In an exercise model this is obviously a very difficult question to address. To indirectly assess possible changes in the renal handling of sodium, attempts have been made to evaluate changes in sodium balance before and after training. The rationale is that a change in sodium balance would reflect an alteration in kidney function. As I will discuss, this approach is futile because it is largely due to a misunderstanding of what sodium balance means.

By definition, if a human or an animal is in sodium balance (steady-state), then sodium output (determined by the kidneys) must equal sodium intake. If one is in sodium balance, total body sodium is constant. The important point is that if a person is in a steady-state with regard to total body sodium, he/she *must* be in sodium balance. Under steady-state conditions, with no progressive loss/gain of total body sodium, measurement of changes in daily urinary sodium excretion do not reflect changes in renal function; differences only represent changes in daily dietary sodium intake. If a person is not in sodium balance, then he/she will be continually changing total body sodium. He/she will continue to do so until such time that a new equilibrium is reached at a new total body sodium (i.e. decreased total body sodium with volume contraction or increased total body sodium with edema). For these reasons, the measurement of daily urinary sodium excretion under steady-state conditions will not provide any information about innate changes in the renal handling of sodium.

To assess changes in renal function after training, one can evaluate the renal responses to specific interventions in non-steady-state situations. Examples would be to determine the renal response to conditions such as: acute dehydration, rehydration, or administration of a sodium load. If changes in kidney function were occurring, they would be represented by alterations in the time course or magnitude of the renal response to a specific intervention. These approaches have been appropriately and successfully used in a small number of studies dealing with the excretory responses of trained versus non-trained individuals to interventions such as water loading, rehydration, and water immersion (Claybaugh et al., 1986; Freund et al., 1988; Skipka et al., 1979). In general, differences in the hormonal responses with training have also been observed (see Chapter 6). A key element of these studies will be to differentiate between an alteration in the renal response due to a systemic factor versus a change within the kidneys themselves.

RENAL COMPLICATIONS WITH EXERCISE

In a classic paper dealing with the "Physiological and Pathological Effects of Severe Exertion (The Marathon Run) . . ." published in 1910 by Barach (Barach, 1910), the following observation was made. Urine was obtained from 24 contestants before the race. After the race it was stated that "we succeeded in getting 19 specimens, and in those the total quantity excreted during the time of the race, which lasted between 3 hours and 14 minutes to five hours, . . . was 220 cc as the largest amount and 35 cc was the smallest." The color "varied from normal to dark smoky; in several it was bloody."

Exercise, especially in conjunction with other factors, such as dehydration and increased ambient temperature, is a profound stress for the kidneys, with significant and potentially deleterious effects. During exercise the renal vasoconstriction and increased rates of renal tubular sodium and water reabsorption significantly decrease tubular flow rate. Tubular luminal fluid solute concentration and acidity are increased, both of which may adversely affect renal tubular epithelial cells. Several major abnormalities in renal function have been associated with strenuous and/or prolonged duration exercise. These would include proteinuria, cylinduria, hematuria, and the occurrence of acute renal failure.

A. Exercise Proteinuria and Hematuria

Exercise proteinuria is the increased urinary excretion of protein after exercise. This transient phenomenon is attributed to the passage of albumin and other large plasma proteins that are normally not filtered, through the glomerular capillary membrane (Poortmans, 1985). In some situations, exercise proteinuria may also be due to a decrease in the renal tubular reabsorption of smaller proteins that are normally filtered and reabsorbed (Poortmans, 1988). Descriptions of the exercise proteinuric response, and the mechanisms believed to be involved, are available in excellent reviews (Castenfors, 1977; Poortmans, 1985). The point is that exercise-induced proteinuria, even though it is considered to be non-pathological, represents a change in the barrier function of the glomerular capillary membrane. This functional alteration that causes this abnormal response is being induced by exercise. Another example of an exercise-induced functional derangement is exercise hematuria. This condition has been reported in several studies of marathon runners (Eichner, 1988; Fred & Natelson, 1977; Hoover & Crombie, 1981; Siegel et al., 1979). This condition is transient, usually resolving in 1-2 days. It is generally believed that adequate hydration may reduce the incidence/magnitude of exercise hematuria.

B. Acute Renal Failure

Acute renal failure is a clinical condition characterized by an abrupt decrease in renal function associated with a significant fall in GFR. With a prolonged decrease in GFR, blood urea nitrogen and plasma creatinine concentration will increase. Cases of acute renal failure, during or immediately after strenuous long term exercise, have been reported (MacSearraigh et al., 1979; Stewart & Posen, 1980).

In normal individuals there are several factors that may lead to acute renal failure, including intravascular volume depletion and hypotension. In addition, extremely high levels of renal sympathetic nerve activity and renin-angiotensin system activity may cause renal ischemia and precipitate acute renal failure. Furthermore, exercise induced rhabdomyolysis and the resultant myoglobinuria may cause renal injury. Fortunately, despite all of these factors having a high probability of being present during long-term endurance exercise, the incidence of exercise induced acute renal failure is low.

Patients with heart failure and cirrhosis are known to be prone to developing acute renal failure. In these patients, a protective role of renal PG has been described that is extremely important (Dunn & Zambraski, 1980). In situations where there is high renal sympathetic nerve activity or increased renin-angiotensin system activity, renal PG serve to attenuate the renal vasoconstriction and thereby maintain RPF and GFR. This is why the indiscriminate use of aspirin or non-steroidal anti-inflammatory drugs, which decrease renal PG synthesis, is not advised.

The issue of whether renal PG are important in attenuating the renal vasoconstriction associated with exercise has been examined in two studies from this laboratory. It was found that the administration of either aspirin on the non-steroidal anti-inflammatory drug, indomethacin did not alter changes in GFR seen with short-term (30–40 minute) exercise (Zambraski et al., 1986; Zambraski et al., 1982). The question of whether renal PG are important in maintaining GFR during long-term exercise, especially when the subjects are dehydrated and exposed to heat, has not been studied. An intact renal PG system may serve to reduce the incidence of exercise-induced acute renal failure.

SUMMARY

Kidney function plays an important role in the body's integrated response to the stress of exercise. With short-term exercise the actual impact of the renal response, whether it be in the amount of renal blood flow redistributed to other sites, or the absolute amount of sodium/water which can be conserved, is limited. However, after prolonged exercise, during the recovery period the renal response is substantially greater and essential in replacing sodium/water deficits.

During acute exercise the sympathetic nervous system appears to be the major control system regulating renal hemodynamics, tubular function, and renin release. In the post-exercise period, with dehydration and accumulated sodium deficits, decreased activity of the sympathetic system with an increased involvement of the renin-angiotension-aldosterone system appears to occur.

There are several situations in which the renal response to exercise and/or fluid imbalance is inappropriate. For reasons which are unclear, in some exercise conditions the kidneys' capacity to concentrate urine is impaired, resulting in increased free water clearance. Secondly, with large fluid/sodium losses incurred during prolonged exercise, and the consumption of large amounts of water, the failure of the kidneys to excrete copious amounts of hypotonic urine may lead to hyponatremia. Lastly, in a dehydrated state, the consumption of large amounts of fluid in an attempt to rapidly rehydrate is associated with an increase in urine flow rate. This renal response occurs before plasma volume or total body water has been repleted, and thus, increases the time required for complete rehydration.

During acute exercise, changes in renal function have systemic implications. With exercise the profound renal vasoconstriction assists in maintaining an increase in arterial pressure by offsetting extensive skeletal muscle vasodilation. The release of renin and the generation of angiotensin II influences the maximal arterial pressure response to exercise. Also, during exercise a large fraction of the increased circulating levels of NE, which has multiple cardiovascular and metabolic effects, may originate from the kidneys. Long-term adaptations of the kidneys to exercise training, or to dehydration, have not been described. Because of the high degree to which extrarenal factors such as circulating hormones or sympathetic nerve activity regulate renal function, adaptations in kidney function with training or dehydration will largely depend upon changes in these factors.

Exercise, particularly in conjunction with hypohydration, sodium deprivation, and/or heat stress, represents a major stress to the kidneys. Changes in renal function (i.e. renal vasoconstriction, antinatriuretic response) are increased in magnitude when dehydration and/or heat stress is added to the exercise stress. The occurrences of exercise proteinuria and hematuria demonstrate that the stresses are of sufficient magnitude to cause dramatic changes in renal function. Fortunately, the incidence of acute renal failure, which has been reported in marathon runners, is relatively small.

BIBLIOGRAPHY

Astrand, P. and K. Rodahl. *Textbook of Work Physiology*. McGraw-Hill, New York, 1986, p. 152.

Aurell, M., M. Carlsson, G. Grimby, and B. Hood. Plasma concentration and urinary excretion of certain electrolytes during suprine work. *J. Appl. Physiol.* 22:633–638, 1967.

Banks, R.O. Effects of a physiological dose of ANP on renal function in dogs. *Am. J. Physiol.* 255: F907–F910, 1988.

Barach, J.H. Physiological and pathological effects of severe exercise (The Marathon Race) on the circulatory and renal systems. *Arch. Intern. Med.* 5:382–405, 1910.

Blair-West, J.R., A.P. Gibson, R.L. Woods, and A.H. Brook. Acute reduction of plasma vasopressin levels by rehydration in sheep. *Am. J. Physiol.* 248:R68–R71, 1985.

Buileau, M., E. Fuchs, J.M. Barry, and C.V. Hodges. Stress hematuria: athletic pseudonephritis in marathoners. *Urology* 15:471–474, 1980.

Bozovic, L., J. Castenfors, and M. Piscator. Effect of prolonged, heavy exercise on urinary protein excretion and plasma renin activity. *Acta Physiol. Scand.* 70:143–146, 1967.

Carlin, M.R., C.B. Mueller, and H.L. White. Effects of exercise on renal blood flow and sodium excretion in dogs. *J. App. Physiol.* 3:291–294, 1950.

Castenfors, J. Effect of ethacrynic acid on plasma renin activity during supine exercise in normal subjects. *Acta Physiol. Scand.* 70:215–220, 1967.

Castenfors, J. Renal clearances and urinary sodium and potassium excretion during supine exercise in normal subjects. *Acta Physiol. Scand.* 70:207–214, 1967.

Castenfors, J. Renal function during prolonged exercise. *Annal. NY. Acad. Sci.* 301:151–159, 1977.

Castenfors, J., F. Mossfeldt, and M. Piscator. Effect of prolonged heavy exercise on renal function and urinary protein excretion. *Acta Physiol. Scand.* 70:194–206, 1967.

Chapman, C.B., A. Henschel, J. Minckler, A. Forsgren, and A. Keys. The effect of exercise on renal plasma flow in normal male subjects. *J. Clin. Invest.* 27:639-644, 1948.

Claybaugh, J.R., D.R. Pendergast, J.E. Davis, C. Akida, M. Pazik, and S.K. Hong. Fluid conservation in athletes: responses to water intake, supine posture, and immersion. *J. Appl. Physiol.* 61:7-15, 1986.

Convertino, V.A., L.C. Keil, E.M. Bernaver, and J.E. Greenleaf. Plasma volume, osmolarity, vasopressin, and renin activity during graded exercise in man. *J. Appl. Physiol.* 50:123-128, 1981.

Convertino, V.A., L.C. Keil, and J.E. Greenleaf. Plasma volume, renin, and vasopressin responses to graded exercise after training. *J. Appl. Physiol.: Respirat Environ. Exercise Physiol.* 54:508-514, 1983.

Delgado, R., T.M. Sanders, and C.M. Bloor. Renal blood flow distribution during steady-state exercise and exhaustion in conscious dogs. *J. Appl. Physiol.* 39:474-478, 1975.

Demers, L.M., T.S. Harrison, D.R. Halbert, and R.J. Santen. Effect of prolonged exercise on plasma prostaglandin levels. *Prostaglandin Med.* 6:413-418, 1981.

DiBona, G.F. The functions of the renal nerves. *Rev. Physiol, Biochem. Pharmacol.* 94:75-181, 1982.

DiBona, G.F. Symposium: Neural control of renal function. *Fed. Proc.* 37:1191-1221, 1978.

Dunn, M.J. Nonsteriodal anti-inflammatory drugs and renal function. *Annu. Rev. Med.* 35:411-428, 1984.

Dunn, M.J., and E.J. Zambraski. Renal effect of drugs that inhibit prostaglandin synthesis. *Kid. Int.* 18:609-622, 1980.

Eichner, E. Other medical considerations in prolonged exercise. *Perspectives in Exercise Science and Sports Medicine* (Indianapolis, Benchmark, 1988, 1:415-442.

Esler, M., G. Jennings, P. Korner, I. Willett, F. Dudley, G. Hasking, W. Anderson, and G. Lambert. Assessment of human sympathetic nervous system activity from measurements of norepinephrine turnover. *Hypertension.* 11:3-20, 1988.

Fagard, R., A. Amery, T. Reybrouck, P. Lijnen, E. Moerman, M. Bogaert, and A. DeSchaepdryver. Effects of angiotensin antagonism on hemodynamics, renin and catecholamines during exercise. *J. Appl. Phyisol.* 43:440-444, 1977.

Fagard, R., A. Amery, T. Reybrouck, P. Lijnen, L. Billiet, M. Bogaert, E. Moerman, and A. DeSchaepdryver. Effects of angiotensin antagonism at rest and during exercise in sodium-deplete man. *J. Appl. Physiol.* 45:403-407, 1978.

Fagard, R., R. Grauwels, D. Grocseneken, P. Lijnen, J. Stacssch, L. Vanhees, and A. Amery. Plasma levels of renin, angiotension II, and 6-Keto-prostaglandin $F_{1\alpha}$ in endurance athletes. *J. Appl. Physiol.* 59:947-952, 1985.

Fasola, A.F., B.L. Martz, and O.M. Helmer. Plasma renin activity during supine exercise in offspring of hypertensive parents. *J. Appl. Phyisol.* 25:410-415, 1968.

Fasola, A.F., B.L. Martz, and O.M. Helmer. Renin activity during supine exercise in normotensives and hypertensives. *J. Appl. Physiol.* 21:1709- 1712, 1966.

Francesconi, R.P., M.N. Sawka, K.B. Pandolf, R.W. Hubbard, A.J. Young, and S. Muza. Plasma hormonal responses at graded hypohydration levels during exercise-heat stress. *J. Appl. Physiol.* 59:1855-1860, 1985.

Freeman, R.H., J.O. Davis, and R.G. Vari. Renal response to atrial natriuretic factor in conscious dogs with caval constriction. *Am. J. Physiol.* 248:R495-R500, 1985.

Fred, H.L., and E.A. Natelson. Grossly bloody urine of runners. *Southern Medical Journal.* 70:1394-1395, 1977.

Freund, B.J., J.R. Claybaugh, G.M. Hashiro, and M.S. Dice. Hormonal and renal responses to water drinking in moderately trained and untrained humans. *Am. J. Physiol.* 254:R417-R423, 1988.

Fujita, T., Y. Sato, K. Ando, H. Noda, N. Ueno, and K. Murakami. Dynamic responses of active and inactive renin and plasma norepinephrine during exercise in normal man. *Jpn. Heart J.* 23:545-551, 1982.

Gardner, K.J. Athletic pseudonephritis-alteration of urine sediment by athletic competition. *J.A.M.A.* 161:1613-1617, 1956.

Gauguelin, G., G. Thibault, M. Cantin, E.L. Schiffrin, and R. Garcia. Glomerular atrial natriuretic factor receptors during rehydration: Plasma NH_2- and COOH-terminal levels. *Am. J. Physiol.* 225:F621-F625, 1988.

Geelen, G., L.C. Keil, S.E. Kravik, C.E. Wade, T.N. Thrasher, P.R. Barnes, G. Pyka, C. Nesvig, and J.E. Greenleaf. Inhibition of plasma vasopressin after drinking in dehydrated humans. *Am. J. Physiol.* 249:R968-R971, 1984.

Goetz, K.L. Physiology and pathophysiology of atrial peptides. *Am. J. Pysiol.* 254:E1-E15, 1988.

Grignolo, A., J.P. Koepke, and P.A. Obrist. Renal function, heart rate, and blood pressure during exercise and avoidance in dogs. *Am. J. Physiol.* 242:R482-R490, 1981.

Grimby, G. Renal clearances during prolonged supine exercise at different loads. *J. Appl. Physiol.* 20:1294-1298, 1965.

Guezennec, C.Y., G. Defer, G. Cazorla, C. Sabathier, and F. Lhoste. Plasma renin activity, aldosterone and catecholamine levels when swimming and running. *Eur. J. Appl. Physiol.* 54:632-637, 1986.

Hansson, B.G., J.F. Dymling, P. Manhem, and B. Hokfelt. Long term treatment of moderate hypertension with the $beta_1$-receptor blocking agent metoprolol. *Europ. J. Clin. Pharmacol.* 11:247-254, 1977.

Hansson, B.G., and B. Hokfelt. Long term treatment of moderate hypertension with penbutolol (Hoe 893d). *Europ. J. Clin. Pharmacol.* 9:9-19, 1975.

Hesse, B., N.J. Christensen, an E.D. Andersen. Renin release in relation to plasma noradrenaline during supine exercise in cardiac patients. *Acta Med Scand.* 204:185–189, 1978.

Hohimer, A.R., J.R. Hales, L.B. Rowell, and O.A. Smith. Regional distribution of blood flow during mild dynamic leg exercise in the baboon. *J. App. Physiol.* 55:1173–1177, 1983.

Hohimer, A.R., and O.A. Smith. Decreased renal blood flow in the baboon during mild dynamic leg exercise. *Am. J. Physiol.* 236:H141–H150, 1979.

Hoover, D.L. and W.J. Cromie. Theory and management of exercise-related hematuria. *Phys. and Sportsmed.* 9:91–95, 1981.

Januszewicz, P., G. Thibault, J. Gutkowska, R. Garcia, C. Mercure, F. Jolicoeur, J. Genest, and M. Cantin. Atrial natriuretic factor and vasopressin during dehydration and rehydration in rats. *Am. J. Phyisol.* 251:E497–E501, 1986.

Jeffries, W.B., Y. Wang, and W.A. Pettinger. Enhanced vasopressin (V_2-receptor)-induced sodium retention in mineralcorticoid hypertension. *Am. J. Physiol.* 254:F739–F746, 1988.

Kachadorian, W.A. and R.E. Johnson. Renal responses to various rates of exercise. *J. Appl. Physiol.* 28:748–752, 1970.

Kattus, A.A., B. Sinclair-Smith, J. Genest, and E.V. Newman. The effects of exercise on the renal mechanism of electrolyte excretion in normal subjects. *Johns Hopkins Hospital Bulletin.* 84:344–368, 1949.

Koch, G., U. Johansson, and E. Arvidsson. Radioenzymatic determination of epinephrine, norepinephrine and dopamine in .l ml plasma samples. Plasma catecholamine response to submaximal and near maximal exercise. *J. Clin. Chem. Clin. Biochem.* 18:367–372, 1980.

Koepke, J., and G.F. DiBona. Blunted natriuresis to atrial natriuretic peptide in chronic sodim-retaining disorders. *Am. J. Physiol.* 252:F865- F871, 1987.

Kosunen, K.J. and A.J. Pakarinen. Plasma renin, angiotensin II, and plasma and urinary aldosterone in running exercise. *J. Appl. Physiol.* 41:26–29, 1976.

Kosunen, K., A. Pakarinen, K. Kuoppasalmi, H. Naveri, S. Rehunen, C.G. Standerskjold-Nordenstam, M. Harkonen, and H. Adlercreutz. Cardiovascular function in the renin-angiotensin-aldosterone system in long-distance runners during various training periods. *Scand. J. Clin. Lab. Invest.* 40:429–435, 1980.

Lammintausta, R., M. Koulu, and H. Allonen. Alpha- and beta-adrenoceptor blocking properties of labetalol in renin release. *Inter. J. Clin. Pharmacol. Biopharm.* 17:240–243, 1979.

Leenen, F.H.H., P. Boer, and C.LG. Geyskes. Sodium intake and the effects of isoproterenol and exercise on plasma renin in man. *J. Appl. Physiol.* 45:870–874, 1978.

Lijnen, P.J., A.K. Amery, R.H. Fagard, T.M. Reybrouck, E.J. Moerman, and A.F. DeSchaepdryver. The effects of β-adrenoreceptor blockade on renin, angiotensin, aldosterone and catecholamines at rest and during exercise. *Br. J. Clin. Pharmac.* 7:175–181, 1979.

Lijnen, P., P. Hespel. J.R. M'Buyamba-Kabangu, M. Goris, R. Lysens, E. Vanden Eynde, R. Fagard, and A. Amery. Plasma atrial natriuretic peptide and cyclic nucleotide levels before and after a marathon. *J. Appl. Physiol.* 62:1180–1184, 1987.

Lijnen, P., P. Hespel, E. Vanden Eynde, and A. Amery. Urinary excretion of electrolytes during prolonged physical activity in normal man. *Eur. J. App. Physiol.* 53:317–321, 1985.

MacSearraigh, E.J.M., J.C. Kallmeyer, and H.B. Schiff. Acute renal failure in marathon runners. *Nephron* 24:240, 1979.

McGrath, B.P., and L.F. Arnolda. Enalapril reduces the catecholamine response to exercise in patients with heart failure. *Eur. J. Clin. Pharmacol.* 30:485–487, 1986.

McLeod, A.A., J.E. Brown, B.B. Kitchell, F.A. Sedor, D.C., Kuhn, R.S. Williams, and D.G. Shand. Hemodynamic and metabolic responses to exercise after $alpha_1$ - $beta_1$ and nonselective beta-adrenoceptor blockade in man. *Am. J. Med.* Feb. 97–100, 1984.

Melin, B., J.P. Eclache, G. Geelen, G. Annat, A.M. Allevard, E. Jarsaillon, A. Zebidi, J.J. Legros, and Cl. Gharib. Plasma AVP, neurophysin, renin activity, and aldosterone during submaximal exercise performed until exhaustion in trained and untrained men. *Eur. J. App. Physiol.* 44:141–151, 1980.

Merrill, D.C., M.M. Skelton, and A.W. Cowley, Jr. Humoral control of water and electrolyte excretion during water restriction. *Kidney Int.* 29:1152–1161, 1986.

Musch, T.I., D.B. Friedman, K.H. Pitetti, G.C. Haidet, J. Stray-Gundersen, J.H. Mitchell, and G.A. Ordway. Regional distribution of blood flow of dogs during graded dynamic exercise. *J. Appl. Physiol.* 63:2269–2277, 1987.

Nelson, P.B., A.G. Robinson, W. Kapoor, and J. Rinaldo. Hyponatremia in a marathoner. *Phys. and Sportsmed.* 16:78–88, 1988.

Nielsen, B., G. Sjogaard, and F. Bonde-Petersen. Cardiovascular, hormonal and body fluid changes during prolonged exercise. *Eur. J. Appl. Physiol.* 53:63–70, 1984.

Noakes, T.D, N. Goodwin, B.L. Rayner, T. Branken, and R.K.N. Taylor. Water intoxication: A possible complication during endurance exercise. *Med. Sci. Sport Exer.* 17:370–375, 1985.

Norsk, P. and M. Epstein. Effects of water immersion on arginine vasopressin release in humans. *J. Appl. Physiol.* 64:1–10, 1988.

Nose, H., G.W. Mack, X. Shi, and E.R. Nadel. Involvement of sodium retention hormones during rehydration in humans. *J. Appl. Phyisol.* 65:332–336, 1988.

Nose, H., G.W. Mack, X. Shi, and E.R. Nadel. Shift in body fluid compartments after dehydration in humans. *J. Appl. Physiol.* 65:318–324, 1988.

Nowak, J. and A. Wennmalm. Effects of exercise in human arterial and regional venous concentrations of prostaglandin E. *Prostaglandin Med.* 1:489–497, 1978.

Okuno, T., T. Yawata, H. Nose, and T. Morimoto. Difference in rehydration process due to salt concentration of drinking water in rats. *J. Appl. Physiol.* 64:2438–2443, 1988.

Peronnet, F., L. Beliveau, G. Boudreau, F. Trudeau, G. Brisson, and R. Nadeau. Regional plasma catecholamine removal and release at rest and exercise in dogs. *Am. J. Physiol.* 254:R663–R672, 1988.

Peronnet, F., J. Cleroux, H. Perrault, D. Cousineau, J. deChamplain, and R. Nadeau. Plasma norepinephrine response to exercise before and after training in humans. *J. Appl. Physiol.* 51:812–815, 1981.

Poortmans, J.R. Exercise and renal function. *Sports Med.* 1:125–153, 1984.

Poortmans, J.R. Postexercise proteinuria in humans. *J.A.M.A.* 253:236- 240, 1985.

Poortmans, J.R., H. Brauman, M. Staroukine, A. Verhiory, C. Decaestecker, and R. Leclercq. Indirect evidence of glomerular/tubular mixed-type post exercise proteinuric in healthy humans. *Am. J. Physiol.* 254:F277–F283, 1988.

Radigan, L.R., and S. Robinson. Effects of environmental heat stress and exercise on renal blood flow and filtration rate. *J. Appl. Physiol.* 2:185–191, 1949.

Raisz, L.G., W.Y.W. Av, and R.L. Scheer. Studies on the renal concentration mechanism. III. Effect of heavy exercise. *J. Clin. Invest.* 38:8–13, 1959.

Rauch, A.L. and W.G. Campbell. Nephrectomy-induced alterations in the synthesis of catecholamines in the sympathetic and central nervous system. *A. J. Hypertension.* 1:50–53, 1988.

Refsum, H.E. and S.B. Stromme. Relationship between urine flow, glomerular filtration, and urine solute concentrations during prolonged heavy exercise. *Scand. J. Clin. Lab. Invest.* 35:775–780, 1975.

Rowell, L.B. Human cardiovascular adjustments to exercise and thermal stress. *Physiol Rev.* 54:75–159, 1974.

Sadowski, J., R. Gellert, J. Kurkus, and E. Portalska. Denervated and intact kidney responses to exercise in the dog. *J. Appl. Physiol.* 51:1618–1624, 1981.

Sanders, M., S. Rasmussen, D. Cooper, and C. Bloor. Renal and intrarenal blood flow distribution in swine during severe exercise. *J. Appl. Physiol.* 40:932–935, 1976.

Siegel, A.J., C.H. Hennekens, H.S. Salomon, and B. VanBoeckel. Exercise-related hematuria. *J.A.M.A.* 241:391–392, 1979.

Shenker, Y. Atrial natriuretic hormone effect on renal function and aldosterone secretion in sodium depletion. *Am. J. Physiol.* 255:R867- R873, 1988.

Skipka, W., D. Boning, K.A. Deck, W.R. Kulpmann, and K.A. Neurer. Reduced aldosterone and sodium excretion in endurance-trained athletes before and during immersion. *Eur. J. App. Physiol.* 42:255–261, 1979.

Smith, J.H., S. Robinson, and M. Pearcy. Renal responses to exercise, heat and dehydration. *J. App. Physiol.* 4:659–665, 1952.

Staessen, J., R. Fagard, P. Hespel, P. Lijnen, L. Vanhees, and A. Amery. Plasma renin system during exercise in normal men. *J. Appl. Physiol.* 63:188–194, 1987.

Stella, A. and A. Zanchetti. Control of renal renin release. *Kid. Int.* 31:589–594, 1987.

Steiner, M., and M.I. Phillips. Renal tubular vasopressin receptors downregulated by dehydration. *Am. J. Physiol.* 254:C404–C410, 1988.

Stewart, P.J., and G.A. Posen. Case Reports: Acute renal failure following a marathon. *Phys. and Sportsmed.* 8:61–64, 1980.

Sundsfjord, J.A., S.B. Stromme, and A. Aakvaag. Plasma aldosterone (PA), plasma renin activity (PRA) and cortisol (PF) during exercise. In: *Metabolic Adaptations to Prolonged Exercise.* Ed. H. Howald, J. Poortmans Switzerland, 1975 p. 308–314.

Thrasher, T.N., J.F. Nistal-Herrera, L.C. Keil, and D.J. Ramsay. Satiety and inhibition of vasopressin secretion after drinking in dehydrated dogs. *Am. J. Physiol.* 240:E394–E401, 1981.

Vapaatalo, H., K. Laustiola, E. Seppala, R. Rauramaa, M. Kaste, M. Hillbom, and M. Kangasaho. Exercise, ethanol and arachidonic acid metabolism in healthy men. *Biomed. Biochina. Acta.* 43:S413–S420, 1984.

Vatner, S.F., C.B. Higgins, and D. Franklin. Regional circulatory adjustments to moderate and severe chronic anemia in conscious dogs at rest and during exercise. *Circ. Res.* 30:731–740, 1972.

Vatner, S.F., C.B. Higgins, S. White, T. Patrick and D. Franklin. The peripheral vascular response to severe exercise in untethered dogs before and after complete heart block. *J. Clin. Invest.* 50:1950–1960, 1971.

Wade, C.E. Response, regulation, and actions of vasopressin during exercise; a review. *Med. Sci. Sports Exer.* 16:506–511, 1984.

Wade, C.E., and J.R. Claybaugh. Plasma renin activity, vasopressin concentration, and urinary excretory responses to exercise in men. *J. Appl. Physiol,* 49:930–936, 1980.

Wade, C.E., R.H. Dressendorfer, J.C. O'Brien, and J.R. Claybaugh. Renal function, aldosterone, and vasopressin excretion following repeated long-distance running. *J. Appl. Physiol.* 50:709–712, 1981.

Wade, C.E., L.C. Hill, M.M. Hunt, and R.H. Dressendorfer. Plasma aldosterone and renal function in runners during a 20-day road race. *Eur. J. Appl. Physiol.* 54:456–460, 1985.

Wade, C.E., S.R. Ramee, M.M. Hunt, and C.J. White. Hormonal and renal responses to converting enzyme inhibition during maximal exercise. *J. Appl. Physiol,* 63:1796–1800, 1987.

Wennmalm, A., and G.A. Fitzgerald. Excretion of prostacyclin and thromboxane A_2 metabolites during leg exercise in humans. *Am. J. Physiol.* 255:H15–H18, 1988.

White, H.L., and D. Rolf. Effects of exercise and of some other influences on the renal circulation in man. *Am. J. Physiol.* 152:505–516, 1948.
Winer, N., W.D. Mason, C.H. Carter, T.L. Willoughby, G.M. Kochak, I. Cohen, and R.M.S. Bell. Effects of atenolol on blood pressure, heart rate, renin, and norepinephrine during exercise. *Clin. Pharmacol. Ther.* 26:315–325, 1979.
Zambraski, E.J., R. Dodelson, S.M. Guidotti, and C.A. Harnett. Renal prostaglandin E_2 and $F_{2\alpha}$ synthesis during exercise: effects of indomethacin and sulindac. *Med. Sci. Sports Exer.* 18:678–684, 1986.
Zambraski, E.J., T.A. Rofrano, and C.D. Ciccone. Effects of aspirin treatment on kidney function in exercising man. *Med. Sci. Sports Exer.* 14:419–423, 1982.
Zambraski, E.J., M.S. Tucker, C.S. Lakas, S.M. Grassl, and C.G. Scanes. Mechanism of renin release in exercising dog. *Am.J. Physiol.* 246:E71– E78, 1984.

DISCUSSION

KACHADORIAN: In humans, renal blood flow decreases with exercise, at least heavy exercise. There apparently are some controversial findings about this in the dog and that, as you mentioned, is not probably pertinent to understanding the case for humans. One point that should be raised here is that diminished renal blood flow during exercise appears to have certain negative consequences that, in some cases, can be very dramatic. In particular, proteinuria, microscopic hematuria, and cyclinduria are regular accompaniments of heavy exercise. These outward effects are yet to be fully appreciated, but suffice it to point out that fatalities in otherwise healthy people have been associated with renal failure during extreme exercise, particularly with dehydration in severe environments. My experience and impression is that these negative effects of exercise on renal function can be attenuated simply by maintaining hydration during exercise.

ZAMBRASKI: I would agree that the hydrated state is probably one of the best defenses against renal injuries. I don't think we should take the position that people should be excessively water loaded before a prolonged endurance event. However, if a person could go into the race and maintain a urine volume of 1.0 mL/min that would be extremely advantageous. It is interesting to note that exercise has been used as a provocative test to induce an excessive proteinuria in young diabetics before they show the onset of the disease. This exaggerated exercise proteinuria has also been reported in blacks with essential hypertension. Studies from my lab have been examining the exercise proteinuria in normotensive and hypertensive miniature swine. The proteinuria response to exercise is 8–10 times greater in hypertensive versus normal animals. This difference in the response appears to involve the renal prostaglandin system.

SCHEDL: I enjoyed your presentation immensely. I would like to ask a question about the exhaustive exercise experiment in which the same water loading was induced. I've done similar experiments with sustained water loading in resting patients with fluid retention that is antidiuretic. The patients were decompensated cirrhotics and people in congestive heart failure. If you do the control water loading intravenously with 4%

fructose or 5% glucose infused at about 15 mL/min, you can establish a urine flow and free water clearance rate. Assume that increased proximal tubular fluid reabsorption determines the antidiuresis. Then repeat the experiment, substituting a non-reabsorbable solute such as mannitol for half the sugar. The mannitol would change intratubular dynamics and deliver more volume to the distal tubule, where dilution occurs. That would be a way to test the mechanism of antidiuresis to see whether you could restore the diuresis even during exercise.

ZAMBRASKI: I agree. There are no data to explain the mechanism of the antidiuretic effect of exhaustive exercise in excessively water loaded subjects. The problem with testing this response in humans is that one must be concerned about causing severe hyponatremia.

TIPTON: With regard to proteins in the urine, you did not mention the lysine infusion studies in which Poortmans showed that tubular protein reabsorption in normals and in diabetic subjects was inhibited. I am concerned about renal damage after dehydration. You did not discuss your research showing a chronic loss of fluids and a state of dehydration in wrestlers during a three-day state tournament. Can a urinary profile indicate total fluid changes as well as when fluid homeostasis has occurred?

ZAMBRASKI: In the competitive situation, you can't use the renal urinary profile to estimate total body fluid status. The rehydration studies show that. In the dehydrated state, if they drink anything, they will induce a natriuresis and diuresis. If you just look at the urine, you would say that they were well hydrated. But clearly, as shown, they are diuresing before the plasma or extracellular volume is restored.

The studies that Tipton is referring to is where we looked at urine profiles of a large number of wrestlers when they weighed in and 5 h later when they knew they were going to step on the mat and wrestle. They knew they were dehydrated and that they were supposed to eat and drink. The problem, and my fear in that study, was that if they ate or drank anything, their urinary profile would have changed, but we would not have known if they were rehydrated. In actual fact, they didn't drink anything. Consequently, the urinary profile was just the way it was 5 h earlier. In that situation, the lack of change in the kidney urinary profile did reflect a negative extracellular volume. But it is not a good test.

Your first point was about assessing kidney damage. We do not have a good test. The problem is the potential damage to the kidneys when we add additional stresses such as dehydration and heat exposure during exercise. The point that is not made very often is that the oxygen requirement of the kidneys is a function of the amount of sodium that the kidneys are required to reabsorb. With hypohydration and prolonged exercise, sodium reabsorption is heightened. Thus, one would expect a higher renal oxygen demand in this situation. As far as the occurrence of renal ischemia, there is no direct evidence.

HARVEY: I'm interested in the diuresis and natriuresis that occurs when you are trying to rehydrate yourself after heavy exercise. Recovery for these athletes is certainly frustrating when they are trying to drink at the same time that they are going to the bathroom. Your manuscript indicates that if you ingest a sodium-containing drink that response may be attenuated a little bit. If the sodium load is increased after these bouts of exercise, do you think we can attenuate this response?

ZAMBRASKI: In the chapter, what I referred to was the fact that when trying to rehydrate after being dehydrated, in the rat studies, ANF or ANP goes up very fast. Also, in the hypohydrated state, the renal receptors to ANP, which can cause dilation and a natriuresis, are upregulated or increased. Maybe with rehydration we release ANP, which in turn induces the natriuresis. The solution we ingest could alter the increase in ANP. In two different human studies with drinking there wasn't a clear cut increase in ANP. A difference may be that these individuals were fully hydrated prior to the fluid consumption. The increase in renal excretion of water and sodium, at the same time that one is trying to restore body fluids, is clearly a problem that must be addressed.

GISOLFI: You have given us the impression that renal function is not severely compromised during acute bouts of exercise, but what about prolonged exercise, especially when performed in a warm environment.

ZAMBRASKI: I didn't mean to de-emphasize the effects of the combined factors of prolonged exercise, hypohydration, and heat stress. Robinson's work back in the early 1950s clearly showed that with the same exercise stress, if subjects are dehydrated or exposed to the heat, their renal blood flow and GFR decrements were about 20–30% greater. These clearly are additional significant stresses. However, these decrements in blood flow and GFR could produce severe consequences. Acute renal failure could occur. I am not as concerned about the proteinuric response. You can get this with very light exercise, and also under conditions where you don't have these additional factors, although it is worse when you combine exercise with heat stress and/or hypohydration.

SUTTON: First, if we look at supra maximal exercise where you are going all out for 15–20 or even 30 seconds, this invariably is followed by many hours of reduced urine output, 5–10 mL/h. I wonder if you might just tell us a little about that. The next question I have concerns the various structures within the kidney and their vulnerability to ischemia. Could you tell me if there is a difference in sensitivity of these different structures to ischemia? For instance, when we hear about problems related to dehydration and heat stress associated with exercise, invariably we hear of a tubular problem. Is this simply something to do with the distribution of blood flow in the kidney? Maybe you could elaborate on that. Finally, a comment. The point that Jerry just made about things like hemaglobin and myoglobin in the urine are simply a reflection of problems elsewhere where you actually get hemolysis or where you get rhabdomyolysis. Presumably both of those things have implications for the deterioration in kidney function.

ZAMBRASKI: On your first point concerning supramaximal exercise, I don't know what the exact mechanism is, but there are large endocrine responses to that type of work. You have a prolonged elevation of aldosterone and ADH. I don't think anyone has measured a prolonged decrease in GFR with this type of exercise.

NADEL: I am impressed by this issue of hyponatremia, especially with respect to the slide you put up showing decreases in renal filtration and blood flow during prolonged exercise, even when drinking. There have been enough reports about hyponatremia that we are all familiar with it. The questions I have are related to this. (1) When someone is drinking water without any solutes at a high rate and the body is not ridding itself of the water, how is the plasma volume changing? Is the plasma volume expanding? If so, why aren't the cardiopulmonary receptors providing the appropriate stimuli to allow renal blood flow to remain elevated? (2) Secondly, we know from Rowell's 1966 paper that splanchnic vascular resistance increases when exercise intensity increases above a certain point. Furthermore, heat exposure combined with exercise causes a shift in splanchnic vascular resistance that is greater than under cool conditions. Is it known whether renal blood flow changes occur in a graded fashion? What you have told us is that renal blood flow decreases during heavy exercise; is this graded with the intensity of exercise? I would expect this to be the case, but is this known?

ZAMBRASKI: I don't know why the kidneys are not responding to the normal volume and plasma osmolality changes that occur with profound fluid consumption during high-intensity exercise. It may relate to the intensity of exercise. If sympathetic drive is high despite fluid loading, it simply may not be inhibited. This could explain why some individuals do not show the required increase in water excretion to prevent hyponatremia.

BUSKIRK: There are two environments you didn't say anything about and people certainly exercise in them; one is a cold environment and the other is at relatively high terrestrial altitudes. The former involves diuresis and the latter involves hypoxia. Can you comment on these?

ZAMBRASKI: As far as the diuretic response to a cold environment, I'm not familiar with the mechanism although I believe there is an increase in GFR.

BUSKIRK: As early as with first exposure?

KACHADORIAN: In earlier studies we compared the effects of cold, temperate, and hot environments on renal function, using healthy young males. Indeed, stimulatory effects of mild exercise tended to be even more so in the cold. Moreoever, reduction in renal function by exercise as exercise intensity increased were to lesser degrees in the cold. Finally, there was virtually no evidence of athletic nephritis in the cold during moderately heavy exercise.

SUTTON: Just a comment on the altitude story. For whatever reason, there have been lots of reported proteinuria in mountainous altitudes, but whether that is related to hypoxia per se, exercise, or however you compound the two, it is very difficult to know. Upon arrival at altitude, subjects that tended to diurese were ostensibly protected from the ravages of high altitude mountain sickness. Those who tended to gain weight over the first 24 or 48 h of altitude, and for what it's worth had a slightly reduced urine output, are the ones tht developed more symptoms of acute mountain sickness. Some of them even went on to have suggestive fluid accumulation in the lungs. And of course, the converse was the case as well.

8

Fluid Replacement During Exercise: Effects on Physiological Homeostasis and Performance

EDWARD F. COYLE, PH.D.

MARC HAMILTON, M.A.

PROLONGED EXERCISE

A. Introduction

Fluid replacement is obviously important to performance during prolonged exercise that causes large body water losses due to heavy sweating. As discussed in Chapter 1, sweating rate, and therefore the amount of dehydration incurred during exercise, is a function of exercise intensity, the environmental conditions, and the duration of exercise. During prolonged exercise at environmental temperatures of 20–25°C, sweating rates frequently exceed 1 L/h and in warmer environments can be as high as 2–3 L/h. The potentially adverse effects of these large fluid losses on physiological homeostasis and exercise performance are influenced by many factors, including body fluid status before exercise, the duration of exercise, and fluid ingestion during exercise.

B. Body Water Loss Prior to Prolonged Exercise Results in Relatively Large Reductions in Plasma Volume

Much of our understanding of the effects of body water loss on physiological homeostasis and exercise performance has developed from studies that induced hypohydration *prior to exercise.* (*Hypohydration* indicates a body water deficit, whereas *euhydration* refers to "normal" body water status.) The term *dehydration* refers to the process by which body water is lost or to the transition from the euhydrated to the hypohydrated state. Typically, hypohydration is produced prior to exercise by methods including: a) deprivation of dietary water, b) heavy sweating from heat exposure in a sauna and/or from mild exercise, and c) drug-induced diuresis. As reviewed in Chapter 1, hypohydration induced by these methods reduces endurance performance primarily by impairing cardiovascular function and thermoregulation. Compared to when exercise is begun in a euhydrated state, hypohydration prior to prolonged submaximal exercise generally produces the events outlined in Table 8–1.

As shown by Sawka et al. (1984b), hypohydration due to water deprivation before exercise lowers plasma volume below euhydrated levels both at rest and during subsequent moderate intensity exercise. Additionally, progressively larger body water deficits that occur before exercise result in progressively lower plasma volumes and increased heat storage during exercise (Sawka et al., 1984a, 1984b, 1985b; Fig. 1–5 in Chapter 1). Therefore, it is clear that the magnitude of hypohydration prior to exercise directly affects plasma volume and apparently the magnitude of cardiovascular dysfunction and hyperthermia during exercise.

The important point to be made by Table 8–2 is that the various methods of producing hypohydration *prior to exercise* produce relatively

TABLE 8-1. *Major physiological effects during exercise of hypohydration before exercise.*

1) Decreased plasma volume and blood volume
2) Increased plasma osmolality (not as evident with iso-osmotic diuresis)
3) Decreased skin blood flow
4) Decreased sweating rate
5) Increased heat storage and increased body temperature
6) Increased heart rate and decreased stroke volume

TABLE 8-2. *Comparison of percentage decline in body weight and plasma volume through various methods of dehydration.*

Study	Dehydration Method	% Reduction in Body Weight	% Reduction in Plasma Volume*
Sawka et al.;	water and food denial}	3%	8%
1985 b	water and food denial}	5%	15%
Caldwell et al.;	diuretics}	4%	14%
1984	sauna}	4%	10%
	prolonged exercise}	4%	1%
Saltin; 1964a	sauna}	4%	18%
	prolonged exercise}	4%	3%
Claremont et al.; 1976	diuretics}	3%	16%

*% reduction in plasma volume, measured during submaximal exercise when hypohydrated, below the plasma volume during submaximal exercise when euhydrated. # Water and food denial for 15 h after exercising in mild heat.

large reductions in plasma volume both at rest and during submaximal exercise. However, when hypohydration is produced by sweating *during prolonged exercise*, relatively large losses of body water can be incurred with little or no reduction in plasma volume.

Sawka et al. (1985) have observed that body water losses due to heat exposure followed by 15 hours of food and water denial, produce 8% and 15% reductions in plasma volume during subsequent exercise when body weight is reduced by 3% and 5%, respectively. Table 8-2 also reports that when sauna-induced sweating or diuretic drugs (i.e., furosemide or thiazides) are used to reduce body weight by 3-4%, plasma volume during exercise is reduced 10-18%. In sharp contrast, however, Caldwell et al. (1984) and Saltin (1964a) found that when body weight was reduced 4% by sweating during prolonged exercise, plasma volume was reduced only 1-3%. Therefore, hypohydration induced by sauna or diuretics produces marked hypovolemia whereas only minor hypovolemia is produced by hypohydration associated with prolonged exercise.

Hypohydration *prior* to exercise is a powerful tool to study the effects of body water loss upon physiological homeostasis during subsequent exercise, and hypovolemia occurs in this process. However, hypovolemia *during* prolonged exercise is usually minimal and therefore is probably not primarily responsible for the sequence of events 2-6 outlined in Table 8-1. Factors other than hypovolemia, e.g., hyperthermia, probably contribute to cardiovascular drift during prolonged exercise (Raven & Stevens, 1988; Rowell, 1986). The salient point of this discussion is that fluid ingestion during prolonged exercise, although minimizing cardiovascular drift and improving some types of performance, should not necessarily be viewed as a means of preventing hypovolemia. This is contrary to widely held beliefs that have arisen from studies of hypohydration *prior* to exercise and not necessarily from studies of dehydration *during* exercise.

In this chapter, we focus upon the physiological and performance effects of beverage ingestion to replace fluids lost *during* prolonged exercise. More specifically, our focus is on the responses of people who begin prolonged exercise in a euhydrated state and then become hypohydrated by sweating.

C. Factors That Influence Blood and Plasma Volume During Exercise

Several review articles (Sawka, 1984a; Harrison, 1985; Senay & Pivarnik, 1985; Sawka, Sawka and Pandolf, Chapter 1) have focused upon the factors that regulate alterations in plasma volume when exercise is initiated from the resting state. The extent to which plasma volume increases or decreases from resting levels is determined by the balance between osmotic, colloid, tissue, and hydrostatic pressures, among others. The conditions that influence these pressures include exercise mode, intensity, environmental conditions, state of training and pre-exercise hydration status (Gaebelein & Senay, 1980; 1982a; 1982b). According to this balance of pressures, fluid shifts responsible for changes in plasma and blood volume are established after only a few minutes of exercise. The important issue at hand is how the progressive dehydration experienced during prolonged exercise (which is begun in a euhydrated state) alters blood volume and fluid volumes in the intracellular space and interstitial space.

It is important to realize that we are defining "nonmovolemia" for this discussion to be that blood volume which is established after 4–10 of exercise that is begun in the euhydrated state (Figure 8-1). This is sufficient time for fluid shifts to occur before a significant amount of *total body water is lost (i.e. still euhydrated)*. Therefore, by our definition, a decrease in blood volume below that observed after 10 min of exercise is considered "hypovolemia," whereas an increase above this early exercise level is "hypervolemia." Our definitions are different from studies that consider the resting pre-exercise condition to be the reference point and thus view blood volume status during exercise as being "hypovolemic" if it is below resting and "hypervolemic" if blood volume increases above resting values. In our opinion, comparisons made relative to the resting state add unnecessary variability and confusion because of the many physiological and methodological factors that have large effects on resting blood volume (Harrison, 1985). When changes in blood volume are made relative to the volume at rest, rather than relative to the euhydrated blood volume established in early exercise, the actual fluid shifts due to the progression of exercise per se tend to be obscured by the fluid shifts occurring in the transition from rest to exercise. We will continue to clarify this point in the discussion to follow.

Another important point for consideration is that it is functionally more appropriate to report alterations in blood volume rather than

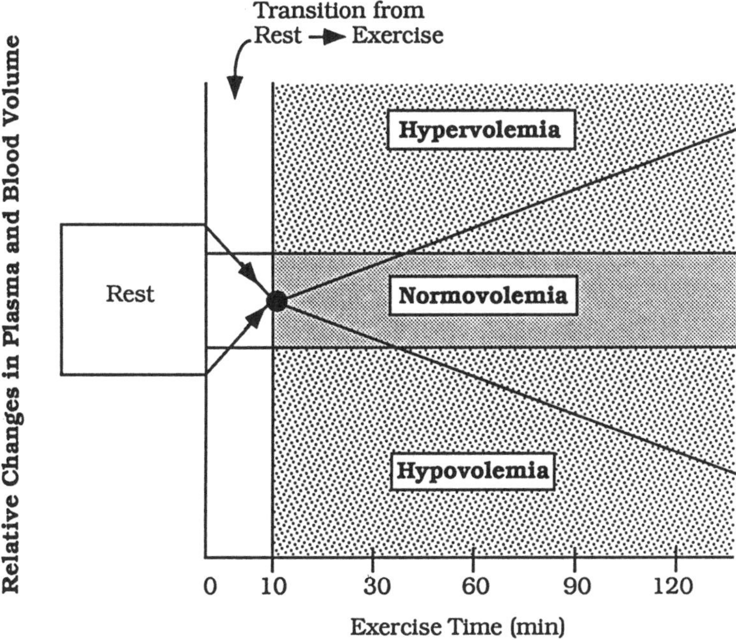

FIGURE 8-1. *Conceptual view that normal blood volume (normovolemia) or plasma volume is established after 10 min of exercise begun in the euhydrated state. This has advantages over comparing changes from rest.*

plasma volume when describing blood fluid changes during dehydration or fluid replacement. Granted, the absolute change in blood volume is often similar to the change in plasma volume. However, alterations in plasma osmolality due to dehydration or ingestion of various fluids can change the size of the red blood cells sufficiently so that alterations in plasma volume may not reflect changes in blood volume of up to several hundred milliliters (Costill et al., 1974a). However, because most studies focus upon alterations in plasma volume, for simplicity of presentation we will do the same, recognizing the limitation to this approach.

D. Plasma Volume And Intracellular Fluid Shifts During Prolonged Exercise In Cold or Neutral Environments Without Fluid Replacement

Before discussing when and why fluid replacement is advisable during exercise, it is important to first understand which fluid compartments undergo dehydration during prolonged exercise. Table 8-3 presents the results from numerous studies reporting the alterations in plasma volume that accompany running or cycling for 1-3 h at intensities from 36-75% $\dot{V}O_2$max. These experiments were performed in the field or laboratory with neutral ambient temperatures of 19-25°C or in the cold at -4.5°C to 15°C. The remarkable point is that after the initial he-

TABLE 8-3. *Plasma volume responses during dehydration induced by prolonged exercise*

Study	Exercise		Environment	Body Weight	Changes In
	Mode	Intensity		Loss	Plasma Volume (PV)
Costill et al. (1970)	running	74% VO_2max	25°C	−4.8% to −6.2%	No change in PV from 10-120 min; no fluids
Sawka et al. (1979)	running	70% VO_2max	22-25°C	−4%	No change in PV from 30 to 160 min
Sawka et al. (1980)	running	65-75% VO_2max	22-25°C	−4%	No change in PV from 30 160 min
Macek et al. (1976)	running	60% VO_2max	24°C		No change in PV from 10-60 min
Costill & Fink (1974)	running and cycling	~65–75% VO_2 max	22°C	−4%	2% reduction in PV from 10-120 min
Astrand & Saltin (1964)	85 km ski race 5-9.5 h		-9 to −4.5°C	−5.5%	No change in PV; fluid consumption - 200-400mL/h
Maron et al. (1975)	42 km run		15-29°C	−4.3%	PV declines 4.3%; fluid consumption - 0.19L/h
Refsum et al. (1973)	90 km ski race			−2.6%	PV increased approximately 6%

moconcentration in the transition from rest to exercise, plasma volume remained stable throughout the remainder of prolonged exercise. This occurred despite reductions in body weight of 3–7%, which represents a 2–5 kg loss of fluid at a rate of 1–1.5 L/h. Since plasma volume is remarkably stable from 10 min through several hours during exercise in a neutral or cold environment, the source of the lost fluid must be primarily the intracellular space (approximately 65% of total body water), with some fluid possibly coming from the smaller interstitial space (25% of total body water) (Kozlowski & Saltin, 1964; Sawka et al., 1984b). Therefore, it is clear that plasma volume is well defended during prolonged exercise in a neutral or cold environment and that fluid losses occur primarily from within some of the cells of the body. This understanding leads to some obvious questions. When ingesting fluids during prolonged exercise to counteract dehydration, into what fluid space does the ingested fluid go? Is dehydration of the intracellular space prevented, and, if so, is it likely that all cells of the body are equally affected? Since "hypovolemia" is either minimal or absent during prolonged exercise in a neutral or cool environment, does fluid replacement increase blood volume and cause hypervolemia? Does the composition of the fluid replacement solution affect these processes?

E. Plasma Volume Shifts During Prolonged Exercise in Hot Environments Without Fluid Replacement

Plasma volume shifts during prolonged exercise in the heat (i.e., > 32°C) are variable, and, as stated by Senay and Pivarnik (1985), results are inconsistent in seemingly similar experiments. Variability in plasma volume shifts are likely due to experimental differences regarding exercise mode, posture, intensity, duration, skin temperature, subjects' state of training and heat acclimation, and the conditions under which the reference or pre-exercise blood sample was obtained. For instance, the blood of acclimated individuals running in the heat is often hemodiluted compared to rest, whereas unacclimated people display a more unstable plasma volume (Sawka, 1984b; Senay and Pivarnik, 1985; Sawka and Pandolf, Chapter 1). Additionally, Harrison et al. (1975) found plasma volume to decline progressively to values 15% below rest during 50 min of cycling in the heat (42°C) at 25% $\dot{V}O_2max$. However, when the cycling intensity was increased to 55% $\dot{V}O_2max$ and the environmental temperature was lowered to 30°C, a 15% hemoconcentration above rest was observed after only 5 min with little change from 5–50 min.

Although plasma volume responses to exercise and heat are variable, some general trends are vaguely apparent. Reductions in plasma volume tend to be greater when cycling compared to running, as the environmental temperature increases, and as the exercise is extended over prolonged periods (Harrison, 1985; Sawka, 1984b; Senay & Pivarnik, 1985).

The question addressed below is: Are the conditions that induce the largest reduction in plasma volume relative to total body water losses, the same conditions under which fluid replacement is most beneficial? Exercise in the heat appears to reduce plasma volume to a greater extent than exercise in a neutral or cold environment. This may be the case even when the reductions in plasma volume are compared at the same absolute volumes of body water loss, in spite of the fact that body water loss occurs more rapidly in the heat. However, we are not familiar with any investigations that have directly tested this hypothesis.

F. Comparison of the Physiological Responses to Prolonged Exercise in a *Neutral or Cool Environment With and Without Fluid Ingestion During Exercise*

1. Plasma volume. As indicated in Table 8-3, during prolonged exercise in a neutral or cold environment, plasma volume remains remarkably stable from the first 5–10 min of exercise throughout several hours when dehydration ranges from 3–7% of body weight and no fluids are ingested. Therefore, it might be expected that fluid ingestion would, if anything, increase plasma volume and result in *hyper*volemia during exercise. To our knowledge, little published data exists regarding this point. When observing men running on a treadmill for 120 min and comparing a no fluid ingestion trial with fluid ingestion (either water or a glucose-electrolyte solution), Costill et al. (1970) did not observe consistent differences in blood hematocrit, hemoglobin, or protein concentration. Essentially, Costill et al. (1970) reported that after the first 10 min of running, plasma volume was not different over time (10–110 min) or, more importantly, plasma volume was not different whether the subjects drank nothing or 0.88 L/h of water or a glucose-electrolyte solution. (See Senay and Pivarnik, 1985, page 355, for a more thorough interpretation of these data.) Plasma volume during running appeared fairly stable regardless of fluid losses due to sweating or fluid replacement via ingestion.

Owen et al. (1986) observed moderately well-trained men during 2 h of running in a cool environment (i.e., 25°C) while they drank 600 mL of water per hour, which represented approximately one-half of the fluid lost. Plasma volume remained very stable during the entire duration of the run. It is clear that drinking water at this rate did not increase plasma volume during 30–120 min of exercise. In another recent study, fluid ingestion of approximately 1 L/h did not increase plasma volume during 30–180 min of running in the heat (i.e., 33°C) (Ryan et al., 1989). Although a no-fluid trial was not included in these studies, these results appear similar to those shown in Table 8-3.

Based upon these observations, we hypothesize that fluid ingested during exercise in a cool (and possibly some hot environments; see below), does not accumulate in the plasma and increase its volume. These data, however are indirect, and as far as we know, the appropriate investigations have yet to be published. The important inference is that fluid ingested during prolonged exercise functions primarily to attenuate the decline of fluid within the intracellular and perhaps the interstitial compartments, but *not* within the blood.

2. Cardiovascular Responses. Prolonged exercise causes "cardiovascular drift," characterized by a progressive increase in heart rate and decrease in stroke volume throughout exercise. As recently reviewed by Raven and Stevens (1988), the rate of "drift" increases with increasing environmental temperature and relative exercise intensity. These observations and a substantial amount of other evidence suggest that the major factor associated with cardiovascular drift is a shift of the circulating blood volume into the circulation of the skin to dissipate heat (Ekelund, 1967; Ekelund et al., 1967; Johnson & Rowell, 1975; Raven & Stevens, 1988; Rowell, 1986).

The extent of "cardiovascular drift" during prolonged treadmill running in a neutral environment (22–25°C) was well documented by Sawka et al. (1979). They observed trained men during two bouts of high-intensity running (each 80 min at 70% $\dot{V}O_2max$) separated by a 90-min rest interval. Fluid ingestion was limited to only 100 mL during each 80-min run and 280 mL of a carbonated soft drink between the runs; thus, the subjects lost 4% of their body weights. When comparing cardiovascular responses during the early part of the first run with the latter portion of the second run, stroke volume declined by 19% while heart rate increased approximately 10%. This "drift" was associated with progressive hyperthermia. Even though the environment was not above 25°C, rectal temperatures reached over 40°C at the end of this intense bout of exercise. Similar observations were made by Davies and Thompson (1986).

3. Hyperthermia. Body heat storage is a function of bodily heat production as well as environmental factors that affect heat loss. Dangerous hyperthermia can occur during exercise in seemingly cool environments (e.g., 25°C) when the exercise intensity elicits a high percentage of $\dot{V}O_2max$ (Hughson et al., 1983, Robinson, 1963). Additionally, endurance athletes capable of performing a given amount of work rapidly are very susceptible to hyperthermia (Adams et al, 1975; Drinkwater, 1984; Hughson et al., 1983; MacDougall et al., 1974; Maughan, 1985; Noakes 1982; Noakes et al., 1988; Robinson, 1963). They not only exercise at a high percentage of $\dot{V}O_2max$, they also are capable of the greatest rates of heat production. Exercise-induced hyperthermia can potentially impair performance, and, more seriously, it can result in severe damage to various bodily organs (e.g., gastrointestinal system, kidneys, liver, and brain) and in death (Leithead and Lind, 1964; Milvy, 1977; Shibolet et al., 1976; Wyndham, 1977). For these reasons, the elevation of core temperature to greater than 40°C is considered dangerous and should be avoided.

It is possible that even lower levels of hyperthermia present dangerous conditions to some individuals who are more susceptible to heat injury.

Based upon the deleterious effects of hyperthermia upon cardiovascular function and performance, we think that an important purpose of fluid replacement during exercise is to attenuate the increase in body temperature so as to optimize performance and minimize heat illness. Other purposes of fluid replacement might include enhancing muscle blood flow and sympathetic drive, as discussed below.

Rowell (1986) suggests that hyperthermia during exercise may be the primary factor causing cardiovascular drift. Exercise-induced hyperthermia causes increased sympathetic stimulation, one manifestation of which is increased heart rate. Additionally, it appears to increase alpha-adrenergic vasoconstriction of the exercising musculature, thus potentially reducing muscle blood flow. At the same time that blood flow to the skin increases, stroke volume decreases due to reduced myocardial filling pressure (Rowell, 1986). Accordingly, a smaller percentage of cardiac output is diverted to the working musculature. It is even possible for cardiac output to decline, e.g., if stroke volume decreases more than heart rate increases.

As exercising people get hotter, two scenarios may occur regarding muscle blood flow (Rowell, 1986; Fig. 13-12, p. 382). In the first, blood flow to the working musculature may decline. This could potentially impair performance by reducing oxygen delivery or possibly by reducing the elimination of metabolic by-products that cause fatigue. In the second scenario, muscle blood flow is maintained (Savard et al., 1988); however, for this to occur, symapthetic drive must be greatly increased, resulting in a high heart rate and cardiac output. Theoretically, performance would be impaired in this second scenario if the required increase in heart rate and cardiac output exceeded the capacity of the individual to respond. This suggests that a greater level of sympathetic drive or a greater sensation of effort or motivation is required to maintain performance when one is hyperthermic. Or stated another way, for a given level of motivation or effort, people do not appear to be able to exercise as intensely when hyperthermic compared to when body temperature is lower. In this light, hyperthermia is viewed as a noxious agent which can potentially can reduce performance.

4. Fluid Replacement and Endurance Performance in a *Neutral or Cool Environment.* We think that the primary purpose of fluid replacement during prolonged exercise in a neutral or cool environment is to prevent the elevation of body temperature that might impair performance and/or endanger organs. Remember, fluid replacement will primarily offset the dehydration of the intracellular and interstitial spaces and *not* of the blood. Although it is clear that fluid replacement attenuates hyperthermia and improves endurance performance during exercise in the heat (see below), little direct evidence is available regarding benefits of fluid replacement during exercise in a neutral or cool environment (i.e., 25°C or less). Because of this scarcity of direct data, we must take a "prospectus" approach to the question.

In a recent provocative article, Noakes et al. (1988) presented the concept that during prolonged exercise in mild environments (<25°C) a fluid intake of 0.5 L/h will prevent significant dehydration and hyperthermia in the majority of athletes. During competitive running and canoeing for durations of 170–340 min, they observed body weight losses to average approximately 0.95 L/h. Therefore, when the athletes ingested 0.5 L/h, net weight loss averaged slightly less than 0.5 L/h, which is in agreement with previous reports regarding the balance between dehydration and *ad lib* fluid intake in mild environments (Table 4 in Noakes et al., 1988).

Noakes et al. (1988) essentially presented two arguments in support of the idea that fluid ingestion at rates greater than 0.5 L/h is not beneficial during prolonged exercise in mild environments. First, because rectal temperature usually remained in the range of 38–39°C and because there was little relationship between the extent of dehydration and degree of hyperthermia when comparing more than 200 athletes, Noakes et al. (1988) concluded that dehydration is not a primary cause of hyperthermia during competition in mild temperatures. They argued instead that the fastest runners usually become the hottest, which we think is correct, and they cited several supportive studies (Maron et al., 1975; Maughan, 1985; Wyndham, 1977). Yet their own data failed to support this hypothesis. Because of the extreme inter-subject variability in Noakes et al. (1988), it is not surprising that nothing appeared to be related to hyperthermia. We think the importance of the article of Noakes et al. (1988) lies not in their data but in the question which they are appropriately restating. That question is: During exercise in a mild environment, should fluid intake equal the rate of weight loss so as to prevent dehydration?, *or*, as they favor, Should endurance athletes keep their *ad lib* fluid intake at approximately 0.5 L/h and thus become somewhat dehydrated? We are not aware of any investigations that directly address these questions regarding the effects of partial compared to total fluid replacement on rectal temperature and performance in cool environments.

The second argument put forth by Noakes et al. (1988) in support of the idea that fluid intake does not have to match fluid loss is that body water losses of 0.5 L/h represent the loss of the water stored with combusted glycogen and therefore does not represent true dehydration. Essentially, this argument contends that the water stored with glycogen inside the cell does not enhance cellular function to any extent, and therefore there is little or no adverse effect when it is removed to balance sweat losses as glycogen is consumed.

5. A "Voice In the Wilderness." From our perspective at this moment, we look back and hear a "Voice in the Wilderness." That voice belonged to Costill, Kammer and Fisher (1974b), who reported some classic data in four "elite" distance runners. On three separate occasions the men ran for 2 h on a laboratory treadmill while ambient temperature was 25°C and they were cooled with a fan. During one trial, no fluids were consumed. During the other two trials they drank approximately 1 L/h of either water or a glucose-electrolyte beverage (4.3 g carbohydrate/100 mL; 20 mM sodium; 15.3 mM chloride and 2.4 mM potassium). As we mentioned before, Costill, Kammer and Fisher (1974b) found no apparent difference in blood volume whether these men drank nothing or water or the glucose-electrolyte drink. Interestingly, they also did not observe large differences in heart rate when comparing the three trials. The only apparent influence of drinking was that rectal temperature leveled off at approximately 38.6°C during the 1–2 h period when either of the solutions was ingested, whereas rectal temperature continued to rise when no fluid was ingested, and it reached 39.4°C after 2 h of running.

These early observations on but a few subjects suggest that during treadmill running at 25°C, fluid replacement attenuates the increase in body temperature. Other purposes of fluid replacement might also include influencing muscle blood flow and sympathetic drive, as presented below. To our knowledge, no "hard data" (i.e., sufficient numbers of subjects with consistent responses) exists at this time regarding the effects of fluid replacement on performance in environments that are not hot.

G. Comparison of the Physiological Responses to Prolonged Exercise in a *Hot Environment With and Without Fluid Ingestion During Exercise*

1. Plasma Volume and Hyperthermia. The ingestion of water during exercise in the heat will attenuate the progressive body heat storage which occurs when fluid replacement is absent (Pitts et al., 1944; Ladell, 1954; Gisolfi & Copping, 1974). Gisolfi and Copping (1974) demonstrated that both 10°C water or water warmed to body core temperature consumed at a rate of 600 mL/h were effective in preventing ~0.7°C of the increase in rectal temperature observed during 2 h of treadmill running. Unfortunately, we are unable to conclude if rehydration benefitted thermoregulation by increasing blood volume because these three studies measured neither hematocrit nor hemoglobin.

We have been led to believe that the plasma volume responses to prolonged exercise in the heat when comparing "no fluid replacement" with "fluid replacement" is usually as described by Costill and Miller (1980; Fig. 10, p. 10). The response they describe is that plasma volume declines by about 3–5% with the transition from rest to exercise and that when prolonged exercise (i.e., cycling at 50% of $\dot{V}O_2max$) in the heat is performed "without fluid replacement," plasma volume continues to decline to levels 9% below the resting state. In contrast, they report that drinking water at rates of 900 mL/h causes plasma volume to continuously increase during the 10–120 min period of exercise such that after 120 min of exercise, plasma volume is much greater when fluids are ingested compared to when no fluids are ingested.

We are not sure of the actual data from which this well known figure has been drawn, but the concept is that exercise in the heat without fluid replacement causes *hypo*volemia, whereas fluid ingestion promotes *hyper*volemia. (Remember that "normovolemia" is that blood volume established after the first few minutes of exercise when euhydrated and before significant fluid is lost by sweating.) This simple concept is a useful teaching aid for students who are first being introduced to this area. Implicit in this concept, however, is that fluid replacement is primarily important to thermoregulation because it increases the volume of blood or plasma. We recognize that increased blood volume has the potential to attenuate hyperthermia during exercise in the heat by increasing sweating rate and skin blood flow (Nadel, 1988; Sawka et al., 1988). However, our salient point is that fluid replacement during exercise often does *not* alter circulating blood volume, and yet hyperthermia is still reduced. This suggests that fluid replacement probably serves other important thermoregulatory functions such as preventing plasma hyperosmolality and/or cellular dehydration (see chapters by Greenleaf and Nadel in this volume). These important points are often forgotten when too much emphasis is placed upon plasma volume.

As discussed in a previous section, the plasma volume responses to prolonged exercise in the heat are variable (Senay and Pivarnik, 1985). Progressive dehydration during prolonged exercise in the heat sometimes causes progressive reductions in plasma volume (Candas et al., 1986; Francis, 1979; Harrison et al., 1975), sometimes plasma volume remains stable (Harrison, 1985; Sawka et al., 1988), and sometimes it increases (Sawka et al., 1984b; Sawka, 1988; Sawka et al., 1988). Fluid ingestion during prolonged exercise in the heat usually causes plasma volume to be higher than observed during exercise without fluid ingestion, and thus it often alleviates hypovolemia and may possibly promote hypervolemia (Candas et al., 1986; Francis, 1979; Harrison et al., 1975). (However, as far as we can tell, in Candas et al. (1986) and Francis (1979), plasma volume change from rest was measured during the rest periods between repeated bouts of exercise and therefore probably does not reflect responses during exercise.)

In contrast, plasma volume sometimes remains stable at normovolemic levels despite drinking large amounts of fluids (> 1 L/h) to replace the majority of body weight losses (Ryan et al., 1988). Therefore, fluid ingestion can have little effect on plasma volume, in which case the subject remains somewhat hypovolemic or normovolemic, or it can reverse hypovolemia and restore plasma volume to normovolemic or even hypervolemic levels. The only generalization that can be made is that the plasma volume is never lower when ingesting fluid compared to not ingesting fluids. Other combinations of effects seem possible. For a more complete discussion of the factors that regulate these responses, the reader should see the excellent reviews by Sawka et al. (1984a), Harrison (1985), and Senay and Pivarnik (1985).

Subjects who would otherwise be hypovolemic during exercise improve thermoregulation when blood volume is increased to normal levels (Fortney et al., 1981; Fortney et al., 1985; Nadel et al., 1980; Sawka et al., 1983; Sawka et al., 1985). However, in subjects who are normovolemic during exercise in the heat, the thermoregulatory advantages of hypervolemia, per se, are less clear-cut (Greenleaf and Castle, 1971; Nadel et al., 1980; Sawka et al., 1983; Sawka et al., 1988b). It is possible that an advantage of fluid replacement during exercise, other than increasing plasma volume, is to reduce plasma hyperosmolality. Plasma hyperosmolality can elevate core temperature during exercise in the heat (Fortney et al., 1985; Sawka et al., 1985) and result in a decreased threshold for sweating onset and a decrease in the rate of sweating for a given increase in core temperature (Fortney et al., 1985; Harrison et al., 1978).

2. Cardiovascular Responses. Rowell has taught us that there are two fundamental challenges to cardiovascular function during exercise in the heat (Rowell, 1974; 1986 p. 363).

> First, skin and muscle compete for blood flow and their combined needs can easily exceed the pumping capacity of the heart. Second, cutaneous vasodilation displaces blood volume into cutaneous veins and lowers cardiac filling pressure and stroke volume. Accordingly, cardiac pumping capacity may be reduced at a time when demands for flow are the greatest that humans ever experience. Clearly the demands for oxygen transport to muscle and for heat transport to skin require more than the heart can provide. Failure to maintain adequate muscle blood flow means that work must stop; failure to maintain adequate cutaneous blood flow means that hyperthermia must occur. It is the consequence of the latter that we fear most.

Progressive hyperthermia appears to promote progressive cardiovascular drift and thus greater increases in sympathetic drive to maintain muscle blood flow and skin blood flow (Rowell, 1986).

3. Hyperthermia and Performance. An important purpose of fluid replacement during prolonged exercise in the heat is to prevent an elevation of body temperature that might impair performance and/or endanger organs. It is clear that fluid replacement attenuates hyperthermia during exercise in the heat, yet we are not sure if it acts primarily to increase blood volume, to reduce hyperosmolality, or to reduce cellular dehydration.

The classic experiments published in 1944 by Pitts, Johnson, and Consolazio as well as the work of Ladell (1954), are the only investigations, to our knowledge, that have exercised people for prolonged periods in the heat to the point of fatigue in an attempt to determine the advantage of ingesting water as compared to becoming progressively dehydrated. These early reports clearly demonstrate an improvement in performance when fluid is consumed *during* exercise. Because these two studies provide *direct* evidence that endurance is improved during exercise in the heat by drinking, the methodology should be discussed. Both studies (Pitts et al., 1944; Ladell, 1954) were conducted on young, healthy, and acclimatized men during leg exercise at environmental temperatures of 32–38°C and relative humidities of approximately 30–80%.

The study performed by Pitts et al. (1944) at the Harvard Fatigue Laboratory is, in our opinion, the clearest study to date addressing the issue of the performance benefits derived from drinking water during prolonged exercise in the heat. The subjects walked at 3.5 mph on a 2.5% incline for up to 6 h with 10 min of rest after every hour. It must be emphasized that the same subjects were not always used in each experiment. In one series of experiments the subjects either drank water from the beginning of exercise which equalled 2/3 of their sweat loss, or they drank nothing. When no fluid was ingested, in 10 of 16 or 62% of the trials, the subjects were unable to complete 2 h of walking. When the subjects drank water (equal to 2/3 of sweat loss), 22 subjects completed at least 2 h of walking; it was not reported if any of the subjects became fatigued before 2 h. When exhaustion occurred in the "no fluid" condition, rectal temperature was greater than 39.4°C, and heart rate was over 170 beats/min compared to 2 h values of 39.1°C and 153 beats/min when drinking water.

Qualitatively, the results of these experiments were described as follows:

> When water was withheld it is found that: rectal temperature and pulse rate rise steadily to uncomfortable levels; the rate of sweating declines steadily; mechanical efficiency decreases as is shown by the increase in oxygen consumption; and serum protein increases. The subject gradually feels worse and worse, and eventually becomes incapacitated from exhaustion of dehydration, no matter how tough or well acclimated he be. Administration of water combats these undesirable changes, and in general, the more nearly water intake approximates sweat loss, the better off the subject remains. (Pitts et al., 1944, p. 256).

Figure 8-2 below is a reproduction of the responses of one of their subjects. He performed six trials; two with no water, two with water *ad*

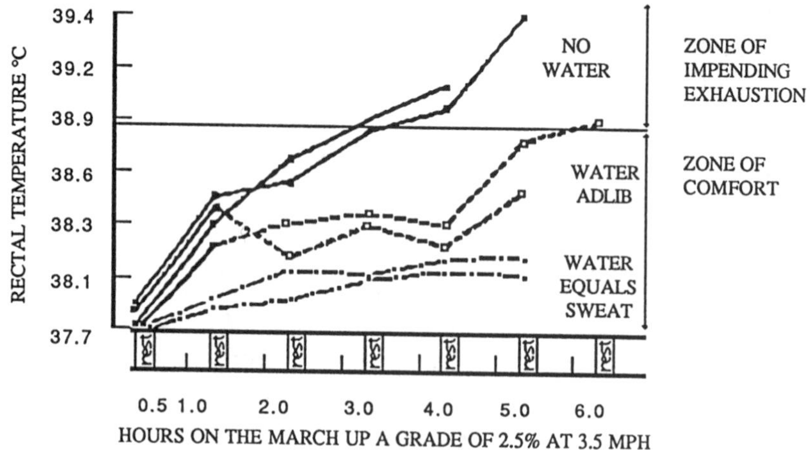

FIGURE 8-2. *Effect of water consumption on marching in the heat. (Six experiments on subject J.S. at temperature 37.7°C, relative humidity 35–45% (Pitts et al., 1944).*

lib, two with water replaced to equal sweat loss. When no water was consumed, rectal temperature increased steadily to the "zone of impending exhaustion," and the subject was exhausted after 4–5 h. When water consumption equalled sweat rate, rectal temperature increased only slightly and remained stable and within the "zone of comfort" during the 6th hour of exercise. During the *ad lib* trial, no water was consumed during the first hour, and then it was consumed at a rate equal to 2/3 of sweat loss. Rectal temperature rose during the first hour and then remained fairly stable at levels intermediate between the other two conditions. In this group of five subjects, the average heart rate response after 4 h was 154, 143 and 132 beats/min for the "no water," "*ad lib*," and "water equals sweat" trials, respectively. It appears that hyperthermia and cardiovascular drift were attenuated by fluid ingestion, and that it is best to replace all the fluid lost through sweating.

Ladell (1954) performed experiments to those of Pitts et al. (1944) by using low-intensity intermittent exercise (which in this case we think was stairstepping). Performance was measured as the number of trials in which the subjects completed the protocol. The criterion for a 'failure' was subjective. Four heat-acclimated subjects were tested 80 times in all. Several important conclusions regarding performance are emphasized by Table 8-4. When no water was provided, 75% of the tests resulted in subjective failure, compared to only a 7% failure rate when sweat losses were completely replaced with water consumption.

Recently the effectiveness of fluid replacement in the heat with beverages containing carbohydrates has been investigated (Murray 1987a). Murray et al. (1987b) and Davis et al. (1988a, 1988b) have demonstrated

TABLE 8-4. *Number and percentage of "failures" to complete 160 min of exercise at 34°C under the various fluid replacement conditions. Summarized from Ladell (1954).*

Condition	Number of Failures	% of Failures
No water	9 of 12	75%
Water Replacement	3 of 41	7%

during prolonged cycle ergometry that rectal temperature and plasma volume are similar when ingesting water or carbohydrate solutions up to 12% in concentration. They additionally have observed that carbohydrate solutions can enhance performance compared to a water placebo.

NEUROMUSCULAR POWER AND STRENGTH

Hypohydration produced by various methods of prolonged fluid restriction or by heavy sweating induced by a sauna or exercise in the heat has varied effects on neuromuscular strength and short-term power. As discussed by Sawka and Pandolf in this book (See chapter 1, Table 1-1) the majority (i.e., 75%) of studies cited indicate that reductions in body weight of up to 7% can be tolerated without a reduction in strength during maximal isometric or isotonic contractions (Ahlman & Karvonen, 1961; Bijlani & Sharma, 1980; Greenleaf et al., 1966; Serfass et al., 1984; Saltin, 1964a; Tuttle, 1943; Singer and Weiss, 1968). Since hypohydration (i.e., $<$7% decrease in body weight) does not usually impair strength, fluid replacement appears to be important to physical performance for reasons other than restoring strength.

Strength or muscular force generation during a particular action is determined by the ability of the nervous system to recruit motor units as well as by the quantity of muscular contractile proteins in cross-section and their ability to convert stored energy into force. It is unlikely that moderate reductions in muscle water alter force generation capability or energy production when maximally stimulated. It is more likely that the infrequently reported reductions in strength following hypohydration are due to a diminished ability of the central nervous to recruit motor units.

Three studies that reported 10–11% reductions in strength, employed prolonged fluid and food restriction to decrease body weight 3, 6, and 8%, respectively (Bosco & Terjung, 1968; Bosco et al., 1974; Houston et al., 1981). It is likely that the somewhat stressful experience of prolonged fluid and food restriction reduces the ability of some people to motivate themselves to produce "true" maximal voluntary muscular contractions. Therefore, food and fluid restriction may reduce strength independent of the degree of hypohydration per se. Unfortunately, these studies (Bosco & Terjung, 1968; Bosco et al., 1974; Houston et al., 1981) that observed reductions in strength following fluid restriction did not determine if strength was restored by feedings and, therefore, if the time course of strength restoration follows that of rehydration.

Although hypohydration does not usually reduce muscular strength, it is prudent to rehydrate and/or eat within comfortable limits prior to events such as weight lifting, wrestling, etc. If the event requires muscular endurance (i.e., wrestling; high-intensity running or cycling) fluid replacement becomes increasingly more important to performance. People can rehydrate a 5% weight loss in 2–4 h and show signs of restored cardiovascular function (Costill & Sparks, 1973; Palmer, 1969; Ribisl and Herbert, 1970).

HIGH-INTENSITY EXERCISE

Many athletic events and recreational activities require people to exercise at high intensities for several minutes to one hour. Although the importance of fluid replacement during prolonged low-intensity exercise (i.e.>1 h) has justifiably received a great deal of attention, the importance of hydration during high-intensity exercise of shorter durations is a more difficult topic to broach. Obviously, the amount of fluid replacement possible during short-term exercise is relatively small (i.e., 10–20 mL/min; see Chapter 3 by Costill). Additionally, drinking during intense exercise is logistically difficult to coordinate; it may detract from performance, and it often produces an uncomfortable stomach fullness. These real considerations, however, should not overshadow the potential importance of adequate hydration to performance during intense, short-term exercise. Although it may be difficult to offset dehydration during short-term, high-intensity exercise, people should make every attempt to be well hydrated at the start of exercise. This is particularly important when performing in a thermally stressful environment. During activities lasting 30–60 min which culminate in a sprint (e.g., 10 km running; 25–40 km bicycling) or heightened action (e.g., tennis, basketball), it may be advisable to replace fluid early in exercise.

A. Rates of energy expenditure, dehydration, and hyperthermia during short-term exercise.

It is helpful to first discuss the rate of dehydration and degree of hyperthermia experienced during high-intensity exercise as well as the effects of hypohydration on short-term performance. Exercise that results in fatigue after 3–5 min can be performed at rates of energy expenditure that elicit $\dot{V}O_2max$. Exercise at 80–95% $\dot{V}O_2max$ can be maintained for approximately 30 min, whereas exercise at 70–80% $\dot{V}O_2max$ can usually be tolerated for approximately 60 min or longer (Coyle et al., 1986; Coyle et al., 1988). Endurance trained individuals are capable of exercising at higher absolute rates of energy expenditure as well as at a higher % $\dot{V}O_2$max for a given duration compared to untrained people (Coyle et al., 1988). Thus, endurance-trained athletes are exposed to a great deal of metabolically generated heat during intense exercise. The intensity of performance in warm or hot environments invariably declines, body core temperature can increase to dangerously high levels (i.e.,>40–41°C) in a relatively short period of time. Severe hyperthermia and heat stroke have often occurred following running events of 15–30 min duration (Adams et al., 1975; Drinkwater, 1984; Hughson et al., 1983; MacDougall et al., 1974; Noakes et al., 1982; Robinson, 1963). Obviously, fluid ingestion during intense activities of approximately 30 min duration is of limited value because it can do little to offset dehydration. Although sweating rates can be high and are critical for cooling, they generally are not incurred for long enough durations to make dehydration of primary concern to health and performance. Hyperthermia is the primary concern. This important point must be realized by sponsors of athletic events, in particular those who organize 5–10 km races to be held under thermally stressful conditions. It does not suffice to simply encourage fluid replacement during exercise. Races should not be conducted in conditions that present thermal dangers. To reduce hyperthermia, people should make certain they are well hydrated prior to exercise, and they must plan on reducing their exercise intensity.

B. Hypohydration Prior to Exercise

As presented by Sawka and Pandolf (Chapter 1), people who begin exercise in the hypohydrated state are particularly prone to hyperthermia (Armstrong et al., 1985; Claremont et al., 1976; Sawka et al., 1984a) and will likely experience impaired performance during high-intensity activities. Interestingly, hypohydration induced by diuretics, sweating in a sauna, or prior exercise in the heat have been reported to have little effect upon $\dot{V}O_2$max or maximal stroke volume (Saltin, 1964a) when measured in a cool or thermally neutral environment, despite reductions in body weight ranging from 2–8% (Armstrong et al., 1985; Buskirk, 1958; Houston, 1981) However, hypohydration reduces the ability to perform short-term, high-intensity exercise in a neutral environment (Armstrong et al., 1985; Saltin, 1964a). Hypohydration markedly reduces performance in a hot environment (Craig and Cummings, 1966). Therefore, hypohydrated individuals should make every attempt to replace fluids prior to high-intensity, short term exercise in a neutral environment, and especially prior to exercise in a hot environment.

SUMMARY

When body water is lost *before* prolonged exercise, large deficits in plasma volume occur during the exercise. On the other hand, when large amounts of body water are lost by sweating *during* exercise, very minor losses of plasma volume typically occur. Most, if not all, of the plasma volume lost during exercise in the euhydrated state is lost in the first 5-10 min of exercise, i.e., before there is any loss of total body water. It is the plasma volume measured after this initial 10 min period of homeostatic adjustment that should be considered as the baseline euhydrated plasma volume ("normovolemia"). Accordingly, contrary to popular opinion, fluid ingestion during prolonged exercise begun in the euhydrated state should not be expected to prevent hypovolemia because there is little or no dehydration-induced hypovolemia in this condition. In fact, most data suggest that fluid ingestion during exercise does not increase plasma volume.

It appears that a major benefit of fluid ingestion during prolonged exercise is the prevention of hyperthermia, perhaps by preventing intracellular dehydration or extracellular fluid hyperosmolality. Dehydration typically has little or no adverse affect on force production during brief maximal muscle contractions (strength performance). However, as the duration of high-intensity exercise increases beyond about 20-30 min, fluid ingestion can be of value to prevent hyperthermia, decreased performance, and heat injury.

BIBLIOGRAPHY

Adams, W.C., R.H. Fox, A.J. Fry, and I.C. MacDonald. Thermoregulation during marathon running in cool, moderate, and hot environments. *J. Appl. Physiol.* 38:1030-1037, 1975.

Ahlman, K. and M.J. Karvonen. Weight reduction by sweating in wrestlers, and its effect on physical fitness. *J. Sports Med. Phys. Fitness.* 1:58-62, 1961.

Armstrong, L.E., R.W. Hubbard, B.H. Jones, and J.T. Daniels. Preparing Alberto Salazar for the heat of the 1984 Olympic Marathon. *Physician Sportsmed.* 14:73-81, 1986.

Armstrong, L.E., D.L. Costill, and W.J. Fink. Influence of diuretic-induced dehydration on competitive running performance. *Med. Sci. Sports Exerc.* 17:456-461, 1985.

Astrand, P.-O. and B. Saltin. Plasma and red cell volume after prolonged severe exercise. *J. Appl. Physiol.* 19:829-832, 1964.

Bijlani, R.L. and K.N. Sharma. Effet of dehydration and a few regimes of rehydration on human performance. *Ind. J. Phyisol. Pharmacol.* 24:255-266, 1980.

Bosco, J.S., J.E. Greenleaf, E.M. Bernauer, and D.H. Card. Effects of acute dehydration and starvation on muscular strength and endurance. *Acta Physiol. Pol.* 25:411-421, 1974.

Bosco, J.S. and R.L. Terjung. Effects of progressive hypohydration on maximal isometric muscular strength. *J. Sports Med. Phys. Fitness* 8:81-86, 1968.

Buskirk, E.R., P.F. Iampietro, and D.E. Bass. Work performance after dehydration: effects of physical conditioning and heat acclimation. *J. Appl. Physiol.* 12:189-194, 1958.

Caldwell, J.E., E. Ahonen, and J. Nousiainen. Differential effects of sauna-, diuretic-, and exercise-induced hypohydration. *J. Appl. Physiol.* 57:1018-1023, 1984.

Candas, V., J.P. Libert, G. Brandenberger, J.C. Sagot, C. Amoros, and J.M. Kahn. Hydration during exercise: effects on thermal and cardiovascular adjustments. *Eur. J. Appl. Physiol.* 55:113-122, 1986.

Claremont, A.D., D.L. Costill, W. Fink, and P. van Handel. Heat tolerance following diuretic induced dehydration. *Med. Sci. Sports* 8:239-243, 1976.

Costill, D.L. and J.M. Miller. Nutrition for endurance sport: Carbohydrate and fluid balance. *Int. J. Sports Medicine* 1:2-14, 1980.

Costill, D.L., and W.J. Fink. Plasma volume changes following exercise and thermal dehydration. *J. Appl. Physiol.* 37:521-535, 1974.

Costill, D.L., L. Branam, D. Eddy, and W. Fink. Alterations in red cell volume following exercise and dehydration. *J. Appl. Physiol.* 37:912-916, 1974a.

Costill, D.L., W.F. Kammer, and A. Fisher. Fluid ingestion during distance running. *J. Appl. Physiol.* 37:679-683, 1974b.

Costill, D.L., W.F. Kammer, and A. Fisher. Fluid ingestion during distance running. *Arch. Environ. Health* 21:520-525, 1970.
Costill, D.L. and K.E. Sparks. Rapid fluid replacement following thermal dehydration. *J. Appl. Physiol.* 34:299-303, 1973.
Coyle, E.F., A.R. Coggan, M.K. Hopper, and T.J. Walters. Determinants of endurance in well-trained cyclists. *J. Appl. Physiol.* 64:2622-2630, 1988.
Coyle, E.F., A.R. Coggan, M.K. Hemmert, and J.L. Ivy. Muscle glycogen utilization during prolonged strenuous exercise when fed carbohydrate. *J. Appl. Physiol.* 61:165-172, 1986.
Craig, F.N. and E.G. Cummings. Dehydration and muscular work. *J. Appl. Physiol.* 21:670-674, 1966.
Davies, C.T.M. and M.W. Thompson. Physiological responses to prolonged exercise in man. *J. Appl. Physiol.* 61:611-617, 1986.
Davis, J.M., W.A. Burgess, C.A. Slentz, W.P. Bartoli, and R.R. Pate. Effects of ingesting 6% and 12% glucose/electrolyte beverages during prolonged intermittent cycling in a warm environment. *Eur. J. Appl. Physiol.* 57:563-569, 1988a.
Davis, J.M., D.R. Lamb, R.R. Pate, C.A. Slentz, W.A. Burgess, and W.P. Bartoli. Carbohydrate-electrolyte drinks: effects on endurance cycling in the heat. *Amer. J. Clin. Nutr.* 48:1023-1030, 1988b.
Drinkwater, B.L. Heat as a limiting factor in endurance sports. *Am. Acad. Phys. Ed.* 18:93-100, 1984.
Ekelund, L.G. Circulatory and respiratory adaptations during prolonged exercise. *Acta Physiol. Scand.* (Suppl. 292) 70:5-38, 1967.
Ekelund, L.G., A. Holmgren, and C.O. Ovenfors. Heart volume during prolonged exercise in the supine and sitting position. *Acta Physiol. Scand.* 70:88-98, 1967.
Fortney, S.M., C.B. Wenger, J.R. Bove, and E.R. Nadel. Effect of hyperosmolality on control of blood flow and sweating. *J. Appl. Physiol.* 57:1688-1695, 1985.
Fortney, S.M., E.R. Nadel, C.B. Wenger, and J.R. Bove. Effect of acute alteration of blood volume on circulatory performance in humans *J. Appl. Physiol.* 50:292-298, 1981.
Francis, K.T. Effect of water and electrolyte replacement during exercise in the heat on biochemical indices of stress and performance. *Aviat. Space Environ. Med.* 50:115-119, 1979.
Gaebelein, C.J. and L.C. Senay, Jr. Vascular volume changes during cycling and stepping in women at two hydration levels. *Eur. J. Appl. Physiol.* 48:1-10, 1982a.
Gaebelein, C.J. and L.C. Senay, Jr. Vascular volume dynamics during ergometer exercise at different menstrual phases. *Eur. J. Appl. Physiol.* 50:1-11, 1982b.
Gaebelein, C.J. and L.C. Senay, Jr. Influence of exercise type, hydration, and heat on plasma volume shifts in men. *J. Appl. Physiol.* 49:119-123, 1980.
Gisolfi, C.V. and J.R. Copping. Thermal effects of prolonged treadmill exercise in the heat. *Med. Sci. Sports Ex* 6:108-113, 1974.
Greenleaf, J.E. and B.L. Castle. Exercise temperature regulation in men during hypohydration and hyperhydration. *J. Appl. Physiol.* 30:847-853, 1971.
Greenleaf, J.E., M. Matter, J.S. Bosco, L.G. Douglas, and E.G. Averkin. Effects of hypohydration on tolerance to $+G_z$ acceleration in man. *Aerospace Med.* 37:34-39, 1966.
Harrison, M.H. Effects of thermal stress and exercise on blood volume in humans. *Physiol. Rev.* 65:149-207, 1985.
Harrison, M.H., R.J. Edwards, and P.A. Fennessy. Intravascular volume and tonicity as factors in the regulation of body temperature. *J. Appl. Physiol.* 44:69-75, 1978.
Harrison, M.H., R.J. Edwards, and D.R. Leitch. Effect of exercise and thermal stress on plasma volume. *J. Appl. Physiol.* 39:925-931, 1975.
Houston, M.E, D.A. Marrin, H.J. Green, and J.A. Thomson. The effect of rapid weight loss on physiological functions in wrestlers. *Physician Sportsmed.* 9:73-78, 1981.
Hughson, R.L., L.A. Staudt, and J.M. Mackie. Monitoring road racing in the heat. *Physician Sportsmed.* 1:94-105, 1983.
Johnson, J.M. and L.B. Rowell. Forearm skin and muscle vascular responses to prolonged leg exercise in man. *J. Appl. Physiol.* 39:920-924, 1975.
Kozlowski, S. and B. Saltin. Effect of sweat loss on body fluids. *J. Appl. Physiol.* 19(6):1119-1124, 1964.
Ladell, W.S.S. The effects of water and salt intake upon the performance of men working in hot and humid environments. *J. Physiol.* 127:11-46, 1954.
Leithead, C.S. and A.R. Lind. *Heat Stress and Heat Disorders.* Davis, Philadelphia, 1964.
MacDougall, J.D., W.G. Reddan, C.R. Layton, and J.A. Dempsey. Effect of metabolic hyperthermia on performance during prolonged exercise. *J. Appl. Physiol.* 36:538-544, 1974.
Macek, M., J. Vavra, and J. Novosadova. Prolonged exercise in prepubertal boys. II. Changes in plasma volume and in some blood constituents. *Eur. J. Appl. Physiol.* 35:299-303, 1976.
Maron, M.B., S.M. Horvath, and J.E. Wilkerson. Blood biochemical alterations during recovery from competitive marathon running. *Eur. J. Appl. Physiol.* 36:231-238, 1977.
Maron, M.B., S.M. Horvath, and J.E. Wilkerson. Acute blood biochemical alterations in response to marathon running. *Eur. J. Appl. Physiol.* 34:173-181, 1975.
Maughan, R.J. Thermoregulation in marathon competition at low ambient temperature. *Int. J. Sportsmed.* 6:15-19, 1985.
Milvy, P. (ed). *The Marathon, Physiological, Medical, Epidemiological, and Psychological Studies.* Ann. NY Acad. Sci. 301, 1977.

Murray, R. The effects of consuming carbohydrate-electrolyte beverages on gastric emptying and fluid absorption during and following exercise. *Sportsmed.* 4:322–351, 1987.
Murray, R., D.E. Eddy, T.W. Murray, J.G. Seifert, G.L. Paul, and G.A. Halaby. The effect of fluid and carbohydrate feedings during intermittent cycling exercise. *Med. Sci. Sports Exerc.* 19:597–604, 1987.
Nadel, E.F. Temperature regulation and prolonged exercise. In *Perspectives in Exercise Science and Sports Medicine Vol. 1 Prolonged Exercise,* D.R. Lamb and R. Murray (eds.). pp. 125–151. Indianapolis: Benchmark Press, 1988.
Nadel, E.R., S.A. Fortney, and C.B. Wenger. Effect of hydration state on circulatory and thermal regulations. *J. Appl. Physiol.* 49:715–721, 1980.
Noakes, T.D., B.A. Adams, K.H. Myburgh, C. Greeff, T. Lotz, and M. Nathan. The danger of an inadequate water intake during prolonged exercise. *Eur. J. Appl. Physiol.* 57:210–219, 1988.
Noakes, T.D. Heatstroke during the 1981 National Cross-Country running championships. *S. Afr. Med. J.* 61:145, 1982.
Owen, M.D., K.C Kregal, P.T. Wall and C.V. Gisolfi. Effects of ingesting carbohydrate beverages during exercise in the heat. *Med. Sci. Sports Exer.* 18:568–575, 1986.
Palmer, W.K. Selected physiological responses of normal young men following dehydration and rehydration. *Res. Quart.* 39:1054–1059, 1969.
Pitts, G.C., R.C. Johnson and F.C. Consolazio. Work in the heat as affected by intake of water, salt and glucose. *Amer. J. Physiol.* 142: 253–259, 1944.
Raven, P.B. and G.H.J. Stevens. Cardiovascular function and prolonged exercise. In *Perspectives in Exercise Science and Sports Medicine Vol. 1 Prolonged Exercise,* D.R. Lamb and R. Murray (eds). pp. 43–74. Indianapolis: Benchmark Press, 1988.
Refsum, H.E., B. Tveit, H.D. Meen, and S.B. Stromme. Serum electrolyte, fluid and acid base balance after prolonged heavy exercise at low environmental temperature. *Scand. J. Clin. Lab. Invest.* 32:117–122, 1973.
Ribisl, P.M. and W.G. Herbert. Effects of rapid weight reduction and subsequent rehydration upon the physical working capacity of wrestlers. *Res. Quart.* 41:536–541, 1970.
Robinson, S. Temperature regulation in exercise. *Pediatrics* 32:691–702, 1963.
Rowell, L.B. *Human Circulation Regulation During Physical Stress.* 308–322, 356–374, 257–286. New York: Oxford Press, 1986.
Rowell, L.B. Human cardiovascular adjustment to exercise and thermal stress. *Physiol. Rev.* 54:75–159, 1974.
Ryan, A.J., T.L. Bleiler, J.E. Carter, and C.V. Gisolfi. Gastric emptying during prolonged cycling exercise in the heat. *Med. Sci. Sport Exerc.* 21:51–58, 1989.
Saltin, B. Aerobic and anaerobic work capacity after dehydration. *J. Appl. Physiol.* 19:1114–1118, 1964a.
Saltin, B. Aerobic work capacity and circulation at exercise in man with special reference to the effect of prolonged exercise and/or heat exposure. *Acta Physiol. Scand. Supp.* 230:1–52, 1964b.
Saltin, B., G. Blomquist, J.H. Mitchell, R.L. Johnson, Jr., K. Wildenthal, and C.B. Chapman. Response to exercise after bed rest and after training. A longitudinal study of adaptive changes in oxygen transport and body composition. *Circulation* 38 (Supp. VII):1–78, 1968.
Saltin, B., and L. Hermansen. Esophageal, rectal, and muscle temperature during exercise. *J. Appl. Physiol.* 21:1757–1762, 1966.
Saltin. B. Circulatory response to submaximal and maximal exercise after thermal dehydration. *J. Appl. Physiol.* 19:1125–1132, 1965.
Savard, G.K., B. Nielsen, J. Lazzcynska, B.E. Larsen, and B. Saltin. Muscle blood flow is not reduced in humans during moderate exercise and heat stress. *J. Appl. Physiol.* 64:649–657, 1988.
Sawka, M.N. Body fluid responses and hypohydration during exercise-heat stress. In *Human Performance Physiology and Environmental Medicine at Terrestrial Extremes.* K.B. Pandolf, M.N. Sawka, and R. R. Gonzalez (eds.) Indianapolis: Benchmark Press, 1988, pp. 227–266.
Sawka, M.N., R.R. Gonzalez, A.J. Young, S.R. Muza, K.B. Pandolf, W.A. Latzka, R.C. Dennis, and C.R. Valeri. Polycythemia and hydration: effects on thermoregulation and blood volume during exercise-heat stress. *Am. J. Physiol.* 255:R456–R463, 1988b.
Sawka, M.N., A.J. Young, R.P. Francesconi, S.R. Muza, and K.B. Pandolf. Thermoregulatory and blood responses during exercise at graded hypohydration levels. *J. Appl. Physiol.* 59:1394–1401, 1985.
Sawka, M.N., R.P. Francesconi, N.A. Pimental, and K.B. Pandolf. Hydration and vascular fluid shifts during exercise in the heat. *J. Appl. Physiol.* 56:91–96, 1984a.
Sawka, M.N., R.P. Francesconi, A.J. Young, and K.B. Randolph. Influence of hydration level and body fluids on exercise performance in the heat. *J.A.M.A.* 252:1165–1169, 1984b.
Sawka, M.N., M.M. Toner, R.P. Francesconi, and K.B. Pandolf. Hypohydration and exercise; effects of heat acclimation, gender and environment. *J. Appl. Physiol.* 55:1147–1153, 1983.
Sawka, M.N., R.G. Knowlton, and R.G. Glaser. Body temperature, respiration and acid-base equilibrium during prolonged running. *Med. Sci. Sports Exerc.* 12:370–374, 1980.
Sawka, M.N., R.G. Knowlton, and J.B. Critz. Thermal and circulatory responses to repeated bouts of prolonged running. *Med. Sci. Sports Exerc.* 11:177–180, 1979.
Senay, L.C. Jr. and J.M. Pivarnik. Fluid Shifts During Exercise. *Exerc. Sports Sci. Rev* 13:335–387, 1985.
Serfass, R.C., G.A. Stull, J.F. Alexander, and J.L. Ewing. The effects of rapid weight loss and attempted

rehydration on strength and endurance of the handgripping muscles in college wrestlers. *Res. Quart.* 55:46–52, 1984.
Shibolet, S., M.C. Landcaster, and Y. Danon. Heat stroke: a review. *Aviat. Space Environ. Med.* 47:280–301, 1976.
Singer, R.N. and S.A. Weiss. Effects of weight reduction on selected anthropometric, physical, and performance measures in wrestlers. *Res. Quart.* 39:361–369, 1968.
Tuttle, W.W. The effect of weight loss by dehydration and the withholding of food on the physiologic responses of wrestlers. *Res. Quart.* 14:158–166, 1943.
Wyndham, C.H. Heat stroke and hyperthermia in marathon runners. *Ann. NY Acad. Sci.* 301:128–138, 1977.

DISCUSSION

SHERMAN: Your chapter is very provocative in establishing a baseline after the initial transition during the first 10 min of exercise. I think this can be justified. You are proposing that the primary advantage of fluid consumption during exercise in the heat is to prevent cellular dehydration and/or osmotic perturbations to help maintain normal cellular function. When fluids are consumed in a cool environment where the plasma volume is unchanged, you suggest that the fluid is going into the intracellular fluid compartment. Is it possible that those cells might expand, become hypo-osmotic to change the relationship between substrates and enzymes, and therefore have a potentially negative influence on metabolism and performance?
COYLE: If fluid ingestion is indeed serving to offset dehydration of the active musculature, I don't think that the amount of fluid uptake would be sufficient to markedly reduce cellular osmolality or affect cellular function. Fluid ingestion probably serves mainly to offset fluid losses and simply return cellular water to normal levels. Secondly, the bodily intracellular water compartment is so large that I don't think a large enough volume of fluid could be ingested to significantly dilute the intracellular fluid, especially since the cells are losing water due to sweating.
COSTILL: Some of the biopsy work we did in the mid 1970s made it fairly clear that the water that initially moves out of plasma and into the active muscle subsequently can serve as a bit of a reservoir. As we progressively lose water through sweating and become dehydrated, that water is drawn back from the cells to maintain plasma volume fairly constant. If an athlete drinks a lot of water, you don't see a rise in plasma volume, and this supports the idea that the fluid is going into the cells. Interestingly, nearly all of the cases of hyponatremia occur after exercise, and that's when all that intracellular fluid comes back to the vascular bed and we get hemodilution. So I think you do have a reservoir available to maintain plasma volume fairly steady. The mechanism that controls that reservoir is an interesting problem.
SAWKA: Getting a handle on blood volume during exercise is a very difficult thing. Your data, particularly in Table 8-3, suggest to me that exercise intensity is an important consideration in analyzing blood vol-

ume changes during exercise. I know of at least two other studies of exercise at about 40% of $\dot{V}O_2$max that showed plasma volume losses. You showed that with dehydration at environmental temperatures of 20–25°C, there is little loss of plasma volume over time. It may be that most of these studies you cited used fairly high exercise intensities. During high-intensity exercise, you don't necessarily see the reduction in plasma volume that you'd expect to occur with water loss. Vic Convertino noted that hormones such as vasopressin and angiotensin, both vasoconstrictors, do increase with exercise intensity and perhaps with dehydration. It may be that with high-intensity work or dehydration, an elevation of these hormones causes vasoconstriction within active muscle masses, so you decrease capillary pressure and therefore get less fluid loss from the capillaries. That is just one thing that may stir up comments.

The other is that I think Tim Noakes' work really needs to be looked at very carefully. There are some problems with his interpretation. One is that he just observed end exercise temperatures and tried to relate them to level of dehydration. It would be extremely surprising to me if he would see a relationship of dehydration and end-exercise temperatures because everyone is running for different durations and intensities. It is known that the rise in core temperature during exercise is mostly a function of exercise intensity.

Third, I was very glad to see that you brought up the importance of osmolality. I do think the relationship between osmolality and hyperthermia is important, because when I look at sweating responses in my subjects, everything fits tightly; it's very easy to find a relationship to changes in osmolality, as have other people, such as Charlie Senay. Often you have to go through at least low levels of hyperthermia and many gyrations to see some sort of relationship.

COYLE: Regarding your first point about the exercise intensity, Dr. Harrison has two papers showing that there may be more of a reduction in plasma volume during prolonged low-intensity exercise than during high-intensity exercise in the heat. In my paper, I was fairly critical of Dr. Noakes. His paper raises important questions. However, because of the variability in the subjects' responses, he criticized the hypothesis that hyperthermia is related to dehydration, and he argued that hyperthermia is most likely dependent upon exercise intensity; yet his own data did not support this latter hypothesis.

SAWKA: He also was under a false impression of what body temperature should be.

COYLE: But he's raising a good question. This is what people do, they drink only 500 mL/h and become dehydrated; what is your justification for doing otherwise, i.e., for suggesting that people replace all the fluid they are losing? Is it acceptable to dehydrate to a certain extent? Noakes says we don't have the data to counter these arguments.

SAWKA: It has been shown by Greenleaf that even a 1% loss of body water will result in an elevation of temperature. Depending on the duration of the event and the ambient conditions, such hyperthermia may or may not be important.

COYLE: These are sports where you observe increases in body temperature up to 39-40°. Runners who are sprinting at the end and therefore exercising very intensely over the last mile are getting very hot. Is this acceptable if they are winning the race or because they perform the best? Does this mean that hyperthermia is not of concern? I don't agree with that proposition at all.

SAWKA: I think there is some truth to it. It gets back to what Dr. Costill stated. I think a lot of it has to do with the conditions of skin temperature, displacement of blood volume, and what kind of internal temperature you can tolerate.

SUTTON: It is important to bring up the importance of environmental conditions such as wind and humidity that can drastically influence thermoregulation, even at a dry bulb temperature of 25°C. We've recorded rectal temperatures of 42–43°C in people who have had severe heat stroke when the environmental temperature was as low as 10–16°C. Just because the temperature doesn't appear to be in the range where one might expect to have everyone dropping like flies, it certainly does not mean that we shouldn't be on guard in terms of the possibility of heat illness occurring. Also, would you justify how you can dismiss the basal blood volume, or the resting measurement, ignore the blood volume changes for the first 5–10 min or more, and propose that only data collected later in exercise should be used to study some of these problems?

COYLE: I agree that one can experience hyperthermia at ambient temperatures of 25°C and lower. A key point is that when one is competing in 5 k or 10 k runs, rectal temperature can get up above 40–41°C. There is not much to be done as far as fluid replacement is concerned because heat is stored so rapidly; you are running intensely for 15–45 min. The only thing one can do to prevent hyperthermia in this case is either reduce the intensity of exercise or avoid those conditions.

My justification for defining normal blood volume as that volume established early in exercise is just to simplify the comparison of exercise responses. The concept is that early in exercise, the body establishes a homeostasis regarding blood volume which is a dynamic balance. That really should be our norm, not what happens at rest. I get very confused with data that focus on the changes from rest to exercise. Those data are fine if you're interested in the transition from rest to exercise. If you're not, don't talk about rest; just determine what the normal values are once exercise has begun and a steady state has been reached. That all is predicated on the assumption that individuals are euhydrated at the start of exercise so that they have adequate fluid to establish a normal homeostasis of the Starling factors that regulate blood volume

HUBBARD: I like the idea of looking at the initial running starting point for changing plasma volume. But if plasma volume is relatively stable, how important can changes in plasma volume be to thirst? This is a very confusing issue.

CONVERTINO: I, too, like your concept, Ed. As you said, it tells us about what the mechanism is during exercise. In fact, one can argue the constancy of plasma volume or the defense of plasma volume during exercise. The thing I am a little bothered about is the use of the term "normovolemia." We usually think of that in the context of the resting state. If, during exercise, plasma volume is defended at a lower level, why isn't it brought back to a resting level and defended there? Perhaps a term such as a "new set point during exercise" is better than "normovolemia."

COYLE: I think there are advantages in some individuals to raising their blood volume and plasma volume above that set point during exercise. We've seen in untrained subjects that an expanded blood volume raises stroke volume and lowers total peripheral resistance. Mike Sawka has done some interesting work in infusing whole blood and seen that certain subjects do benefit by blood volume expansion, as far as thermoregulation is concerned. I think that more functionally we might define normal blood volume within a certain range.

NADEL: Like Roger Hubbard, I find your concept intriguing, Ed; but like John Sutton, I am relatively dubious about the usefulness of the concept. In other words, I agree mostly with John. The reason I am dubious about this concept is that if we use temperature regulation or blood pressure regulation during exercise as an analogy for blood volume regulation, dissimilar events are occurring. Temperature is regulated around 37°C, and the body is attempting to get back to 37°C in the transition from rest to exercise and during exercise. The fact that there is a tremendous amount of heat production during exercise provides for maintenance of an elevated temperature, and achievement of this new temperature occurs when heat dissipation balances heat production. With blood pressure regulation, I think it is generally accepted that there is a regulated elevation of blood pressure during exercise. With blood volume regulation during exercise, it seems to me that the body is trying to regulate blood volume at the initial resting level. The offset that occurs during exercise is due to changes in the Starling forces at the muscle capillary level such that the changes in filtration forces outweigh the changes in the absorption forces in the muscle capillaries. I think that to talk about that as normovolemia is probably a misnomer.

COYLE: Give my position time; it will grow on you.
NADEL: Why would having blood volume reductions below resting values—as occurs during exercise—be considered "normal?"
COYLE: You can look at it the other way; why don't you keep a high blood volume during exercise? It's a dynamic balance. That's what is appropriate for the conditions of hydrostatic forces and osmotic gradients. I'm agreeing with you 100% saying that for the set of conditions, there is an appropriate blood volume. As exercise intensity increases during cycling, your blood volume goes down the same as your blood pressure goes up. To me, it's the same concept.
NADEL: There may be another factor here which you touched on and that is that blood volume displacement or distribution is important. Blood volume displacement occurs during exercise in the heat.
BUSKIRK: There is such a thing as progressive dehydration. I don't know if you've looked at some of the old studies that were done in the Minnesota lab. But there, when the people were drinking 900 mL of water per day and they had regular bouts of exercise, their temperatures on a daily basis continued to escalate day by day as they exercised in this thermally stressing environment. Also, their plasma volumes over time decreased day by day, as did the total body water.
COYLE: I suspect that, based upon Sawka's work, when exercise is begun in a hypohydrated condition, there will be a greater increase in body temperature, and plasma volume will be lower.
NADEL: I think that cardiovascular drift is due to hyperthermia, where blood pools in the large capacity venules. The way to get the blood out of these venules is to keep the person cool. That's the most effective way of maintaining filling pressures and reducing cardiovascular drift. I think that in the heat, cooling the body is of much greater priority than maintaining blood volume. In a cool environment, the priorities are very different, obviously.
COYLE: I believe there is an optimal plasma volume and distribution of blood volume, i.e., a volume and distribution that will maintain an adequate filling pressure to the heart to maintain an adequate stroke volume. If plasma volume is elevated too much above that level, hemodilution will occur and oxygen-carrying capacity will be reduced. There is an optimal plasma volume established early on in exercise which must be maintained for stroke volume and for thermoregulation throughout the event.

If supine resting plasma volume were maintained during running, that would be advantageous for an untrained person. He would be "hypervolemic" by 400 mL. It is not advantageous, in my opinion, for a trained person, who is already somewhat hypervolemic, to maintain his supine resting plasma volume during prolonged running because the hemoglobin would be too dilute. This contention is based on the fact that when we volume expanded subjects using dextran solutions, untrained people raised their plasma volumes and their maximal oxygen uptakes, despite the fact that we reduced hemoglobin concentration. The increase in stroke volume was greater than the reduction in hemoglobin concentration. In the trained individual, a further increase in plasma volume did not increase stroke volume; they just became hemodiluted. Hemodilution without increased stroke volume is counterproductive for maximal oxygen uptake and for endurance performance.

9

Importance of Fluid Homeostasis for Optimal Adaptation to Exercise and Environmental Stress: Acceleration

JOHN E. GREENLEAF, PH.D.

INTRODUCTION

Integrated physiological responses during adaptation to changes in the force of gravity are paramount because humans presumably evolved from a continuously horizontal posture to an intermittently upright posture. This posture change increased hydrostatic pressure within the cardiovascular system and required more complex neuromuscular and cardiovascular coordination to maintain upright posture and balance. Humans exploring space undergo a nearly complete negation of the natural force of gravity (microgravity), unless inertial or rotational acceleration is provided, or large planetary masses are encountered. This microgravity, or weightlessness, during an orbital mission is produced when the gravitational force is exactly counterbalanced by the centrifugal force imparted to a spacecraft as it travels in a tangential direction to the

Earth's surface. One major question about space travel is whether to provide "artificial" gravity, using an onboard centrifuge and/or total spacecraft rotation, during prolonged space voyages. This question has focused terrestrial research on the mechanisms of acute, long-term (adaptive) responses to microgravity.

Hypo- and microgravity simulations utilize horizontal and head-down bed rest, thermoneutral water immersion, and lower body *positive* pressure (LBPP). Hypergravity research involves radial acceleration on a centrifuge, application of lower body *negative* pressure (LBNP), and orthostasis testing on a tilt table. Hypergravity research is necessary because astronauts are subjected to moderately increased acceleration during lift-off (two $+3.0G_x$ peaks in 8 min) and deceleration during reentry ($+1.2\ G_z$ for 17 to 20 min) (Waligora 1979) (Figure 9-1), and they experience orthostatic intolerance after landing. These stresses can attenuate performance if they exceed normal flight levels, especially when they are imposed on a microgravity-adapted (deconditioned) astronaut. Since Russian cosmonauts have survived spaceflights of 1 year with few, if any,

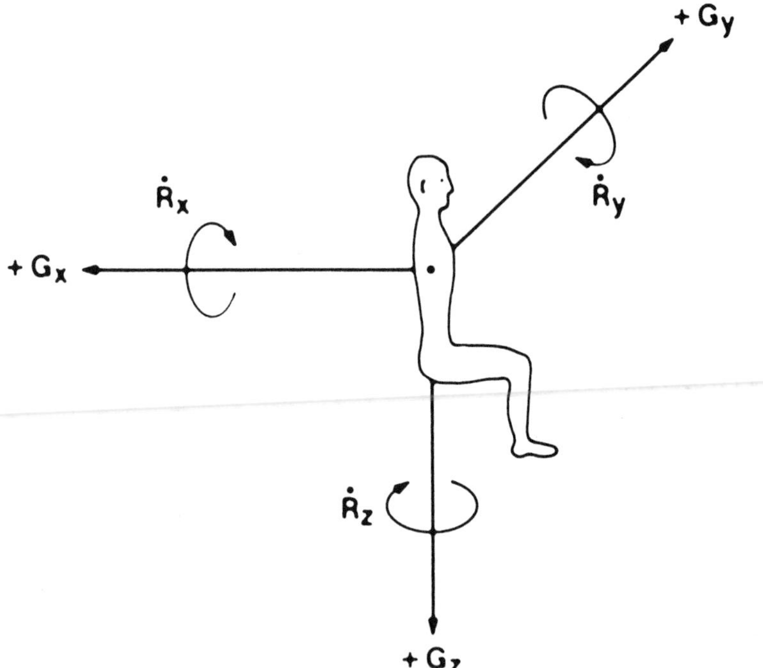

FIGURE 9-1. *AGARD physiological acceleration force terminology system:* $+G_x$ *is chest to back,* $+G_y$ *is left lateral, and* $+G_z$ *is positive (head to foot) acceleration;* $-G_x$ *is back to chest,* $-G_y$ *is right lateral, and* $-G_z$ *is negative (foot to head) acceleration. Tolerance is the* $+G_x$ *vector is 2–3 times greater than that in the* $+G_z$ *vector.* $\pm R_x$ *is roll,* $\pm R_y$ *is pitch, and* $\pm R_z$ *is yaw. From Gell (1961) with permission.*

chronic infirmities, research efforts are being directed toward understanding adaptation to microgravity exposures of 2 to 3 years' duration.

Water comprises about two-thirds of the human body mass and is a major raw material for cellular and vascular functions. Changes in the anatomy of the fluid-electrolyte system occur very early during the transition fron eugravity to microgravity and during the reverse reentry exposure. In fact, it appears now that fluid-electrolyte redistribution is the initial step in the microgravity adaptation syndrome. To understand the mechanism of these fluid-electrolyte responses, it is necessary to employ real or simulated transitions from eugravity to hypogravity and from eugravity to hypergravity. Because few data on the fluid-electrolyte-system responses are available from astronauts for the transition to and reentry from microgravity, this review will focus on fluid-electrolyte regulation during bed rest and heat-to-foot ($+G_z$) acceleration.

General reviews including fluid-electrolyte regulation during gravitational stress have been prepared by Amberson (1943), Blomqvist and Stone (1983), and Rowell (1986).

BODY-FLUID COMPARTMENT ANATOMY AND PHYSIOLOGY

For ease of discussion, total body water is arbitrarily divided into two major compartments (Table 9-1): inside the cells (cellular water, 33 L for a resting, 80-kg man) and outside the cells (extracellular water, 20 L). The latter is further subdivided into vascular (plasma water, 4 L) and interstitial water (16 L) located approximately between the vascular and cellular compartments (Greenleaf and Harrison 1986). Water content of the major body tissues is presented in Table 9-2. Striated muscle, the skeleton, and adipose tissue account for about 60% of the body weight and these

TABLE 9-1. *Fluid Compartment Volumes of a Resting 80 kg MAN**

COMPARTMENT	VOLUME, liters	BODY WEIGHT, percent
EXTRACELLULAR		
PLASMA	4	5
INTERSTITIAL	16	20
	20	25
CELLULAR	33	41
TOTAL	53	66

*MODIFIED FROM GREENLEAF AND HARRISON (1986).

TABLE 9-2. *Weight and Water Content of Body Tissue From a 70.6 kg MAN**

TISSUE	PERCENT OF BODY WEIGHT	PERCENT WATER CONTENT
STRIATED MUSCLE	31.6	79.5
SKELETON	14.8	31.8
ADIPOSE TISSUE	13.6	50.1
SKIN	7.8	64.7
LUNGS	4.2	83.7
LIVER	3.4	71.5
BRAIN AND SPINAL CORD	2.5	73.3
ALIMENTARY TRACT	2.1	79.1
ALIMENTARY TRACT CONTENTS	0.8	–
HEART	0.7	73.7
KIDNEYS	0.5	79.5
SPLEEN	0.2	78.7
PANCREAS	0.2	73.1
BILE	0.2	–
TEETH	0.1	5.0
HAIR	0.1	–
REMAINING TISSUES		
LIQUID	3.7	93.3
SOLID	13.5	70.4
TOTAL BODY	100.0	67.2

*MODIFIED FROM OSER (1965).

components contain about 25%, 5%, and 7%, respectively, of the total body water. Most major organs contain 73% to 84% water.

Normal cation and anion composition of the extracellular and cellular fluid spaces is presented in Table 9-3. Sodium and chloride are the major cation and anion, respectively, in the extracellular fluid. These two ions account for about 95% of the extracellular fluid osmolality. Potassium is the major cellular cation, also present in small quantities in the extracellular fluid; phosphates and proteins comprise the major cellular anions. The total extracellular osmolality (155 + 155 = 310 mosmol/kg H_2O), is theoretically equal to the total cellular osmolality (175 + 135 = 310 mosmol/kg H_2O) so equal total osmotic concentrations between the extracellular and cellular fluid compartments can be maintained in spite of widely different constituent compositions. In reality the normal osmolality of the extracellular compartment is 285-290 mosmol/kg H_2O because of the variable content of its multicharged ions and the binding state of the ions to larger molecules, e.g., proteins (Greenleaf and Harrison 1986).

In resting subjects fluid is shifted and homeostasis is maintained

TABLE 9-3. *Normal Composition of Fluid Spaces in Men**

	CATIONS				ANIONS			
FLUID SPACE	Na^+ mEq/l	K^+ mEq/l	Ca^{+2}, Mg^{+2}, and $Other^+$ mEq/l	$Osmols^+$ mosmol/kg	Cl^- mEq/l	HCO^{-3} mEq/l	PO_4^{-3}, PRO^-, and $Other^-$ mEq/l	$Osmols^-$ mosmol/kg
EXTRA-CELLULAR	142	5	8	155	103	27	25	155
CELLULAR	10	145	20	175	2	8	190	135
TOTAL	152	150	28	330	105	35	215	290

*FROM GREENLEAF AND HARRISON (1986).

mainly by changes in osmotic pressure between the plasma and red blood cell fluid compartments, and between the interstitial and other cellular fluid compartments. But the shift from the interstitial to the plasma fluid compartment is by osmotic and oncotic (protein) pressures (Figure 9-2). Protein, including that which "leaks" from the plasma to the interstitial space, is returned to the vascular space in lymph via the thoracic duct, which joins the venous system at the jugular-subclavian vein junction. With increased gravitational force in the head-to-foot ($+G_z$) direction or change in posture from horizontal to standing, plasma filtrate moves to the interstitial space through the capillaries mainly from increased hydrostatic pressure.

The control mechanisms of the peripheral circulation are complicated and redundant. There are neural, humoral, metabolic, and myogenic components involved in the maintenance of plasma volume (PV) and blood pressure, particularly with increased hydrostatic pressure in the head-to-foot direction. Most of the control appears to reside with the sympathetic nervous system with its vasoconstrictive action on the smooth muscle of the capillary network. Hormones (e.g., atrial natriuretic peptide) promote vasodilation; vasopressin in high concentrations and angiotensin cause vasoconstriction; tissue metabolites (e.g., potassium) influence local vascular tone; and the myogenic mechanism, where blood vessel distension exerts a direct stimulating action on vascular smooth muscle (Mellander et al. 1987), influences vasoregulation, transcapillary fluid shifts, and blood pressure.

The microcirculation between arteries and veins is composed of arterioles, an arterio-venous capillary bridge, and venules. This large-diameter vascular system is connected in both series and parallel with smaller true capillaries. Arteriolar smooth-muscle activity controls

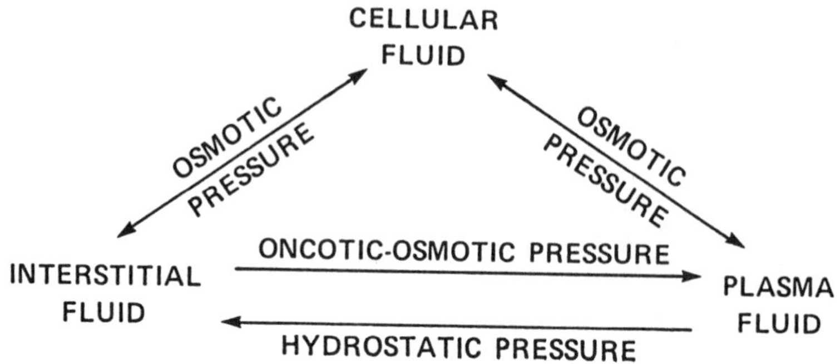

FIGURE 9-2. *Major fluid-driving forces between the cellular and extracellular (plasma and interstitial) fluid compartments. From Greenleaf and Harrison (1986) with permission.*

mainly tissue blood flow, and precapillary sphincter smooth-muscle activity controls the blood flow within the capillary vascular system. Smooth muscle in arterioles and in postcapillary venules is controlled by active sympathetic vasoconstriction. Precapillary resistance appears to be regulated by local metabolites and myogenic factors. Capillary hydrostatic pressure can be calculated (Hargens 1987) by

$$P_c = [P_a(R_{post}/R_{pre}) + P_v]/[1 + (R_{post}/R_{pre})]$$

where P_c is capillary hydrostatic pressure in mmHg, P_a is arterial pressure, P_v is venous pressure, R_{pre} is precapillary resistance, and P_{post} is postcapillary resistance.

Increased precapillary resistance will decrease capillary hydrostatic pressure, and increased postcapillary resistance will increase capillary hydrostatic pressure. Changes in venous pressure will affect capillary hydrostatic pressure to a greater extent than similar changes in arterial pressure. The level of capillary hydrostatic pressure is a major determinant of net absorption or filtration of fluid. Capillary blood pressure in the human toe is 80 to 90 mmHg when the human is standing and only 30 mmHg when the toe is at the level of the heart (Hargens 1987). Net transcapillary fluid transport (J_c), in mL/min·cm^2), can be calculated from the Starling equation:

$$J_c = K_f[(P_c - P_i) - \sigma_p(\pi_c - \pi_i)]$$

where K_f = capillary filtration coefficient in mL/(min·cm^2·mmHg) = L_pA, where L_p is the hydraulic conductivity for the capillary basement membrane, and A is capillary surface area. $L_p = \psi Nr^4/\zeta t$ where ψ is a constant, N is number of pores per unit area, r is pore radius, ζ is ultrafiltrate viscosity, and t is capillary membrane thickness.

P_c is capillary hydrostatic pressure and ranges from 20 to 40 mmHg in skeletal muscle. P_i is interstitial fluid pressure, which may be 0 to 4 mmHg and can rise to 570 mmHg with isometric muscular contractions (Sejersted 1984).

π_c is capillary blood colloid osmotic pressure, which is identical to systemic colloid osmotic pressure and ranges from 20 to 35 mmHg.

π_i is interstitial fluid colloid osmotic pressure and is 40% to 60% of the plasma protein concentration. With a mean π_c of 29 mmHg, π_i is 15 mmHg in the thorax and 10 mmHg in the ankle (Hargens 1987).

σ_p is the capillary membrane reflection coefficient, which ranges from 0 to 1 (dimensionless). It would be 1 if membrane were a perfect osmometer, so colloid osmotic pressure in blood and interstitial fluid must be multiplied by σ_p, which characterizes a given tissue or tissues. Calculated values range from 0.70 to 0.95.

FLUID-ELECTROLYTE REGULATION DURING ACCELERATION

In ambulatory people on Earth, many body responses are designed to counter the force of gravity. When the integration of the cardiovascular and neuromuscular systems fail, gravity intercedes and the upright person is forced into a horizontal position, one of reduced hydrostatic pressure (Figure 9-3). Gravity is an important factor in essentially all volitional movements. Gravireceptors in the vestibular apparatus respond mainly to the force of terrestrial gravity, with a small contribution from linear acceleration of the body and its appendages. But with negation of the effects of gravity during weightlessness, stimuli to the gravireceptors emanate exclusively from linear acceleration (movements) of the body.

Gauer and Haber (1950) have calculated the acceleration required to reach parabolic velocity (11.2 km/sec at the Earth's surface) for various time intervals; that is, the acceleration required to carry a rocket out of the Earth's gravitational field (Figure 9-4). It is clear from Figure 9-4 that shorter acceleration times require higher acceleration levels, so a compromise between rocket performance and human tolerance for accelera-

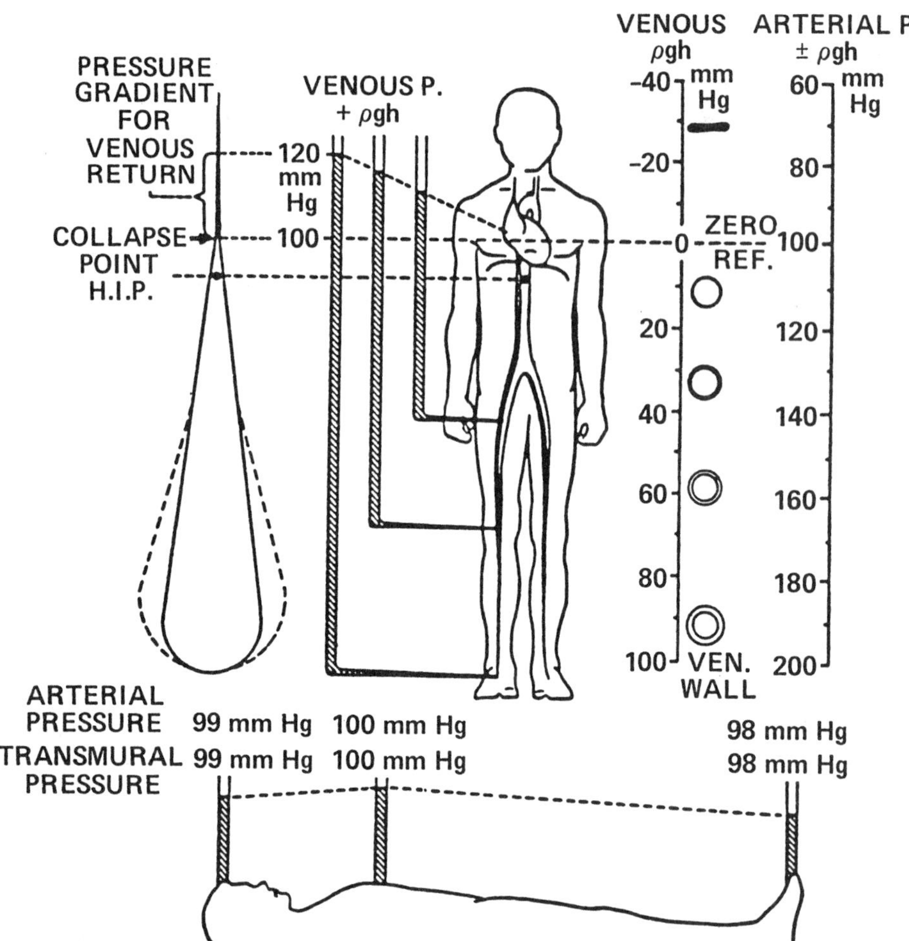

FIGURE 9-3. *"Distribution of pressures in upright and supine humans. Pressure scales on right are arterial pressures, including dynamic pressure generated by the heart plus the hydrostatic pressure (ρgh). Venous hydrostatic pressure (ρgh) is without additional driving pressure. Ellipses and circles show shape and wall thickness of veins (VEN WALL) relative to distance from the heart. Heart level is the zero pressure reference level (Zero Ref). On the person's left, water-filled tubes show measured venous pressure (driving pressure + ρgh), showing a 20-mmHg gradient (120–100 mmHg),* the pressure gradient for venous return. *Veins collapse at Zero Ref. (Collapse Point) as illustrated by the water-filled, thin-walled, rubber tube on the left. Note insensitivity of collapse point to added volume (dashed line around tube). Hydrostatic indifferent point (H.I.P.) is below collapse point—at approximately diaphragmatic level. Supine human below shows distribution of dynamic arterial driving pressure and transmural pressure in this posture." Figure and caption from Rowell (1986) with permission.*

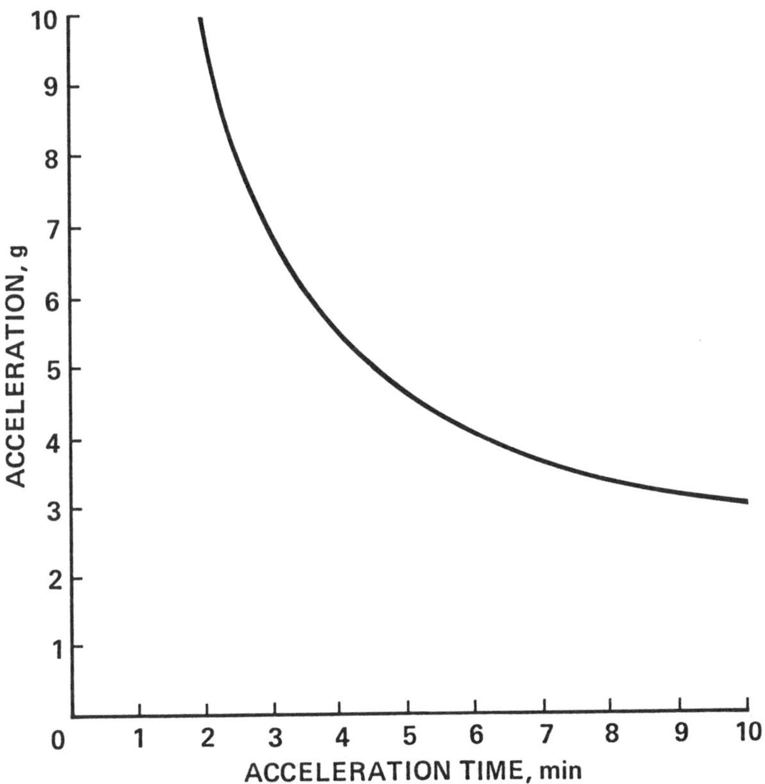

FIGURE 9-4. *Time required at various accelerations to carry a rocket beyond the Earth's gravitational field and reach parabolic velocity of 11.2 km/sec.*

tion is necessary. Tolerance for chest-to-back acceleration on Earth (+9 to +11 G_x) is about three times greater than tolerance for head-to-foot acceleration (+3 to +5 G_z). While all G-levels during actual lift-offs and reentries have been well within the limits of human tolerance, the acceleration intensity has decreased with successive flight programs. A typical launch profile for the Mercury-Atlas vehicle produced accelerations of +6.0 to +6.4 G_x for 89 sec with a peak level of +8 G_x. Peak acceleration during launch of the Apollo-Saturn rocket was +7.2 G_x for 1 min. The Space Shuttle reaches a peak launch acceleration of only +3.4 G_x; and maximal reentry acceleration is only +1.2 G_z, but the increased force acts for 17 to 20 min. (Waligora, 1979). Because the astronauts have acclimatized (deconditioned) to microgravity, during reentry an acceleration stress of +1.2 G_z is approximately equivalent to at least +2.2 G_z in normal astronauts.

The point of tolerance (the time of useful consciousness during $+G_z$ acceleration) occurs when central vision is lost (grayout) but the subject is not yet unconscious. At that point blood pressure in the retinal vessels drops to about 20 mmHg, just below intraocular pressure (Lambert and Wood, 1946). The resulting "excess" intraocular pressure compresses the retinal arteries so blood flow ceases and vision is lost, even though blood perfusion to the rest of the brain is adequate to maintain consciousness. If acceleration continues, unconsciousness will occur and then death from, presumably, cerebral hypoxia.

Because blood pressure is influenced by cardiac output and peripheral resistance, coordinated changes in flow and resistance act during acceleration to maintain pressure. Total leg blood flow measured at midcalf with impedance plethysmography is reduced by about half: from 6 to 9 mL/min per 100 mL tissue to about 3 to 4 mL/min per 100 mL tissue at the tolerance point after 5 to 6 min of $+G_z$ acceleration at a rate of +0.5 G/min (Greenleaf et al. 1977b). The fact that application of LBPP with a G-suit (Wood et al. 1961) and water immersion (Wood et al. 1963) will prolong acceleration tolerance indicates that reduced cardiac output and decreased blood transit time from the legs and splanchnic regions contribute to the lowering of retinal blood pressure and visual acuity. A more important effect of LBPP is to increase systemic resistance rather than to increase ventricular filling (Gaffney et al. 1981). It is likely that LBPP acts in much the same manner as exposure to water immersion by increasing postcapillary resistance and facilitating filtration from the vascular compartment causing hypovolemia. The increased venous pressure, however, could assist in maintaining atrial filling (central venous) pressure (Kravik et al. 1986). Thus, a major mechanism for reducing acceleration tolerance appears to be the hypotensive effect of increased hydrostatic pressure, which increases capillary filtration, resulting in hypovolemia and reduced atrial filling.

The relative distribution of pressures in the cardiovascular system in standing and supine humans has been clearly illustrated by Rowell (1986) in Figure 9-3. The total pressure within blood vessels is the algebraic sum of three major components: 1) a static pressure at zero blood flow that is a function of the blood volume (fullness of the system); 2) a dynamic pressure, from the pumping action of the heart, that is a function of flow and resistance; and 3) a hydrostatic pressure, from the force of gravity, that is a function of fluid density (p), the acceleration due to gravity (g), and the height of the hydrostatic column (h). Accelerative forces acting on the body in the $+G_z$ direction influence all three components via reduced fullness of the circulatory system (hypovolemia) caused by a shift of fluid from plasma to the interstitial space; increased heart rate and peripheral resistance; and increased hydrostatic pressure, mainly from the increasing accelerative force. Fluid density and the height of the hydrostatic column are essentially unchanged during acceleration. The discussion of fluid-electrolyte regulation during acceleration will emphasize factors influencing the fullness of the cardiovascular system, that is, the maintenance of the plasma volume and its distribution.

Dehydration, Fluid-Electrolyte Shifts, and Acceleration Tolerance

If the volume of blood transferred from the head and thorax to the lower extremities is an important determinant for control of blood pressure, then total body dehydration with its concomitant reduction in plasma volume should have a deleterious effect on $+G_z$ acceleration tolerance. Beetham and Buskirk (1958) first measured the effect of body dehydration (loss of 5% of weight by resting overnight at 46° C DBT) on cardiovascular responses to 70° head-up tilt for 4 min. In comparison with normal hydrated responses, they found that dehydrated subjects had significant increases in pulse rate during tilting, but no significant changes in systolic, diastolic, or pulse pressures. Also, 3 weeks of daily cross-country running with or without additional heat acclimation (consisting of alternating 30-min periods of walking and resting for 4 h/day), which should have increased plasma volume, did not improve the pulse rate or blood pressure responses to tilting after dehydration, although in the short 4-min tilt period meaningful physiological changes were unlikely. It appears that hypovolemia induced deleterious responses, but probable acclimation-induced hypervolemia was without effect.

From 1962 to 1965 the Mercury and Gemini astronauts returned to Earth after flights of 15 to 35 h and 44 to 198 h, respectively, with excessive weight losses ranging from 1.4% to 4.6% (Figure 9-5). The weight loss was, in part, a result of dehydration caused by warm capsule temperatures. At that time it was suggested (Noble and Taylor 1953) that physiological responses to orthostasis (tilting) were qualitatively but not quantitatively similar to those responses during acceleration. This was later confirmed by Greenleaf et al. (1985).

The first two studies on the effect of dehydration on $+G_z$ acceleration tolerance were conducted in 1964. The first (Greenleaf et al. 1966b) investigated a group of five men (25-33 years old) dehydrated by 3.4% of their body weight by acute exposure in a sauna bath (50°-80° C) for 3-4 h ($\Delta PV = -12.7\%$). A second group of eight men (22-36 years old) was dehydrated chronically by fluid restriction for 48 h; they lost 3.8% of body weight, and PV decreased by 10.2%. Passive (no muscular contraction) acceleration tolerance, measured at a rate of $+3.7\ G_z/min$ and held at 6.0 G until grayout (loss of peripheral vision) occurred, decreased from a control (hydration) time of 105 sec to 89 sec ($\Delta time = 15\%, P < 0.05$) in the acute dehydration group, and from 104 to 83 sec ($\Delta time = 20\%, P < 0.05$) in the chronic dehydration group. There was no difference in mean toler-

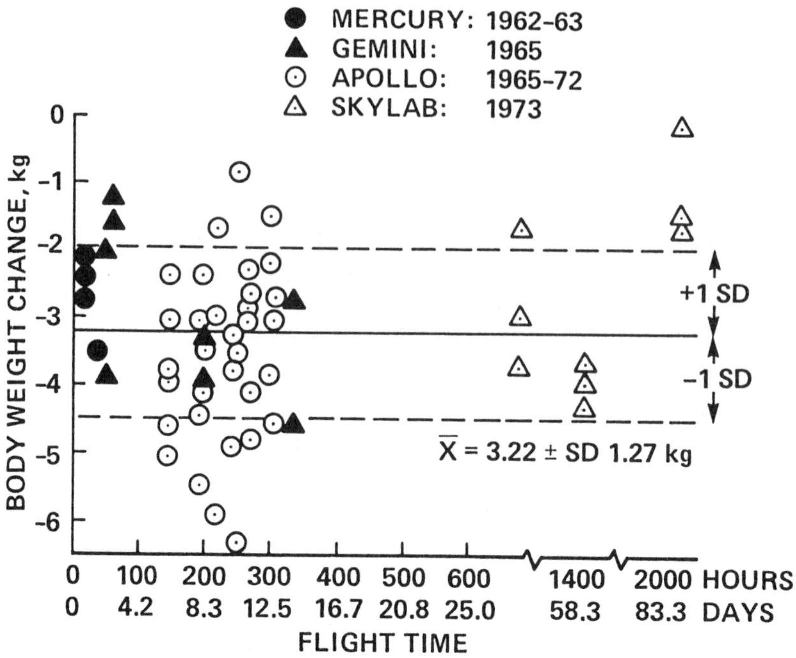

FIGURE 9-5. *Individual body-weight losses of Mercury (MA 6,7,8,9); Gemini (GT 3,4,5,7); Apollo (AS 7-17); and Skylab (SS II, III, IV) astronauts (54 men) during their missions. Data from Berry et al. (1966), Catterson et al. (1963), Minners et al. (1962), and Thornton and Ord (1977).*

ance times or in the levels of plasma volumes (hypovolemia) between the two groups. Thus, there were similar significant decreases in tolerance in moderately dehydrated subjects, with similar levels of hypovolemia that were independent of the method or time for induction of hypohydration.

Taliaferro et al. (1965) dehydrated eight men (21-29 years old) by resting them at 52° C (20% to 30% rh). One group was hypohydrated by 2.8% of their body weight ($\Delta PV = -10.0\%$, $n = 4$) and another was hypohydrated by 1.1% ($\Delta PV = -4.2\%$, $n = 3$). Body temperatures were allowed to return to normal, and the subjects were accelerated at the rapid rate of $+18\ G_z$/min. Compared with tolerance times from normohydration control runs, tolerance-time decrements of 18% ($P < 0.05$) at 2.8% hypohydration and of 14% ($P < 0.05$) at 1.1% hypohydration were found.

Results from these two studies suggested that moderate hypovolemia of 4% to 13%, induced by water restriction or by heat exposure and associated with minimal body weight losses of 1.1% to 3.8%, results in significant reduction in $+G_z$ acceleration tolerance. These findings were confirmed in a subsequent study in which fluid restriction causing a weight loss of 4.3% ($\Delta PV = -13.8\%$) in nine men (21–29 years old) resulted in an 11.2% reduction in tolerance time with acceleration of $+3.0\ G_z$/min (Greenleaf et al. 1966a)

In these studies, low correlation coefficients between the levels of pre-acceleration hypovolemia and the subsequent tolerance times suggested a lack of direct cause and effect. However, combining $+G_z$ acceleration-tolerance data from studies of ambulatory control and ambulatory recovery, after 15 days of horizontal bed rest, in 12 women (23-34 years old) produced a correlation coefficient of 0.72 ($P < 0.01$) between acceleration tolerance and the percent change in PV during centrifugation. Post-bed rest tolerance time was reduced by 49% (Greenleaf et al. 1977c) (Figure 9-6). This coefficient indicates that at least half of the variability in tolerance times must be accounted for by factors other than the level of hypovolemia. The tolerance curve in Figure 9-6 reaches the asymptote at a decrease in PV of 19.4%, indicating one physiological limiting factor. A comparison of changes in PV that occurred during bed rest and during subsequent $+G_z$ acceleration (Table 9-4) indicated that the tolerance point was reached when the combined hypovolemia reached 17% to 20% with acceleration levels held between +3.0 and +3.2 G_z. Exercise training during bed rest (68% $\dot{V}O_{2max}$ for 1 h/day for 14 days) had no significant effect on combined hypovolemia; decreased tolerances of -24% and -28% with isometric and isotonic training, respectively, resulted in combined hypovolemia of -16.4% and -14.7% respectively.

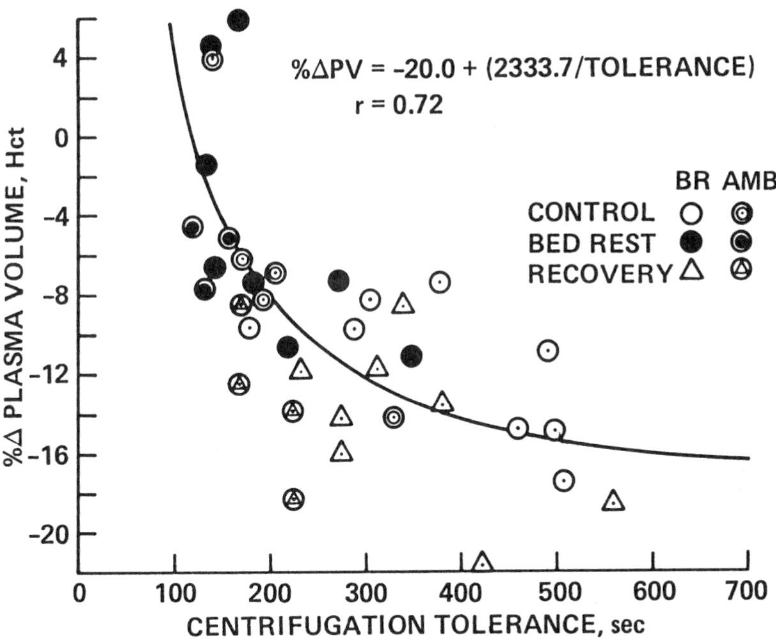

FIGURE 9-6. *Change in plasma volume and centrifugation tolerance in women when ambulatory and after bed rest. From Greenleaf et al. (1977c) with permission.*

TABLE 9-4. *Mean Centrifugation Tolerance, Maximal Heart Rate, and Plasma Volume Changes During Bed Rest and Acceleration in Men and Women*

STUDY	CENTRIFUGATION				BED REST	TOTAL
	TOLERANCE		MAX HR, beats/min	PV, %Δ		
	MEAN, %Δ	RANGE, %Δ			PV, %Δ	PV, %Δ
GREENLEAF ET AL. 1973 (3.2 G) ♂						
BR-1	-30	(0 to -61)	163	-6.8	-10.6	-17.4
BR-2	-29	(+5 to -40)	154	-5.4	-11.9	-17.3
GREENLEAF ET AL. 1975 (3.2 G) ♂						
BR-1	-33	(+4 to -72)	127	-6.3	-14.9	-21.2
GREENLEAF ET AL. 1977C (3.0 G) ♀						
BR-1	-40	(-20 to -71)	172	-4.1	-12.6	-16.7

(Van Beaumont et al. 1974). Different acceleration profiles result in different levels of hypovolemia at the tolerance point (Greenleaf et al. 1977b), as discussed below.

To gain more insight into the mechanism of the effects of dehydration and hypovolemia, a study was done in two phases (Greenleaf et al. 1977b). In Phase I, tolerance to $+0.5\ G_z$/min continuous acceleration rate was measured in six men (21-27 years old) after hemorrhage of 400 mL of blood and after blood reinfusion. In Phase II, tolerance was measured again after a second hemorrhage, and then after oral rehydration with 800mL of 0.9% NaCl (Figure 9-7). In confirmation of previous findings, hemorrhage hypovolemia (Phase I) reduced tolerance times in all subjects from a mean of 6.4 +0.4 min to 5.4 +0.2 min (Δtol = –15.1%, $P<0.05$). The shift of PV during the hydrated control run (Cl) was –8.0% (Figure 9-7, heavy lines); in addition to hemorrhage hypovolemia (H1), the extravascular PV shift in the subjects during acceleration was –8.4%, not different from the hydrated control shift. After reinfusion (I), tolerance times increased in all subjects to hydrated control levels of 6.1 +0.2 min (ΔPV = –7.9%). Phase II hemorrhage (H2) tolerance time was 5.7 +0.2 min (ΔPV = –5.8%) and tolerance time following oral hydration increased in every subject to a mean level of 6.4 +0.3 min (Δtol = +11.3%, $P<0.05$), not different from the Phase I hydration tolerance time of 6.4 +0.4 min. Change in PV during these drinking runs (D) was –7.0%. With significant

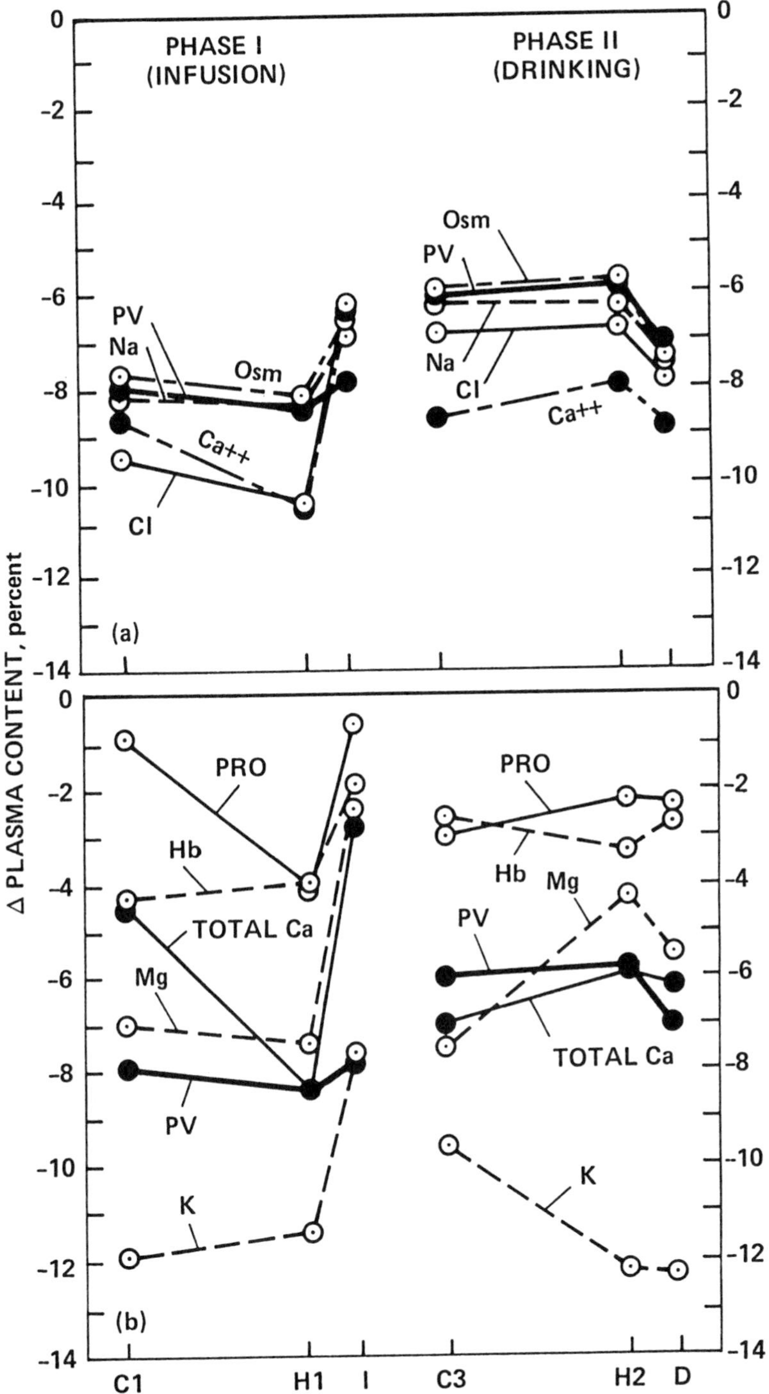

FIGURE 9-7. *Mean percent changes in PV (heavy lines) and plasma contents at grayout during* $+0.5\ G_z$ *acceleration in the phase I (infusion) and phase II (drinking) experiments. C = control, H = hypovolemia from hemorrhage, I = infusion, D = drinking. Top panel: variables that shifted with PV. Bottom panel: variables that did not shift with PV. From Greenleaf et al. (1977b) with permission.*

changes in tolerance time from hemorrhage and fluid restoration (a range of -15.1% to +11.3%), the extravascular shift of PV during acceleration was remarkably constant (a range of -5.8% to -8.4%).

Vartbaronov et al. (1987) reported an 11.1% decrease in PV during exposure to +7 G_z. Thus, it appears that the increased hydrostatic force, not the initial level of PV, determines the magnitude of the PV shift at one particular rate of acceleration. Lack of important changes in the mean corpuscular volume (+1.7% to +2.0%) and in the mean corpuscular hemoglobin concentration and content indicate the plasma is shifted into the extravascular fluid compartments and not into the red blood cells (Greenleaf et al. 1977b, 1977c). With a range in plasma osmolality of -1 to +13 mosmol/kg H_2O, the red blood cell in vivo is resistant to volume changes induced by a variety of exercise and environmental stresses (Greenleaf et al. 1979). Factors that do not influence red cell volume (RCV) are the level of exercise metabolism, heat exposure at rest, and short-term +G_z acceleration. Factors that probably influence RCV are high-altitude exposure and head-up tilting for more than 1 h. Factors that definitely change RCV are prior dehydration and periods of exposure to stress greater than 2 h (Greenleaf et al. 1979). Some of these factors may degrade work performance; for example, during extended extravehicular activity (EVA), where the astronauts are probably hypovolemic, hyperthermic, and exposed to an 8-psi atmosphere in the EVA suit. These findings emphasize the important function of changes in PV as a determining factor for acceleration tolerance. It would seem that blood pressure change during slow onset acceleration is controlled to a great extent by the rate of loss PV interacting with the baroreceptors.

During acceleration, the extracellular (plasma) calcium, sodium, and chloride ions are shifted from the plasma isosmotically, i.e., in proportion to their normal plasma concentrations (Figure 9-7, top panel). This shift was probably the result of the increased hydrostatic pressure and capillary filtration. Plasma constituents that did not shift isosmotically are shown in Figure 9-7, bottom panel. In general, total protein content and hemoglobin shifted least as would be expected, although they lost 1% to 4% of their content; total calcium and magnesium content made intermediate shifts; and potassium content shifted the most, by 8% to 12%. The decreased shifts of all constituents (Figure 9-7, both panels) in the infusion run (I) were due to the addition of these substances with infusion. On the other hand, there was a greater decreasing trend for shifts in PV and all constituents except protein and hemoglobin during acceleration after drinking isotonic saline. Plasma potassium (intracellular ion) has its own response pattern with a much greater loss of content than the extracellular cations. In a subsequent +G_z acceleration study (Greenleaf et al. 1985) a similar exaggerated loss of plasma potassium was observed during accleration in men but not in women, for no apparent reason.

This acceleration-induced loss of plasma potassium-ion content is the opposite of the shift that occurs during acute physical exercise. During exercise, plasma K^+ concentration and content *increase*, indicating loss from muscle, while Na^+, Cl^-, Osm, total protein, and Ca^{++} respond much as they do to the PV shift during acceleration (Convertino et al. 1980a; Covertino et al. 1980b; Greenleaf et al. 1980b). It should be mentioned that during our acceleration studies the subjects were trained to ride the centrifuge without muscular contraction to eliminate confounding effects of exercise on fluid-electrolyte shifts. Sjogaard (1986, 1988) has suggested that the relatively large loss of intracellular potassium during muscular contraction may be responsible for muscular fatigue because of a decreased excitability of the cellular membrane. It is interesting to speculate that the reverse exaggerated shift of potassium ions from the vascular to extravascular (perhaps intracellular) space during acceleration may contribute to the grayout threshold by changing the cellular function of baroreceptors.

Vasoactive and Fluid-Electrolyte Hormone Responses During Acceleration

Many hormones that act to maintain fluid and electrolyte homeostasis also possess vasoactive properties. These hormones are potent vasoconstrictors and will increase the pre- to postcapillary resistance across the capillary, resulting in enhanced reabsorption of fluid from the interstitial space to maintain the PV. Plasma vasopressin (PVP), the antidiuretic hormone, and plasma renin activity (PRA), which is used to estimate angiotensin II activity, are the two important fluid-electrolyte controlling factors that have been studied most extensively during acceleration. Atriopeptins (AP), secreted mainly but not exclusively by the atria in response to atrial distension, play important roles in fluid-electrolyte homeostasis, but their precise functions at physiological concentrations are not clear (Goetz 1988). They antagonize the action of angiotensin II and they inhibit the secretion of vasopressin in the central nervous system. They are also vasoactive and act to decrease arterial blood pressure, cardiac filling pressure, and cardiac output. They promote vasodilation of the aorta and renal vessels, as well as fluid shifts from the plasma to the interstitial space (Goetz 1988). Apparently AP have not been studied during acceleration; since plasma AP increase during exercise (Freund et al. 1987; Nishikimi et al. 1986; Tanaka et al. 1986), water immersion (Epstein et al. 1989), and body tilting (Ogihara et al. 1986), it is likely they would also increase during $+G_z$ acceleration.

The human vasopressin molecule is an octapeptide that has arginine in position 8, hence the name arginine vasopressin. It is also called plasma vasopressin because of its effect on blood pressure. It is produced in magnocellular neurosecretory cells in the supraoptic and paraventricular nuclei of the hypothalamus and stored in the posterior pituitary gland (Share 1988). Its normohydration physiological range in plasma is 0.5 to

3.0 pg/mL and one major function is to promote reabsorption of water in collecting ducts and distal tubules in the kidney. Vasopressin responds to less than a 1% change is plasma osmolality, and also to changes in the activity of volume (pressure) receptors in blood vessels and possibly in the heart. Its pressor effect, which increases blood pressure via constriction of vascular smooth muscle, occurs at plasma concentrations above 10 pg/mL, and PVP concentrations greater than 500 pg/mL have been measured at syncope (J. Greenleaf, personal observation). In addition to its secretion by hyperosmotic stimuli, it responds to a variety of emotional and physical stresses, including venipuncture, pain, hypovolemia (hemorrhage, dehydration), postural fainting (Kravik et al. 1986), and vagus nerve and supraoptic nuclei stimulation (Noble and Taylor 1953). It also increases during $+G_z$ acceleration (Greenleaf et al. 1977b, 1985). Vasopressin secretion is inhibited by hypervolemia, hyposmotemia, epinephrine, and cold exposure, and by drinking water (Geelen et al. 1984) or ethyl alcohol (Goodman 1980).

Noble and Taylor (1953) found no evidence of biological vasopressin activity in the form of inhibition of water-induced diuresis in rats, following injection of urine from nine men who became unconscious (blackout) during acceleration at levels of +4.0 to +6.5 G_z. Other men were subjected to venisection; postural fainting (unconsciousness) occurred in seven experiments and no fainting occurred in seven other experiments. There was no quantitative correlation between the volume of blood withdrawn and the occurrence of fainting. All subjects who fainted excreted detectable quantities of vasopressin in their urine. No vasopressin was found in the urine of the nonfainters (the assay may have been too insensitive), in the control urine of the fainters, or in the urine collected before or after acceleration-induced unconsciousness. The authors' very interesting conclusion was that vasopressin excretion was related directly to the incidence of postural unconsciousness, and indirectly to the stimuli that initiated the faint or to cerebral anoxia (blackout); thus posture-induced unconsciousness and acceleration-induced unconsciousness would seem to be basically *different* reactions. Support for this hypothesis comes from a comparison of hormonal responses in men and women at the point of tolerance during 70° head-up tilting and +0.5 G_z/min acceleration (Greenleaf et al. 1985). During tilting there were significant increases in plasma epinephrine, norepinephrine, renin activity, and vasopressin, but with acceleration, only norepinephrine and vasopressin increased significantly.

Urine Flow

Urine formation and excretion are controlled by renal plasma flow in the afferent and efferent arterioles in the nephron, by the filtration rate through the glomerular membrane, and by reabsorption of fluid and solutes by the nephron tubules. During $+G_z$ acceleration there is a marked reduction in urine flow ($\dot{V}$) in previously hydrated subjects (Piemme et al. 1966; Stauffer and Errebo-Knudsen 1950) that is not caused by changes in renal plasma flow (RPF) or glomerular filtration rate (GFR) (Piemme et al. 1966; Meehan and Brandt (1960). GFR is estimated from the creatinine clearance (C_{cr}):

$$C_{cr} = U_{cr} \times \dot{V}/P_{cr}$$

This suggests a minor effect of the adrenergic nervous system on RPF. The hydropenia is not caused by changes in osmotic clearance ($C_{osm}=U_{osm} \times \dot{V} / P_{osm}$), but is the result mainly of reduced free water clearance ($C_{H_2O}=\dot{V}-C_{osm}$). This was postulated by Stauffer and Errebo-Knudsen (1950) and shown clearly by Piemme et al. (1966) to occur at $+3.0\ G_z$, but not at $+1\ G_z$ or $+2\ G_z$ (Figure 9-8). The slow rate of onset of acceleration (0.10 G/sec) and the 90-min centrifugation time of Piemme et al.'s five subjects probably allowed the urine flow reductions to be measured without interference from stimuli associated with the acute stress of a

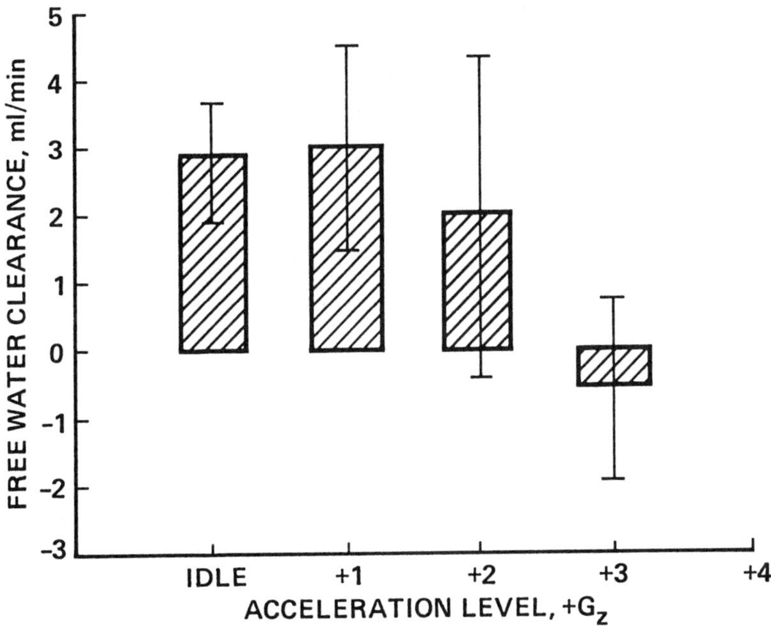

FIGURE 9-8. *Mean (±SD) free water clearance in 5 men at rest and during 3 levels of $+G_z$ acceleration. From Piemme et al. (1966) with permission.*

rapid acceleration rate. The 1-min centrifugation runs of Stauffer and Errebo-Knudsen with, presumably, higher rates of onset resulted in little change in urine flow during the run, but the reduced outputs became evident by 30 min into the recovery period. These findings strongly suggest action of a hormonal system, i.e., PVP, on the kidney tubules as the primary mechanism for the hydropenia. Since C_{osm} was unchanged, any action of factors that could change sodium excretion (e.g., the renin-angiotensin-aldosterone system or atrial natriuretic peptides) was not apparent.

During chest-to-back acceleration there is a shift of blood from the legs into the thorax. Watson and Rapp (1962) accelerated six men for 10 min at +4.0 G_x and found a significant increase in GFR during acceleration and an increased GFR, RPF, and urine flow 30 min after acceleration. These responses were accompanied by small but significant reductions in C_{osm} and C_{H_2O} only during the first 45 min of recovery, by no changes in plasma osmolality or urinary sodium clearance, but by significant reduction in urinary potassium clearance. The decreased potassium clearance suggests a modest inhibition of the renin-aldosterone system. Thus, the accentuated urine flow after $+G_x$ centrifugation, with the modest increases in RPF and GFR and the greater increases in $C_{H_2O,}$ suggested the diuretic effect of PVP inhibition in response to the increased right atrial pressure (Wood et al. 1961). Similar but not identical fluid, electrolyte, and hormonal responses occur during application of LBPP (60 mmHg applied to the legs and 30 mmHg to the abdomen) for 4.5 h of 70° head-up tilt (Geelen et al. 1989). Glomerular filtration rate was unchanged, and the increased urine flow, $C_{osm,}$ $C_{H_2O,}$ and fractional sodium excretion ($U_{Na}\dot{V}$) were associated with increased blood pressure and effective RPF. Attenuation of PVP contributed to the increased $C_{H_2O,}$ and to suppression of PRA and aldosterone-enhanced C_{osm} and $U_{Na}\dot{V}$; a combination free water and osmotic diuresis was the result. Thus fluid-electrolyte-hormonal responses to LBPP are qualitatively similar to those during $+G_x$ acceleration. The differences are due to the various levels of acceleration and LBPP employed.

Plasma Vasopressin and Renin-Angiotensin II-Aldosterone Activity

Rogge et al. (1967) subjected nine men to +2 G_z and +2 G_x accelerations for 30 min at a slow rate (0.05 G/sec) of onset and deceleration and measured peripheral venous PVP activity by bioassay. Plasma vasopressin increased significantly from resting levels by 2.97 μU (7.42 pg/mL) during the $+G_z$ runs and tended to decrease (nonsignificantly) by 0.86 μU (2.15 pg/mL) during $+G_z$ acceleration with a G-suit inflated to 60 mmHg. During $+G_x$ acceleration blood PVP decreased significantly by 0.89 μU (2.22 pg/mL). These findings show clearly that the rise in PVP is a response to shifts, or lack of shifts, of blood to and from the central circulation.

Mean PVP levels in hydrated men at the tolerance point during $+G_z$ acceleration at +0.5 G/min range from 4 to 12 pg/mL (Figure 9-9, top panel); after hemorrhage of 400 mL, PVP levels at the tolerance point increased from 22 to 35 pg/mL. The magnitude of these responses was a reflection of the hemorrhage-induced hypovolemia because the acceleration-induced plasma fluid shifts were essentially the same as during the corresponding hydration control run (Figure 9-7). Keil and Ellis (1976) found that PVP was elevated greatly to 52 pg/mL at the point of tolerance in male subjcts whose PV had been reduced by 12.6% after 14 days of horizontal bed rest. The correlation coefficient between postacceleration PVP and tolerance time was +0.67 ($P<0.05$). The assumption is that changes in central venous pressure, resulting from hypovolemia combined with previous hemorrhage or from hypovolemia alone caused by prior bed rest or acceleration, stimulate secretion of PVP, thereby inhibiting C_{H_2O} to preserve vascular volume and inducing peripheral vasoconstriction to counteract hypotension. The effect of acceleration on cerebral-spinal fluid pressure and on circulatory dynamics needs further investigation.

Renin is secreted by the juxtaglomerular (JG) cells in the renal afferent arteriole. Renin is released osmotically by the JG cells because of reduced concentrations of sodium and chloride at the macula densa cells in the JG area. Decreased stimulation of vascular stretch receptors in the renal afferent arteriole and increased catecholamine and sympathetic nerve activity on the JG cells cause the release of renin via changes in calcium (Goodman 1980). Renin may stimulate secretion of aldosterone and vasopressin via an increase in angiotensin II. Aldosterone (a mineralocortcoid) is an adrenal steroid, derived from cholesterol, that is released from the zona glomerulosa cells of the adrenal cortex by angiotensin II which, in turn, is activated by renin in response to a fall in blood pressure. Its only known action is to preserve extracellular fluid volume and acid-base balance by promoting the reabsorption of sodium and the excretion of potassium and hydrogen ions in the kidneys' distal tubules, the intestines, and the ducts of sweat and salivary glands (Goodman 1980).

Normal resting plasma renin activity (PRA) in men and women is 0.5 to 0.8 ng AngI/mL·h. For accelerations between +3.0 and +3.5 G_z, PRA tends to increase slightly at the tolerance point by about 0.2 ng AngI/mL·h. Pre-acceleration hemorrhage elevates PRA further to about 1.0 ng AngI/mL·h (Figure 9-9, bottom panel). Plasma epinephrine and norepinephrine tend to increase by 60% to 70% (N.S.) during acceleration (Greenleaf et al. 1985). Rogge et al. (1967) observed PRA increases of 0.4 to 0.8 ng during 20 to 30 min of centrifugation at $+2\ G_z$ with or without a G-suit inflated to 60 mmHg. Epstein et al. (1974) reported a doubling of

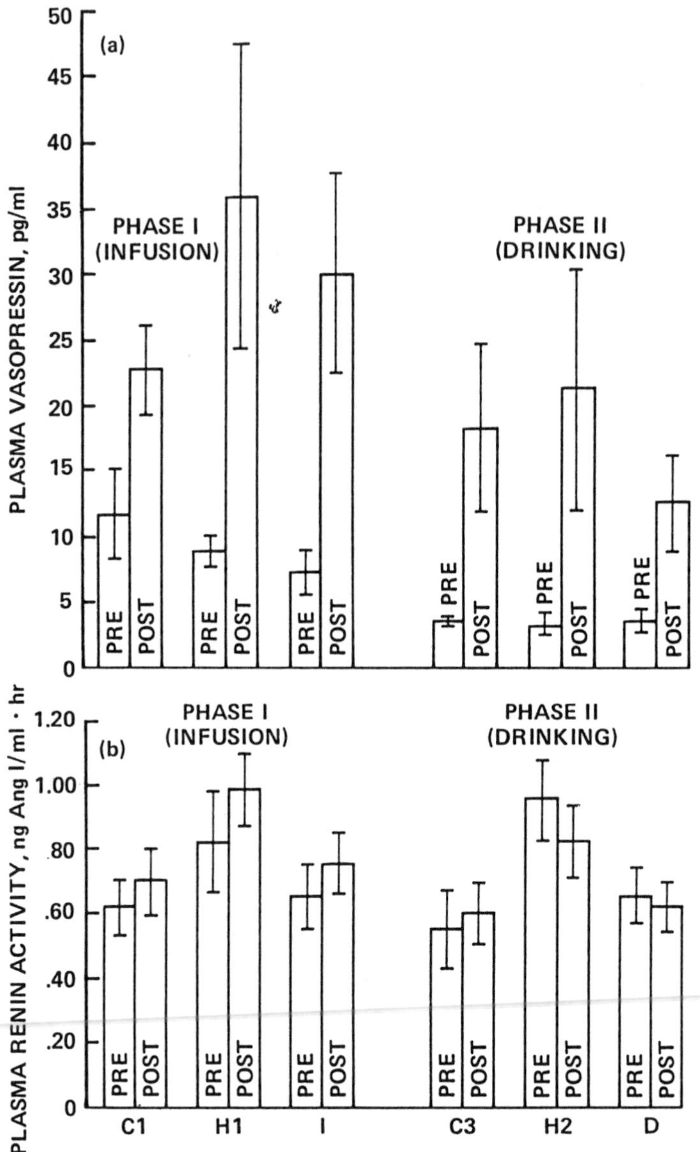

FIGURE 9-9. *Mean (±SD) PVP concentrations (top panel) and plasma renin activity (bottom panel) at the tolerance point during* $+0.5\ G_z$*/min acceleration in the phase I (infusion) and phase II (drinking) experiments. From Greenleaf et al. (1977b) with permission.*

PRA after 30 min at $+2.0\ G_z$; this was associated with a significant decrease in natriuresis caused by a significant reduction in GFR (Shubrooks et al. 1974). G-suit inflation to 125 mmHg during centrifugation did not change the magnitude of the natriuresis. Thus, while the antinatriuresis was associated with increased PRA, the latter probably did not cause the reduced sodium excretion because GFR was also reduced proportionally. This finding suggests that other factors (hemodynamic) alter renal function. Because the application of LBPP and $+G_z$ acceleration induces competing physiological stimuli, the net response depends on the magnitudes of the competing stimuli. Failure of the G-suit to maintain increased central venous pressure during acceleration leads to the conclusion that while G-suit inflation of 100 to 125 mmHg probably induces a significant increase in peripheral arterial resistance, the increased counterpressure is unable to resist blood redistribution into the lower extremities during centrifugation.

After 14 days of bed rest deconditioning, PRA levels at tolerance during $+3.0\ G_z$ acceleration (0.03 G/sec onset) in women were only slightly higher than those in ambulatory men (Keil and Ellis 1976); PRA levels in the women reached about 1.5 ng after bed rest compared to 1.0 ng in the men during the ambulatory control period (Figure 9-10). The

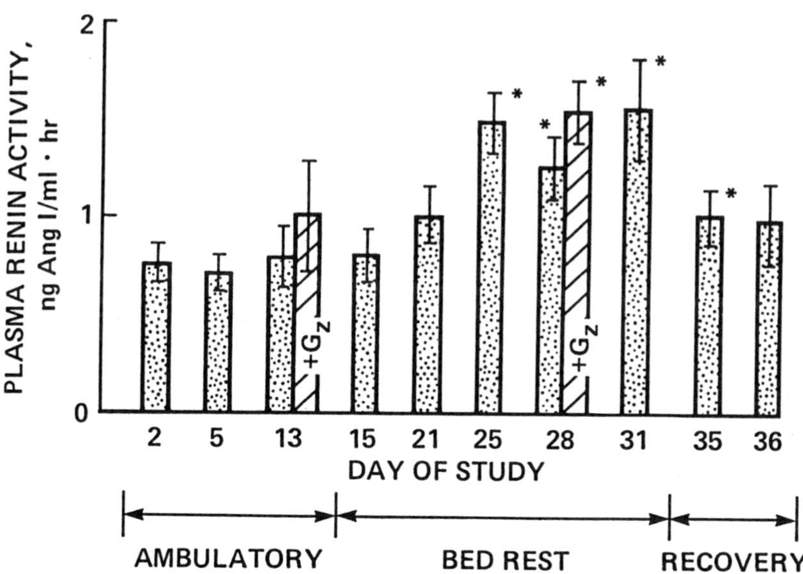

FIGURE 9-10. *Mean (±SD) plasma renin activity at the tolerance point during $+3.0\ G_z$ acceleration in 8 women during the ambulatory control period, after 14 days of bed rest, and during recovery. $^*P < 0.05$ when compared to either day 2 or day 5 of the ambulatory control period. From Keil and Ellis (1976) with permission.*

mean reduction in PV in the men during bed rest was 12.6%; this, plus the additional post-bed rest, acceleration-induced PV shift of -4.1%, equaled a total hypovolemic level of 16.7% (Greenleaf et al. 1977a). This reduction in PV had little effect on PRA during acceleration runs of 6- to 7-min duration. Thus, although PRA increased typically by 25% to 50%, and sometimes by 100% during $+G_z$ acceleration lasting from 6 to 30 min, its major effect appears to be associated with attenuated natriuresis. Bed rest deconditioning with its attendant hypovolemia does not influence the normal 0.2-ng increase in PRA during centrifugation. During acceleration, it appears that the hemodynamic (hypertensive) effects of vasopressin and renin are more pronounced than are their fluid and electrolyte actions.

EFFECTS OF FLUID REPLACEMENT AND HYPERHYDRATION ON ACCELERATION AND ORTHOSTATIC TOLERANCES

With very few exceptions, space travelers return to Earth with moderate to severe body weight loss (Figure 9-5). Mean (±SD) weight loss of the astronauts of projects Mercury 6–9 (4 men), Gemini 3, 4, 5, and 7 (8 men), Apollo 7–17 (33 men), and Skylab II, III, IV (9 men) was 3.22±1.27 kg. The range of loss was 0.09 kg (~0.1%) on the longest Skylab flight (84 days) to 6.36 kg (~9.1%) on Apollo 12 (10.2 days). Weight measurement was often delayed a few hours after landing so the measured weight changes underestimate the true loss. It is interesting that the lowest mean weight loss during any mission was on Skylab IV, where the astronauts performed the most exercise training (1.5 h/day). Sweating from exposure to high capsule temperatures contributed to the weight losses on the shorter Mercury and Gemini flights.

Mean (±SD) percentage changes in measured fluid-compartment volumes during some Gemini and Apollo flights and all Skylab flights are presented in Table 9-5. The larger RCV losses on the Gemini flights were due to the capsule atmosphere of 100% oxygen, and RCV loss was nearly zero in the Skylab flights that had sea-level oxygen content in the spacecraft. The greatest decreases in PV occurred on the consecutive Skylab flights, in which exercise training increased from 0.5 to 1.0 to 1.5 h/day. Apparently the varied types of isotonic and isometric exercise regimens could not maintain normovolemia even though body-weight losses were minimal. The 13% to 16% losses in PV (432 to 529 mL) would account for the 1% (600 mL) losses in total body water with essentially no change in interstitial volume.

Usually, plasma and interstitial volumes change in proportion to their normal volumes, maintaining their 1:4 ratio (Greenleaf et al. 1980a) (Table 9-1). Leach et al. (1975) have reported a 4.4% loss of PV with only a 2.2% loss of interstitial volume in the three Apollo 17 astronauts. This

TABLE 9-5. *Mean (±SD) Changes in Measured Body Weight and in Plasma, Red-Cell, Blood, and Fluid Volumes in Crewmen on Some Gemini (2-Man Crews), Apollo (3-Man Crews), and Skylab (3-Man Crews) Missions*

MISSION	$\overline{X}$ TIME, DAYS	$\overline{X}$ ΔWt, kg	ΔPV, %	ΔRCV, %	ΔBV, %	ΔECV, %	ΔTBW, %
GEMINI 4	1.8	-2.95±1.29	-9	-13*	-22		
GEMINI 5	8.2	-3.64±0.32	-7	-21	-28		
GEMINI 7	13.8	-3.64±1.29	+11	-14	-3		
APOLLO 7-8	8.5±3.3	-2.99±0.64	-8	-2	-10		
APOLLO 9	10.0	-4.03±0.78	-9	-7	-16		
APOLLO 14-17	11.2±1.6	-3.31±1.32	-4±2	-10±1	-14		
APOLLO 15-17	12.0±0.8	-3.23±1.10	-5	-3⁺	-8	-4	-2
SKYLAB II	28.0	-2.77±1.06	-9	-2⁺	-11	0	-3
SKYLAB III	59.5	-3.94±0.26	-13	0⁺	-13	-5	-1
SKYLAB IV	84.0	-1.06±0.84	-16	+3⁺	-13	0	-1
MEAN±SD		-3.16±0.85	-7±7	-7±7	-14±7	-2±3	-2±1

⁺ΔRCV = ΔBV - ΔPV

* CALCULATED

FROM: BERRY et al. 1966, CATTERSON et al. 1963, JOHNSON 1979, KIMZEY et al. 1975, LEACH et al. 1975, MINNERS et al. 1962, RAMBAUT et al. 1975, and THORNTON AND ORD 1977.

observation and those in Table 9-5 suggest a reduced loss or a greater-than-normal shift of fluid into the interstitial space in astronauts in microgravity, in the presence of a reduced PV. This shift may have contributed to the astronauts' head fullness; puffy faces; distended jugular veins; and distended veins of the temple, forehead, arm, and hand (Gazenko et al. 1979; Thornton et al. 1977). A similar "excessive" interstitial fluid volume has been measured in men between the 4th and 13th days of horizontal bed rest; this was independent of the exercise training regimens performed during bed rest (Greenleaf et al. 1977a). There is no obvious reason to assume that interstitial fluid crystalloid or colloid osmotic pressures would increase significantly, so the most likely explanation is an increased hydrostatic pressure. The question remains, why the persistent vascular distension only in the head, neck, and arms? That this upper-body fullness persists for so many days (84 in Skylab IV) is difficult to reconcile with the much shorter time necessary for the general fluid balance to reach equilibrium in microgravity; i.e., there is no progressive loss of weight or water as flight duration lengthens (Figure 9-5). The mechanism of this vascular distension and head fullness needs further study.

Eugravity

Essentially all investigators who have utilized water (Asyamolov et al. 1974; Dlusskaya and Khomenko 1985; Grigor'yev et al. 1978; Kotovskaya et al. 1987); hypo-, iso-, or hypertonic saline (Greenleaf et al. 1973, 1977b; Grigor'yev et al. 1978; Hyatt and West 1977; Kotovskaya et al. 1987); or blood reinfusion (Greenleaf et al. 1977b) have found a positive effect on cardiovascular responses or an increased tolerance to orthostasis, to LBNP, or to radial acceleration. In general, fluid loading for 2 to 3 h prior to exposure to these stresses is better than loading just prior to exposure, and an iso- or hypertonic fluid composition seems generally better than plain water.

An early study concerning the effects of fluid-electrolyte replacement on acceleration tolerance (Greenleaf et al. 1973) was performed on eight men, bed-rested for 14 days, who were hypovolemic by 15.2±2.0%. The hypothesis being tested was that hypovolemia was an important determinant of acceleration tolerance, and its restoration would attenuate the reduction in tolerance after bed rest deconditioning. The rehydration fluid was composed of 5 parts 0.9% saline and 1 part frozen grapefruit juice concentrate, and it contained 143 mEq/L sodium, 31 mEq/L potassium, and a total osmolality of 620 mosmol/kg H_2O. The drink (1.0 to 1.9 L) was administered over a 3-h period before acceleration to replace the estimated loss of extracellular fluid volume. Because of urinary loss and gastric distension, the volume consumed was only about 59% of the calculated deficit (Greenleaf et al. 1983). Rehydration restored 64% of the tolerance time lost after bed rest deconditioning at +2.1 G_z, but there was no change in tolerance times at accelerations of +3.1 G_z and +3.8 G_z, which lasted about one-third the duration of the +2.1 G_z acceleration. This suggests that oral rehydration is less effective with accelerations of higher intensity and shorter duration, which are accompanied by greater levels of hydrostatic pressure. Hyatt and West (1977) found, in men bed-rested for seven days, that continuous exposure to LBNP at −30 mmHg for 4 h, in conjunction with consumption of 1 L of slightly hypertonic saline (beef bouillon), restored ambulatory-control heart rates and systolic blood pressure for about 18 h. But 20 h after this treatment the hypervolemia remained, while tolerance to −50 mmHg had decreased to post-bed-rest levels (Johnson 1979). In addition, Hoffler (1977) found a significant correlation of only 0.54 between percent changes in spaceflight blood volume and heart rate during -50 mm Hg LBNP, indicating that only 30% of the variance in LBNP heart rate, used as a measure of tolerance, could be accounted for by the changes in blood volume.

Drinking hyperosmotic fluids maintains plasma volume by at least two means: its hyperosmotemic effect and its hypervolemic effect. The former can influence the latter. Firstly, hyperosmotemia stimulates vasopressin secretion, which increases tubular reabsorption of water if the hypervolemia is 10% or less. Secondly, since the rate of plasma shift from increased hydrostatic pressure is relatively constant during head-up tilting (Convertino et al. 1984) and $+G_z$ acceleration (Greenleaf et al. 1977b), hypervolemia induced before acceleration by a PV increase brought on by drinking and exercise training (acclimatization), should keep the absolute level of PV higher at any given time during acceleration. This hypervolemia should help to attenuate the decrease in tolerance.

Microgravity

After these fluid-loading countermeasures were extensively tested on the ground, they were utilized by cosmonauts and astronauts to increase their tolerance to moderate $+G_z$ acceleration levels during reentry and to ameliorate the immediate postflight orthostatic intolerance.

The first microgravity test of fluid loading apparently occurred on the 53rd day (July 15, 1975) of the second crew's stay aboard the Salyut-4 space station (Gazenko et al. 1979). The two cosmonauts consumed an additional 4 g of NaCl and 600 to 800 mL of water with two meals, and another 300 to 400 mL of water 20 to 30 min prior to the LBNP exposure (2 min at -25 mmHg and 3 min at -35 mmHg), which was conducted 3 h after the last meal. Although the two cosmonauts responded somewhat differently to the LBNP test, both exhibited reduced heart rates and blood pressures compared with those on the 44th day of that flight. Consequently, both cosmonauts were given 9.0 g NaCl and 1 to 2 L of water in three equal portions at the three meals prior to reentry. Postflight orthostatic stability was greatly improved (Grigoriev 1983). At present there is no way to measure the effects of fluid replacement and hypervolemic treatments on $+G_z$ tolerance during reentry separately from orthostatic tolerance after landing because the latter is influenced by the former.

When does the dehydration-induced hypovolemia become normovolemia during exposure to microgravity? Clearly, crew members in microgravity for 1 yr are not hypohydrated as long as they remain in orbit. Rehydrating a dehydrated person probably requires a drink of a different composition from one used to rehydrate a normohydrated person, such as the microgravity-adapted astronaut with a reduced total body water.

Russian and American research teams have investigated combinations of countermeasures that included exercise training, $+G_z$ acceleration with prolonged (3 to 13 days) water immersion with and without fluid loading prior to acceleration, and intermittent LBNP training with and without fluid loading prior to the LBNP stress. Johnson (1979) concluded that the Hyatt and West (1977) protocol of 1 L of saline ingestion during 4 h of LBNP at −50 mmHg was optimal for the lowest increment in heart rate, and found that the hypervolemia was stabilized after 2 h of combined treatment. Because of the difficulty in providing LBNP treatment for entire Space Shuttle crews 24 h before reentry, it was decided to provide only oral rehydration (8 × 1 g NaCl tablets and 912 mL of water; 0.9% saline) starting 2 h before reentry for 17 crew members on the first eight Shuttle flights (Bungo et al. 1985). Some crew members substituted fruit juices for the water. Fluid consumption varied from 0.5 L of hypotonic solution to 1.0 L of isotonic solution. Compared with responses from nine crew members who did not consume the rehydration solution, fluid loading reduced the heart-rate increment by 29% during a quiet standing orthostatic tolerance test, and the cardiovascular index of deconditioning (CID $=\Delta HR - \Delta SBP + DBP$) from 49 units in the control group to 21 units ($P < 0.003$) in the rehydration group. It is clear that hypovolemia plays a major role in the etiology of postflight orthostatic intolerance.

SUMMARY

Accelerative forces of slow onset, acting on the body in the $+G_z$ (head-to-foot) direction, affect the three major components controlling blood pressure. The increased hydrostatic pressure promotes hypovolemia via increased capillary filtration, which is associated with the decreased cardiac output and decreased right atrial pressure that stimulates increased peripheral resistance (decreased leg blood flow).

The magnitude of hypovolemia induced before acceleration and the rate of plasma loss during acceleration can account for at least half the variance in acceleration tolerance time. In addition to norepinephrine, hypovolemia is a major stimulus for secretion of vasoactive substances (renin and vasopressin). Hyperosmotemia is not. During acceleration, the hemodynamic (hypertensive) effects of renin and vasopressin are more important than their effects on fluid-electrolyte homeostasis.

Acceleration tolerances depressed by negative water balance can be returned to normal by blood reinfusion or oral fluid loading in ambulatory subjects, but usually not in those who have been deconditioned by prolonged bed rest of exposure to microgravity. Better acceleration and orthostatic countermeasures employ a combination of exercise-training (in-heat) induced hypervolemia plus oral fluid loading during application of LBNP. Additional work is needed to determine the effects of acceleration on colloid osmotic pressure, interstitial fluid pressure, central venous pressure, and peripheral blood flow, and on their interactions with the vasoactive hormones.

Amberson, W.R. Physiologic adjustments to the standing posture. *Bull. Univ. Maryland Sch. Med.* 27:127–145, 1943.

Asyamolov, B.F., V.S. Panchenko, and I.D. Pestov. Water load as a method for changing the orthostatic reaction in man after brief hypodynamia. *Kosm. Biol. Aviakosm. Med.* 8:80–82, 1974.

Beetham, W.P., Jr., and E.R. Buskirk. Effects of dehydration, physical conditioning and heat acclimatization on the response to passive tilting. *J. Appl. Physiol.* 13:465–468, 1958.

Berry, C.A., D.O. Coons, A.D. Catterson, and G.F. Kelly. Man's response to long-duration flight in the Gemini spacecraft. In: *Gemini Midprogram Conference: Including Experiment Results.* NASA Special Publication 121, 1966, p. 235–261. National Aeronautics and Space Administration, Washington, DC.

Blomqvist, C.G., and H.L. Stone. Cardiovascular adjustments to gravitational stress. In: *Handbook of Physiology. The Cardiovascular System. Peripheral Circulation and Organ Blood Flow.* J.T. Sheperd, F.M. Abboud, and S.R. Geiger, eds. Bethesda, MD: American Physiological Society. Sect. 2, vol. III, part 2, chap. 28, 1983, p.1025–1063.

Bungo, M.W., J.B. Charles, and P.C. Johnson, Jr. Cardiovascular deconditioning during space flight and the use of saline as a countermeasure to orthostatic intolerance. *Aviat. Space Environ. Med.* 56:985–990, 1985.

Catterson, A.D., E.P. McCutcheon, H.A. Minners, and R.A. Pollard. Aeromedical observations. In: *Mercury Project Summary, Including Results of the Fourth Manned Orbital Flight, May 15 and 16, 1963.* NASA Special Publication 45, 1965, p. 299–326. National Aeronautics and Space Administration, Washington, DC.

Convertino, V.A., P.J. Brock, L.C. Keil, E.M. Bernauer, and J.E. Greenleaf. Exercise training-induced hypervolemia: role of plasma albumin, renin, and vasopressin. *J. Appl. Physiol.* 48:665–669, 1980a.

Convertino, V.A., J.E. Greenleaf, and E.M. Bernauer. Role of thermal and exercise factors in mechanism of hypervolemia. *J. Appl. Physiol.* 48:657–664, 1980b.

Convertino, V.A., L.D. Montgomery, and J.E. Greenleaf. Cardiovascular responses during orthostasis: effect of an increase in $\dot{V}O_2$ max. *Aviat. Space Environ. Med.* 55:702–708, 1984.

Dlusskaya, I.G., and M.N. Khomenko. Distinctions in reactions to active orthostatic water-loading tests of subjects differing in tolerance to $+G_z$ accelerations. *Kosm. Biol. Aviakosm. Med.* 19:22–27, 1985.

Epstein, M., P. Norsk, and R. Loutzenhiser. Effects of water immersion on atrial natriuretic peptide release in humans. *Am. J. Nephrol.* 9:1–24, 1989.

Epstein, M., S.J. Shubrooks, Jr., L.M. Fishman, and D.C. Duncan. Effects of positive acceleration ($+G_z$) on renal function and plasma renin in normal man. *J. Appl. Physiol.* 36:340–344, 1974.

Freund, B.J., J.R. Claybaugh, M.S. Dice, and G.M. Hashiro. Hormonal and vascular fluid responses to maximal exercise in trained and untrained males. *J. Appl. Physiol.* 63:669–675, 1987.

Gaffney, F.A., E.R. Thal, W.F. Taylor, B.C. Bastian, J.A. Weigelt, J.M. Atkins, and C.G. Bloomqvist. Hermodynamic effects of the medical anti-shock trousers (MAST garment). *J. Trauma* 21:931–937, 1981.

Gauer, O. and H. Haber. Man under gravity-free conditions. In: *German Aviation Medicine, World War II,* vol. I. New York: Scholium International, Inc., 1950, p. 641–644.

Gazenko, O.G., A.I. Grigor'yev, V.A. Degtyarev, L.I. Kakurin, G.I. Kozyrevskaya, N.A. Lapshina, Yu.V. Natochin, I.P. Neumyvakin, A.S. Nekhayev, and A.A. Savilov. Stimulation of fluid-electrolyte metabolism as a means of preventing orthostatic instability in the crew of the second expedition aboard the Salyut-4 station. *Kosm. Biol. Aviakosm. Med.* 13:10–15, 1979.

Geelen, G., L.C. Keil, S.E. Kravik, C.E. Wade, T.N. Thrasher, P.R. Barnes, G. Pyka, C. Nesvig, and J.E. Greenleaf. Inhibition of plasma vasopressin after drinking in dehydrated humans. *Am. J. Physiol.* 247:R968–R971, 1984.

Geelen, G., S.E. Kravik, A. Hadj-Aissa, G. Leftheriotis, M. Vincent, C.-A. Bizollon, C.W. Sem-Jacobsen, J.E. Greenleaf, and C. Gharib. Antigravity suit inflation: kidney function and cardiovascular and hormonal responses in men. *J. Appl. Physiol.* 66:792–799, 1989.

Gell, C.F. Table of equivalents for acceleration terminology. *Aerospace Med.* 32:1109–1111, 1961.

Goetz, K.L. Physiology and pathophysiology of atrial peptides. *Am. J. Physiol.* 254:E1–E15, 1988.

Goodman, J.M. Endocrine glands, part XIII. In: *Medical Physiology,* vol. 2, V.B. Mountcastle, ed. St. Louis: C.V. Mosby Co., 1980,p.1459–1673.

Greenleaf, J.E., E.M. Bernauer, H.L. Young, J.T. Morse, R.W. Staley, L.T. Juhos, and W. Van Beaumont. Fluid and electrolyte shifts during bed rest with isometric and isotonic exercise. *J. Appl. Physiol.* 42:59–66, 1977a.

Greenleaf, J.E., P.J. Brock, R.F. Haines, S.A. Rositano, L.D. Montgomery, and L.C. Keil. Effect of hypovolemia, infusion, and oral rehydration on plasma electrolytes, ADH, renin activity, and $+G_z$ tolerance. *Aviat. Space Environ. Med.* 48:693–700, 1977b.

Greenleaf, J.E., P.J. Brock, L.C. Keil, and J.T. Morse. Drinking and water balance during exercise and heat acclimation. *J. Appl. Physiol.* 54:414–419, 1983.

Greenleaf, J.E., P.J. Brock, D. Sciaraffa, A. Polese, and R. Elizondo. Effects of exercise-heat acclimation on fluid, electrolyte, and endocrine responses during tilt and $+G_z$ acceleration in women and men. *Aviat. Space Environ. Med.* 56:683–689, 1985.

Greenleaf, J.E., V.A. Convertino, and G.R. Mangseth. Plasma volume during stress in man: osmolality and red cell volume. *J. Appl. Physiol.* 47:1031-1038, 1979.
Greenleaf, J.E., R.F. Haines, E.M. Bernauer, J.T. Morse, H. Sandler, R. Armbruster, L. Sagan, and W. Van Beaumont. $+G_z$ tolerance in man after 14-day bedrest periods with isometric and isotonic exercise conditioning. *Aviat. Space Environ. Med.* 46:671-678, 1975.
Greenleaf, J.E., and M.H. Harrison. Water and electrolytes. In: *Nutrition and Aerobic Exercise,* D.K. Layman, ed. Washington, DC: American Chemical Society, 1986,p.107-124.
Greenleaf, J.E., M. Matter, Jr., J.S. Bosco, L.G. Douglas, and E.G. Averkin. Effects of hypohydration on work performance and tolerance to $+G_z$ acceleration in man. *Aerospace Med.* 37:34-39, 1966a.
Greenleaf, J.E., M. Matter, Jr., L.G. Douglas, S.A. Raymond, J.S. Bosco, E.G. Averkin, and R.H. St. John, Jr. Effects of acute and chronic hypohydration on tolerance to $+G_z$ acceleration in man: I. Physiological results. *NASA Technical Memorandum X-1285,* 1966b.
Greenleaf, J.E., E. Shvartz, S. Kravik, and L.C. Keil. Fluid shifts and endocrine responses during chair rest and water immersion in man. *J. Appl. Physiol.* 48:79-88, 1980a.
Greenleaf, J.E., H.O. Stinnett, G.L. Davis, J. Kollias, and E.M. Bernauer. Fluid and electrolyte shifts in women during $+G_z$ acceleration after 15 days' bed rest. *J. Appl. Physiol.* 42:67-73, 1977c.
Greenleaf, J.E., W. Van Beaumont, E.M. Bernauer, R.F. Haines, H. Sandler, R.W. Staley, H.L. Young, and J.W. Yusken. Effects of rehydration on $+G_z$ tolerance after 14-days' bed rest. *Aerospace Med.* 44:715-722, 1973.
Greenleaf, J.E., W. Van Beaumont, P.J. Brock, L.D. Montgomery, J.T. Morse, E. Shvartz, and S. Kravik. Fluid-electrolyte shifts and thermoregulation: Rest and work in heat with head cooling. *Aviat. Space Environ. Med.* 51:747-753, 1980b.
Grigoriev, A.I. Correction of changes in fluid-electrolyte metabolism in manned space flights. *Aviat. Space Environ. Med.* 54:318-323, 1983.
Grigor'yev, A.I., B.S. Katkovskiy, A.A. Savilov, V.S. Georgiyevskiy, B.R. Dorokhova, and V.M. Mikhaylov. Effects of hyperhydration on human endurance of orthostatic and LBNP tests. *Kosm. Biol. Aviakosm. Med.* 12:20-24, 1978.
Hargens, A.R. Interstitial fluid pressure and lymph flow. In: *Handbook of Bioengineering,* R. Skalak and S. Chien, eds. New York: McGraw-Hill, 1987, p.19.1-19.25.
Hoffler, G.W. Cardiovascular studies on U.S. space crews: an overview and perspective. In: *Cardiovascular Flow Dynamics and Measurements,* N.H.C. Hwang and N.A. Normann, eds. Baltimore: University Park Press, 1977,p.335-363.
Hyatt, K.H., and D.A. West. Reversal of bedrest-induced orthostatic intolerance by lower body negative pressure and saline. *Aviat. Space Environ. Med.* 48:120-124, 1977.
Johnson, P.C. Fluid volume changes induced by spaceflight. *Acta Astronautica* 6:1335-1341, 1979.
Keil, L.C., and S. Ellis. Plasma vasopressin and renin activity in women exposed to bed rest and $+G_z$ acceleration J. Appl. Physiol. 40:911-914, 1976.
Kimzey, S.L., C.L. Fischer, P.C. Johnson, S.E. Ritzmann, and C.E. Mengel. Hematology and immunology studies. In: *Biomedical Results of Apollo,* R.S. Johnston, L.F. Dietlein, and C.A. Berry, eds. NASA Special Publication 368, 1975, p. 197-226. National Aeronautics and Space Administration, Washington, DC.
Kotovskaya, A.R., S. Baranski, D. Gembizka, M. Voitkowjak, I.F. Vil-Vilyams, and N.I. Kokova. Improvement of human tolerance to head-pelvis ($+G_Z$) accelerations by increasing hydration. *Kosm. Biol. Aviakosm. Med.* 21:14-18, 1987.
Kravik, S.E., L.C. Keil, G. Geelen, C.E. Wade, P.R. Barnes, W.A. Spaul, C.A. Elder, and J.E. Greenleaf. Effect of antigravity suit inflation on cardiovascular, PRA, and PVP responses in humans. *J. Appl. Physiol.* 61:766-774, 1986.
Lambert, E.H., and E.H. Wood. The problem of blackout and unconsciousness in aviators. *Med. Clin. N. Am.* 30:833-844, 1946.
Leach, C.S., W.C. Alexander, and P.C. Johnson. Endocrine, electrolyte, and fluid volume changes associated with Apollo missions. In: *Biomedical Results from Apollo,* R.S. Johnston, I.F. Dietlein, and C.A. Berry, eds. NASA Special Publication 368, 1975,p. 163-184. National Aeronautics and Space Administration, Washington, DC.
Meehan, J.P., and W. Brandt. Para-amino hippurate and endogenous creatinine clearances in positive acceleration. *Aerospace Med.* 31:220-224, 1960.
Mellander, S., M. Maspers, J. Bjornberg, and L.-O. Andersson. Autoregulation of capillary pressure and filtration in cat skeletal muscle in states of normal and reduced vascular tone. *Acta Physiol. Scand.* 129:337-351, 1987.
Minners, H.A., W.K. Douglas, E.C. Knoblock, A. Graybiel, and W.R. Hawkins. Aeromedical preparation and results of postflight medical examinations. In: *Results of the First U.S. Manned Orbital Space Flight,* February 20, 1962, p.83-92. Manned Spacecraft Center, Houston, TX. National Aeronautics and Space Administration, Washington, DC.
Nishikimi, T., M. Kohno, T. Mastuura, K. Akioka, M. Teragaki, M. Yasuda, H. Oku, K. Takeuchi, and T. Takeda. Effect of exercise on circulating atrial natriuretic polypeptide in valvular heart disease. *Am. J. Cardiol.* 58:1119-1120, 1986.
Noble, R.L., and N.B.G. Taylor. Antidiuretic substances in human urine after haemorrhage, fainting, dehydration, and acceleration. *J. Physiol.* 122:220-237, 1953.

Ogihara, T., J. Shima, H. Hara, Y. Kumahara, K. Kangawa, and H. Matsuo. Changes in human plasma atrial natriuretic polypeptide concentration in normal subjects during passive leg raising and whole-body tilting. *Clin. Sci. Lond.* 71:147-150, 1986.

Oser, B.L. (ed.). *Hawk's Physiological Chemistry.* New York: McGraw-Hill, 1965.

Piemme, T.E., M. McCally, and A.S. Hyde. Renal response to $+G_z$ gradient acceleration in man. *Aerospace Med.* 37:1253-1256, 1966.

Rambaut, P.C., M.C. Smith, Jr., and H.O. Wheeler. Nutritional studies. In: *Biomedical Results of Apollo,* R.S. Johnston, L.F. Dietlein, and C.A. Berry, eds. NASA Special Publication 368, 1975,p.277-302. National Aernautics and Space Administration, Washington, DC.

Rogge, J.D., W.W. Moore, W.E. Segar, and A.F. Fasola. Effect of $+G_z$ and $+G_x$ acceleration on peripheral venous ADH levels in humans. *J. Appl. Physiol.* 23:870-873, 1967.

Rowell, L.B. Adjustments to upright posture and blood loss. In: *Human Circulation Regulation During Physical Stress,* by L.B. Rowell. New York: Oxford University Press, 1986, p.137-173.

Sejersted, O.M., A.R. Hargens, K.R. Kardel, P. Blom, Ø. Jensen, and L. Hermansen. Intramuscular fluid pressure during isometric contraction of human skeletal muscle. *J. Appl. Physiol.* 56:287-295, 1984.

Share, L. Role of vasopressin in cardiovascular regulation. *Physiol. Rev.* 68:1248-1284, 1988.

Shubrooks, S.J., Jr., M. Epstein, and D.C. Duncan. Effects of an anti-G suit on the hemodynamic and renal responses to positive ($+G_z$) acceleration. *J. Appl. Physiol.* 36:345-349, 1974.

Sjogaard, G. Water and electrolyte fluxes during exercise and their relation to muscle fatigue. *Acta Physiol. Scand.* 128, Suppl. 556: 129-136, 1986.

Sjogaard, G. Muscle energy metabolism and electrolyte shifts during low-level prolonged static contraction in man. *Acta Physiol. Scand.* 134:181-187, 1988.

Stauffer, F.R., and E.O. Errebo-Knudsen. Positive acceleration and urine output. *J. Aviat. Med.* 21:500-506, 1950.

Taliaferro, E.H., R.R. Wempen, and W.J. White. The effects of minimal dehydration upon human tolerance to positive acceleration. *Aerospace Med.* 36:922-926, 1965.

Tanaka, H., M. Shindo, J. Gutkowska, A. Kinoshita, H. Urata, M. Ikeda, and K. Arakawa. Effect of acute exercise on plasma immunoreactive-atrial natriuretic factor. *Life Sci.* 39:1685-1693, 1986.

Thornton, W.E., G.W. Hoffler, and J.A. Rummel. Anthropometric changes and fluid shifts. In: *Biomedical Results from Skylab,* R.S. Johnston and L.F. Dietlein, eds. NASA Special Publication 377, 1977, p.330-338. National Aeronautics and Space Administration, Washington, DC.

Thornton, W.E., and J. Ord. Physiological mass measurements in Skylab. In: *Biomedical Results from Skylab,* R.S. Johnston and L.F. Dietlein, eds. NASA Special Publication 377, 1977, p. 175-182. National Aeronautics and Space Administration, Washington, DC.

Van Beaumont, W., J.E. Greenleaf, H.L. Young, and L. Juhos. Plasma volume and blood constituent shifts during $+G_z$ acceleration after bed rest with exercise conditioning. *Aerospace Med.* 45:425-430, 1974.

Vartbaronov, R.A., G.D. Glod, N.N. Uglova, and I.S. Rolik. Human and animal hypovolemia reactions to increasing $+G_z$ accelerations. *Kosm. Biol. Aviakosm. Med.* 21:35-39, 1987.

Waligora, J.M. Physical forces generating acceleration, vibration, and impact. In: *The Physiological Basis for Spacecraft Environmental Limits,* J.M. Waligora, ed. NASA Reference Publication 1045, 1979, p. 71-107. National Aeronautics and Space Administration, Washington, DC.

Watson, J.F., and R.M. Rapp. Effect of forward acceleration on renal function. *J. Appl. Physiol.* 17:413-416, 1962.

Wood, E.H., E.F. Lindberg, C.F. Code, and E.J. Baldes. Effect of partial immersion in water on response of healthy men to headward acceleration. *J. Appl. Physiol.* 18:1171-1179, 1963.

Wood, E.H., W.F. Sutterer, and H.W. Marshall. Effect of headward and forward accelerations on the cardiovascular system. Wright Air Development Division *Technical Report* 60-634, 1961.

DISCUSSION

TIPTON: It was appropriate that John Greenleaf was selected to address the role of fluid and electrolytes with conditions of acceleration because he has been one of the few physiologists conducting research in this area. Unfortunately, the main concern of NASA and the military has been on interventions rather than mechanisms. Until recently, the focal point has been on G-tolerance and the selection of individuals who can achieve a tolerance of 9 G's.

In conjunction with Bernauer and others, John has been able to demonstrate an improved G-tolerance with isometric exercise training. Interestingly, females are as capable as males to tolerate high G-forces although we know very little about how age and disease will alter the process. Since elevated blood pressures appear to be an advantage against syncope, it is likely that hypertensive individuals would have an advantage when subjected to increasing acceleration forces.

Although Burton has shown that acceleration can cause cardiac a-v dissociation, we know very little about the responsible mechanism or about related aspects. I was surprised that none of the recent Russian literature was cited as it appears that G-tolerance is improved if plasma volume is expanded. Other than a possible increase in AVP release, there is very little information to explain this observation. Because of these and related matters, I hope that the presentation by Greenleaf will stimulate those present to initiate more research in this area so that our degree of understanding can achieve the level demonstrated in other topics discussed at this meeting.

GREENLEAF: One of the problems is that not everyone has a human centrifuge in their laboratory and there aren't too many operational machines in the United States. We are beginning to examine the effects of exercise during acceleration on fluid-electrolyte-endocrine responses under those conditions. There is an increase, of course, in the hydrostatic pressure and it may be easier to increase the level of plasma volume when you exercise under an increased hydrostatic load.

HARVEY: In conversation with a couple of flight surgeons, I learned that many fighter pilots have given up late night beer drinking and womanizing for endurance exercise. Many of these people are stationed at places that are hot and humid like Mearmar or a carrier in the Coral Sea. They tend to be highly competitive people, they go out for heavy duty runs, and from what has been said, it sounds like these people are frequently dehydrated. Since the state of hydration certainly relates to their ability to withstand these G-forces, has anyone looked at these people over several days of their sitting around in ready rooms and alternately endurance training in the heat? The other question is, would they be better off in the weight room doing heavy resistance exercise rather than running all the time?

GREENLEAF: I'm not familiar with all the literature involving pilots because NASA is interested mainly in slow onset and low levels of acceleration. I know that there have been at least three investigations on the influence of heavy endurance weight training exercise on high-onset acceleration tolerance. At the present time, fighter pilots utilize alternating isometric contractions during periods of increased acceleration, so that procedure becomes kind of an endurance exercise. When they utilize these isometric-isokinetic training routines on the ground, they can increase their in-flight acceleration tolerance. Every pilot knows that those with the greater acceleration tolerance survive longer in air combat. So perhaps increased survival potential indicates that they shouldn't be out all night. Of course, we still have the problem with the effect of aerobic exercise training on orthostatic tolerance. I'm not sure we want to get into that at this moment. But it's quite interesting that some athletes, some long distance runners for instance, have low orthostatic tolerance. One of the questions we haven't actually answered is whether or not we should ask astronaut pilots to engage in strenuous endurance training that might result in lower orthostatic tolerance on re-entry. Our work indicates that there is no relationship between these two factors; because some athletes have lower orthostatic tolerance doesn't mean that it's because of the exercise training; it could be due to a number of other things.

TIPTON: I have some information that might provide some insight on the nature of your question. Within the past year, the Armed Forces held a conference on the topic of physical fitness and the fighter pilot. Matters of training, acceleration G-forces, and injuries were discussed in some detail before a conference manual was written and distributed to fighter pilots in the respective services (USAFSAM-SR-881 and NAMRL-1334; *Physical Fitness Program to Enhance Aircrew G Tolerance*). It was the consensus of those present that the exercise prescription for fighter pilots should be one that advocates muscle power activities and maximum isometric contractions rather than long-term endurance exercises of events. The rationale was that the responsiveness of the baroreceptors are altered by endurance training and that muscle pressor responses are enhanced by isometric contractions and power activities.

Although the ideal hydrostatic position for a fighter pilot is to fly while in a horizontal position (on his back), they refuse to do so because of the difficulty in determining whether the "enemy" is behind them. Hence, pilots fly in a seated position so they can rapidly turn to look in all directions. Because of these factors, they experience an excessive number of neck injuries, are prone to syncope, and must combine valsalva maneuvers and isometric contractions to prevent loss of consciousness during high G-forces.

SUTTON: You mentioned the importance of the valsalva maneuver to counteract the effects of the added G-forces. The actual gain in pressure from that is rather modest compared with what you would gain by doing isometric contraction.

GREENLEAF: The valsalva maneuver is a near maximal isometric contraction of all trunk and limb muscles held during the increased G-stress, then released. So they don't have to endure the increased G's too long at any one time.

SUTTON: What is the effect of training on orthostatic hypotension? If you train a group of average people do they develop orthostatic intolerance?

CONVERTINO: Peter Raven with co-workers have recently reported the incidence of syncopal episodes in a cross-sectional comparison of three fitness groups: 1) a high fitness group of competitive runners with $\dot{V}O_2max$ over 65–70 mL/kg/min; 2) a middle fitness group; and 3) very sedentary subjects with $\dot{V}O_2max$ less than 30 mL/kg/min. As many subjects in the low fitness group fainted as in the high fitness group with no fainters in the middle fitness group. We have recently completed a series of studies that address this issue. In a longitudinal endurance exercise training study, we purposely selected subjects with middle fitness levels because that represents the level of fitness of the average astronaut population, i.e., average $\dot{V}O_2max$ of about 45 mL/kg/min. We trained 16 subjects with an average $\dot{V}O_2max$ of 40 Ml/kg/min using endurance-type activity (30 min/day, 4 days/week for 10 weeks of cycling at 70%–80% $\dot{V}O_2$ max), which increased their $\dot{V}O_2$ max by 20%. We observed no change in the high pressure baroreflex response, but found a reduction in the low pressure baroreflex control of vascular resistance which was correlated with the increase in plasma and blood volume. This work was conducted in collaboration with Ethan Nadel and Gary Mack at the John Pierce Foundation. In a subsequent study, we found that acute hypovolemia of the magnitude that astronauts experience during spaceflight (about 15%) reduces the reserve capacity for vasoconstriction controlled by the low pressure baroreflexes. These data suggest that an important role of the hypervolemic response to training is its effect of increasing vasoconstrictive reserve capacity under any particular orthostatic stress and helps defend against the development of hypotension. Against expectations, orthostatic tolerance was increased following this endurance exercise training, which is contradictory to some of the published cross-sectional data. However, our results are consistent with previous data that demontrate that half of the longitudinal training studies reported in the literature (10 total) resulted in no change in orthostatic tolerance while the other half showed an increase (reported in Volume 15 of *Exercise and Sport Science Reviews*). All of the studies that demonstrated increased orthostatic tolerance used cycle ergometry as the mode of training while those that did not change tolerance used running for their training regimen. Some interesting trends are developing. Clearly, our data demonstrate that individuals with average fitness levels can undertake an endurance training regimen that significantly increases their aerobic capacity without compromising blood pressure control mechanisms and their orthostatic tolerance. We now believe that there may be a U-shaped relation between fitness ($\dot{V}O_2max$ as the independent variable) and incidences of fainting (dependent variable). The incidence of fainters appears to increase with very sedentary individuals, is small with average fit subjects, and increases again with individuals who are endurance athletes with high aerobic capacities.

SUTTON: You've used the end point of syncopy in this particular scenario.

GREENLEAF: That is a very important point; i.e., syncopy.

SUTTON: That is obviously the clinical end point that is most relevant. Is there a difference in the drop in arterial pressure that is required to produce syncopy in these groups? In other words, is there a change in sensitivity of the brain to blood pressure change or the level to which blood pressure falls?

CONVERTINO: I don't think so. If systolic blood pressure falls below 80mmHg, we observe them very carefully. That is about the point that most subjects experience syncopy.

GREENLEAF: During the tilt-table test, we measure blood pressure with the cuff technique over a 30-sec period of time. We tried to measure it at the time the individual exhibited presyncopal symptoms, so there is considerable variability. If one looks at the mean data, syncope occurs at a mean arterial pressure of about 60 mmHg. We do all the laboratory testing of syncopy on the centrifuge with the subjects riding without muscular contraction. With muscular contraction, the subject can alter the end point almost any way you like. Under flight conditions, pilots employ muscular contraction to increase their tolerance, but that is not the way to do the testing.

SCHEDL: I thought that there may be some special value to the calcium and magnesium measurements that you made during those hemorrhage experiments. With reinfusion, you get a very large increase in ionized and total calcium and you also get a nice increase in magnesium, all of which might be important. Could that relate to the kind of anticoagulant you use in the blood that was drawn or is there some other explanation?

GREENLEAF: We used Na-Heparin as the anti-coagulant.

SCHEDL: Was it citrated?

GREENLEAF: It was not citrated. Obviously the hemorrhage removed some ions over a period of 20–45 minutes concurrent with some inflow of interstitial fluid. So the plasma volume was changing continually; i.e., increasing following hemorrhage. Reinfusion probably resulted in some hypervolemia, so the ion content would be higher when compared with control levels.

SCHEDL: It really seemed to give a very positive retroaction of those ions.

GREENLEAF: Actually, we were adding additional ions.

NADEL: Actually, I wanted to make an observation that this is one discipline where the engineers seem to be way ahead of the physiologist; the use of G-suits seems to be protecting the fighter pilots to a much greater extent than the physiological incidence. Is that true or not true?

GREENLEAF: One G? Perhaps 1 1/2. Probably not true, but a clear answer is difficult. G-suits add 1.0-1.5 G's to $+G_3$ tolerance in hydrated pilots. Isometic contractions about the same amount. Dehydration lowers $+G_2$ tolerance by 20-30% in ambulatory subjects and up to 40% in bed-rested subjects.

NADEL: I'd also add something. In our cross-sectional study published by Gary Mack two years ago, we found that the cardiopulmonary baroreflex sensitivity to changes in central venous pressure induced by lower body negative pressure was lower in fit poeple than in unfit people. What this means practically is that as gravitational stress is increased, fit people constrict the peripheral vascular bed less to a given decrease in CVP than unfit people. This would seem to put them at a disadvantage. Vic implied that fit people have a much larger blood volume. The trade-off then was that the elevated blood volume compensated for the decreased sensitivity to some extent. A longitudinal study now has provided more information about this. The question is whether the decreased cardiopulmonary baroreflex sensitivity is a response to elevated blood volume or a response in some way to training. This is still, in my view, an open question. We have preliminary data from a study that Brian Quigley just finished in our lab that speaks to the former hypothesis . . . that the change in sensitivity is a response to the elevated blood volume. But there is no way to predict where the advantages lie. Expansion of blood volume may be advantageous in some domains, but the change in cardiopulmonary baroreflex sensitivity may counteract the advantage.

GREENLEAF: To some degree. But I always advocate that we should increase plasma volume to the highest level possible to have some reserve.

NADEL: I tend to agree with you on this point.

GREENLEAF: I just want to add one more comment. Three years ago, we tested tilt-table tolerance in middle-aged men, the astronaut type, before and after 6 months of physical training of progressively increasing intensity. Maximal oxygen uptake increased by about 18%, but tilt tolerance was unchanged.

WADE: One point is that it did not change their plasma volume.

GREENLEAF: True. We did not see an increase in plasma volume. If plasma volume did rise, the increase was eliminated by the time we reached the end of the experiment.

BUSKIRK: We talked about the acceleration problem, and you alluded to the role of rehydration prior to re-entry. Since we are interested in rehydration, what happens to blood volume after rehydration and during re-entry? What is the thinking with respect to fluid replacement both during the flight and prior to re-entry?

GREENLEAF: I hesitate to offer an answer, but perhaps for a few hours ahead of reentry, salt tablets and water. That's not the best rehydration fluid, but it seems to work and the astronauts will use it. The other question is whether the astronauts are dehydrated according to Earth standards if they are in microgravity long enough; do they reach some level of adaptation? When does this particular hypohydration level become the ordinary euhydration level? When we think about a hydration regimen for astronauts in flight, we must hyperhydrate someone who is already adequately hydrated, even though his total body water is reduced. That indicates we would need a drink composition of something other than what we ordinarily use for someone who is dehydrated on Earth.

GISOLFI: As a follow-up to that question; didn't you and William Van Beaumont develop a fluid replacement beverage for space flight and re-entry?

GREENLEAF: That was during preparation for a bed rest study in 1971. We wanted to find a good rehydration drink to overcome the hypohydration induced by prolonged bed rest. We tried Gatorade, but the hydrated subjects diuresed it after about 15 minutes. The final drink was isotonic saline in grapefruit juice concentrate with an osmolality of about 600 mosm. At the end of best rest, we had a number of hours of rehydration, so we gave them about 1.5 L over these hours, put them on centrifuge, and restored about 3/4 of the loss in $+G_z$ acceleration tolerance. It seemed to work even though its osmolality was very high. The probable reason that Gatorade caused diuresis was the loss of osmols due to metabolism of the carbohydrate content; that eliminated the higher osmolality and it then acted much like water.

TIPTON: In response to Buskirk's question on the Russian research, recent reports show they are ingesting a saline solution before entry and re-entry conditions.

BUSKIRK: Is anything being done in terms of nutritional guidance concerning the diets of the astronauts including the salt in their food products? In the military, I know, there is a serious problem with salt in many of the rations because salt is used as a preservative.

GREENLEAF: The astronauts' diet is formulated at Johnson Space Center. I assume that they have almost normal intake of all necessary foodstuffs, and the daily caloric content is about 3,100 kcal. However, the astronauts will not always eat everything, so we never quite know their daily intake. That could be one aspect of the problem with maintaining hydration because food and fluid intake go together.

HARVEY: I think it's interesting how salt tablets keep cropping up; they're starting to sneak into our scientific research and the guys in the field are using them. I gave Nadel the prescription off the labels for the salt tablets of how they are to be used and I have to admit that the way I got those was that I walked into our football training room and there they were right on the table; our coaches and trainers use them. I try to discourage it, but I have as much effect as you do in discouraging it in your astronauts. It's interesting. Football coaches find that if people use them, they maintain their weight; it also worked for the astronauts. One of the things I've learned from this conference is that we may be bringing salt tablets back out of the closet, with the appropriate water use I hope.

GREENLEAF: Hopefully the concentration is below isotonic so any current hyperosmolality is not accentuated. The problem with allowing free access to salt tablets and water is that the subjects during or after a stress will take the salt, but involuntary dehydration may inhibit consumption of an adequate volume of fluid to dilute the salt to at least isotonicity. That is why premixed drinks are better.

10

Brain Mechanisms in the Control of Body Fluid Homeostasis

ALAN KIM JOHNSON, PH.D.

INTRODUCTION: THE BIOLOGICAL PROBLEM OF INTERMITTENT SUPPLY AND FLUCTUATING DEMAND

Under normal conditions animals eat and drink intermittently. Between the post-absorptive phase when hydro-mineral balance is optimum and the next period of repletion, both intrinsic and behavioral controls operate to optimize and restore body water and sodium. The processes that minimize the effects of fluid and salt loss and ensure periodic restoration involve the coordinated participation of endocrine, neural, and behavioral mechanisms. Orchestration of the multiple control systems involved in the maintenance of fluid balance requires the integrative action of the central nervous system (see Figure 10-1).

The regulatory processes that maintain hydro-mineral homeostasis operate in the face of a wide range of environmental challenges. Immediately after the theoretical moment of homeostatic balance, animals begin to endure water and ionic losses to the environment through the nephron, skin, gastrointestinal tract, and lungs. The kidneys are the only route of dissipation on which appreciable physiological control can be exercised. The rate of water and sodium loss can be reduced by the renal action of water- and sodium-retaining hormones and through modulation of efferent sympathetic renal nerve activity.

Total body sodium and water may be excessive at various times. Accordingly, mechanisms that increase the loss of solute and water are activated. If the balance between sodium and water becomes disturbed, a pattern of neural and hormonal mediators is generated to effect a disproportionate loss of one versus the other in an attempt to restore an appropriate sodium concentration. Although intrinsic or reflexive water and sodium conservation and balancing mechanisms may provide a temporizing action, it is only through mobilization of motivated behaviors of seeking and consuming water and salt that repletion occurs. The activation of renal, sudomotor, and behavioral defenses to ensure fluid balance requires sensing and responding to intrinsic stimuli that function as signals to the brain of the organism's hydrational status. The nature of these stimuli, their receptors, the signaling modality from these receptors to the brain, and the processing of receptor-derived information by the central nervous system are the topics of this review.

CELLULAR AND EXTRACELLULAR FLUID COMPARTMENTS AND THEIR SIGNALING MECHANISMS

Environmental challenges produce water loss from both the cellular and the extracellular fluid compartments. An animal at rest in a thermoneutral setting loses water and sodium to the environment. Exercise and

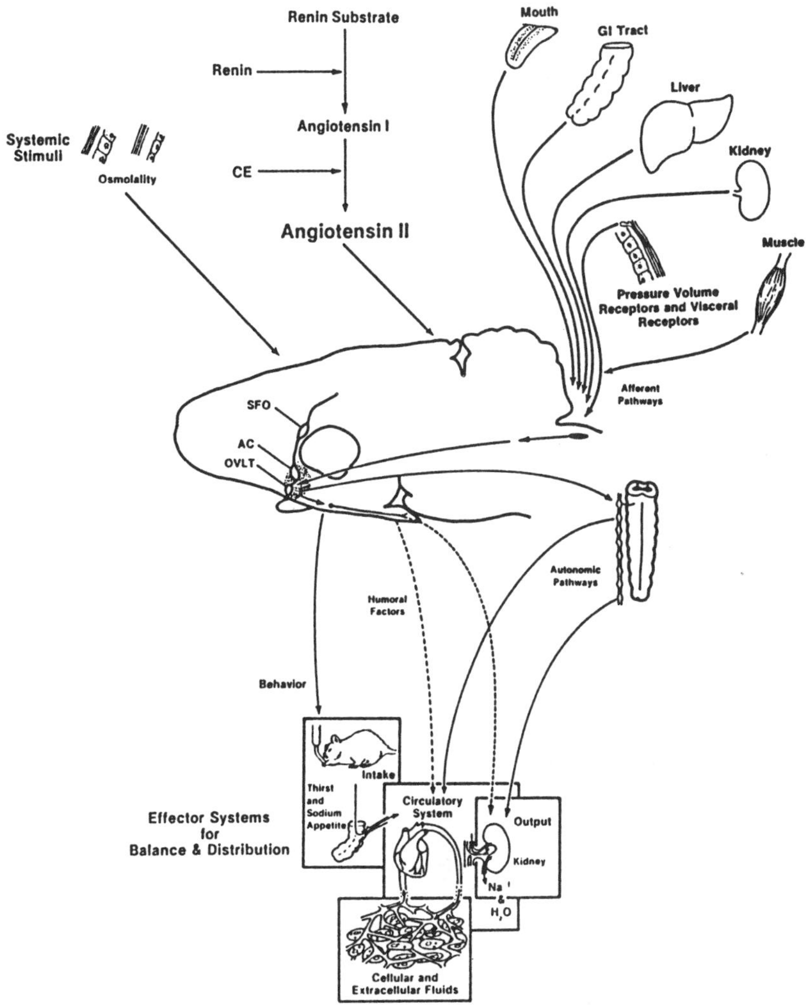

FIGURE 10-1. *A representation of the major behavioral, endocrine and neural mechanisms involved in the control of body fluid balance. The brain receives information about hydrational status in the form of both humoral and neural input. Humoral input includes changes in extracellular osmolality and/or sodium concentration and plasma angiotensin II levels. Neural input arises from various visceral sources including the gastrointestinal tract and cardiovascular system. Body water and sodium losses are repleted by the activation of drinking and salt ingestive behaviors. In states of sodium and water deficits both neural and hormonal mechanisms act on the kidneys to promote optimum retention of these substances. Conversely, if water and sodium are in excess, neural and hormonal processes facilitate their loss.*

The humoral and neural information reflecting body hydro-mineral status converges in the central nervous system and is integrated so that, in light of momentary conditions, an appropriate pattern of effector activity is generated to optimize available resources and restore body fluid homeostasis.

environmental challenges act to accelerate dehydration and sodium depletion. Since the ratio of salt to water loss is variable, depending on a host of factors (e.g., momentary hydrational state, humidity, renal function, rate of sweat or saliva loss, etc.), the relative depletion of the cellular and extracellular body fluid compartments at any moment is variable. As fluid loss proceeds, efferent controls act through the kidneys to determine the ratio of sodium to water loss and to establish the relative amount of dehydration suffered by each compartment. The cellular space can be spared at the expense of extracellular fluid by the induction of a natriuresis. Conversely, retention of sodium causes a shift of water out of the cells into the extracellular space (Figure 10-2). Because of the high degree of coupling between the cellular and extracellular fluids and the unique homeostatic requirements of each, it is not surprising to find that both spaces generate unique stimuli that serve as signals to enable the CNS to receive unconfounded appraisals from each compartment.

Studies of the mechanisms underlying the generation of thirst and drinking behavior led investigators nearly 20 years ago to the formulation of the *double depletion hypothesis* (Epstein, 1973). This hypothesis stated that water intake results from a sufficient (i.e., above threshold) dehydration of *either* the cellular fluid compartment *or* the extracellular fluid compartment of the body. Although the double depletion hypothe-

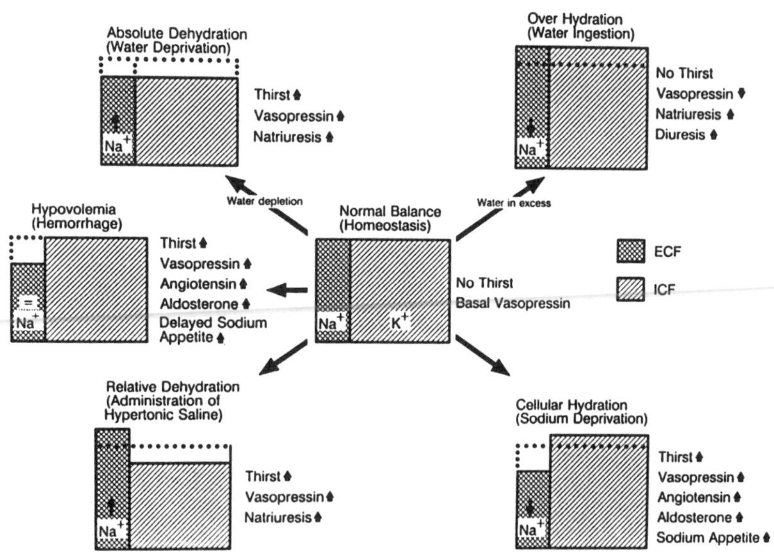

FIGURE 10-2. *Diagrams of changes in body fluid distribution and composition as a result of manipulations that produce negative and positive water and sodium balances. Above each diagram is a description of the body fluid status and an example of a manipulation used to induce it. To the right of the diagram is an indication of the control actions elicited attempting to compensate for or correct the disturbance. ECF=extracellular fluid compartment; ICF=intracellular fluid compartment; thirst=drinking water; sodium appetite =ingestion of sodium (adapted from Andersson, 1971; and Rolls & Rolls, 1982).*

sis was more formally articulated as a heuristic to account for thirst, it has also been applied to the study of various control mechanisms (e.g., antidiuretic hormone) involved in body fluid regulation (e.g., see Robertson, 1977).

The tactical use of the double depletion hypothesis in the analysis of the physiological controls of body fluid homeostasis makes it possible to specify a momentary hydrational state in terms of the status of the cellular and extracellular compartments. An important corollary of the double depletion hypothesis is that the regulatory responses of the body to correct dehydration depend only upon the existence of compartmental deficits and not how these deficits were induced. Various experimental strategies have been developed to manipulate both independently and in combination the hydrational status of each fluid compartment (see Figure 10-2). These experimental manipulations make it possible to investigate the various types of internal stimuli, which indicate the hydrational status of respective fluid compartments and activate systemic and central receptors that mediate the regulatory responses.

The experiments of Gilman (1937) demonstrated that the property of solutions to create an effective osmotic gradient across cells was the critical variable that produced drinking in dogs infused with hypertonic solutions. Hypertonic NaCl caused the dehydration of cells and drinking, whereas equiosomolar urea, which is not excluded from cells, was notably less effective as a stimulus for water intake. Studies by Gilman and Goodman (1937) also defined dehydration induced by water deprivation and by hypertonic saline in the control of the antidiuretic response that results from the action of pituitary-released vasopressin (VP) on the kidneys.

The nature and general location of the receptors hypothesized to mediate the responses to increased osmolality were first hypothesized by Verney (1946; 1947) as a result of experiments employing arterial injections to the head and brain. Verney proposed the existence of a cephalic receptor that was sensitive to osmotic changes, that is, an osmoreceptor. Although the cephalic osmoreceptor has enjoyed the most theoretical and experimental attention over the years, it should be noted that there are also many receptors located in the periphery that are sensitive to osmolality and/or sodium concentration.

Rydin and Verney (1938) were the first to provide evidence that hemorrhage is a potent stimulus for VP release. In comparison to hyperosmolality, hypovolemia induced by blood loss is a markedly more potent stimulus for elevating plasma levels of VP (Share, 1974). Hemorrhage is an effective stimulus for release of this antidiuretic hormone even in the absence of hypotension and vice versa (Share, 1974). Both neural and humoral afferent mechanisms have been hypothesized to mediate the release of VP in response to hypovolemia/hypotension. The best characterized neural afferent signals derive from receptors located in both the high and low pressure sides of the vascular system (see below).

In addition to releasing VP, reduced input from pressure/volume receptors also activates the renin-angiotensin system. Elevated levels of circulating angiotensin (ANG) II may contribute to VP release in the hypovolemic/hypotensive animal. Bonjour and Malvin (1970) demonstrated that systemic infusions of ANG II in pharmacological doses release VP. Although some investigators have not replicated this observation (Claybaugh, Share & Shimizu, 1973), others have reported reliability (Ramsay, Keil, Sharpe & Shinasko, 1978).

The question of whether ANG II participates in VP release when administered at physiological doses remains unresolved. However, particular atention must be paid to the status of extracellular volume (Ramsay, 1982) and blood pressure (Mitchell et al., 1982). Ramsay (1982) has suggested that the reason some studies do not demonstrate VP release by ANG II is that the presence of an inadvertent volume expansion will markedly inhibit VP secretion to large doses of ANG II. The effects of "contradictory" pressor input on VP release have been deduced from observations made in electrophysiological recording studies. Supraoptic magnocellular neurons (putatively vasopressinergic) are activated by low, non-pressor doses of intravenous ANG II, whereas pressor doses cause brief activation of the cells followed by an inhibition of neuronal firing as pressure begins to rise (Mitchell et al., 1985) (Figure 10-3). Furthermore, removal of high pressure feedback by deafferentation of the arterial baroreceptors produces only excitation of the magnocellular neurons, even to pressor doses of intravenous angiotensin (Mitchell, et al., 1982). These results suggest that in states of dehydration/hypovolemia, when pressure is in the normotensive to hypotensive range (but certainly not hypertensive), there is no conflicting information arising from pressure/volume components in which case a contribution to VP release from elevated ANG II may be realized.

Another hormonal response to hemorrhage is the activation of the pituitary-adrenal axis. Hypovolemia and/or hypotension is a potent releaser of ACTH (Gann, Ward & Carlson, 1978). Corticotropic releasing hormone (CRF) is released into pituitary portal vessels in response to blood loss (Plotsky & Vale, 1984). Both adrenal mineralocorticoids (e.g., aldosterone) and glucocorticoids (e.g., cortisol) are stimulated by ACTH (see Muller, 1988, for review). Aldosterone acts on the kidneys to promote sodium retention (Gross, 1974; see below). Cortisol, among its many actions, acts to affect the distribution of fluids between the cellular and extracellular compartments (Swingle et al., 1959) and maintains vascular reactivity to pressor hormones (Espiner, 1987).

For many years the question of whether thirst (operationally defined as drinking) was generated by pure hypovolemia remained unanswered.

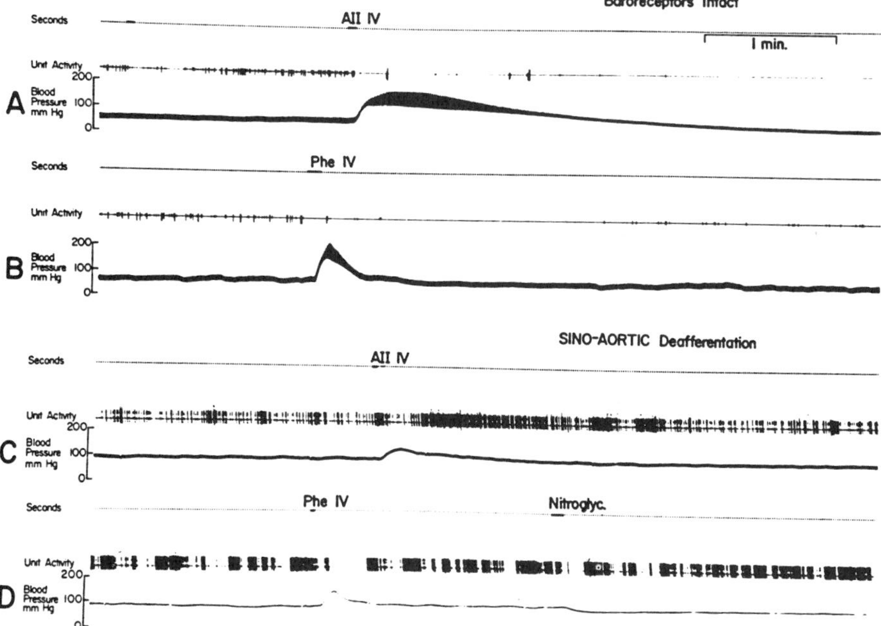

FIGURE 10-3. *The effect of systemic angiotensin II (AII) and phenylephrine (Phe) on activity of identified magnocellular neurons in the supraoptic nucleus in intact rats and in rats without high pressure baroreceptors (e.g., sino-aortic deafferentation—SAD). A. In intact animal, AII administered to raise blood pressure by 50 mmHg caused inhibition of a magnocellular neuron. B. In intact animal, Phe titrated to raise blood pressure by same amount also inhibited a magnocellular neuron. C. In SAD rat, AII (12 ug/kg) raised blood pressure by about 50 mmHg and caused excitation of a magnocellular neuron. D. In SAD rat Phe (0.6 ug/kg) raised blood pressure to the same level (140 mmHg) without excitation of the magnocellular neuron. Nitroglycerine (Nitroglyc) reduced blood pressure but did not affect the neuron's activity (from Mitchell et al., 1982).*

Experiments studying the effects of hemorrhage on drinking had produced equivocal results. Considering the fact that hemorrhaged animals are anemic and as a consequence likely to manifest a non-specific disruption of behavior, it is easy to realize why hypovolemia induced in this manner may not reliably generate thirst. By administering hyperoncotic colloids (e.g., gum acacia; polyethylene glycol) into the interperitoneal cavity to sequester isotonic plasma, Fitzsimons (1961) was able to definitely demonstrate the efficacy of hypovolemia as a dipsogenic stimulus. Drinking generated by producing an isotonic-hypovolemia is highly correlated with the size of the reduction of extracellular fluid volume (Stricker, 1966).

The afferent stimuli that mediate the drinking response to hypovolemia are in all likelihood the same as those involved in VP release. Beginning with the insightful work of Fitzsimons (1969), there has been a steady progression of experiments that have implicated circulating ANG II as one of the participating contributors to increased thirst associated with hypovolemia or hypotension (Fitzsimons & Simons, 1969; Houpt & Epstein, 1971; Hsiao, Epstein & Camardo, 1977; Mann, Johnson & Ganten, 1980; Johnson, et al., 1981; Rettig, Ganten & Johnson, 1981; Johnson, Robinson & Mann, 1986; Mann et al., 1987) (Figure 10-4). Although Fitzsimons (1970) speculated that ANG acts to sensitize systemic baroreceptors, the discovery of the potent dipsogenic action of ANG when applied directly to the brain (Booth, 1968; Epstein, Fitzsimons, & Rolls, 1970) placed the immediate focus of attention on the central nervous system (CNS).

Because nephrectomized rats drink nearly as much water in response to hypovolemia as intact animals (Fitzsimons, 1961), it has been

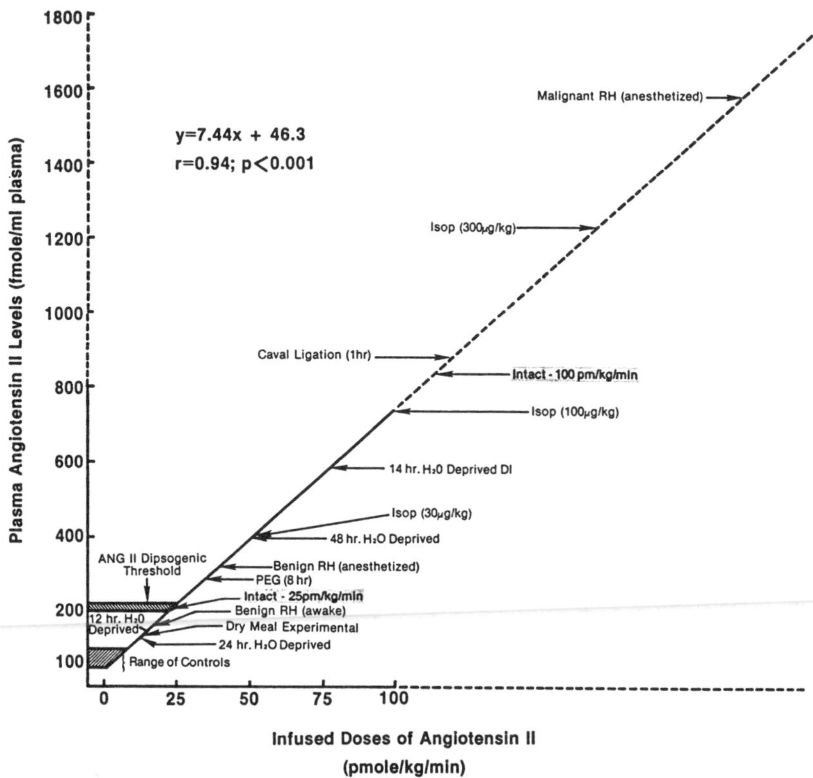

FIGURE 10-4. *Relationship between infused doses of ANG II (abscissa) and ANG II concentrations measured in plasma (ordinate) with plasma levels of ANG II produced by various thirst stimuli indicated along the regression line. Intact 25 pmol/kg/min and 100 pmol/kg/min indicates level of circulating ANG II after 60-min infusion into unanesthetized rats with kidneys intact. Upper shaded area represents approximate ANG II plasma level at dipsogenic threshold. The threshold at which ANG II induces drinking with iv infusion was established by Hsaio, Epstein & Camardo (1977). As can be seen from the regression line, plasma ANG II levels surpass the dipsogenic threshold for ANG II after between 24 and 48 h of water deprivation. Abbreviations: DI=diabetes insipidus; RH=renal hypertension; PEG=polyethylene glycol; ISOP=isoproterenol (from Mann et al., 1980; Johnson et al., 1986).*

presumed that vascular pressure/volume receptors are important in mediating extracellular depletion-induced thirst (Fitzsimons, 1972). There is also evidence that nephrectomized animals drink to controlled hypotension in the absence of hypovolemia (Hosutt, Rowland & Stricker, 1978, Rettig et al., 1981).

As indicated earlier, the volume and distribution of water throughout the body is markedly influenced by the total amount and also the concentrations of extracellular sodium. As is the case for a water deficit, sodium reduction activates both renal and behavioral defenses to minimize loss and achieve a restoration of balance. Sodium conservation, in part, arises from activation of the renin angiotensin system (RAS) to enhance synthesis and release of aldosterone (Davis, 1974). ANG II at low concentrations as well as aldosterone acts on the kidneys to promote sodium reabsorption (Harris & Navar, 1985).

Hydro-mineral balance can be directly affected through alterations in autonomic outflow. Renal sympathetic efferent nerve activity is one of the important controlling mechanisms of renin release (see DiBona, 1982, for review). Efferent renal nerves also contribute to the control of reabsorption of sodium by the kidneys. Increases in nerve activity produce a parallel increase in renal tubular water and sodium reabsorption which are mediated by adrenergic nerve terminals in contact with the renal tubular epithelial cells (DiBona, 1982, for review).

Sodium deficiency generates an appetite that is specific for sodium. This hunger becomes manifest with the animal's first experience with sodium deficiency (Denton, 1982). Although sodium deficiency-induced avidity for salt can be modified by experience, it is not a learned preference (Denton, 1982). Various humoral and neural peripheral-CNS signaling mechanisms have been proposed as afferent stimuli facilitating and inhibiting sodium appetite. These include both hormonal mechanisms and the response of sodium receptors to changes in sodium concentration (see Denton, 1982 for review). Recent experimental findings suggest important roles for the action of ANG II and aldosterone (Epstein, 1982; Fregly & Rowland, 1985). Epstein (Epstein, 1982; Epstein & Sakai, 1987) has emphasized that there is a synergistic action between the peptide and steroid hormones in the induction of sodium appetite. Because ANG II and aldosterone are elevated in states of sodium deficiency, their contributions to sodium appetite seem to provide a biologically consistent behavioral response complementing the renal actions of these hormones.

Overingestion of water or salt in the face of impaired excretion has the potential for dire consequences. Dilution of the fluid matrix can produce water intoxication if excretion is not appropriately brisk. For example, rats with renal mechanisms "clamped" with exogenous VP have been shown to ingest sufficient quantities of a palatable saccharine solution to induce severe hyponatremia and osmotic dilution (Rolls, Wood &

Stevens, 1978). Water and sodium administered at rates inappropriately high for the capacity of the kidneys to excrete them has been demonstrated repeatedly to result in arterial hypertension (Guyton et al., 1974; Hall et al., 1986). Under normal circumstances both osmotic and extracellular pressure-related mechanisms operate to inhibit water intake (Stricker, 1969; Robinson & Evered, 1987). Similarly, VP secretion is inhibited by decreased osmolality or volume expansion (Gauer & Henry, 1963; Share, 1974; Robertson, 1977).

It has long been hypothesized (Smith, 1957) that elevated total body sodium increases the levels of a "third factor" to enhance the excretion of sodium; in other words, a natriuretic factor. Many established hormones, such as VP, oxytocin, adrenocorticotrophic hormone (ACTH), and gamma-melanocyte stimulating hormone (γ-MSH), have been proposed as natriuretic substances from experiments where pharmacological doses were usually employed. In addition, several substances that have been extracted or partially isolated seemed to hold promise of being "the" natriuretic agent (Buckalew & Gruber, 1984). Many of these known and unknown factors are still under serious investigation as candidates for humoral mediators of sodium loss. It is worth pointing out that several of the potential natriuretic substances are neurohormones that are often released in conjunction with one another. Because some combinations of these hormones (e.g., oxytocin and VP; Balment, et al., 1986) show potentiation of their natriuretic capacity when co-administered, natriuresis may in fact be managed by a patterned hormonal release rather than a single factor.

Within the last decade a substance has been discovered that is a serious contender to be considered as a natriuretic hormone. deBold (1982) was the first to draw attention to the natriuretic action of extracts of heart atria which have now become identified as atrial natriuretic peptide (ANP), among other names. With the power of modern peptide and molecular biochemistry the extraction, biochemical identification, synthesis, identification of messenger RNA, and mode of release of ANP quickly ensued (Needleman et al., 1985). The role of this material in the control of sodium and water balance under physiological and pathophysiological conditions is presently a topic of major research commitment. At the present time there is no strong evidence that release of ANP is under control of the nervous system. However, ANP or a related peptide, brain natriuretic peptide (Saper et al., 1989) may have actions in the CNS (Saper et al., 1985).

Clearly, the volumes of the cellular and the extracellular compartments play both joint and independent roles in the excitation and inhibition of the major controls of fluid balance. Differential loss of salt and water over time is influenced greatly by the immediate antecedent conditions, the behavioral state (e.g., exercise) of the animal and its environment (e.g., ambient temperature). The precise mix of cellular vs. extracellular hydration varies greatly and, in turn, different control actions are initiated. A better understanding of how the brain receives the information required to activate appropriate patterns of control responses to achieve this end and an appreciation of the different receptor systems and afferent routes to the central nervous system will be useful.

TARGET ISSUES, RECEPTORS, AND AFFERENT SIGNALING

A. Gastrointestinal Tract

Water and salt enter the body through the mouth of mammals. It is not surprising to find afferent mechanisms that appraise the organism of the nature of what it is ingesting. The hedonic quality of liquids and food markedly influences the quantities consumed (Young, 1967). Palatable substances evoke response patterns characterized by approach behaviors and oral responses consistent with ingestion and swallowing. Unpalatable substances, when placed in the mouth, evoke a behavioral sequence of aversive responses (Grill & Berridge, 1985). Specific taste receptors and the coding of afferent input for salty, sweet, sour, and bitter, participate to provide appropriate positive or negative feedback to influence the quantity consumed which, depending upon the amount of water and salt contained in ingesta, can influence hydro-mineral intake (Figure 10-5). There is also evidence for afferent nerves from the mouth being specifically activated by salt (Pfaffman & Bare, 1950) and water (Cohen, Hagiwara & Zotterman, 1955).

Ora-pharyngeal mechanisms play a significant role in controlling the volume ingested by a mechanism which appears to compute the volume consumed. Oral metering of water has been shown to be most remarkable in animals that are rapid drinkers, such as the dog (rats and man are slow drinkers). Adolph (1939) demonstrated that a water-deprived dog drinks in 5 min a quantity sufficient to restore the fluid deficit, even though minimal systemic effects of the rehydration are realized within that short time (Thrasher et al., 1981).

In addition to the influences on ingestive responses, substances that stimulate the oral cavity can rapidly alter the response of other physiological controls of body fluid homeostasis. For example, Nicolaidis (1969) demonstrated in humans an immediate increase in perspiration and increased urine flow after placing water in the oral cavity. More recently, Thrasher and colleagues (1981) have found that water-deprived dogs reduce VP levels almost immediately after they begin to drink. The reduction in circulating VP occurs even when the ingested water is immediately removed from the animal via a stomach fistula. The results indicate that rapid inhibition of VP is dependent solely on oral-pharyngeal factors. It is interesting to note that in contrast to the effects on VP secretion, water intake does not immediately suppress water

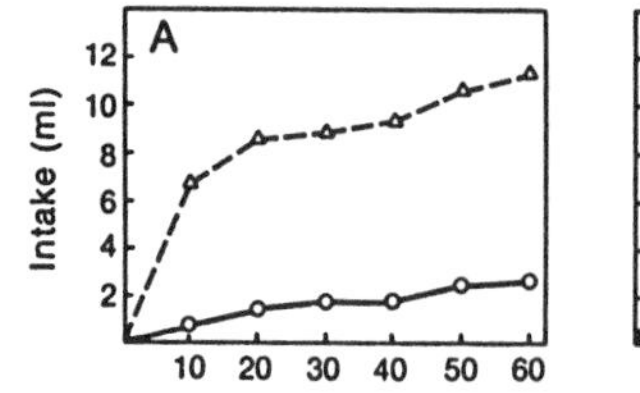

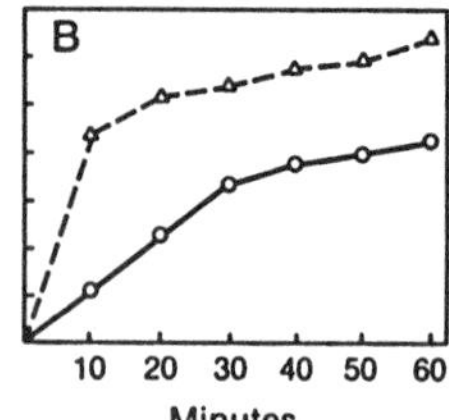

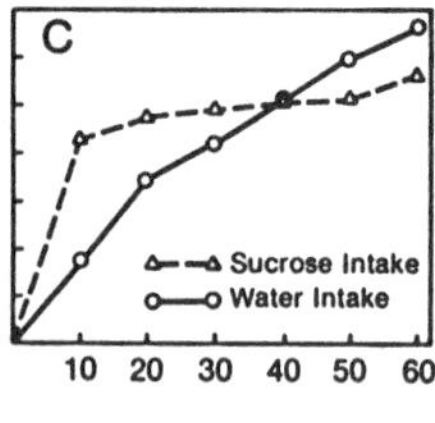

FIGURE 10-5. *An example of the interaction of fluid palatability and gastrointestinal inhibitory factors that determine the drinking pattern and fluid preference after 1 h of access to a 27% w/V sucrose solution and distilled water in rats deprived of water (but not food) for 11 (panel A), 23 (panel B), and 47 (panel C) h. After water deprivation, rats (n=12) were exposed to a 2-bottle choice test of water and sucrose solution. Nearly all the water-deprived rats began the drinking session by ingesting the sucrose solution. After a sustained bout of sucrose solution intake (i.e., of about 10 min duration), the animals began to switch to water probably because of gastric inhibition due to the osmolality of the sucrose solution (Mook, 1963). The sucrose intake is asymptotic after approximately 10 min and animals tend to restore their remaining fluid deficit by ingesting water. The greater the period of water deprivation the more likely an animal will show a "water preference", as typically defined, at the conclusion of the test period (Johnson & Fisher, 1973).*

deprivation-induced elevations of plasma renin activity in either dog (Thrasher et al., 1981) or sheep (Blair-West et al., 1979).

The stomach and lower gastrointestinal tract contain receptors that are sensitive to volume and osmolality. Such receptors have been shown to be especially effective in the reflex release of numerous digestive and metabolic hormones. Consequently, it is likely that such receptors may also modulate the intake of sodium and water (see Chapter 3 by Costill and Chapter 4 by Gisolfi in this volume). Inhibitory effects are clearly apparent, because water placed directly into the stomach immediately decreases subsequent water intake in fluid-deprived animals (Adolph, 1939).

Under *ad libitum* conditions, animals consume a disproportionately large amount of water in conjunction with feeding. The rat, for example, consumes 70-80% of total daily water in conjunction with meals (Fitzsimons & Le Magnen, 1969; Bealer & Johnson, 1980) (Figure 10-6). The quantity of water consumed as periprandial drinking (i.e., drinking immediately before and after a meal) in neurologically intact animals is highly correlated with the meal size (Fitzsimons & Le Magnen, 1969; Bealer & Johnson, 1980). The correlated relationship between meal size and amount of water consumed raises the speculation that the meal-associated consequences of cellular dehydration due to the osmotic load and/or relative hypovolemia-induced by movement into the gastrointestinal tract may be the stimuli for meal-associated drinking. Abdominal vagotomy, which impairs water intake to systemic administration of hypertonic saline (Kraly, Gibbs, & Smith, 1975; Jerome & Smith, 1982a), ANG II (Rowland, 1980; Jerome & Smith, 1982b), and histamine (Kraly & June, 1982), also reduces drinking in association with food intake (Kraly, Smith & Carty, 1978). Although receptors which respond to hydration-

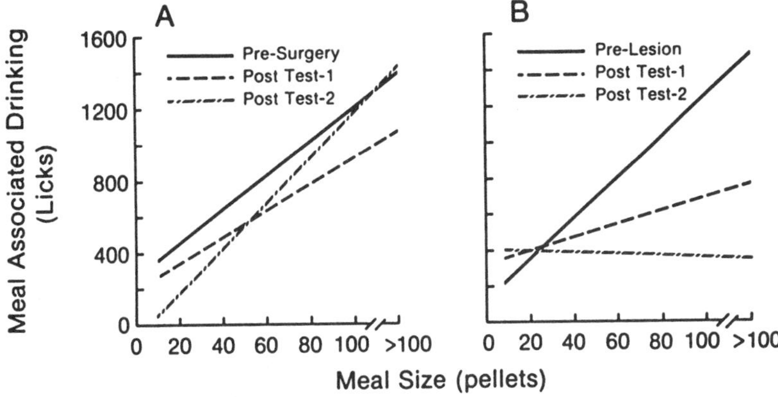

FIGURE 10-6. *Regression lines demonstrating the high correlation between meal size and amount of water consumed and the disruptive effects of a brain lesion on this relationship. Regression lines for the amount of water consumed (licks) versus meal size (pellets) in sham-lesion (control) rats (n=4; panel A) and in rats receiving lesions of the periventricular tissue surrounding the anteroventral third ventricle (AV3V) (n=5; panel B) are shown prior to surgery and on days 6, 7, and 8 (post-test 1) and on days 19, 20, and 21 (post-test 2) post-surgery. After surgery, 24 h* ad libitum *water intake had returned to normal in both groups prior to the first post-test. The correlation coefficients for the relationship between meal size and the amount of meal-associated drinking were highly significant for all animals prior to surgery (range of Pearson product-moment r values = .36 to .73). Post-surgery all of the sham-lesion rats demonstrated the highly correlated relationship between meal size and drinking, but in 4 of the 5 animals with AV3V lesions the significant correlation was abolished (from Bealer & Johnson, 1980).*

associated stimuli may be located in the gastrointestinal tract, it is also likely that transduction mechanisms related to sodium-water balance are located in portions of the splanchnic region.

B. Mesenteric and Hepatic Receptors

The work of Haberich and colleagues (see Haberich, 1968 for review) conducted in the 1960s was the first to direct attention to the role of hepatic and hepatic portal mechanisms in the control of fluid balance. Haberich (1968) demonstrated that relative to administrations into the vena cava, infusions of water into the portal vein were more effective in producing diuresis and that hypertonic NaCl portal injections were more effective in producing an antidiuretic response. Electrophysiological recordings of vagal afferent activity indicates the presence of altered firing induced by hyper- or hypo-osmotic solutions applied to the liver through the portal vein (Niijima, 1969; Adachi, Niijima, & Jacobs, 1976; Andrews & Orbach, 1974; Rogers, Novin, & Butcher, 1979). The firing rate of fibers in the hypothalamohypophyseal tract is increased by administration of hypertonic solutions into the portal vein (Baertschi & Vallet, 1981) and portal vein infusions of hypertonic saline elevate plasma VP (Chwalbinska-Moneta, 1979; Baertschi & Vallet, 1981).

Administration of hyperosmotic solution into the hepatic portal system also affects ingestive behavior. Blake & Lin (1978) found that the amount of isotonic saline consumed after 24 h of water deprivation was reduced by hepatic portal vein infusion. In sodium-depleted animals, Tordoff, Schulkin & Friedman (1986) demonstrated that sodium appetite was reduced by saline infusion with concentrations as low as 0.15M into the portal vein.

In spite of a growing number of studies that report results consistent with a hepatic sodium/osmoreceptor mechanism, there have also been a reasonable number of reports of failure to find effects with hepatic portal vein infusion (Schneider et al., 1970; Glasby & Ramsay, 1974; Kapteina et al., 1978; Liard, Dolci, & Vallotton, 1984). Vallet and Baertschi (1980) have argued that the hepatic-related receptors are located in the portal vein and that the discrepancies may have occurred when investigators who obtained negative results bypassed the osmosensitive region of the portal vein with the infusion cannula or inadvertently destroyed osmosensitive areas or their associated afferent nerves. Transection of the hepatic branch of the vagus (Haberich, 1968; Adachi et al., 1976; Andrews & Orbach, 1974; Rogers et al., 1979; Contreras & Kosten, 1981; Chwalbinska-Moneta, 1979) has been shown to alter sodium-related neural, hormonal, and behavioral responses. Vallet and Baertschi (1982) suggest that spinal afferents may also play a role in responses to hyperosmotic stimuli of the hepatic portal vein.

Teleologically, the implication of splanchnic osmo-/sodium-sensitive mechanisms among the controls of fluid balance is appealing. Haberich (1968) perceived the portal circulation as "an advanced post in the 'dangerous' front line between the enteral and parenteral space of the body." At the same time, consideration should be given to other regions of the splanchnic circulation that may also have osmo-/sodium-sensing capabilities that are in the "front line." Arsenijevic and Baertschi (1985) have found that superfusion of the duodenal and jejunal mesenteric veins alter hypothalamohypophyseal activity in a manner similar to that seen with osmotic stimulation of the portal vein (Baertschi & Vallet, 1981).

C. Vascular Pressure and Volume Receptors

At several locations within the vascular tree, deformation of the vessel wall resulting from distention by the blood is sensed by specialized receptors responding to shear (Brown, 1980). Information derived from such receptors is proportional to pressure in the vessel. Most notable of these receptor systems are the high pressure receptors or baroreceptors located in the aortic arch and the carotid sinus and the low pressure receptors (also referred to as cardiopulmonary receptors) positioned in the great veins, atria, and pulmonary circulation, and which sense blood volume. Afferent information from the aortic arch and carotid sinus is carried to the brain over cranial nerves IX and X and input from cardiopulmonary receptors is relayed over the vagus.

The role of both the baro- and volume- receptors in the control of vasopressin release has been studied extensively. Several studies have shown that conditions that increase the stretch of the areas containing baroreceptors or volume receptors inhibit VP release and that unloading of these receptors facilitates release (see Share, 1974 for review). There are a number of important interactions between the high pressure and volume-sensing systems that occur when "contradictory" information is presented to each, simultaneously. For example, in the dog, bilateral carotid occlusion, which stimulates high pressure receptors, will not induce vasopressin release unless the afferents from the low pressure receptors are interrupted (Share & Levy, 1962).

In contrast to the role of high and low pressure afferents in the control of VP release, the importance of these sensory systems in the facilitation and inhibition of thirst remains generally unexplored. Whereas it has been possible to study the role of pressure/volume afferents in VP release in either anesthetized preparations or under relatively acute conditions, investigation of drinking and sodium appetite requires a behaviorally competent animal. Although chronic interruption of high pressure input by sinoaortic denervation is feasible, bilateral vagotomy is poorly tolerated by most species.

Sino-aortic denervation in the rat induces an immediate suppression of *ad libitum* water intake which may be due to surgical trauma; however, normal water intake does recover within 1 to 2 weeks. Rats with chronic deafferentation of high pressure receptors respond normally to thirst challenges associated with the control of extracellular fluid volume, specifically systemic ANG II treatment, isoproterenol injections, and hypovolemia induced with subcutaneous polyethylene glycol (Rettig & Johnson, 1986). Interestingly, animals with either chronic sinoaortic deafferentation or aortic baroreceptor denervation manifest a specific impairment in drinking in response to cellular dehydration on initial tests (Rettig & Johnson, 1986).

The inhibition of drinking by stimulating cardiopulmonary volume receptors has been demonstrated by stretch of the atria and by systemic hypertension. In rats, stretch of the right atrium (a treatment that does not reduce cardiac output in the rat) will inhibit drinking to hypovolemia and isoproterenol treatments but not to cellular dehydration (Kaufman, 1984). The peripheral afferent nerve(s) mediating this inhibition in rat has not been defined. However, Moore-Gillon (1980) has reported that unilateral (either left or right) cervical vagotomy increases water intake after hypertonic saline, isoproterenol, sodium nitrite, and hypovolemia induced by polyethylene glycol.

High pressure afferent input also appears to inhibit drinking. Normalization of arterial pressure elevated by intravenous ANG II infusion enhances drinking to this dipsogenic peptide (Robinson and Evered, 1987) and elevation of systemic pressure attenuates drinking induced by cellular dehydration (Robinson, 1987).

In addition to sinoaortic and cardiopulmonary receptors, pressure receptors have been reported in mesenteric circulation (Sarnoff & Yamada, 1959; Morrison, 1973; Tuttle & McCleary, 1975). Reflex changes in systemic arterial pressure, heart rate, and skeletal muscle and skin blood flow can be evoked by changing perfusion pressure in the mesenteric circulation. To the author's knowledge, such receptor systems have not been investigated for their direct influences on the control of fluid balance. However, changes in mesenteric blood flow accompanying behavioral states such as feeding might be expected to trigger afferents from the mesenteric circulation to influence thirst and antidiuretic mechanisms.

D. Renal Nerves

Renal nerves also carry pressure and chemoreceptor-derived input into the CNS. Renal efferent activity arises form renal mechanoreceptors that respond to renal hypotension and venous congestion. Renal chemoreceptors of different classes respond to renal ischemia and to back flow of urine, but not to isotonic saline, into the renal pelvis (Moss, 1982). Afferent renal nerve stimulation activates neurons in many hypothalamic nuclei (Ciriello & Calaresu, 1980). Stimulation of renal afferents alters the firing of putative supraoptic VP neurons but has no effect on oxytocin cells (Day & Ciriello, 1985). Section of the renal nerves reduces drinking to hypovolemia induced with polyethylene glycol (Sharpe, Mogenson & Calaresu, 1978). Although this effect might be a result of reduced renin release as suggested by the authors, renal afferent nerves should also be considered in the interpretation of this effect.

E. Muscle Receptors

The contraction of skeletal muscle can reflexly activate multiple efferent autonomic and hormonal mechanisms (Coote, Hilton & Perez-Gonzalez, 1971; McCloskey & Mitchell, 1972; Yamashita et al., 1984). An "exercise pressor reflex" includes all of the cardiovascular changes reflexly induced by the contraction of skeletal muscle (see Mitchell, Kaufman, & Iwamoto, 1983, for review). The increase in pressure to exercise appears to be mediated by group III (myelinated) and group IV (unmyelinated) afferent nerves (Mitchell, et al., 1983). Reflex activation from the contraction of skeletal muscle activates hormonal and neural efferent limbs that have the potential to alter renal water and sodium losses (see Chapter 6 by Wade and Freund and Chapter 7 by Zambraski in this volume).

The literature on the effects of exercise on drinking is relatively old, and very little is known about the effects of exercise or the activation of afferents from exercising muscle on thirst. Thirst sensations have been reported to be less intense during exercise (Adolph, 1947). With the same water deficit in the same environment, a man at work sweating rapidly is reported to be more content without drink than when at rest sweating slowly (Wolf, 1958). There is a clear need for data collected with objective contemporary behavioral and physiological methods to definitively evaluate the effects of exercise on thirst and sodium appetite.

F. Central Nervous System

1. Fluid Compartments of the Central Nervous System: The composition of the brain and spinal cord is the most heterogenous component of any system of the body. This statement is true not only as it applies to cell types, structural organization, and functional roles, but also in terms of the access of plasma constituents and the partitioning of extracellular fluids. Problems of access and fluid dynamics in the brain become important considerations when discussing the locus of tissues and receptor systems sensitive to the signals of body hydro-mineral status. Therefore, some prefatory comments about the nature of body-brain fluid relationships and about the distribution of fluids within the brain itself are appropriate prior to a consideration of questions of central targets, tissues, and receptors.

Throughout most of the brain, neurons are separated from capillaries by an astroglial sheath. Processes from astroglia are flattened to produce pericapillary end feet which form tight junctions with each other. In addition, the capillaries of much of the brain are different than other tissues of the body in that the endothelial cells of the capillaries overlap and are sealed. These two sets of tight junctions serve to constitute the structural features of the blood-brain barrier. The capillary endothelium is probably the principal component of the barrier for limiting access to the brain, whereas, the astroglia function to facilitate selective transport into and out of brain (McGeer, Eccles & McGeer, 1987).

The insulation of the parenchyma of the central nervous system from the systemic circulation by the blood-brain barrier is far from absolute. Virtually all substances administered systemically will find their way into the extracellular space of the brain provided that levels in plasma are sufficiently high and maintained (Davson, 1970). It is not only possible to ensure movement of substances into the brain by manipulating systemic levels, but egress of substances from the brain to the periphery can also occur. Furthermore, manipulations in the periphery can cause shifts of substances out of the brain into the systemic compartment. For example, hyperosmotic solutions given in the periphery will dehydrate the brain from the outward movement of water across the blood-brain barrier (Davson, 1970). Clearly, one consideration in evaluating the role of deep parenchymal structures as target tissues for circulating stimuli is whether the agent accessed the tissue under physiological rather than pharmacological conditions.

A blood-brain barrier is not present in several brain-associated structures. The barrier-deficient or extra-blood-brain barrier structures are known as circumventricular organs (CVOs). They are the: 1) subfornical organ (SFO); 2) organum vasculosum of the lamina terminalis (OVLT); 3) median eminence; 4) intermediate lobe of the pituitary; 5) posterior lobe of the pituitary; 6) subcommissural organ; 7) area postrema (AP); and 8) pineal body (Figure 10-7). The "efferent" role of the pituitary in "brain to body" communication has long been appreciated. In contrast, the case for "body to brain" information transfer through the CVOs has gained support only in recent years (see below).

The choroid plexuses, cerebrospinal fluid (CSF), brain ventricles, ventricular empendyma, subarachnoid space, and arachnoid villi comprise another set of related central elements that need special consideration in discussions of function and critical evaluations of experiments on brain and body fluid homeostasis. The ventricular system has the potential to play an important signaling and communication function in various physiological processes (Rodriguez, 1976). In addition, the ventricular system, either knowingly or unknowingly, has provided a major route of experimental delivery of substances to the CNS in many experimental analyses (Johnson & Epstein, 1975).

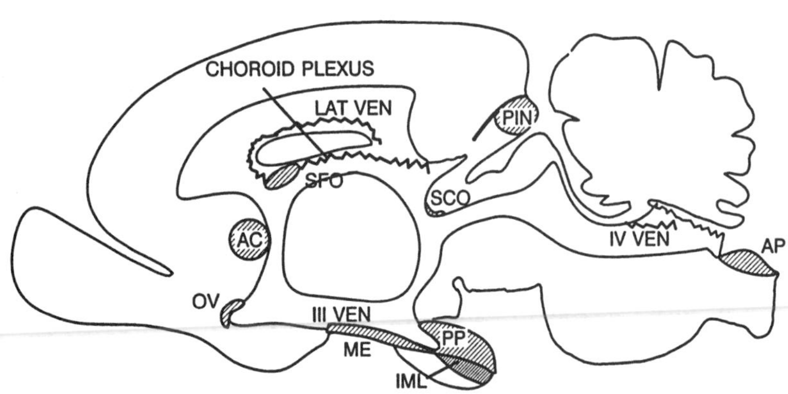

FIGURE 10-7. *The circumventricular organs (CVOs) and cerebroventricular system represented on a sagittal section of the brain. The lateral ventricle is represented in a phantom view since it is located off of the midline. All of the other structures are located on the midline. Cerebrospinal fluid (CSF) is secreted from the choroid plexuses and has a flow pattern from lateral ventricles to third ventricle, through the cerebral aqueduct, into the fourth ventricle and then either into the subarachnoid space or into the central canal. In addition to periventricular sites, CSF can access chemosensitive areas on the exterior of the brain such as those on the ventral surface of the medulla. Abbreviations: OV=organum vasculosum of the lamina terminalis; AC=anterior commissure; SFO=subfornical organ; LAT VEN=lateral ventricle; SCO=subcommissural organ; PIN=pineal; AP=area postrema; PP=posterior pituitary; IML=intermediate lobe; ME=median eminence; III VEN=-third ventricle; IV VEN=fourth ventricle.*

The bulk of cerebrospinal fluid production occurs from components of ultrafiltered plasma being selectively transported across the epithelial sheet of the choroid plexuses. The controlled process of CSF formation by transport is effective in providing a barrier between blood and CSF. The dual processes of ultafiltration across choroidal capillaries combined with carrier-mediated transport function to exclude large blood-borne molecules provides a relative consistency of ionic composition of nascent CSF in the face of variations in blood constituents.

The blood-CSF barrier is as important as the blood-brain barrier in isolating brain parenchyema from the systemic circulation. The flow of CSF through the ventricular system is brisk so that substances delivered upstream (e.g., lateral ventricles) appear within seconds in the fourth ventricle and the cisterna magna (Johnson & Epstein, 1975). CSF flows from the ventricular-cisternal system into the subarachnoid space to eventually enter the venous system through the arachnoid villi. Except for a limited amount of tissue overlying some of the circumventricular organs, most of the ependymal lining of the ventricles affords no restriction for the diffusion from the ventricles and throughout the intercellular matrix. Consequently, materials appearing in CSF can have ready access to most of the CNS.

2. Central Receptors for Hypertonic Solutions: Verney's (1947) classic experiments using close arterial injections to deliver hyperosmotic solutions to the brain provided evidence for the existence of a central osmotic mechanism for the control of VP secretion. Within a few years of Verney's report, Andersson (1953) made the remarkable, serendipitous discovery that the direct injection of hypertonic saline into the hypothalamus produced vigorous drinking in the goat. Further support for involvement of a basal forebrain site emerged from work by Jewell & Verney (1957) in which carotid injections were made into dogs with various branches of their internal carotids ligated. From these studies, the existence of an osmosensitive region in the anterior hypothalamic/preoptic region was deduced. Strangely, the question of brain osmoreception received little attention for more than a decade when finally Andersson (1971) and colleagues addressed the nature of the receptor and when others (Peck & Novin, 1971; Blass & Epstein, 1971) attempted more definitive localizations of the critical sensitive tissue.

Changing concepts on the nature of the blood-brain barrier prompted Andersson (1971) to suggest that the Verney osmoreceptor was in reality a sodium receptor. Andersson argued that systemic administration of hypertonic solutions, regardless of what solute was used, resulted in an increase in the concentration of brain extracellular sodium. In support of this idea, intraventricular (ivt) infusions of hypertonic glucose and sucrose were shown to be ineffective as osmotic agents in stimulating thirst and antidiuresis (Andersson, Olsson & Warner, 1967; Olsson,

1969). However, in response to these data, McKinley, Denton and Weisinger (1978) pointed out that solutions composed only of hyperosmolar glucose or sucrose would dilute the extracellular fluid and reduce the concentration of sodium, an ion clearly important for normal neuronal function. In support of this, McKinley and colleagues (1978) demonstrated that a hypertonic solution constituted by adding sucrose or fructose to artificial CSF (ACSF) was a potent ivt osmotic stimulus. However, a hypertonic solution composed of sucrose or fructose in ACSF was a less potent stimulus than one made of equiosmolar NaCl in ACSF. Consequently, these investigators have argued for the existence of both brain osmoreceptors and sodium receptors.

Part of Peck and Novin's (1971) approach to identifying the locus of osmoreceptors of the rabbit was to map central sites from which drinking could be elicited with intracranial injections of hypertonic solutions. The testing of central injection sites indicated that placements in the lateral preoptic area were osmoreceptive by the criteria that hypertonic saline and sucrose produced reliable water intake but that equiosmolar urea did not. In the same report, lesions of the lateral preoptic region abolished drinking to systemic hypertonic saline. In similar studies in the rat, Blass and Epstein (1971) demonstrated that cannula terminating in the lateral preoptic region generated drinking to hypertonic saline but not urea and that lesions of the lateral preoptic area selectively abolished drinking to subcutaneous hypertonic saline but not to hypovolemia induced by polyethylene glycol. In a joint study of intracranial mapping, Peck and Blass (1975) conducted a broader survey of the anterior hypothalamic-preoptic region to evaluate osmosensitivity of sites eliciting drinking and antidiuresis in the rat. Their results indicated that the distribution of sites eliciting drinking was not identical to that which encompassed placements that reduced urine flow. Although the finding of a dissociation of thirst and VP related sites may be important, a more provocative aspect appears in this more extensive mapping study.

An examination of the effective drinking and antidiuretic sites in the Peck and Blass (1975) study indicates that the epicenter of osmosensitive tissue may be located more medially than the lateral preoptic area. The projections of the histologically verified cannula placements indicated that many sensitive sites were located within 1 mm of the midline. The significance of the osmoreceptive role of the lateral preoptic area as deduced from initial lesion studies has also been called into question by other investigators (Almli & Weiss, 1974; Coburn & Stricker, 1978) who found that rats still drink to hypertonic saline treatments after ablation of this region. Collectively, these points make it seem likely that the lateral preoptic area is not the center of an osmosensitive region. The osmosensitive tissue in the preoptic region seems to lie closer to the midline—within tissue surrounding the ventral third ventricle. In accordance with this interpretation of the Peck and Blass (1975) data, studies comparing the osmosensitivity of central cannulae sites indicated that injections made into the rostral portion of the third ventricle were more effective in eliciting drinking and VP release than those made into the lateral preoptic area (Buggy et al., 1979).

Also, consistent with the idea of osmosensitive tissues lying within the periventricular tissue surrounding the anteroventral third ventricle (AV3V) is the observation that electrolytic destruction of this region in rats produced immediate adipsia (Johnson & Buggy, 1978) and permanent deficits in drinking (Johnson & Buggy, 1977; Buggy & Johnson, 1978), antidiuresis, (Johnson, Hoffman & Buggy, 1978), antidiuretic hormone release (Johnson, 1985a), and pressor responses (Johnson et al., 1978) elicited to hypertonic saline. The results support the conclusion that the AV3V contains a significant proportion of the osmosensitive tissue of the body (Buggy & Johnson, 1977a).

Electrolytic lesions provide the means for conducting both acute and chronic functional studies on the effects of removing the AV3V region of the brain on drinking, antidiuretic, and cardiovascular responses. At this point it should be made clear that in the rat the periventricular lesion which produces a global disruption in the controls of body fluid balance (described in more detail in a later section) is not restricted to a single periventricular structure. The AV3V lesion (Figure 10-8) as defined from functional studies destroys the periventricular tissue between the anterior commissure and optic chiasm. It encompasses several ventral lamina terminalis-associated structures, the OVLT, and the ventral portion of the median preoptic nucleus (MePO). It also destroys the preoptic periventricular nuclei (PPO), including the anteroventral periventricular nuclei (AVPV), and extends into the anterior hypothalamic periventricular nuclei. The medial preoptic (MPO) and anterior hypothalamic nuclei (AH) are not usually damaged beyond their medial borders with their respective periventricular nuclei (Buggy & Johnson, 1977a; Johnson & Buggy, 1978). Larger lesions in the goat (Andersson, Leksell & Lishajko, 1975), and dog (Witt et al., 1952) which disrupt fluid balance and drinking encompass the area defined as the AV3V but are more extensive. Since the initial functional investigations of the AV3V, many studies have been conducted to fractionate the region by relating morphological features and neurochemical systems to more specific hydro-mineral balance/cardiovascular mechanisms.

Of the structures located within the AV3V region, the OVLT with its unique morphological features and lack of blood-brain barrier makes it a provocative choice for consideration as a receptive region. McKinely and colleagues employing intraventricular and intravenous osmotic challenges (1978) studying sheep, and Thrasher and associates (1980) working with dogs hypothesized that osmoreceptors for drinking and VP release reside within a circumventricular organ. Thrasher, Keil, & Ramsay (1982) and Thrasher & Keil (1987) have provided strong support for this

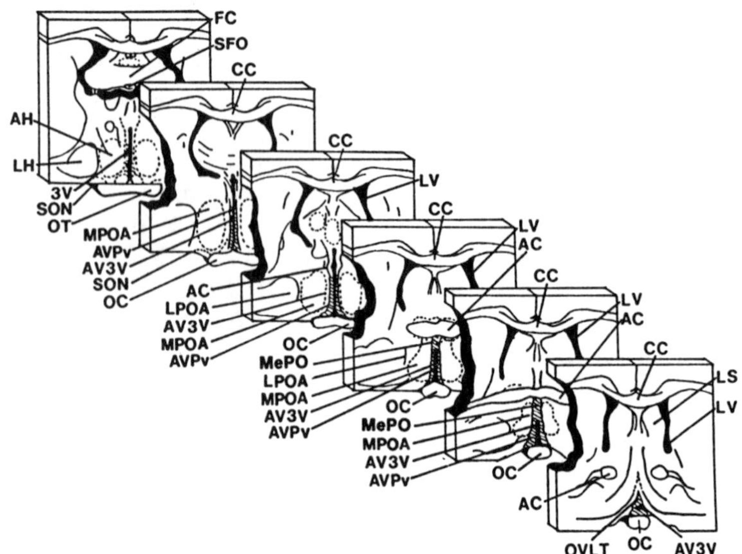

FIGURE 10-8. *Diagram of a portion of the basal forebrain depicting the periventricular region of the AV3V. The diagonal lines depict the extent of a typical AV3V lesion. Abbreviations: AC=anterior commissure; AH=anterior hypothalamic nucleus; AV3V=anteroventral third ventricle; AVPv=anteroventral periventricular nucleus; CC=corpus callosum; FC=fornical commissure; LH=lateral hypothalamus; LPO=-lateral preoptic area; LS=lateral septal nucleus; LV=lateral ventricle; MePO=median preoptic nucleus; MPOA=medial preoptic area; OC=optic chiasm; OT=optic tract; OVLT=organum vasculosum of the lamina terminalis; SFO=subfornical organ; SO=supraoptic nucleus; 3V=third ventricle.*

hypothesis by demonstrating that in dogs electrolytic lesions limited to the OVLT produce deficits in drinking responses and VP release to osmotic stimulation. Findings from *in vitro* studies conducted with hypothalamo-hypophyseal explants taken from rats with chronic AV3V lesions are consistent with the OVLT lesion results in dogs. Explants from rats that had chronic AV3V lesions did not release VP to hyperosmotic NaC1 (Sladek & Johnson, 1983) (Figure 10–9).

In vivo, in the rat, it has always been necessary to ablate more than just the OVLT to induce reliable impairments in drinking to hyperosmotic stimuli (Johnson, 1982) (Figure 10-10). Lesion overlap studies to define the critical tissue indicate that a ventral portion of the MePO region along with the OVLT must be destroyed for drinking deficits to hyperosmotic stimulation to ensue. In sheep it is necessary to make extensive lesions of the structures of the ventral lamina terminalis to obtain marked impairments in VP release to hyperosmotic stimuli (McKinley et al., 1988). Because there is both functional evidence (Hosutt, Rowland, & Stricker, 1981; Lind, Thunhorst, & Johnson, 1984) and electrophysiological evidence (Sibbald, Hubbard & Sirett, 1988) for osmosensitivity of the SFO in the rat and because a significant portion of the projections from

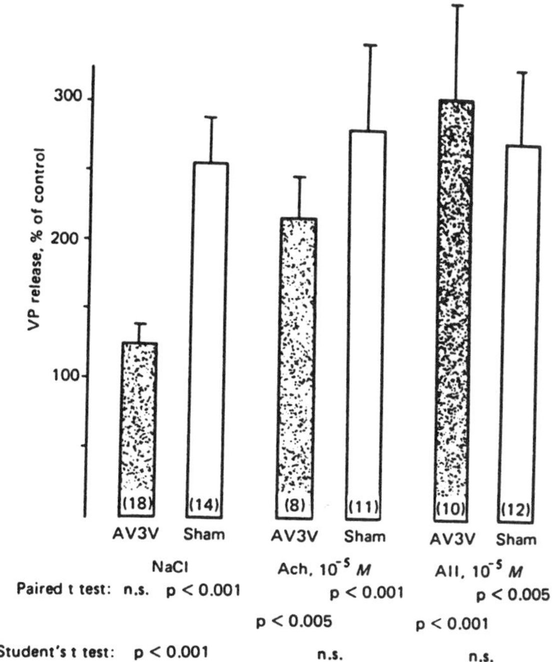

FIGURE 10-9. *Vasopressin (VP) release from explants obtained from rats with AV3V or sham lesions following exposure to either an osmotic stimulus (NaCl sufficient to increase medium osmolality from 295 to 315 mosm/kg H_2O), acetylcholine (Ach, 10^{-5}M), or angiotensin II (AII) (10^{-5}M) during the 1-h test period on either day 3 or 4 of culture. Mean ± SEM. Number of explants in each group is given in parentheses. n.s.-p $\geqslant 0.05$, and therefore the responses are not significantly different from each other (from Sladek & Johnson, 1983).*

the SFO run into and through the MnPO (see below), by extending the lesions more dorsally along the lamina terminalis it may be possible to interrupt important descending fibers that could possibly carry additional information from SFO osmoreceptors (see further discussion of the anatomy of the lamina terminalis region below). Ablation of just the MePO region in rat produces deficits in drinking and VP secretion (Mangiapane et al., 1983). Although it has been assumed that such effects are the result of interruption of input from the circumventricular organs, it is also possible that the osmosensitive zone extends beyond the OVLT and the SFO to include other tissues of the ventral lamina terminalis-AV3V region which are inside the blood-brain barrier. At the present time it is impossible to distinguish between these two possibilities.

Among the sites considered as likely loci for the osmoreceptors by Jewell and Verney (1957) were the magnocellular neurons themselves. In recent years Leng and colleagues (Leng, 1980; Mason, 1980; Leng, Mason, & Dyer, 1982; Leng, Dyball, & Mason, 1985; Leng, Dyball & Russell, 1988) have championed this concept. Electrophysiological studies indi-

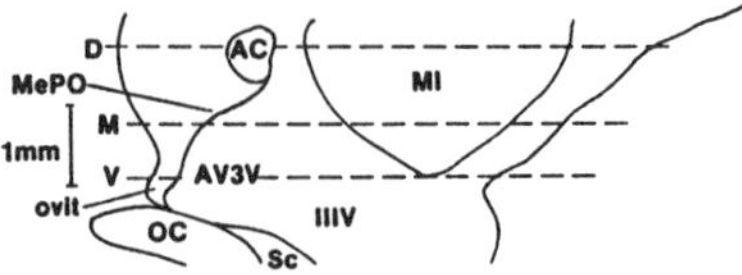

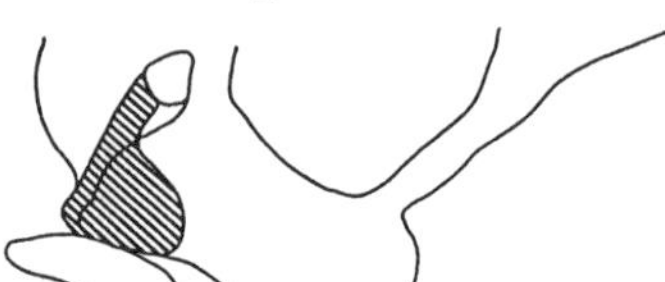

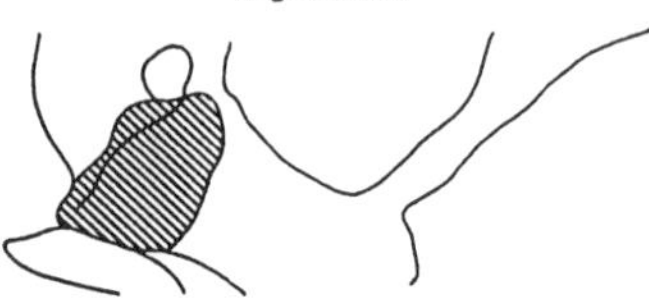

FIGURE 10-10. *Above: A midsagittal view of an intact rat brain depicting the AV3V region and major surrounding regions and structures. Also depicted are 3 planes, dorsal (D), medial (M), and ventral (V), from which horizontal sections were taken for assessment of critical damage. Below: profiles of the area of common overlap (diagonal lines) of lesions in rats in which water intake could not be elicited by a hypertonic saline thirst challenge (n=12) or ANG II (n=6). Animals with comparable damage at the ventral level of the lesion, but little or no damage at the medial and dorsal levels, responded normally to these thirst challenges. Thus, the median preoptic nucleus damage must be critical for the thirst deficits to the challenges studied here (Lind et al., 1979). Abbreviations: MI=mass intermedia of the thalamus; AC=anterior commissure; MePO=median preoptic; OVLT=organum vasculosum of the lamina terminalis; OC=optic chiasm; Sc=supra chiasmatic nucleus of the anterior hypothalamus; III V=third ventricle; AV3V=anteroventral third ventricle (based on Lind et al., 1979; from Johnson, 1982).*

cate that hyperosmotic solutions depolarize supraoptic magnocellular units (Leng, 1980). However, such depolarization does not result in additional action potentials as long as the osmotic changes are in the physiological range (Mason, 1980; Bourque, 1987). Leng and colleagues (1988) suggest that although magnocellular neurons are intrinsically osmoceptive, osmoreceptor input from sources either originating in or passing through the AV3V is necessary for activation of the neurohypophyseal tract and VP release.

3. Central Sites of Action for Angiotensin: Shortly after Fitzsimon's (1969) provocative implication of the renin-angiotensin system in the mediation of thirst, he instigated studies with Epstein and Rolls (Epstein et al., 1970) that directed attention toward the brain as the site of action for the dipsogenic effect of ANG II. Intracranial injections of ANG II produced drinking in a dose range approximately three orders of magnitude less than that required to effect the same response when administered peripherally (Epstein et al., 1970). The central tissues that appeared to be sensitive to the octapeptide appeared to be fairly extensive and included the septal region, the anterior thalamus, and the preoptic area/anterior hypothalamic area (Epstein et al., 1970). Although the extent of the sites from which ANG II seemed to evoke drinking in and of itself was not too surprising, it was difficult to reconcile the large number of central sites with the results of autoradiographic studies conducted in Epstein's laboratory in 1971 and early 1972 (Johnson, 1975; Epstein & Hsaio, 1975; Shrager et al., 1975). In these experiments, tritiated ANG II of high specific activity was administered intravenously and autoradiograms made of 4 u tissue sections taken throughout the brain. In the sections of tissue taken from brains of animals guillotined 2 min after injection of the label, there was evidence of increased radioactivity in the pituitary, AP, choroid plexuses, SFO, median eminence, and cerebrospinal fluid. The puzzling result of these early observations was that there was no increased labeling visible within the tissue parenchyema proposed as the target for ANG II—induced drinking. This apparent paradox was resolved when later in 1972, it was recognized that conventional methods employed at that time for intracranial injections often afforded access of injectate from tissue sites to the cerebral ventriclar system, especially if the injection cannula traversed a ventricle en route to a tissue (Johnson, 1975; Johnson & Epstein, 1975). As a result of these observations, it was proposed that ANG II—induced drinking resulted from an action of the peptide at a periventricular site (Johnson & Epstein, 1975).

The studies by Simpson and Routtenberg (1973) identified a particular periventricular structure, the SFO, as the likely target for the action of ANG II to induce thirst. These experiments demonstrated that the SFO was exquisitely sensitive to locally injected peptide. In addition, SFO lesions appeared to abolish drinking elicited from ANG II injected into other brain sites. The SFO seemed ideally suited to act as a target for circulating ANG II, because tracer studies had indicated the limited access of ANG II to tissues located inside the blood-brain barrier (Johnson, 1975). In addition, other research (Joy & Lowe, 1970; Ueda, Katayama & Kato, 1972; Ferrario, Gildenerg, & McCubbin, 1972) had recently implicated another extra-blood-brain barrier structure, the AP, as a central target for blood-borne ANG II to alter circulatory reflexes.

Although the question of the target for the central action of angiotensin seemed to be resolved, certain inconsistencies incompatible with a complete story started to emerge. Specifically, these were that: 1) with repeated testing to intracranial ANG II rats with SFO lesions, recovered their drinking; 2) after SFO lesions that abolished drinking there was an interruption of CSF flow from the lateral ventricles to the rest of the ventricular system; furthermore, when the peptide-induced dipsogenic response recovered there was a restoration in CSF flow from the lateral ventricles to the rest of the ventricular system; and 3) regional obstruction of the ventricular spaces prevented drinking and pressor responses to CSF-borne ANG II only when access to the periventricular tissues of the AV3V region was prevented (Buggy et al., 1975; Hoffman & Phillips,

1976; Buggy & Fisher, 1974). There clearly seemed to be a brain-related site of action for the dipsogenic effect of ANG II in addition to the SFO. The periventricular tissue of the AV3V seemed like a reasonable target. This hypothesis received further confirmation when AV3V lesions were found to permanently abolish the drinking response to both systemic and central ANG II (Buggy & Johnson, 1977a, 1977b; Johnson & Buggy, 1977; Buggy & Johnson, 1978). In addition, AV3V lesions significantly attenuated the antidiuretic and pressor responses to the centrally injected octapeptide (Johnson et al., 1978; Bealer et al., 1979).

Consistent with the concept of ANG II sensitive tissue within the AV3V are electrophysiological studies showing ANG II sensitive units in the periventricular preoptic nucleus, the OVLT, and MePO (Gronan & York, 1978; Felix & Phillips, 1979; Knowles & Phillips, 1980; Thornton et al., 1985; Nelson & Johnson, 1985). It appears that ANG II sensitive elements are dispersed throughout the AV3V.

In the reports from our laboratory we have never been inclined to identify one specific structure within the AV3V as *the* ANG II target. In functional studies conducted in the rat, ablation of a single structure within the AV3V (e.g., OVLT) is not sufficient to produce drinking deficits to ANG II administered either systemically or centrally. In addition, lesion overlap studies defining the critical area of destruction necessary to obtain deficits in ANG II-induced thirst indicate that the lesion must not only include the OVLT, but also must extend up the lamina terminalis to incorporate the ventral tissue of the MePO as well (Lind et al., 1979; Shrager, 1981; Lind & Johnson, 1982b) (see Figure 10-10). Although it is possible that structures within the AV3V (e.g., in particular the OVLT) are involved in sensing blood-borne ANG II, functional evidence for this is not at present available from studies conducted in the rat. The most parsimonious explanation to account for the mechanism of action of elevated levels of blood-borne ANG II in inducing drinking and VP release in the rat is that the peptide acts primarily on the SFO (Simpson, Epstein & Camardo, 1978; Simpson, 1981). In this species, the profound effects of ANG II on the AV3V produced with ivt injections are in all likelihood a reflection of the role of the AV3V in the integrative control of fluid balance rather than its role as a sensor of blood-borne peptide. This concept will be developed in more detail in later sections.

As with the case of osmoreceptors/sodium receptors, there are apparent species differences in the distribution of sensitive elements for ANG II that putatively monitor blood-borne peptide. In the dog, restricted lesions of either the SFO (Thrasher, Simpson & Ramsay, 1982) or OVLT produce drinking deficits to blood-borne ANG II. In sheep, SFO lesions have no effect on drinking to the systemic administration of the dipsogenic peptide (McKinley et al., 1986). The species differences observed for rat, dog, and sheep may reflect the fact that structures of the dorsal and ventral lamina terminalis function as an entire complex in the control of fluid balance and act collectively to achieve a similar end. Differences may be more apparent than real and that seeming species differences may reflect a slightly different "seeding" of receptors within the OVLT and SFO rather than critical differences.

CENTRAL INTEGRATION AND THE CONTROL OF BODY FLUID HOMEOSTASIS

Although there is clearly much to be learned about fluid balance related signals, receptors, and input to the CNS, it is clear that the brain receives multiple types of information which it integrates to effect control responses. The central processing of hydration-related input involves all levels of the neuraxis. Visceral neural input arrives in the hindbrain and ascends the nervous system. Blood-borne and humoral stimuli exert their influence by an initial action on brain chemosensitive zones that include at least several of the circumventricular organs. Integration requires the convergence of information derived from both neural and humoral sources. Therefore, it is important to understand what central pathways are involved in conducting these two types of afferent input—both neural and humoral. In addition, because chemical messengers play such a significant role in the coding and integration of information in the CNS, the specification of putative neurotransmitter/modulator systems subserving fluid balance is another important dimension to consider when discussing processing of information in central systems.

The areas of the CNS where humoral inputs impinge and where first order visceral afferents synapse are logical starting points to begin the consideration of the processes of central integration and fluid balance. A large percentage the first order visceral input entering the CNS projects to the nucleus of the solitary tract (NTS). This region lies in the medulla in close association with the AP. In addition to its presumed capacity to monitor plasma, the AP also receives first order visceral afferents and is in intimate neuronal contact with the NTS. Several types of evidence suggest that the AP and the NTS function as a complex to perform primary processing and integration of blood-borne and neural input as it enters the CNS.

In the previous section, the importance of the circumventricular structures of the lamina terminalis has been introduced. The SFO and the OVLT have been implicated as targets for blood-borne ANG II and hypothesized to house osmoreceptors/sodium receptors. Other periventricular tissues in the region of the lamina terminalis, which lie inside the blood-brain barrier (i.e., portions of the AV3V), have been demonstrated to be sensitive to ANG II. This area inside the blood-brain barrier may also be sensitive to changes in osmotic and/or sodium concentration.

Lamina terminalis CVO output passes into the AV3V, and the area collectively appears to be important in the early integration of humoral signals in the CNS.

Over recent years, with the advent of new neuroanatomical tract tracing methods, a close relationship between hindbrain and forebrain has become even more apparent. Communication between the AP/NTS and SFO/AV3V complexes, as well as the many "centers" which lie between, affords the opportunity for central integration of both blood-borne and neural CNS input. The next sections will discuss these hindbrain and forebrain integrative complexes, the respective ascending and descending flow of neural information from each, and the putative neurochemical character of these neuronal channels of communication.

A. Hindbrain Integrative Mechanisms and the Control of Body Fluids

1. The Area Postrema/Nucleus of the Solitary Tract Complex: The receptive fields of the facial (VIIth), glossopharyngeal (IXth), and vagus (Xth) nerves encompass large areas of the oral and body cavities but terminate in a very restricted area of the CNS. The nucleus of the solitary tract (NTS) receives the great majority of this visceral input. In addition, the AP receives some of these terminals of primary afferents as well as parts of the spinal trigeminal nucleus in the medulla and the first few segments of the spinal cord (Norgren, 1981). Recently there has been increased effort to describe the terminal distribution of primary visceral afferent projections, particularly those to the NTS. One early motivation for such effort was the demonstration that destruction of the NTS produces fulminating hypertension, presumably because of interruption of the afferent limb of the baroreceptor reflex (Doba & Reis, 1973; Nathan & Reis, 1977). The opportunity for thorough anatomical characterization of visceral afferents that is afforded by new tracer methodologies has permitted the demonstration of a distinct topographic organization of projections to the NTS (e.g., Kalia & Sullivan, 1982; Miselis, Hyde & Shapiro, 1986).

Because of the compact nature of the NTS, the intermingling of its vital elements, and its location at a point of flexion of caudal medulla and spinal cord, it has been difficult, if not impossible, to conduct functional studies of the entire NTS in unanesthetized, behaving preparations. One region that has received some attention in relation to fluid balance, however, is the medial portion of the NTS (cmNTS) that is subjacent to the AP (Hyde & Miselis, 1983; 1984). The AP and medial NTS both receive terminal projections of the vagus (Kalia & Sullivan, 1982; Miselis et al., 1986). Miselis and colleagues describe afferent projections of the subdiaphragmatic vagus that terminate in the AP, the commissural subnucleus of the NTS (which is a portion of the NTS subjacent to the AP), and the subnucleus gelatinosus (which is anterior and slightly lateral to AP).

Although earlier the AP was reported not to receive second order input from the NTS (Norgren, 1978), more recent studies indicate that NTS efferents project into the AP (Shapiro & Miselis, 1985; Edwards, personal communication). Injections of fluorescent microbeads that are confined to the AP show evidence of retrograde transport into the adjacent NTS (Edwards, personal communication). Tracing studies give evidence of efferents from the AP that project into NTS (Shapiro & Miselis, 1984). Miselis et al. (1986; 1987) have pointed out the importance of the intimate association of the AP with the NTS and that the AP/NTS serves as the origin of projections to various regions involved in maintenance of vegetative functions.

Earlier studies have demonstrated that cells immediately adjacent to the AP of cat were activated with systemic infusions of hypertonic NaCl (Clemente, Sutin & Silverstone, 1957) and that stimulation of the area postrema in dog increased water and sodium excretion (Wise & Ganong, 1960). Several functional studies appearing in recent years more thoroughly implicate the AP and subjacent NTS in fluid balance.

Rats with lesions of the AP show a unique pattern of overresponsiveness to various experimental dipsogens. Edwards and Ritter (1982) demonstrated that AP-lesioned rats overdrink when challenged with systemic ANG II, the beta-adrenoceptor agonist isoproterenol, and hypovolemia induced with subcutaneous administration of polyethylene glycol. The rats did not overrespond to hypertonic saline. Thus, AP-lesioned animals appear to have an inhibitory deficit to thirst-generating treatments that are related to stimuli reflecting the status of extracellular fluid volume.

Contreras and Stetson (1981) found that rats with lesions that destroyed the AP without causing appreciable damage to the surrounding NTS had increased consumption of NaCl solutions in 2-bottle preference tests as well as chronic hyperdipsia. The capacity of the AP-lesioned rats to retain sodium was tested by placing them on low sodium diets. The brain-dramaged rats retained sodium as effectively as control rats. However, these animals still maintained a hyperdipsia while on the sodium deficient diet.

Sodium and water metabolism in rats with lesions that include the AP and subjacent NTS have been studied by Hyde and Miselis (1984). When sodium loss was examined over 24 h of total food and water deprivation, these investigators found that rats with AP-subjacent NTS lesions evidenced increased sodium and water loss. Such results suggest that sodium appetite may follow as a consequence of an impairment in the capacity to maintain extracellular volume. That is, the turnover of water and sodium appears to be greater in the AP-lesioned rat. Recent studies (Edwards, Beltz & Johnson, 1988) indicate rats with chornic AP lesions show enhanced excretion of intragastric sodium loads but give no indication of imparired V secretion. Alterations in water and sodium handling that tend to mitigate against an animal effecting extracellular volume expansion might, in part, account for the observations by Mangiapane, Fink and colleagues (Fink, Bruner, & Mangiapane, 1987; Fink et al., 1987) that several forms of experimental and genetic hypertension are prevented by AP lesions.

The AP has received considerable attention for its role in hypertension and cardiovascular control. It was the first circumventricular organ implicated as a central site of action of ANG II (Joy & Lowe, 1970; Ueda et al., 1972; Ferrario et al., 1972). The cardiovascular effect of ANG II action on the AP is to reduce the gain of the baroreceptor reflex, thereby, potentiating the systemic action of pressor agents (Ferrario et al., 1972). In contrast to ANG II, bloodborne VP acts to enhance the gain of the baroreflex (Montani et al., 1980; Cowley, Monos & Guyton, 1974). VP does so in part through its action on the AP. In rabbit, the effects of VP to enhance the reflex gain that is manifest by a great bradycardia and larger fall in renal sympathetic nerve activity for a given rise in pressure is abolished by AP lesions (Undesser et al., 1985). In addition to playing a role in influencing body fluid homeostatis through general cardiovascular actions, a more specific role of the AP in controlling fluid balance might be through a modulating action on sympathetic outflow to the kidneys and by neural efferent projections to forebrain structures controlling pituitary hormone secretions.

2. Efferent Projections of the AP and the NTS: Ricardo and Koh's (1978) anatomical demonstration that monosynaptic projections from the NTS ascend to midbrain and forebrain structures had a great conceptual impact on thinking about the way that visceral information might be conducted through the neuraxis. The visible evidence from these and other tract tracing studies that followed conveyed the impression that visceral information can be communicated to what has been presumed to be the highest levels of autonomic integration over direct routes rather than tedious multisynaptic pathways. Such evidence has had the conceptual effect of elevating the relevance of ascending visceral input in considerations of the role in the processing of fluid-balance information in the CNS. Summarized in Figure 10-11B is a composite of many of the major projections from the NTS defined by various investigators (e.g., Ricardo & Koh, 1978; Loewy & Burton, 1978). Some of these direct pathways terminate in areas of the brain and spinal cord that have been long recognized to be involved in the control of autonomic outflow (e.g., dorsal motor nucleus of the vagus, nucleus ambiguus; intermediolateral cell column). Several of the more rostral projections are to areas known to influence secretion of anterior and posterior pituitary hormones (e.g., parvocellular paraventricular nucleus (pPVN), magnocellular paraventricular nucleus (mPVN), and supraoptic nucleus (SON), areas implicated in autonomic control (PVN), and areas more recently implicated in the control of thirst (AV3V; MePO; SFO).

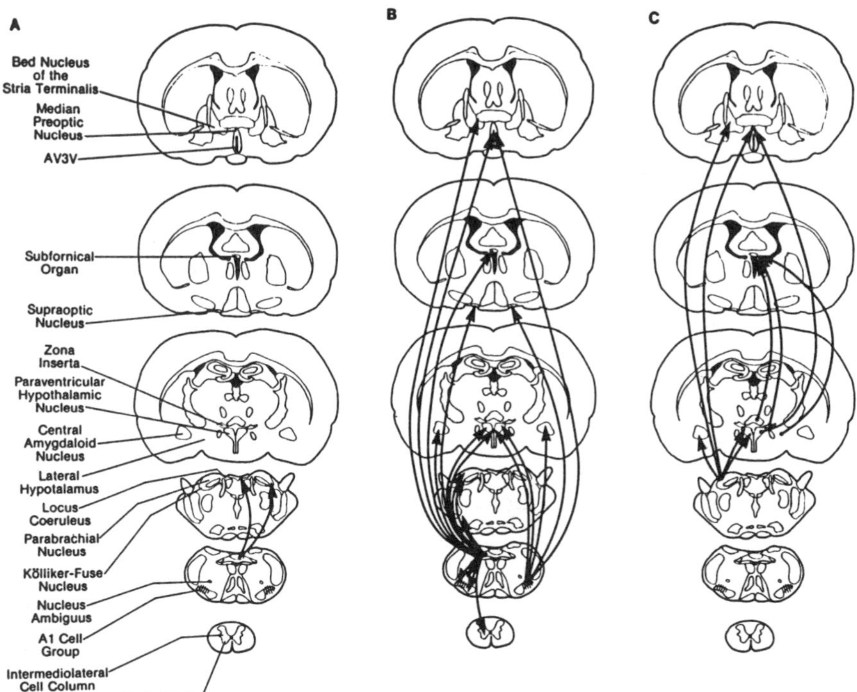

FIGURE 10-11. *Central visceral pathways from the area postrema and nucleus of the solitary tract and "higher order" projections from the caudal ventrolateral medulla and parabrachial nucleus. Panel A, Left: Identification of most of the central targets which receive major visceral afferent input. Panel A, Right: efferents of the area postrema. Panel B, Left: The major spinal and ascending projections of the nucleus of the solitary tract. Panel B, Right: Ascending efferents of the caudal ventrolateral medulla. Panel C, Left: Ascending efferents of the parabrachial nucleus. Panel C, Right: Ascending inputs from diencephalic structures to the structures along the lamina terminalis. (Drawing after components of Loewy, 1982, and based on Miselis, 1986; Miselis et al., 1987; Loewy & Burton, 1978; Ricardo & Koh, 1978; Saper & Loewy, 1980; Zardetto-Smith & Gray, 1987; Lind & Ganten, 1990).*

Ascending projections from the AP, or even the AP/cmNTS, do not appear to project as widely to diencephalic regions as the other parts of the NTS (Van der Kooy & Koda, 1983; Shapiro & Miselis, 1985) (see Figure 10-11A). However, there are ascending hindbrain projections to areas, which, in turn, project to the diencephalic structures involved in autonomic and body fluid control.

3. Hindbrain Regions Receiving Projections from the AP and NTS and that Project to Diencephalon: Two regions in the hindbrain that receive ascending projections from the AP/NTS complex have functionally been implicated in the control of fluid balance. These are the cells located within the ventral lateral region of the medulla (VLM) and the lateral parabrachial nucleus (LPBN). The rostral portion of the VLM (RVLM) contains cells that are influenced by arterial baroreceptor afferents and that are thought to directly descend to the intermediolateral cell column (IML) of the spinal cord (Ross et al., 1984). Other cells located in the caudal VLM (CVLM) are implicated in a more direct manner in the control of body fluids for their likely role in influencing VP secretion. Electrolytic lesions of the Al area produce fulminating hypertension accompanied by VP release (Imaizumi et al., 1985). The release of VP by these lesions probably occurs as a result of the release of transmitter into the magnocellular VP containing regions of the hypothalamus. The CVLM has been implicated in the control of VP secretion by several lines of evidence, specifically: 1) electrical stimulation or application of l-glutamate in CVLM activates identified magnocellular neurons and causes the release of VP into the circulation (Day & Renaud, 1984; Blessing & Willoughby, 1985a; Tanaka et al., 1985; 2) injection of muscimol (a GABA receptor agonist) into the CVLM inhibits neural activity in the PVN and reduces VP secretion (Blessing & Willoughby, 1985b); and 3) neurons in the CVLM that project to the SON increase their firing rate in response to reduced central venous and arterial pressure (McAllen & Blessing, 1987).

Both the A1/C1 cell groups reside within the VLM. It has been proposed that the epinephrine-containing cells in the RVLM exert a major descending excitatory influence on the activity of the autonomic preganglionics of the IML (Ross et al., 1984). The ascending facilitory projection from the CVLM to the magnocellular neurons has been proposed to be norepinephrine (NE) (Blessing & Willoughby, 1988) (see Figure 10-11B). The role of NE in VP secretion will be discussed in more detail in a subsequent section.

The parabrachial nucleus receives major input from the NTS (Norgren, 1978). Lesions of the far lateral region of the lateral parabrachial nucleus (LLPBN) have been shown to produce overdrinking to ANG II and isoproterenol (Ohman & Johnson, 1986) (Figure 10-12). However, rats with LLPBN damage do not consume more water than normal controls when challenged with hypertonic saline. In many ways the rats resemble the AP-lesioned animals of Edwards & Ritter (1982) described in the preceding section. The parallels between the two preparations are even more striking because recent studies conducted in the same laboratory indicate that both LLPBN-lesioned and AP-ablated rats also overdrink to ivt ANG II but do not show significant increases in water intake to ivt carbachol (Ohman & Johnson, 1989).

The anatomical studies of Shapiro & Miselis (1985) indicate that there is a heavy projection from the AP/cmNTS to the LLPBN. Functional studies using the "specific' cytotoxin, ibotenic acid, to preferentially destroy cells in the LLPBN have been conducted to further clarify the NTS-LPBN projection. (Edwards & Johnson, 1987). Ibotenic acid lesions in the LPBN also produce the phenomenon, which indicates that the LLPBN lesion-produced overdrinking is primarily the result of destruction of cells in the nucleus rather than damage to fibers of passage. Be-

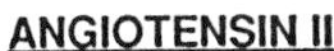

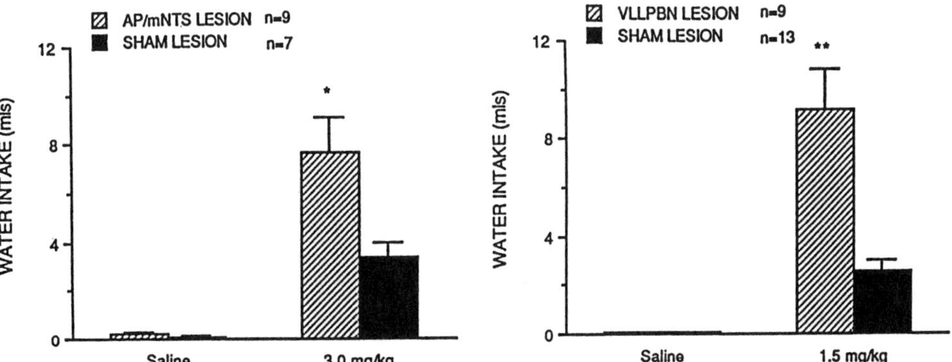

FIGURE 10-12. *The effects of area postrema/medial nucleus of the solitary tract and lateral lateral parabrachial nucleus lesions on drinking to ANG II. Left: Mean water intake at 2 h after subcutaneous administration of ANG II (3.0 mg/kg; Hypertensin, CIBA) and isotonic saline in area postrema and medial region of the nucleus of the solitary tract lesion (AP/mNTS) and sham lesion groups. Right: Mean water intake at 2 h after subcutaneous injection of ANG II (1.5mg/kg) and isotonic saline in ventrolateral region of the lateral parabrachial nucleus (VLLPBN) and sham lesion groups. Values are means +/-SE. *P< 0.05; **P< 0.01. Note the similarity in the overdrinking response to the systemic ANG II treatment in both of the groups of animals that have lesions. (From Ohman & Johnson, 1989).*

cause, as discussed in the previous section, the AP/NTS receives a substantial input of cranial nerve X afferents, a reasonable working hypothesis is that AP/NTS and the LLPBN are central components of a vagal inhibitory system that prevents overhydration (i.e., excessive vascular volume). This idea is supported by studies indicating that inflation of a balloon in the right atrium is no longer effective in inhibiting water intake induced by isoproterenol treatment in rats with LLPBN lesions (Ohman & Johnson, 1987). Recent studies on the effects of LLPBN lesions indicate a similar role for this region in the inhibitory control of VP release (Ohman, Shade & Haywood, 1988).

The functional evidence indicating that cVLM influences VP secretion and that LLPBN lesions affect drinking is clarified by anatomical evidence. Both the cVLM and the LPB project directly to diencephalic areas implicated in cardiovascular/fluid balance control. Some of the major "second order" ascending projections are depicted in Figure 10-11C. In particular, it is important to note that both areas as well as the AP/NTS project to the regions of the nervous system that are literally located at the end of the brain. These are the structures lying along the lamina terminalis.

B. Forebrain Integrative Mechanisms: The SFO/AV3V Complex

1. The Forebrain Sites of 'Afferent' Input: Humoral Targets and Primary Processing: During embryogenesis the rostral end of the neural tube closes and becomes the lamina terminalis. As development proceeds in the mammalian brain, the telencephalon grows enveloping the rostral end of the neural tube. The lamina terminalis is the rostral wall of the third ventricle. The two lamina terminalis associated CVOs, the SFO and OVLT, have been implicated in one species or another as housing sodium/osmoreceptors and sensors of blood-borne ANG II. Also, as described, other periventricular tissues in the proximity of the lamina terminalis are ANG II-sensitive to CSF-borne peptide and may also be responsive to osmotic or sodium concentration changes. The lamina terminalis tissues comprising the SFO and AV3V are in many ways similar to the region containing the AP and NTS. Both regions contain extra-blood-brain barrier organs that have the potential for sampling plasma and, in the rat, both are midline structures with specialized ependymal surfaces facing the ventricular system. However, the two regions at opposite ends of the brain are different in that the AP/NTS receives first order visceral input whereas all neural input received by the SFO/AV3V has passed one or more synapses. Thus, the humoral input into the SFO/AV3V is introduced into the CNS at a higher level. A better understanding of the role of this region in fluid balance can be achieved by examining the changes in hydro-mineral homeostasis produced by AV3V lesions.

2. The AV3V Lesion: Destruction of the small amount of periventricular tissue surrounding the AV3V with an electrolytic lesion or by isolating the region with an encephalatome produces an abrupt cessation of water intake. There are no other overt signs of behavioral disruption. (see Johnson & Buggy, 1977; Johnson, 1979; Johnson, 1982; Johnson, 1985a, 1985b; Brody & Johnson, 1980; 1981; Johnson & Cunningham, 1987; Johnson & Wilkin, 1987; Buggy & Bealer, 1987 for reviews of various aspects of AV3V lesions.) That is, the ingestion of water ceases without signs of motor impairment or reduced food intake beyond that normally observed for a water-deprived animal. The behavioral change is specific for water. For example, if an adipsic animal is given the opportunity to ingest a liquid diet, 5% sucrose or saccharine solutions in place of water, they readily drink the palatable libation. If water is placed in the mouth of a rat with an AV3V lesion during the post-lesion adipsic period, it shows the pattern of oral behaviors comparable to a normal animal receiving an aversive concentration of a bitter quinine solution; that is, the animal behaves as animals described by Grill & Norgren (1978) that are rejecting an aversive substance.

During this period of acute adipsia, the animals show other signs of impaired hydrational controls (Table 10-1). As compared to neurologically intact, water-deprived animals, they lose weight more rapidly, become severely hypernatremic, and both plasma protein concentration and hematocrit increase indicating marked dehydration. While adipsic, VP levels do not rise despite every sign of severe cellular and extracellular fluid losses. Electron microscopic examination of the neurohypophyseal tract indicates that during this acute dehydrated state rats with AV3V lesions do not show the typical signs of increased VP synthesis in magnocellular soma (see Carithers and Johnson, 1988, for review). They do, however, evidence the presence of increased neurosecretory material in axon terminals of the posterior lobe which immunocytochemical staining indicates is VP-like (Wilkin, Gruber, & Johnson, 1986). However, extraction and HPLC characterization of the material in the neurohypophysis indicates that it is not intact VP but most likely unreleased peptide fragments undergoing autolysis (Gruber, Wilkin, & Johnson, 1986). VP synthesis proceeds in magnocellular nuclei as ascertained from pulse-chase studies (Gruber et al., 1986), and VP is transported down the hypothalamo-hypophyseal tract, but is apparently not released. To all intents and purposes, the thirst-related behaviors and the activity of the soma of VP neurons give the appearance that rats with acute AV3V lesions are responding as if they "perceive" themselves as overhydrated rather than dehydrated.

TABLE 10-1. *The Acute and Chronic Effects of AV3V Lesions*

Acute	
Drinking	— adipsia
Vasopressin release	— impaired
Hypernatremia	— severe
Weight loss	— severe
Extracellular Fluid loss	— severe
Chronic	
Drinking	— mean 24 hr intakes recover
	— impaired to challenges
Vasopressin release	— impaired to humoral stimuli
	— intact to extracellular depletion
Hypernatremia	— due to impaired thirst and vasopressin release
Natriuretic Response	— impaired to volume expansion
Natriuretic Factor(s)	— low circulating levels after volume load
Blood Volume	— increased
Plasma Renin	— increased
Basal Arterial Pressure	— normal
Pressor Responses	— attenuated to centrally acting agents
Experimental Hypertension	— blocked or attenuated in most models

If most rats with AV3V lesions are neither hydrated by the investigator nor given a palatable solution (e.g., sucrose), they will usually die of dehydration within 5 to 9 days post-surgery. However, occasionally a lesioned animal will "spontaneously" recover water drinking, and nearly all animals will recover if they are provided adequate hydration either by gavage or by offering them sweetened solutions to drink. The adipsic (for water, that is) animal drinking sweetened solutions during this early period can gradually be "weaned" from hydrational supplementation to water so that by 10 to 14 days post-surgery the average water intake of "recovered" rats with AV3V lesions is comparable to that of sham lesion animals. However, throughout the chronic phase after AV3V lesions, that is the remainder of the animal's life, there are multiple signs of disruption in many hydrational control systems (see Table 10-1). Such deficits are determined by comparing the responses of lesioned and control animals. Rats with AV3V lesions are impaired in their drinking, VP release, and pressor responses to increased extracellular osmolality and ANG II. In contrast to responses evoked by purely humoral stimuli, those having a substantial neural input from visceral receptors (e.g. those responsive to hypovolemia or hypotension) show a degree of recovery (Buggy & Johnson, 1977a; Lind & Johnson, 1983; Johnson, 1985a; Carithers & Johnson, 1988). For example, there are individual rats with chronic AV3V lesions that do not drink to systemic treatments with hypertonic saline or ANG II that will respond to hypovolemia induced by polyethylene glycol (Buggy & Johnson, 1977a; however also see Lind & Johnson, 1983). "Recovered" AV3V lesioned animals will concentrate urine to water deprivation (Fink, Buggy, Johnson & Brody, unpublished observations) and show a normal elevation of VP to hypovolemia (Johnson, 1985a). Examination of electron micrographs of the nuclei containing the magnocellular neurons in animals with chronic AV3V lesions indicates evidence of greater recovery of function in the PVN than in the SON in the response to water deprivation (Carithers & Johnson, 1988). Perhaps the reason for this is because there is greater ascending visceral input from systemic/pressure volume receptors into the PVN as compared to the SON (Carithers & Johnson, 1988).

In addition to impairments in acquiring and retaining water, rats with chronic AV3V lesions are compromised in their capacity to excrete sodium and water. Animals with the periventricular lesion do not effect an appropriate diuresis and natriuresis when volume is expanded (Johnson et al., 1978; Bealer et al., 1983). The impairment in the capacity to increase renal sodium excretion has been suggested to be due to a lack of a natriuretic factor that is an inhibitor of sodium-potassium ATPase activity (Pamnani et al,, 1981; Songu-Mize, Bealer & Caldwell, 1982; Bealer et al., 1983; Buggy et al., 1984).

Collectively, the impairments in function of several of the individual controls of fluid balance "summate" in the rat with chronic AV3V lesions to produce a global pattern of disturbed fluid and cardiovascular regulation. AV3V-lesioned rats remain chronically hypernatremic. In many ways they resemble human patients with brain damage to an area homologus to the AV3V who are diagnosed as having essential or neurogenic hypernatremia (see Ross & Christie, 1969 for review of human essential/neurogenic hypernatremia) (Table 10-2). It is important to note that patients with neurogenic hypernatremia often report impoverished thirst sensations. From an anecdotal description of such an hypernatremic patient, there is reason to believe that water may be perceived as aversive by these dehydrated patients (Skultety & Joynt, 1963). Neurogenic hypernatremia occurs only when *both* thirst and VP mechanisms are impaired (Ross & Christie, 1969).

Rats with AV3V lesions show many indications of altered autonomic function. Attention has been drawn to this fact largely because the chronic rat preparation is remarkably protected against all forms of experimental hypertension studied thus far, and all but one form of genetic hypertension (Table 10-3; see Brody & Johnson, 1980, 1981; Brody, 1988 for reviews). The reasons for the "protective" effects of AV3V lesions against the genesis of high blood pressure are obviously complex and the source of many hypotheses regarding the role of various neural and homeostatic systems involved in the normal and pathophysiological control of blood pressure (e.g., Brody & Johnson, 1980, 1981; Hartle & Brody, 1984; Phillips, 1984, 1987; Brody, 1988; Sanders, Knardahl, & Johnson, 1989). The global alterations in fluid balance and distributive mechanisms that are attendant in the rat with AV3V lesions require an interpretation of the role of this area of the brain in the neural control of these homeostatic processes.

3. A Neurological Interpretation of the AV3V Lesion: The rat with chronic AV3V lesion has little difficulty surviving in the benign environment of the laboratory. The fact that these brain-damaged rats even-

TABLE 10-2. *Parallels between Patients with the Syndrome of Essential Hypernatremia and Rats with Lesions of the Anteroventral Third Ventricle*

	Patients with Essential Hypernatremia	Animals with AV3V Lesions
Hypothalamic Damage	YES	YES
Chronically Elevated Serum Sodium	YES	YES
Reduced or Absent Thirst	YES	YES
Elevated Plasma Renin	YES	YES
Elevated Aldosterone	NO*	NO
Reduced Blood Volume	NO	NO

*1 Patient

TABLE 10-3. *Effects of AV3V Lesions on Experimental Hypertention*

Model	Prevents or attenuates	Reversed
1 kidney, 1 wrap Grollman hypertension	Yes[1]	Yes (water restricted)[2] No (free access conditions)
2 kidneys, 1 clip Goldblatt hypertension	Yes[3]	Yes[3]
Aortic ligation between the renal arteries	Yes[4]	—
Sinoaortic denervation	Yes[5]	—
Lesions of the nucleus of the solitary tract	Yes[5]	—
DOC-salt hypertension	Yes[6]	—
Conflict stress in borderline hypertensive rats (BHR)	Yes[7]	—
Dahl S strain rats	Yes*[8]	—
Spontaneously hypertensive rats	No*[9]	No[2]
Spontaneously hypertensive, stroke-prone rats	No*[10]	—

*Lesion placed at 4 weeks of age.

[1]Buggy et al., 1977
[2]Buggy et al., 1978
[3]Haywood et al., 1978
[4]Hartle et al., 1979
[5]Mow et al., 1978
[6]Fink et al., 1977
[7]Sanders et al, 1989
[8]Brody and Johnson, 1980
[9]Gordon et al., 1982
[10]Gordon et al., 1979

tually recover *ad libitum* water drinking and sufficient VP release to maintain themselves within viable homeostatic boundaries indicates that compensatory changes or reorganization occurs. However, the new or altered mechanisms are not as effective in maintaining homeostasis as those in the intact animals. Under uniform vivarium conditions, as a group, rats with chronic AV3V lesions show intakes that are on the average comparable to the means of sham-lesioned animals. However, the intake of an individual AV3V-lesioned rat shows greater variability in day to day, 24-h water intake, which suggests that these animals probably have less consistency in their hydro-mineral balance (Lind & Johnson, 1983) (Figure 10-13).

The subtle nature of the changes in the controls of fluid balance can be appreciated by examining the disruption in *ad libitum* drinking patterns found in lesioned rats. Normal rats drink the majority of the water they consume daily in conjunction with their meals. In intact animals, meal size and volume of water consumed are highly correlated (Fitzsimons & Le Magnen, 1969; Kraly, 1984). Animals with AV3V lesions still drink in conjunction with meals; however, the relationship between meal size and quantity of water consumed is abolished (Bealer & Johnson, 1980) (see Figure 10-6). Eating is likely to generate stimuli that trigger drinking (Kraly, 1984). Food in the gut or the process of absorption may elevate plasma osmolality and/or ANG II (Johnson et al., 1981) which in turn

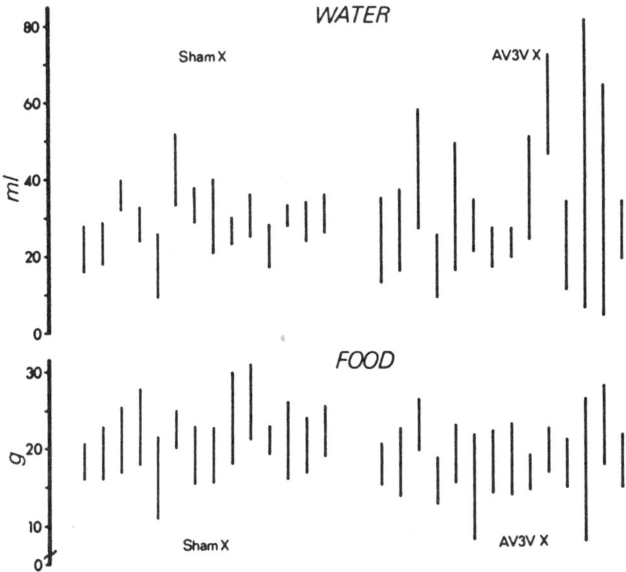

FIGURE 10-13. *The variability of daily food and water intake in "recovered" rats with AV3V lesions. The range of intakes during an 11-day observation period beginning 165 days after surgery in rats that received either sham lesions (Sham X) or AV3V lesions (AV3V X). Water intake for a given rat is depicted directly above its food intake. Rats with AV3V lesions had significantly greater ranges than sham lesion animals in the amounts drunk each day ($P < 0.01$). Variability of food intake was not different for the 2 groups (from Lind & Johnson, 1983).*

serves to signal the brain of a relative dehydration. In other words, it may be that the relationship between meal size and volume of water ingested is a result of the dehydration that is produced by food intake. Because AV3V-lesioned rats are impaired in their responses to humoral stimuli (i.e., ANG II and hyperosmolality), it might be expected that signals accompanying meal-associated dehydration do not act on the brain in rats "blinded" to constituents of the extracellular fluid.

Another indication of the deleterious cumulative effects of subtly compromised function can be detected by assessing the mobilization of defenses against a stressor. When subjected to hypotensive hemorrhage, the chronic AV3V-lesioned animal generates elevated levels of plasma renin, catecholamines, and vasopressin that are only slightly less (i.e., not significantly different with reasonable n's) than neurologically intact rats. However, significantly more lesioned animals die as a result of the hypotensive/hypovolemic challenge (Feuerstein et al., 1984). One interpretation of this finding is that subtle impairments in each of several pressor/volume expansion systems may have a cumulative effect in the brain-damaged animal, causing reduced ability to cope with a severe stress. An animal with an intact AV3V maintains a more consistent internal milieu over a wider range of environmental and endogenous changes and is therefore better adapted.

After recovery, the rat with an AV3V lesion appears to be an excellent example of Jackson's (1884) concepts of neurological organization of function. John Hughlings Jackson espoused the idea that function is represented at multiple levels of the nervous system. Higher levels exert control over and achieve expression through lower levels. The advantages that higher levels of control confer to a given function is increased consistency and enhanced adaptability. That is, the contribution to higher levels of nervous system function is to provide a more consistent internal environment through the addition of mechanisms capable of exercising finer control over the regulated end point (Satinoff, 1978; Lind & Johnson, 1983). The animal with an AV3V lesion appears to be deprived of high level input and/or processing of humoral information that acts on or through structures associated with the lamina terminalis.

4. A Neurobiological Interpretation of The AV3V Lesion: The functional studies of the mid 1970s implicating the periventricular tissues along the rostral wall of the third ventricle were difficult to interpret because there was so little known about the anatomy of the region at that time. The SFO and OVLT had attracted some attention from morphologists because of a unique deficiency in their blood-brain barrier and because of their similarities to the median eminence and posterior pituitary which hinted at neurosecretory function (see Koella & Sutin, 1967, and Weindl, 1973, for early reviews). Only the most prophetic anatomists had suggested a role for this region in the control of salt and water balance (Dietrickx, 1963; Palkovits, 1966) and little was known about communication of these structures with each other or the rest of the brain except for a provocative description of a hypothesized vascular link between the SFO and OVLT (Spoerri, 1963). An early report using degeneration and Golgi techniques presented modest evidence of connections from MePO to SFO and OVLT (Hernesniemi et al., 1972). However, it was not until the application of newly developed tract tracing methods by Miselis and colleagues (Miselis, Shapiro, & Hand, 1979; Miselis, 1981) that data became available to provide insights into the relationship of the structures lying along the lamina terminalis. Efferents were described to project from SFO into MePO, OVLT, and SON (Miselis et al., 1979). Subsequent studies (Camacho & Phillips, 1981b; Miselis, 1981; Lind, Van Hoesen & Johnson, 1982) described the heavy interconnections among the SFO, OVLT, and periventricular preoptic area. Additional studies indicated that AV3V lesions produced terminal degeneration in the SON and degeneration of soma and terminals in the SFO (Carithers et al., 1980).

A distinct bundle of fibers extends from the ventral stock of the SFO along the lamina terminalis and into the AV3V. Many of the fibers in this tract appear to terminate within the AV3V, whereas others sweep through the AV3V in a ventral-caudal direction (Lind et al., 1982). Cutting this descending bundle abolishes blood-borne ANG II-induced drinking but does not block icv ANG II-induced drinking (Lind & Johnson, 1982a, 1982b). In other words, the systemic ANG II-sensitivity of the SFO can be conveniently separated from the central ANG II-sensitivity of the AV3V (Lind & Johnson, 1982a, 1982b).

The SFO sends efferents to several regions implicated in fluid balance in addition to those located along the lamina terminalis. Of particular importance are projections to SON, parvocellular paraventricular nucleus (pPVN), magnocellular paraventricular nucleus (mPVM), reuniens nucleus of the thalamus, zona inserta, medial preoptic nucleus (MPO), and arcuate nucleus of the hypothalamus, (Miselis, 1981; Lind et al., 1982; Miselis et al, 1987). Also, efferents from the OVLT and MePO have been described by Phillips and Camacho, (1987) and by Brown, Standaert and Saper (1985), respectively, that project to many of the same targets (see Figure 10-14B). The lamina terminalis structures receive projections from several areas (some of which were described in previous sections) including NTS, parabrachial nucleus, dorsal and medial raphe, ventrolateral medulla, dorsomedial and lateral hypothalamus, PVN, and reuniens nucleus of the thalamus (Phillips & Camacho, 1987; Lind & Ganten, 1990; Saper & Levishon, 1983). (see Figure 10-11).

Of the structures that comprise the AV3V, the only periventricular tissue in addition to the OVLT and MePO that has received reasonable anatomical consideration is the AVPV. The AVPV contains atrial natriuretic-like peptide and has been described as projecting to PVN (Standaert, Needleman & Saper, 1986). The efferents of the periventricular nuclei, which are medial to the MPO and AH nuclei proper, have received little individual attention and have usually been described collectively with more lateral regions. That is, available anterograde tracing studies do not differentiate the source of efferents of the periventricular preoptic/periventricular anterior hypothalamic nuclei as distinct from the medial MPO/medial anterior hypothalamic nucleus *per se* (Conrad & Pfaff, 1976). Efferent tracing from points in this periventricular/MPO region (Conrad & Pfaff, 1976) or a bit more laterially in the MPO (Swanson, Kucharczyk, & Mogenson, 1978) describe two pathways that descend to the central gray and the ventral tegmental area (see Figure 10-14C).

As previously discussed, there is excellent evidence that the SFO/AV3V complex contains osmo-/sodium and ANG II-sensitive tissue. In addition, neurons within the AV3V have been shown to be activated by stimulation of baroreceptors (Knuepfer, Gebhart, & Brody, 1985). Functional studies indicate that in addition to thirst and VP secretion, autonomic outflow is influenced by activation of the SFO/AV3V. Electrical

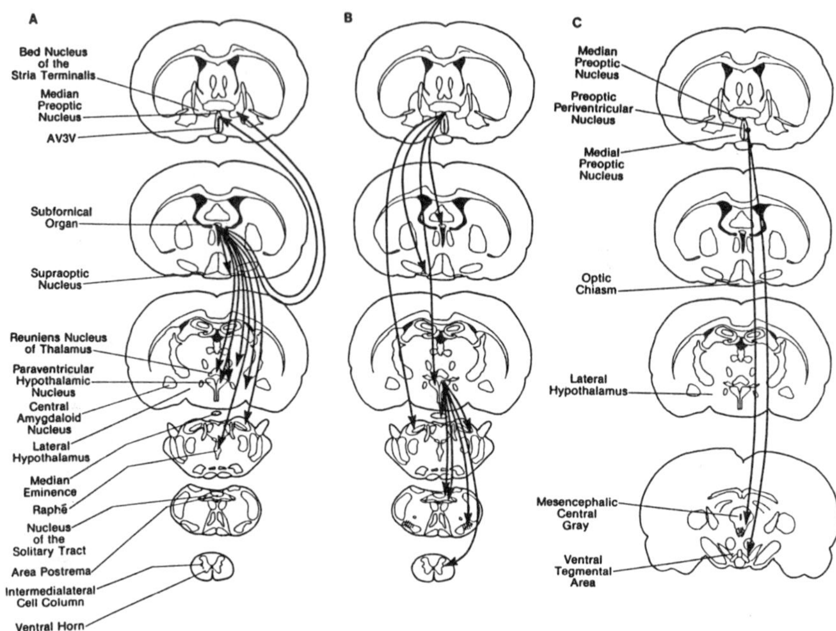

FIGURE 10-14. *Descending projections from the lamina terminalis and hypothalamus. Panel A, Left: Identification of many of the regions associated with descending output of the SFO/AV3V region and of the parvocellular paraventricular nucleus. Panel A, Right: Efferent projections of the SFO. Panel B, Left: Efferents of the median preoptic nucleus. Panel B, Right: Efferents of the parvocellular paraventricular nucleus. Panel C, Efferents from the medial portion of the medial preoptic nucleus and the periventricular preoptic nucleus to the ventral tegmental area and the mesencephalic central gray. (Panels A and B based on Miselis et al., 1986, 1987; Lind et al., 1982; Lind & Ganten, 1989; Swanson & Sawchenko, 1982; Panel C based on Conrad & Pfaff, 1976; Swanson, Kucharczyk & Mogenson, 1978).*

stimulation of the AV3V with relatively large electrodes (Fink et al., 1978; Knuepfer, Johnson, & Brody, 1984; Berecek & Brody, 1982) and of SFO, MePO, OVLT, or periventricular preoptic individually with smaller devices (Mangiapane & Brody, 1987) produces changes in regional blood flows, heart rate and blood pressure.

From the results of a series of studies using electrolytic lesions and knife cuts, Hartle and Brody (1982; 1984) have concluded that the descending projection from the ANG II sensitive SFO, MePO, and OVLT departs from the MePO by a midline course. Interruption of this projection with a medial coronal knife cut blocks the centrally mediated component of the pressor response of ANG II and ANG II-dependent forms of hypertension but not ANG II-independent forms of hypertension (Hartle & Brody, 1982, 1984). Parasagittal knife cuts separating the AV3V from the medial forebrain bundle blocks non-renin dependent forms (i.e., vascular volume- or sodium-dependent) of hypertension but not renin-dependent forms of hypertension (Bealer, 1984; see Hartle & Brody, 1984, and Buggy & Bealer, 1987, for reviews). As of yet, very little is known about the precise origin, neurochemical nature, and terminations of these projections.

Many of the descending projections of the SFO/AV3V terminate in different medial and lateral nuclei of the hypothalamus. The projections to hypothalamic magnocellular PVN and SON have obvious implications in the control of VP release. Other diencephalic regions also are implicated in other fluid-related functions. Of all hypothalamic nuclei, the PVN has received the most attention over the past decade as a major integrative hub influencing endocrine and autonomic function (Swanson & Sawchenko, 1983; Porter & Brody, 1986). In addition to the "descending" projections from the SFO/AV3V, important influences on pPVN arise from hindbrain structures. Both endocrine and autonomic function are likely to be modulated by pPVN. Anterior pituitary function is influenced by PVN cells containing releasing factors that project to the median eminence (see below). In addition, efferents from other components of pPVN project to regions such as parabrachial nucleus rVLM, cVLM, dorsal motor nucleus of X, NTS, and IML (Swanson, 1977; Ono et al., 1978) (see Figure 11-14B). Electrical stimulation of pPVN alters blood pressure, heart rate, and regional blood flow (Porter & Brody, 1985, 1986). Such autonomic changes may be the result of activating descending projections that either 1) act directly or multisynaptically on the final common path of autonomic outflow (i.e., either the sympathetic or parasympathetic preganglionic neurons in the vagal motor complex or IML); 2) act at sites in the baroreceptor or similar reflex pathways to modulate the baroreceptor reflex (Ciriello and Calaresu, 1980); or 3) both. pPVN contains cells responsive to changes in arterial blood pressure and which project to dorsomedial medulla (Kannan & Yamashita, 1983). Several peptides such as VP, oxytocin, and ANG II (see below) have been identified in the projections that descend from pPVN to the dorsal motor complex of X, the VLM, and the IML. Several of these peptides, when injected ivt, produce sympathetic activation (Severs & Daniels-Severs, 1973; Pittman, Lawrence & McLean, 1982). Direct injection of VP (Matsuguchi et al., 1982) and ANG II (Casto & Phillips, 1986; Rettig, Healy & Printz, 1986; Andreatta et al., 1988) into the NTS or VLM produces pressor responses and/or changes in baroreceptor reflex gain.

Figure 10-15 represents a functional composite of the major ascending and descending projections represented in Figures 10-11 and 10-14. Contemplation of Figures 10-11, 10-14, and 10-15 in light of the present discussion should lead to at least two conclusions at this point. The first is related to the overall topic of this paper—the principles of the organization of neural systems involved in the integrative control of body fluid homeostasis. The structures and pathways connecting the AP/NTS and SFO/AV3V constitute the essence of what Miselis and colleagues have termed the *visceral neuraxis* (Miselis et al., 1986; Miselis et al., 1987). That is, this is the major central network representing the diverse inputs of the

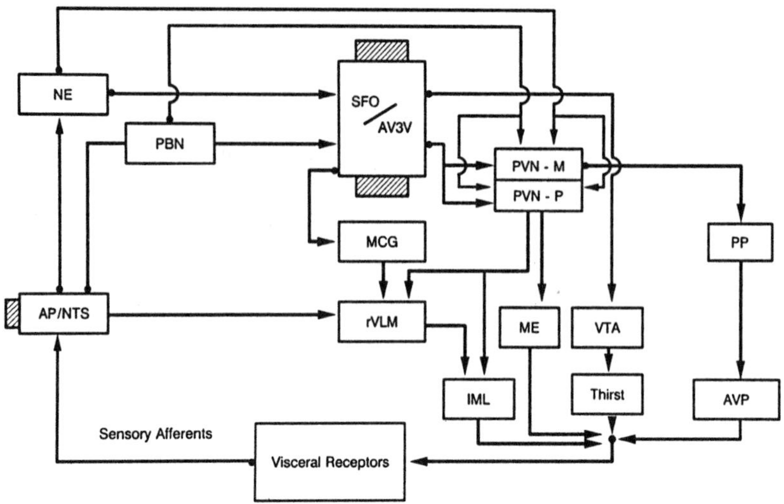

FIGURE 10-15. *Schematic depicting major structures and pathways involved in the neural control of body fluid homeostasis. Bottom, center of the figure, visceral receptors are depicted. Visceral chemo-and mechanoreceptors distributed throughout the body deliver neural input into the CNS over afferent pathways that terminate largely in the region of the area postrema (AP) and nucleus of the solitary tract (NTS). From the AP/NTS ascending input projects to hindbrain norepinephrine cell groups (NE) and to the parabrachial nucleus (PBN; of particular importance in fluid balance is the lateral PBN or LPBN). Efferents from NE and PBN ascend to forebrain regions, including the structures along the lamina terminalis — the subfornical organ (SFO) and the periventricular tissue around the anteroventral third ventricle (AV3V). The SFO and AV3V (as does the AP) contain chemoreceptors which monitor extracellular fluid and blood-borne agents. Pathways descend from the SFO/AV3V complex to innervate several hypothalamic nuclei such as the supraoptic nucleus (SON, not shown) and paraventricular nucleus (PVN; both magnocellular, M, and parvocellular, P, components) and several hindbrain regions such as the mesencephalic central gray (MCG) and ventral tegmental area (VTA). The projections to VTA have been implicated in the control of thirst. The SON and PVN-M vasopressin (AVP) neurons are the "final common path" to the posterior pituitary (PP) and release antidiuretic hormone into the circulation. PVN-P neurons project to the median eminence (ME) and are likely to influence the release of hormones from the anterior pituitary that alter vascular and renal function. Also "autonomic" pathways which influence sympathetic outflow to the vasculature and the kidneys descend to areas such as the rostral ventrolateral medulla (rVLM) which, in turn, influences activity of preganglionic neurons which have their cell bodies in the interomediolateral cell column (IML).*

viscera of the body. Blood-borne information in all likelihood reaches this articulated group of "centers" through the AP, SFO and OVLT; neural input from systemic receptors enters this network primarily through the NTS. At each synapse the potential for imparting or extracting information exists. This is where the primary business of integrative control of fluid balance occurs.

The second conclusion to be drawn relates to the function of the structures of the rostral basal forebrain and control of fluid homeostasis, or: why should an AV3V lesion produce such extensive alterations in fluid balance? The organization of the *visceral neuraxis* indicates that blood-borne input targeting the SFO/AV3V enters this information processing network at a high level and thereby asserts a prepotent role in the control of fluid homeostasis.

Considering currently available anatomical and functional information, a reasonable working hypothesis is that AV3V lesions: 1) destroy elements that function as sensors of concentration and/or other blood-borne agents of extracellar fluids; 2) interrupt fibers of passage originating in the SFO which project to diencephalic structures outside the AV3V; and 3) disrupt processing elements intrinsic to the AV3V that are involved in control of fluid balance. There are many different hydration-related functions played by the SFO/AV3V. The results of early lesion reconstruction studies indicated that it is possible to fractionate the AV3V, that is, dissociate the complex of fluid-related disruptions produced by the typical AV3V lesion. Discrete knife cuts of inflow and outflow of the region, specific neurotoxins, and pharmacological agonists and antagonists are a few of the strategies employed thus far to tease out the functional organization of the region.

One SFO/AV3V function that has been analyzed in more detail than others is the control of extracellular depletion-induced thirst. Our current understanding can best be described by discussing a model of some of the neural systems that interact within the AV3V.

5. A Model of a SFO/AV3V Function In the Control of Extracellular Thirst: Figure 10-16 presents a current model to account for much of the neurobiological and functional data available which indicates that among the many roles of the SFO/AV3V region, it functions in the reception and early processing of information important for the generation of a normal drinking response to extra-cellular fluid depletion. As originally proposed (Lind & Johnson, 1982b), the model stated that blood-borne ANG II, acting on ANG II receptive neurons, increased the activity of a descending bundle of peptide-containing neurons that release ANG II from their terminals into the MePO, in turn, to stimulate higher order neurons involved in the transmission of information in a system controlling extracellular depletion-induced drinking. The model incorporated several pieces of experimental data available at that time, which included demonstrations: 1) of the existence of a major efferent bundle of fibers issuing from the ventral stock of the SFO and running into the AV3V (Miselis et al., 1979; Miselis, 1981; Lind et al., 1982); 2) that cutting this descending bundle abolished the drinking response to systemic ANG (Eng & Miselis, 1981; Lind & Johnson, 1982a), but no CSF borne ANG II (Lind & Johnson, 1982a) ANG II; 3) That drinking induced by blood-borne ANG II was blocked by the presence of CSF-borne ANG II receptor antagonist (Johnson & Schwob, 1975), but that CSF-borne ANG II did not act on the SFO for its dipsogenic effect (Buggy et al., 1975; Buggy & Fisher, 1976); and 4) that cold cream plugs placed in the AV3V while abolishing drinking to CSF-borne ANG II did not impair, but actually

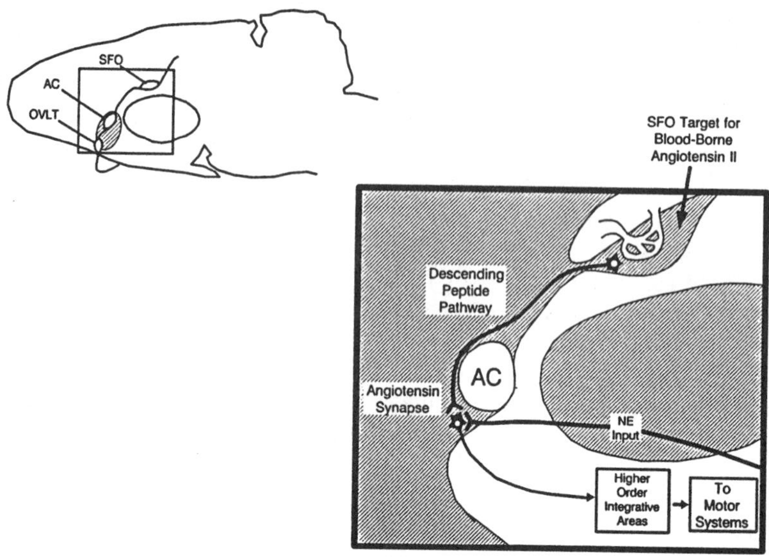

FIGURE 10-16. *A sagittal schematic representation of the interaction of angiotensinergic and noradrenergic inputs into the median preoptic (MePO) nucleus that are involved in the mediation of extracellular thirst. The model is derived from one proposing a dual role for angiotensin (ANG) in thirst (Lind & Johnson, 1982a; 1982b). Blood-borne angiotensin penetrates the fenestrated capillaries of the subfornical organ (SFO) and activates receptors. A "descending" pathway conducts information derived from the action of angiotensin in the SFO down the lamina terminalis and into the AV3V (particularly the MePO). The "descending" pathway contains and uses angiotensin as a peptidergic neurotransmitter. Ascending noradrenergic input into the MePO arises from the A1, A2, and A6 noradrenergic cell groups in the brainstem. It is proposed that norepinephrine (NE) availability in the MePO is inversely proportional to the systemic blood volume and/or blood pressure. Increased synaptic NE in the MePO modulates the action of increased ANG II to facilitate neural output to higher order neurons and regions involved in the control of water intake.*

appeared to enhance (perhaps by sequestration of endogenous brain ANG released into the AV3V) drinking to systemic ANG.

In a subsequent version of the model (Johnson, 1985, 1985b), an ascending modulatory adrenergic input carrying information from pressure/volume receptors into the AV3V was incorporated into the hypothesis to account for the effects of catecholamine depletion-produced impairments in drinking to systemically and icv injected ANG II (Gordon et al., 1979; Gordon, Brody & Johnson, 1985; McRae-Degueurce et al., 1986; Bellin, Bhatnagar & Johnson, 1987a; Bellin, Landas & Johnson, 1987b, 1988; Cunningham & Johnson, 1989). Since the initial presentation of the model, experimental results from several laboratories have presented data that have confirmed all of the fundamental concepts that are included in the hypothesis. "Although the model was proposed to account specifically for the control of drinking to stimuli accompanying extracellular fluid depletion, the basic aspects of the model, particularly the roles played by the brain renin-angiotensin system (BRAS) and by brain norepinephrine (NE), may reflect a common mechanism used in the neural control of other effector systems that defend against hypovolemia (Johnson, 1985a, 1985b; Johnson & Wilkin, 1987; Johnson & Cunningham, 1987; Cunningham & Johnson, 1988). At the heart of the SFO/AV3V model for the control of extracellular dehydration-induced drinking is the interaction of the brain BRAS and of NE. An evaluation of the model in light of current data and an appraisal of its generalizability to other fluid balance controls can be conducted best in light of an understanding of the BRAS and central NE system and the data that implicate their roles in the control of body fluid homeostasis.

C. Neurochemical Systems Controlling Extracellular Volume

1. The Brain Renin-Angiotensin System (BRAS) and Body Fluid Homeostasis: The finding that drinking was induced by the injection of ANG into the CNS (Booth, 1968; Epstein et al., 1970) coincided with the discovery that components of the RAS were present in the brain (Fischer-Ferraro et al., 1971; Ganten et al., 1971) and the formulation of the hypothesis that the brain synthesized the components of this enzyme-peptide system *de novo* (Ganten et al., 1972; Ganten et al., 1976). Although not without healthy skepticism (see Reid, 1979 for review of concerns), there has been a steady marshalling of experimental evidence in support of the presence of a BRAS with a functional role. Through the efforts of several laboratories there is now a substantial body of biochemical literature supporting the concept of a BRAS (see Ganten et al., 1982; Printz et al., 1982; Phillips, 1984, 1987; Moffett, Bumpus & Husain, 1987, for reviews). The development of physiological investigations to complement biochemical approaches has largely stemmed from the known volume and cardiovascular regulatory actions ascribed to the peripheral RAS. Functional evidence indicates that in addition to drinking, centrally injected ANG II produces increased sodium intake (Buggy & Fisher, 1976; Epstein, 1982); vasopressin release (Keil, Summy-Long & Severs, 1975); natriuresis (Andersson et al., 1972); ACTH release (Maran & Yates, 1977); and increases in mean arterial blood pressure mediated by both VP release and sympathetic activation (Severs et al., 1970). The general picture of the central actions of ANG II are consistent with its "traditional" systemic role of optimizing and restoring fluid and cardiovascular homeostasis.

The biochemical characterization of extracted components of the RAS metabolic cascade from the brain do not provide absolute proof that the substances are in fact synthesized in the CNS; that is, they may have been taken up from plasma and sequestered in the brain. Therefore, the recent application of techniques of molecular biology have proved valuable. The cloning of cDNA for angiotensinogen (Ohkubo et al., 1983) and for renin (Rougeon et al., 1981) has led to the identification of the mRNAs of these proteins in brain tissue (Dzau et al., 1986; Ohkubo et al., 1986; Campbell & Habener, 1986; Lynch et al., 1986).

Presently, BRAS-related questions are focusing on concerns of processing brain angiotensinogen and compartmentalization of brain enzyme and substrate (Moffett, Bumpus & Husain, 1987; Richoux et al., 1988). Although components of the renin-angiotensin system have been found in cultured neurons (Hermann et al., 1988; Hermann, Phillips & Raizada, 1989), it has been questioned whether renin and angiotensinogen both exist in neurons *in vivo*. It has been suggested that glia may be the major source of angiotensinogen and that neurons release renin to generate brain ANG II in the extracellular space (Moffett, Bumpus & Husain, 1987). However, recent localization of angiotensinogen mRNA in brain (Lynch, Hawelu-Johnson, & Guyenet, 1987) and immunocytochemical staining (Richoux et al., 1988) for angiotensinogen in neurons may obviate some of the concerns about localization of the components of the BRAS and suggest that the brain uses a more conventional mode of peptide processing for the formation of ANG II.

Other current questions about the BRAS deal with the nature of the "true" effector ANG II-like peptide in the brain. There has been considerable discussion as to whether the heptapeptide ANG III is the endogenous ligand (e.g., see Wright et al., 1985). [Also, although the ANG-like material extracted from brain has been shown to be very similar or even identical to ANG I, II, and III (Hermann et al., 1982; Phillips & Stenstrom, 1985), it has been suggested (Meyer, Phillips, & Eiden, 1982; Pohl et al., 1988) that a higher molecular weight peptide (i.e., weight of 5,000 to 6,000 instead of 1,046) may be another or the true endogenous ligand for the brain angiotensin receptor]. As for any other neurochemical system, the "proof" of existence of the BRAS will require the cumulative weight of many converging lines of evidence.

Recently, Lind and Ganten (1990) have pointed out that ANG in the brain has been characterized with essentially all the tools of modern biology. Among the various strategies used to study the BRAS, the morphological approach has been especially helpful in developing concepts to further understanding about its functional organization as related to fluid homeostasis. Several groups of investigators (e.g., Fuxe et al., 1976; Weyhenmeyer & Phillips, 1982; Healy & Printz, 1984) have identified ANG-like staining throughout the CNS. In extensive immunocytochemical tracer studies, Lind and his colleagues (reviewed in Lind & Ganten, 1990) have identified more than 70 fiber networks and 50 cell groups containing angiotensin immunoreactivity in the CNS. Many of these are associated with the SFO/AV3V and other regions implicated in body fluid regulation. Lind and colleagues have identified a major descending projection of ANG-like fibers from the SFO with terminal fields in the

MePO, PVN, and midbrain raphe to name a few (see Figure 10-17). Combined retrograde tracing and immunocytochemistry show evidence of transported tracer from injection sites in the PVN, MePO (Lind & Ganten, 1990), and SON (Wilkin et al., 1989) back to cell bodies that stain for ANG-like material in the SFO. "Higher order" pathways originating in the MePO and PVN, in turn, project to median eminence, posterior pituitary, dorsal vagal complex, midbrain raphe, and spinal chord—all areas that have been repeatedly implicated in neural/humoral control of fluid and cardiovascular homeostasis (Lind, 1987; Lind & Ganten, 1990).

The SFO-MePO projection (Figure 10-17) is the angiotensinergic pathway in the SFO-AV3V model hypothesized to conduct information about blood-borne ANG from the SFO into the AV3V (Lind & Johnson, 1982b). Angiotensin sensitive units in the MePO have been shown to be activated by electrical stimulation of the SFO using *in vitro* and *in vivo* electophysiological methods (Nelson & Johnson, 1985; Tanaka et al., 1987). Similarly, the functional role for ANG-like fibers arising from SFO and MePO and projecting into putative VP secreting PVN neurons is also supported by electrophysiological evidence of magnocellular acti-

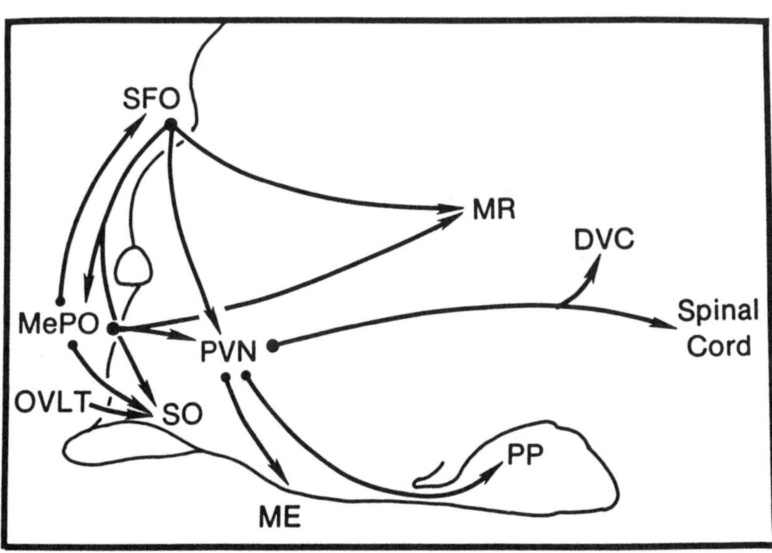

FIGURE 10-17. *A summary of angiotensin-immunoreactive projections from the structures of the lamina terminalis. Pathways represented have been verified with anterograde transport and by retrograde transport combined with angiotensin immunocytochemistry. The majority of the work depicted was conducted by Lind et al. (1984a; 1984b; 1985a; 1985b) and Lind & Ganten, (1990). Wilkin et al. (1989) confirmed the ANG II projection from the SFO to the supraoptic nucleus and identified an ANG-like projection from the OVLT to the supraoptic nucleus (SON) (figure adapted from Lind & Ganten, 1990). Abbreviations: SFO=subfornical organ; MePO=median preoptic nucleus; OVLT=organum vasculosum of the lamina terminalis; PVN=paraventricular nucleus; MR=Midbrain Raphe; ME=median eminence; PP=posterior pituitary; DVC=dorsal vagal complex; sc=spinal cord.*

vation mediated by ANG when these regions are electrically stimulated (Tanaka, Saito, & Kaba, 1987). Blood-borne ANG has been demonstrated to enhance the activity of putative PVN VP cells by acting through SFO (Tanaka et al., 1987).

The SFO-PVN projection terminates in pPVN as well as mPVN (Miselis, 1981; Sawchenko & Swanson, 1983; Swanson & Lind, 1986), and ANG-immunoreactive fibers and varicosities appear also in this region (Lind & Ganten, 1990). Corticotropin-releasing factor (CRF) containing cells in the pPVN project to the portal capillaries of the median eminence. Following adrenalectomy some putative CRF cells show increased ANG-like (Lind et al., 1984a) and vasopressin-like (Sawchenko, Swanson & Vale, 1984; Kiss, Mezey & Skirboll, 1984) staining and increased mRNA for vasopressin (Wolfson, Manning, Davis, Arentzen & Baldino, 1985). Thus, there is the possibility of the SFO influencing the pituitary-adrenal axis through an angiotensinergic SFO-pPVN—pPVN-median eminence projection which, in turn, alters delivery of the three principal ACTH secretagogues (CRF, VP, ANG) to the fenestrated capillaries of the median eminence (Lind et al., 1985a; Lind & Ganten, 1990). Administration of the converting enzyme inhibitor, captopril, ivt blocks the release of ACTH and VP to hemorrhagic stress in sheep (Cameron et al., 1986).

Other ANG containing pPVN cells contribute a small number of fibers to dorsal vagal complex and spinal regions containing autonomic preganglionic cells (Lind, 1987). Stimulation of SFO excites PVN cells that, in turn, project to dorsal medulla (Ferguson, Day, & Renaud, 1984). Angiotensinergic projections from PVN may be responsible for modulating autonomic outflow by altering cardiovascular reflex gain at the NTS (Casto & Phillips, 1986).

In addition to the "descending" ANG-like projections, it is interesting that Lind and colleagues (see Lind & Ganten 1990 for review) have described a set of ANG-like projections that originate in several diencephalic nuclei and project rostrally terminate in the SFO. The cell bodies of these SFO afferents reside in the lateral hypothalamic area, reuniens nucleus of the thalamus, the zona inserta, and MePO. Each of these areas has been implicated in the control of fluid balance, particularly drinking, (see Teitelbaum and Epstein, 1962; Fisher & Coury, 1964; Grossman, 1984; Lind & Johnson, 1982b, respectively, for each region). It is possible that the SFO may be activated by ANG not only from the periphery but also from brain sources.

Recent advances in quantitative autoradiography have provided a means to examine the distribution of ANG receptors in the brain (Mendelsohn et al., 1984; Plunkett et al., 1987). Unlike many peptide systems where there is a mismatch between terminal regions and receptors, there is excellent coincidence for these two elements of the brain (Lind, 1988). In addition there is a remarkable concentration of receptor labeling distributed along the lamina terminalis and throughout the AV3V region (Mendelsohn et al., 1984; Plunkett et al., 1987).

With the use of *in situ* hybridization, it has recently become possible to verify the presence of angiotensinogen mRNA in many sites in the CNS (Lynch, Hawelu-Johnson, & Guyenet, 1987). Angiotensinogen message is distributed throughout the brain with localized high concentrations limited to the number of nuclear boundaries. Strong signals are detected throughout the AV3V, as well as the NTS and parabrachial nucleus (Lynch et al., 1987). Angiotensinogen message has also been reported to be high in the mPVN (Aronsson et al., 1988).

a. *Summary—"Descending" ANG Projections and Fluid Balance*: Since the model to account for the SFO and AV3V in the mediation of ANG-induced drinking was first proposed (Lind & Johnson, 1982b), several basic points of the hypothesis have been confirmed. Specifically: 1) the existence of an angiotensinergic projection from the SFO into the AV3V has been demonstrated with tract tracing and combined immunocytochemical methods; 2) ANG-sensitive cells exist in the AV3V that are activated by SFO stimulation; 3) a high density of ANG receptors resides throughout the AV3V; and 4) a high concentration of mRNA for angiotensinogen is found along the lamina terminalis and within the AV3V.

In addition to SFO projections to the AV3V there are descending pathways that terminate in hypothalamic magnocellular nuclei as well as in the pPVN. An accumulating body of evidence implicates the release of ANG from the projections descending from the lamina terminalis structures with VP release; with control of the ACTH-releasing factors—CRF, VP, and ANG; and with descending pathways modulating autonomic outflow.

2. Central Noradrenergic Mechanisms and the Control of Fluid Balance: The application of the formaldehyde-condensation histochemical method of Falck and colleagues (1962) to brain and spinal cord demonstrated the existence of dopamine-(DA), norepinephrine-(NE), and serotonin-(5-HT) containing neurons in the CNS. The specification of amine trajectories as a result of "chemical neuroanatomy" and the capacity of pharmacological and surgical techniques to activate, inhibit, and destroy amine systems prompted studies on the role of NE, DA, and 5-HT in nearly every conceivable behavioral and physiological system. The mechanisms controiling the distribution and balance of body fluids has not escaped the same type of scrutiny.

One of the useful tools for the analysis of central amine function is the neurotoxin 6-hydroxydopamine (6-OHDA), which with reasonable specificity destroys DA- and NE-containing neurons. When the neurotoxin 6-OHDA is injected ivt, the rats manifest a set of signs that resemble those described for AV3V lesions. The similarities between the two types of lesions are presented in Table 10-4. Given the parallels between AV3V and 6-OHDA lesions on fluid homeostasis, it is reasonable to con-

TABLE 10-4. *Parallels Between Rats with AV3V Lesions and Rats Following 6-Hydroxydopamine Treatment*

Transient adipsia
Permanent deficits to thirst challenges
Prevents the development of many forms of chronic experimental hypertension
Pressor deficits to central angiotension II and hypertonic saline injections
Chronic impairments in vasopressin release
Chronic reduction in body weight

sider whether the two manipulations exert their effects through similar mechanisms. In other words, is a common tissue or neurochemical system insulted by the two treatments?

a. *Thirst:* The results of a series of experiments (Gordon et al., 1979; Gordon et al., 1985; Bellin et al., 1987a) indicate that the presence of NE in a periventricular site is critical for normal drinking responses to ANG. This periventricular site has been further specified by using localized interparenchymal injections of 6-OHDA and was found to lie within a portion of the AV3V region (Bellin et al., 1987b; Bellin et al., 1988). Injections of 6-OHDA into the tissues lying along the ventral lamina terminalis (i.e., the ventral MePO and OVLT), which produce localized depletions of both NE and DA, attenuate drinking and pressor responses to ANG but produce no impairments in drinking to icv carbachol or cellular fluid depletion (Bellin et al., 1988). To be effective, the 6-OHDA treatment along the ventral lamina terminalis must deplete NE; depletion of DA alone within this region has no effect on the ANG-induced responses (Bellin et al., 1988, Cunningham & Johnson, 1989).

Ascending adrenergic input into the MePO arises from the brain stem, in particular from the A1/C1 region of the ventrolateral medulla and from the A2/C2 region in the dorsomedial medulla (Saper, Reis, & Joh, 1983). Relative to NE, the concentration of epinephrine (E) along the ventral lamina terminalis is so low that it is unfeasible to analyze with electrochemical detection-chromatographic methods (Cunningham & Johnson, 1989). Other lines of evidence indicate the importance of NE rather than E in the AV3V in the control of extracellular fluid depletion-related drinking.

If a reduction of NE in the ventral lamina terminalis is the critical aspect of the 6-OHDA induced deficits, then repleting NE should restore function. The use of dispersed fetal cell transplants containing catecholamine cells provides a means for restoring NE to the ventral lamina terminalis. When viable catecholamine cells taken from the fetal (17 day) anlage (i.e., precursor) of the A6 or the A1A2/C1C2 brain regions are placed into the AV3V of a rat previously treated with 6-OHDA, recovery of ANG-induced drinking and pressor responses occurs (McRae-Degueurce et al., 1986; McRae-Degueurce et al., 1987) (Figure 10-18). Because the A6 region contains NE but no E cells, the restoration of func-

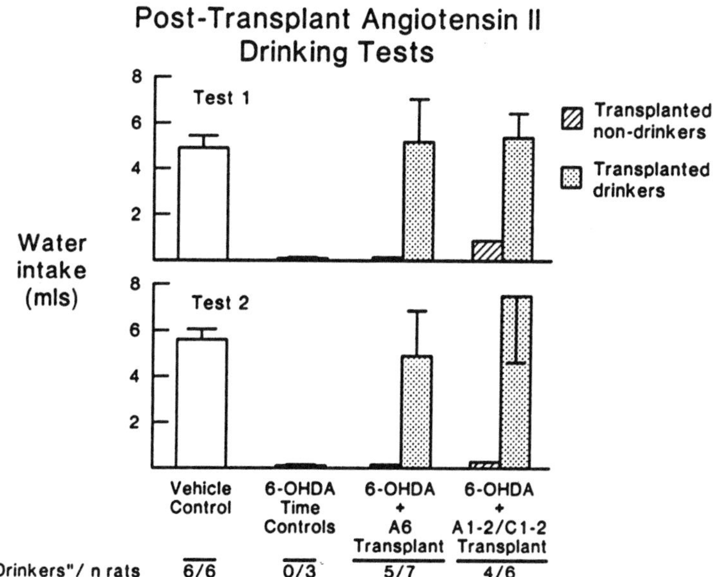

FIGURE 10-18. *Water intake in 2-h drinking tests to subcutaneously injected angiotensin II in a vehicle control group, in a 6-hydroxydopamine-treated time control group, and in two 6-hydroxydopamine-treated plus transplanted groups. The transplanted animals received dissociated 17-day-old fetal cell suspension transplants from either the locus coeruleus (A6) or the hindbrain catecholamine cell groups (A_1,A_2/C_1,C_2). Test I was conducted 2 weeks post-transplant and Test II was conducted on the same animals 3 weeks post-transplant. An isotonic saline challenge (2.0 ml/kg; s.c.) did not stimulate significant drinking responses in any group of animals. (From McRae-Degueurce et al., 1986; Johnson & Cunningham, 1987).*

tion with cells from A6 argues that NE is the more critical of the two catecholamines. More recently, NE replacement in 6-OHDA-depleted animals has been examined directly. When rats with 6-OHDA-induced drinking response deficits are infused ivt with NE, drinking is significantly increased to ivt ANG (Cunningham & Johnson, 1989). Intraventricular infusion of the same dose of NE alone or in combination with ANG in control (i.e., non-6-OHDA treated) rats does not increase drinking. Together, the results of localized and specific depletions and the demonstration that recovery of function can be produced by NE indicate that NE plays an important role interacting with the actions of ANG within the AV3V.

NE innervation of the forebrain originates from a relatively small number of cell bodies in the medulla and pons. As the system ascends the neuraxis, it branches and splays out to influence virtually all of the forebrain. Investigations of the locus coeruleus and its NE projections has led to the hypothesis that NE primarily modifies the throughput of sensory transmission and increases the signal to noise ratio, when other transmitters are released (Woodward et al., 1979; Jahr & Nicoll, 1982; Foote, Bloom, & Aston-Jones, 1983). In the SFO/AV3V model, the descending ANG pathway from the SFO is a sensory input carrying information about blood-borne ANG. The level of NE released into regions of the AV3V therefore would act to set the gain for the transfer of information across nuclei such as the MePO. Under what types of conditions might the gain be enhanced? An obvious condition would be hypovolemia/hypotension. This hypothesis has recently been tested. NE activity was evaluated in alpha-methyl-para-tyrosine treated animals subjected to hypovolemia. Alpha-methyl-para-tyrosine was used to block NE synthesis so that the decline in NE levels in a given brain region can be considered as an index of the activity of the catecholamine over the time course of the treatment. Hypovolemia induced with polyethylene glycol treatment significantly increased NE turnover in the MePO (Wilkin et al., 1987; see Figure 10-19). In other words, more NE was probably released into the region of the AV3V as a result of the hypovolemia. The results of preliminary *in vitro* electrophysiological studies indicating that bath administration of NE enhances the responses from MePO neurons to either SFO electrical stimulation or to ANG II application (Graham, Nelson, & Johnson, 1985) is consistent with the proposed role of NE in the SFO/AV3V model.

b. *Vasopressin:* Both the PVN and SON receive noradrenergic input. From earlier studies it was concluded by Sawchenko and Swanson (1983) that both nuclei have a major input from the A1 region of the

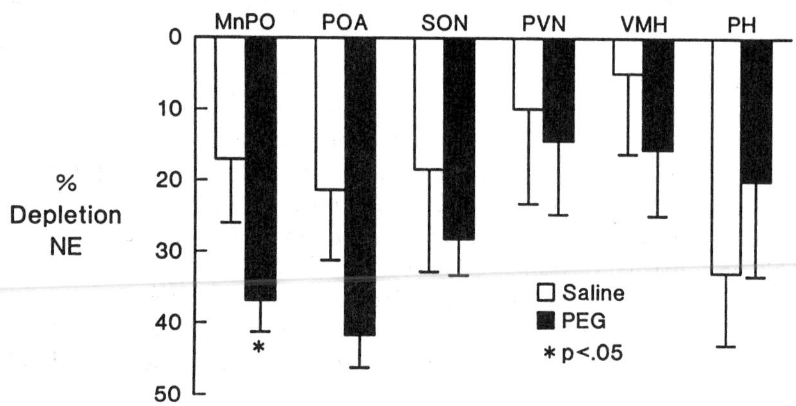

FIGURE 10-19. *The effect of hypovolemia on norepinephrine (NE) turnover in several diencephalic regions. Hypovolemia was induced by subcutaneous injection of 5 mL of 30% polyethylene glycol (PEG). Relative changes in NE levels are shown 240 min following alpha-methyl paratyrosine (aMPT) treatment in saline and PEG treated groups. The changes are expressed as percent depletion +/- SEM of 0-time controls. The relative turnover of NE is indicated by depletion of NE levels following aMPT administration as compared to NE levels in untreated control animals. Larger percent depletions indicate higher NE turnover levels. *P< 0.05 compared to Saline. Micropunches were taken from the median preoptic nucleus (MnPO), preoptic area (POA), supraoptic nucleus (SON), paraventricular nucleus (PVN), ventromedial hypothalamus (VMH), and posterior hypothalamus (PH). Although several of the fluid-related regions in the hypothalamus (e.g., MnPO, SON, PVN) tended to show an increase in NE turnover, only the MnPO was significant at the time interval tested.*

caudal ventrolateral medulla, and that the PVN receives relatively greater input from the A2 and A6 regions than does the SON. More recent experiments using doxorubicin as a retrograde tracer provide evidence for NE input into the SON that originates from the A2 and A6 NE cell groups as well as from the A1 area (Wilkin et al., 1989).

Although NE appears to be in the appropriate regions to affect VP release, many functional studies have generated what appear to be equivocal outcomes. Intraventricular administrations of adrenergic agonists have been reported to either increase (e.g., Kuhn, 1974; Brooks, Share, & Crofton, 1986) or decrease (Kimura et al., 1981) plasma levels of the antidiuretic hormone. *In vitro* studies have yielded the same types of inconsistencies with reports of little effect (Bridges, Hillhouse, & Jones, 1976) or of inhibition of release by NE (Armstrong, Sladek, & Sladek, 1982). As concluded in earlier literature reviews (Share, 1983; Sklar & Schrier; 1983), such discrepancies apparently are due to either methodological or species differences.

An illuminating insight into a methodological problem that appears to account for some of the equivocal findings on NE and VP release has recently emerged from electrophysiological investigations. Early recording studies pointed to an inhibitory effect of NE. Barker, Crayton, and Nicoll (1971) and Moss, Urban, and Cross (1972) observed that iontophoretic application of NE onto antidromically identified SON neurons was primarily inhibitory. Similarly, Arnauld and colleagues (1983) usually saw inhibition with iontophoresis. However, it was also noted in the later study that NE applied with low currents was occasionally excitatory. A clarification of such apparent descrepancies in the electrophysiological findings has been proposed by Renaud and colleagues (1985). These investigators suggest that the iontophoretic method of drug application may lead to variable and/or high levels of NE near the pipet tip. In the presence of NE in low concentrations alpha-adrenoceptors are preferentially activated, but at high levels, beta-adrenergic receptors also may be stimulated. The use of pressure injection methods for micro application of NE has produced results consistent with this explanation. When delivery of NE has been more effectively controlled by pressure injection, low doses of NE produce excitation and high doses inhibition (Randle, Bourque, & Renaud, 1984). *In vivo* and *in vitro* recordings from SON neurons indicate that alpha-1 adrenoceptor agonists excite and beta adrenoceptor agonists inhibit firing of putative VP magnocellular neurons (Randle et al., 1984; Wakerley, Noble, & Clarke, 1983). Thus, the concentration of NE at adrenergic receptors on magnocellular neurons in the PVN or SON determines the response. It should be noted that the concentration of an agent at receptors is likely to be influenced by the route of delivery as well as the dose applied. Recent functional confirmation of the role of alpha-versus beta-adrenoceptors has been provided by

Willoughby and colleagues (1987) who have shown that alpha-1, but not alpha-2 nor beta-adrenoceptor agonist applications to the SON elicit vasopressin release.

As previously indicated, ivt 6-OHDA injections impair vasopressin release (see Table 10-4). The activation of putative VP SON neurons by stimulation of the A1 region of the ventral lateral medulla is blocked by injection of 6-OHDA into the SON (Day & Renaud, 1984). Neurotoxin injections have been made into the dorsal ascending noradrenergic bundle that arises from the A6 cell group (i.e., the locus coereleus) or into and the ventral bundle that carries ascending input from the A1 and A2 cell groups (Lightman, Todd, & Everitt, 1984). 6-OHDA injections into the dorsal bundle produce a significant impairment in vasopressin release to hemorrhage, whereas injections into the ventral bundle results in an attenuation but to a lesser degree (i.e., not statistically significant).

Current evidence suggests that A1 neurons receive pressure/volume information from the NTS and, in turn, project to magnocellular neurons to release NE and increase VP levels (Blessing & Willoughby, 1988). This hypothesis is supported by the demonstration that both catecholamine metabolism in the A1 and VP release are increased by nitroprusside-induced hypotension or by hemorrhage (Quintin et al., 1987). However, central or systemic administration of adrenergic receptor antagonists are not as effective in blocking activation of the VP magnocellular system as would be expected (Blessing & Willoughby, 1988). Thus, there are reasons to believe that there are alternative ascending pathways from NTS to magnocellular neurons or that other transmitters (e.g., NPY) in addition to NE are present in the VLM-magnocellular projection (Blessing & Willoughby, 1988). In addition, it is possible that "descending" influences (e.g., ANG from the SFO/AV3V) may play an important role even when ascending pathways are blocked.

c. *Autonomic Efferent Pathways*: Central NE mechanisms have been repeatedly implicated in the control of autonomic outflow. The majority of this research has focused on the role of adrenergic mechanisms in the control of blood pressure. Destruction of central catecholamines with 6-OHDA prevents the development of hypertension of many different etiologies (see Brody, 1988 for review).

There is good evidence that autonomic outflow is influenced by the interaction of brain ANG and central NE. Pressor responses to ivt ANG, carbachol, or hypertonic saline are significantly attenuated in rats which have central catecholamine depletions after ivt 6-OHDA treatments (Hoffman, Phillips, & Schmid, 1977; Gordon et al., 1979). Furthermore, blockade of adrenergic receptors with phentolamine attenuates the pressor response to ivt ANG (Camacho & Phillips, 1981a). An important component of the tissues involved in centrally evoked pressor responses involves the tissue of the AV3V because, as described above, local depletion of NE along the ventral lamina terminalis attenuates the pressor response to ivt ANG II (Bellin, et al., 1987b). Although there is research showing that manipulation of NE has profound effects on heart rate, blood pressure, and hemodynamics, there are few, if any, experimental investigations of the role of such mechanisms on renal sympathetic activity and renal function controlling hydration *per se*. However, there is good reason to think that such effects can be demonstrated. Koepke and colleagues (1986) have shown that the local injection of a beta 2-adrenoceptor antagonist into the posterior hypothalamus blocked an air stress-induced increase in sympathetic nerve activity and antinatriuresis in spontaneously hypertensive rats.

d. *Endocrine Efferent Pathways*: The role of central NE in the release of homones from the anterior pituitary is of major interest. Especially pertinent to the control of fluid balance is the release of potential secretagogues of ACTH into the portal vessels of the median eminence. Recent experimental evidence suggests that brain adrenergic mechanisms may serve as a link between brain stem and the secretion of ACTH releaser(s) into the portal system.

Similar to the case for VP, early work on the role of NE in the control of ACTH release generated equivocal results (see Weiner and Ganong, 1978, for review). Species differences and routes of administration may account for some of the differences (Jones et al., 1987). However, it appears (as was the case for VP) that the actual concentration of the hormone receptor site is likely to be a very critical variable. Plotsky (1987) has shown in rats that ivt NE applied in low doses releases CRF and in high doses inhibits CRF release.

Electrical stimulation of the A1 region in the CVLM activates tuberoinfundibular neurons in the PVN (Day, Ferguson, & Renaud, 1985; Kannan et al., 1987). Alpha-1 adrenergic receptor antagonist treatment blocks the increase of CRF release into pituitary portal vessels that is induced by electrical stimulation of the ventral noradrenergic bundle (Plotsky, 1987). In man the release of ACTH that occurs in response to a meal is enhanced by the alpha-1 adrenoceptor agonist methoxamine and inhibited by the alpha-1 adrenoceptor antagonist thymoxamine (Al-Damluji et al., 1987). Kasai and Yamashita (1988), recording *in vitro*, have shown that tuberoinfundibular pPVN neurons that were excited by bath application of NE showed a cortisol-related suppression of the NE-induced increase.

Local depletion of NE by injection of 6-OHDA into the PVN produces an attenuation in the increase of plasma coritcosterone levels to various so-called "neural stimuli" (i.e., photic stimulation, acoustic stimulation, sciatic nerve stimulation) (Feldman, Conforti, & Melamed, 1986).

Taken together, the data are consistent with the hypothesis that, in response to some stressors, the secretion of ACTH is mediated by release of NE in the PVN.

3. Generalization of the Interction Between the BRAS and Noradrenergic System: In the previous two sections, research findings were reviewed suggesting that a "descending" BRAS and ascending NE pathways facilitate the generation of thirst and VP release. A reasonable body of evidence currently indicates that extracellular depletion-induced drinking as well as VP and CRF release employ "descending" angiotensinergic and "ascending" noradrenergic pathways to act on common structures in the basal forebrain (e.g., MePO, mPVN, SON). In addition, there is circumstantial evidence from anatomical and electrophysiological studies that analogous "descending" angiotensinergic and ascending noradrenergic mechanisms may influence autonomic outflow to the kidneys through their actions on the pPVN. It is reasonable to take as a working hypothesis the essential components of the model for the role of the SFO/AV3V in extracellular depletion induced thirst and apply it to other fluid control mechanisms that are mobilized to defend against hypovolemia (see Figure 10-20). Again the essential components are: 1) a descending angiotensinergic input from the SFO/AV3V which is activated by increased plasma levels of ANG II, and 2) ascending NE which is activated by visceral afferents from systemic pressure/volume receptors.

SUMMARY, CONCLUSIONS, AND FUTURE DIRECTIONS

The problem of maintaining constancy of the volume and distribution of fluids within the body is one of the most fundamental homeostatic problems confronting an organism. The solution involves using multiple stimuli, sensors, and afferent pathways and relying on the integrative capacity of the central nervous system. Since the identification of effective osmolality as a putative stimulus for thirst by Gilman more than 50 years ago, some important advances have been made pertinent to the understanding of the neural control of body fluid homeostasis. Among these are: 1) development of the concept of an osmoreceptor; 2) the discovery that humoral stimuli act directly on the brain to evoke the action of control systems (e.g., drinking, VP release); 3) the implication in the control of fluid balance of multiple systemic receptors including vascular pressure/volume receptors; 4) implication of circulating ANG as an afferent signal to the CNS; 5) discovery that ANG acts on CVOs to activate the CNS; 6) discovery that components of the renin-angiotensin system are formed *de novo* in the brain; and 7) the elucidation of the nature of CNS noradrenergic mechanisms and pathways.

In recent years new neuroanatomical and functional techniques

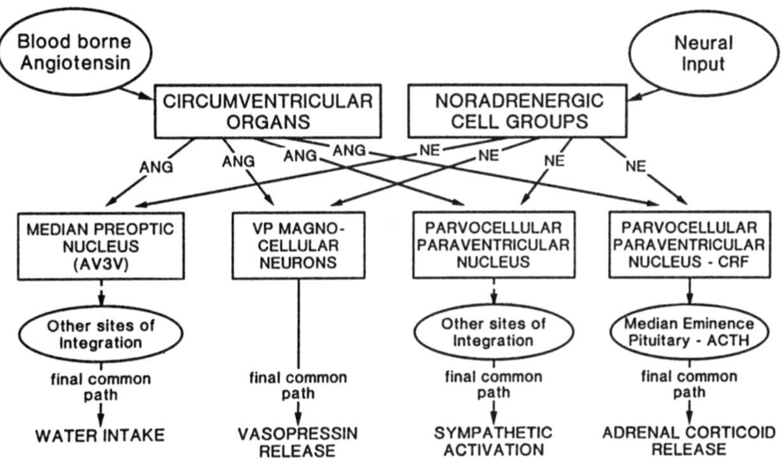

FIGURE 10-20. *A generalized model for the interaction of descending angiotensinergic and ascending noradrenergic inputs into the AV3V, supraoptic nucleus, and parvocellular and magnocellular components of the paraventricular nucleus. Within the AV3V, the median preoptic region has been implicated in the control of exracellular depletion-induced drinking. The magnocelular neurons of the SON and PVN contain VP cell bodies. The pPVN contains projections to brain stem and spinal cord regions involved in controlling autonomic outflow and fibers to the median eminence which contain releasing factors influencing anterior pituitary trophic hormones. The descending angiotensinergic input derives from the SFO/AV3V region and the ascending noradrenergic input arises in the A1, A2, and A6 noradrenergic cell groups. Hypovolemia/hypotension generates elevated plasma levels of ANG II and activates systemic vascular volume/pressure afferents. Circulating ANG acts on the SFO to activate descending antiotensinergic pathways. Pressure/volume afferents activate ascending NE pathways projecting to AV3V and VP-containing neurons and to pPVN. NE is proposed to enhance the action of ANG within the specified nuclei to amplify the action of the peptide.*

have permitted the preliminary investigation of how neural input reflecting hydrational status gains access to the CNS and where such information is likely to be processed. Two neurochemical substrates implicated in the control of extracellular fluid volume are the BRAS and the brain noradrenergic pathways. Brain ANG pathways implicated in fluid balance are primarily descending projections from structures located along the lamina terminalis (i.e., SFO/AV3V). Many of the structures located in the medial basal forebrian that have been implicated in the control of fluid balance receive ascending input from medullary and pontine regions containing NE cell bodies. Functional evidence indicates that disruption of either the descending ANG pathways or ascending NE projections disorders the controls of body fluid homeostasis, particularly those related to extracellular fluid volume.

Although there is an emerging consensus that the OVLT houses cells that are likely to be the "Verney osmoreceptors," such cells are yet to be unequivocally characterized either electrophysiologically or morphologically. In addition, at present no especially strong candidates as neurochemical mediators between the osmoreceptor and respective final common paths for the various effectors of fluid balance have emerged.

Also of major importance for future work will be to identify the locus or loci of the interface between the neural systems involved in control of extracellular and cellular fluid volumes. Clearly, functional evidence indicates that the two systems interact to facilitate and inhibit effector responses.

The sites and mechanisms discussed in this review are high on the afferent limb. Certainly, much will be learned as work progresses toward the "final common path." Although what lies between early processing areas of the medial basal forebrain and the mesencephalic regions involved in the generation of locomotor patterns has been a subject of creative and insightful hypothetical discussion (Swanson & Mogenson, 1981), much work is required before the complexities involved in the neural organization of motivated behaviors (i.e., drinking and sodium appetite) are comprehended. In contrast, it is fortunate that the locus of the final site of integration for the control of the release of the antidiuretic hormone is the magnocellular VP neuron. At the present time many outstanding research groups are focusing on the SON and mPVN to investigate the neural and neurochemical processes of integration involved in the control of VP release (see Sladek and Armstrong, 1987 for review).

It is an exciting and optimistic time to be involved in the investigation of the neural control of body fluid homeostasis. The questions are challenging and difficult but new concepts and a growing body of experimental methodology provide a means to understand the biological processes that keep a degree of calm within the life's restless internal seas.

BIBLIOGRAPHY

Adachi, A., A. Niijima, & H.L. Jacobs. (1976). An hepatic osmoreceptor mechanism in the rat: Electrophysiological and behavioral studies. *American Journal of Physiology, 231*(4), 1043–1049.

Adolph, E.F. (1939). Measurements of water drinking in dogs. *Am. J. Physiol., 125*, 75–86.

Adolph, E.F. (1947). *Physiology of Man in the Desert*, E.F. Adolph, ed. New York: Interscience.

Al-Damluji, S., T. Iveson, J.M. Thomas, D.J. Pendlebury, L.H. Rees, & G.M. Besser. (1987). Food-induced cortisol secretion is mediated by central alpha$_1$-adrenoceptor for modulation of pituitary ACTH secretion. *Clinical Endocrinology, 26*, 629–636.

Almli, R.C., & C.S. Weiss. (1974). Drinking behaviors: Effects of lateral preoptic and lateral hypothalamic destruction. *Physiology and Behavior, 13*, 537–538.

Andersson B. (1953). The effect of injections of hypertonic NaCl-solutions into different parts of the hypothalamus of goats. *Acta Physiologica Scandinavica, 28*, 188–201.

Andersson, B. (1971). Thirst and brain control of water balance. *Am. Scientist, 59*, 408–415.

Andersson, B., L. Eriksson, O. Fernandez, C.G. Kolmodin, & R. Oltner. (1972). Centrally mediated effects of sodium and angiotensin II on arterial blood pressure and fluid balance. *Acta Physiologica Scandinavica 85*, 398–407.

Andersson, B., L.G. Leksell, & F. Lishajko. (1975). Perturbations in fluid balance induced by medially placed forebrain lesions. *Brain Research, 99*, 261–275.

Andersson, B., K. Olsson, & R.G. Warner. (1967). Dissimilarities between the central control of thirst and the release of antidiuretic hormone (ADH). *Acta Physiologica Scandinavica, 71*, 57–64.

Andreatta, S., D.B. Averill, R.A.S. Santos, & C.M. Ferrario. (1988). The ventrolateral medulla; A new site of action of the renin-angiotensin system. *Hypertension, 11* (Suppl. I, I-163-I-166).
Andrews, W.H.H., & J. Orbach. (1974). Sodium receptors activating some nerves of perfused rabbit livers. *American Journal of Physiology, 227,* 1273-1275.
Armstrong, W.E., C.D. Sladek, & J.R. Sladek, Jr. (1982). Characterization of noradrenergic control of vasopressin release by the organ-cultured rat hypothalamo-neurohypophyseal system. *Endocrinology, 111,* 273-279.
Arnauld, E., M. Cirino, B.S. Layton, & L.P. Renaud. (1983). Contrasting actions of amino acids, acetycholine, noradrenaline and leucine enkephalin on the excitability of supraoptic vasopressin-secreting neurons. *Neuroendocrinology, 36,* 187-196.
Aronsson, M., K. Almasan, K. Fuxe, A. Cintra, A. Harfstrand, J.-A. Gustafsson, & D. Ganten. (1988). Evidence for the existence of angiotensinogen mRNA in magnocellular paraventricular hypothalamic neurons. *Acta Physiologica Scandinavica, 132,* 585-586.
Arsenijevic, Y., & A.J. Baertschi. (1985). Activation of the hypothalamo-neurohypophysial system by hypertonic superfusion of the rat mesentery. *Brain Research, 347,* 169-172.
Baertschi, A.J., & P.G. Vallet. (1981). Osmosensitivity of the hepatic portal vein area and vasopressin release in rats. *Journal of Physiology, 314,* 217-230.
Balment, R.J., M.J. Brimble, M.L. Forsling, L.P. Kelly, & C.T. Musabayane. (1986). A synergistic effect of oxytocin and vasopressin on sodium excretion in the neurohypophysectomized rat. *Journal of Physiology, 381,* 453-464.
Barker, J.L., J.W. Crayton, & R.A. Nicoll. (1971). Noradrenaline and acetycholine responses of supraoptic neurosecretory cells. *Journal of Physiology, 218,* 19-32.
Bealer, S.L. (1984). Hypothalamic knife cuts attenuate maintenance of deoxycorticosterone acetate-salt induced hypertension, *Brain Research, 309,* 192-195.
Bealer, S.L., J.R. Haywood, K.A. Gruber, V.M. Buckalew, G.D. Fink, M.L. Brody, & A.K. Johnson. (1983). Preoptic-hypothalamic periventricular lesions reduce natriuresis to volume expansion. *American Journal of Physiology, 244,* R51-57.
Bealer, S.L., & A.K. Johnson. (1980). Preoptic-hypothalamic periventricular lesions alter food-associated drinking and circadian rhythms. *Journal of Comparative and Physiological Psychology, 94,* 547-555.
Bealer, S.L., M.I. Phillips, A.K. Johnson, & P.G. Schmid. (1979). Anteroventral third ventricle lesions reduce antidiuretic response to angiotensin II. *American Journal of Physiology, 236,* E610-E615.
Bellin, S.I., R.K. Bhatnagar, & A.K. Johnson. (1987a). Periventricular noradrenergic systems are critical for angiotensin-induced drinking and blood pressure responses, *Brain Research, 403,* 105-112.
Bellin, S.I., S.K. Landas, & A.K. Johnson. (1987b). Localized injections of 6-hydroxydopamine into lamina terminalis-associated structures: Effects on experimentally-induced drinking and pressor responses. *Brain Research, 416,* 75-83.
Bellin, S.I., S.K. Landas, & A.K. Johnson. (1988). Selective catecholamine depletion of structures along the ventral lamina terminalis: Effects on experimentally-induced drinking and pressor responses, *Brain Research, 456,* 9-16.
Berecek, K.H., & M.J. Brody. (1982). Evidence for a neurotransmitter role for epinephrine derived from the adrenal medulla. *American Journal of Physiology, 242,* H593-H601.
Blair-West, J.R., A.H. Brook, A. Gibson, M. Morris, & P.T. Pullan. (1979). Renin, antidiuretic hormone and the kidney in water restriction and rehydration. *Journal of Physiology*-London, *294,* 181-194.
Blake, W.D., & K.K. Lin. (1978). Hepatic portal vein infusion of glucose and sodium solutions on the control of saline drinking in the rat. *Journal of Physiology, 274,* 129-139.
Blass, E.M., & A.N. Epstein. (1971). A lateral preoptic osmosensitive zone for thirst in the rat. *Journal of Comparative and Physiological Psychology, 76,* 378-394.
Blessing, W.W., & J.O. Willoughby. (1985a). Excitation of neuronal function in rabbit caudal ventrolateral medulla elevates plasma vasopressin. *Neuroscience Letters, 58,* 189-194.
Blessing, W.W., J.O. Willoughby. (1985b). Inhibiting the rabbit caudal ventrolateral medulla prevents baroreceptor-initiated secretion of vasopressin. *Journal of Physiology, 367,* 253-265.
Blessing, W.W., & J.O. Willoughby. (1988). Adrenoreceptor agents and baroreceptor-initated secretion of vasopressin. In A.W. Cowley, Jr., J.-F. Liard & D.A. Ausiello (Eds.), *Vasopressin: Cellular and integrative functions* (349-353). New York: Raven Press.
Bonjour, J.P., & R.L. Malvin (1970). Stimulation of ADH release by the renin angiotensin system. *American Journal of Physiology, 218,* 1555-1559.
Booth, D.A. (1968). Mechanism of action of norepinephrine in eliciting an eating response on injection into the rat hypothalamus. *Journal of Pharmacology and Experimental Therapeutics, 160,* 336-48.
Bourque, C.W. (1987). Osmotic induction of bursting in magnocellular neuroendocrine cells: in vitro analysis using perfused hypothalamic explants. *Neuroscience Letters,* Suppl. *29,* S16.
Bridges, T.E., E.W. Hillhouse, & M.T. Jones (1976). The effect of dopamine on neurohypophysial hormone release *in vivo* and from the rat neural lobe and hypothalamus *in vitro. Journal of Physiology, 260,* 647-666.
Brody, M.J. (1988). Central nervous system and mechanisms of hypertension. *Clinical Physiology and Biochemistry, 6,* 230-239.

Brody, M.J. & A.K. Johnson (1980). Role of the anteroventral third ventricle region in fluid and electrolyte balance, arterial pressure regulation and hypertension. In L. Martini & W.F. Ganong (Eds.). *Frontiers in Neuroendocrinology*, Vol. 6 (pp. 249–292). New York: Raven Press.

Brody, M.J., & A.K. Johnson (1981). Role of forebrain structures in models of experimental hypertension. In F.M. Abboud, H.A. Fozzard, J.P. Gilmore, & D. Reis (Eds.) *Disturbances in the neurogenic control of the circulation* (pp. 105–117), Clinical Physiology Series, American Physiological Society. Baltimore: Williams & Wilkins Co.

Brooks, D.P., L. Share, & J.T. Crofton (1986). Central adrenergic control of vasopressin release. *Neuroendocrinology, 42*, 416–420.

Brown, A.M. (1980). Receptors under pressure. *Circulation Research, 46*, 1–10.

Brown, E.R., D.G. Standaert, & C.B. Saper (1985). Efferent connections of the medial preoptic region in the rat. *Society for Neuroscience Abstracts, 11*, 827.

Buckalew, V.M. Jr., & K.A. Gruber (1984). Natriuretic hormone. *Annual Review of Physiology, 46*, 343–358.

Buggy, J. & S.L. Bealer. Physiological regulation by the AV3V region. In P.M. Gross (Ed.), *Circumventricular Organs and body fluids* (Vol. 1, pp. 172–190). Boca Raton, Florida: CRS Press, Inc.

Buggy, J., G.D. Fink, J.R. Haywood, A.K. Johnson, & M.J. Brody (1978). Interruption of the maintenance phase of established hypertension by ablation of the anteroventral third ventricle (AV3V) in rats. *Clinical and Experimental Hypertension I*, 337–353.

Buggy, J., G.D. Fink, A.K. Johnson, & M.J. Brody (1977). Prevention of the development of renal hypertension by anteroventral third ventricular tissue lesions. *Circulation Research, 40*, I-110–I-117.

Buggy, J. & A.E. Fisher (1974). Evidence for a dual central role for angiotensin in water and sodium intale. *Nature*, (London) *250*, 733–735.

Buggy, J. & A.E. Fisher (1976). Anteroventral third ventricle site of action for angiotensin induced thirst. *Pharmacology, Biochemistry and Behavior, 4*, 651–660.

Buggy, J., A.E. Fisher, W. Hoffman, A.K. Johnson, & M.I. Phillips (1975). Ventricular obstruction: Effect on drinking induced by intracranial injection of angiotensin. *Science, 190*, 72–74.

Buggy, J., W.E. Hoffman, M.I. Phillips, A.E. Fisher, & A.K. Johnson (1979). Osmosensitivity of rat third ventricle and interactions with angiotensin. *American Journal of Physiology, 236*, R75–R82.

Buggy, J., S. Hout, M. Pamnani, & F. Haddy (1984). Periventricular forebrain mechanisms for blood pressure regulation. *Federation Proceedings, 43*, 25.

Buggy, J., & A.K. Johnson (1977a). Preoptic-hypothalamic periventricular lesions: thirst deficits and hypernatremia. *American Journal of Physiology, 233*, R44–R52.

Buggy, J., & A.K. Johnson (1977b). Anteroventral third ventricle periventricular ablation: Temporary adipsia and persisting thirst deficits. *Neuroscience Letters, 5*, 177–182.

Buggy, J. & A.K. Johnson (1978). Angiotensin-induced thirst: Effects of third ventricular obstruction and periventricular ablation. *Brain Research, 149*, 117–128.

Camacho, A., & M.I. Phillips (1981a). Separation of drinking and pressore responses to central angiotensin by monoamines. *American Journal of Physiology, 240*, R106–R110.

Camacho, A., & M.I. Phillips (1981b). Horseradish peroxidase study in rat of the neural connections of the organum vasculosum of the lamina terminalis. *Neuroscience Letters, 25*, 201–204.

Cameron, V.A., E.A. Espiner, M.G. Nicholls, M.R. MacFarlane, & W.A. Sadler (1986). Intracerebroventricular captopril reduces plasma ACTH and vasopressin responses to hemorrhagic stress. *Life Sciences, 38*, 553–559.

Campbell, D.J., & J.F. Habener (1986). Angiotensinogen gene is expressed and differentially regulated in multiple tissues of the rat. *Journal of Clinical Investigation, 78*, 31–39.

Carithers, J., S.L. Bealer, M.J. Brody, & A.K. Johnson (1980). Fine structural evidence of degeneration in supraoptic nucleus and subfornical organ of rats with lesions in the anteroventral third ventricle. *Brain Research, 201*, 1–12.

Carithers, J.R., & A.K. Johnson (1988). Fine structural studies of the effects of AV3V lesions on the hypothalamo-neurohypophyseal neurosecretory system. In A.W. Cowley, J.-F. Liard, & D.A. Ausiello (Eds.), *Vasopressin*, pp. 301–320. New York: Raven Press.

Casto, R., & M.I. Phillips (1986). Angiotensin II attenuates baroreflexes at nucleus tractus solitarius of rats. *American Journal of Physiology, 250*, R193–R198.

Chwalbinska-Moneta, J. (1979). Role of heptatic portal osmoreception in the control of ADH release. *American Journal of Physiology, 236*(6), E603–E609.

Ciriello, J., & F.R. Calaresu (1980). Hypothalamic projections of renal afferent nerves in the cat. *Canadian Journal of Physiology and Pharmacology, 58*, 574–576.

Claybaugh, J.R., L. Share, & K. Shimizu (1972). The inability of infusions of angiotensin to elevate plasma vasopressin concentration in the anesthetized dog. *Endocrinology, 90*, 1647–1652.

Clemente, C.D., J. Sutin, & J.T. Silverstone (1957). Changes in electrical activity of the medulla on the intravenous injection of hypertonic solutions. *American Journal of Physiology, 188*, 193–198.

Coburn, P.C., & E.M. Stricker (1978). Osmoregulatory thirst in rats after lateral preoptic lesions. *Journal of Comparative & Physiological Psychology, 92*, 350–361.

Cohen, M.J., S. Hagiwara, & Y. Zotterman (1955). The response spectrum of taste fibres in the cat: A single fibre analysis. *Acta Physiologica Scandinavica, 33*, 316–332.

Conrad, L.C.A., & D.W. Pfaff (1976). Efferents from medial basal forebrain and hypothalamus in the rat: An autoradiographic study of the medial preoptic area. *Journal of Comparative Neurology, 169*, 185–220.

Contreras, R.J., & T. Kosten (1981). Changes in salt intake after abdominal vagotomy: Evidence for hepatic sodium receptors. *Physiology and Behavior, 26,* 575–582.
Contreras, R.J., & P.W. Stetson (1981). Changes in salt intake after lesions of the area postrema and the nucleus of the solitary tract in rats. *Brain Research, 211,* 355–366.
Coote, J.H., S.M. Hilton, & J.F. Perez-Gonzalez (1971). The reflex nature of the pressor response to muscular exercise. *Journal of Physiology (Lond)., 215,* 789–804.
Cowley, A.W., E. Monos, and A.C. Guyton (1974). Interaction of vasopressin and the baroreceptor reflex system in the regulation of arterial blood pressure in the dog. *Circulation Research, 34*: 505–514.
Cunningham, J.T. & A.K. Johnson (1988). Models for the integration of humoral and neural factors critical to body fluid homeostasis. In S. Yoshida & L. Share (Eds.), *Recent progress in posterior pituitary hormones* (pp. 97–105). Amsterdam: Elsevier.
Cunningham, J.T., & A.K. Johnson (1989). Decreased norepinephrine in the ventral terminalis region is associated with Angiotensin II drinking response deficits following local 6-hydroxydopamine injections, *Brain Research, 480,* 54–71.
Davis, J.O. (1974). The renin-angiotensin system in the control of aldosterone secretion. In I.H. Page and F.M. Bumpus (Eds.) *Angiotensin*. Berlin, Heidelberg: Springer-Verlag.
Davson, H. (1970). *Physiology of the cerebrospinal fluid*. London: J. & A. Churchill, Ltd.
Day, T.A., & J. Ciriello (1985). Afferent renal nerve stimulation excites supraoptic vasopressin neurons. *American Journal of Physiology, 249,* R368–R371.
Day, T.A., A.V. Ferguson, & L.P. Renaud (1985). Noradrenergic afferents facilitate the activity of tuberoinfundibular neurons of the hypothalamic paraventricular nucleus. *Neuroendocrinology, 41,* 17–22.
Day, T.A., & L.P. Renaud (1984). Electrophysiological evidence that noradrenergic afferents selectively facilitate the activity of supraoptic vasopressin neurons. *Brain Research, 303,* 233–240.
deBold, A.J. (1982). Tissue fractionation studies on the relationship between an atrial natriuretic factor and specific atrial granules. *Canadian Journal of Physiology and Pharmacology, 60,* 324–330.
Denton, D. (1982). *The hunger for salt*. Springer-Verlag: Berlin, Heidelberg.
DiBona, G.F. (1982). The functions of the renal nerves. *Reviews of Physiology, Biochemistry and Pharmacology, 94,* 76–181.
Dietrickx, K. (1963). The subfornical organ, a specialized osmoreceptor. *Naturwissenschaften, 50,* 163–164.
Doba, N., & D.J. Reis (1973). Acute fulminating neurogenic hypertension produced by brainstem lesions in the rat. *Circulation Research, 32,* 584–593.
Dzau, V.J., J. Ingelfinger, R.E. Pratt, & K.E. Ellison (1986). Identification of renin and angiotensinogen messenger RNA sequences in mouse and rat brains. *Hypertension, 8,* 544–548.
Edwards, G.L., & A.K. Johnson (1987). Neuronal loss in the lateral parabrachial nucleus causes enhanced drinking to extracellular thirst challenges. *Neuroscience Abstracts,* (Suppl. 22), S332.
Edwards, G.L., T.G. Beltz, & A.K. Johnson (1988). Enhanced secretion of Sodium by area postrema-lesioned rats after intragastric saline loads. Society for Neuroscience Abstracts, 14, 316.
Edwards, G.L., & R.C. Ritter (1982). Area postrema lesions increase drinking to angiotension and extracellular dehydration. *Physiology and Behavior, 29,* 943–947.
Eng., R., & R.R. Miselis (1981). Polydipsia and abolition of angiotensin-induced drinking after transections of subfornical organ efferent projections in the rat. *Brain Research, 225,* 200–206.
Epstein, A.N. (1973). Epilogue: Retrospect and prognosis. In A.N. Epstein, H.R. Kissileff, & E. Stellar (Eds.). *The Neuropsychology of Thirst: New Findings and Advances in Concepts,* 315–332, New York: Wiley.
Epstein, A.N. (1982). Mineralocorticoids and cerebral angiotensin may act together to produce sodium appetite. *Peptides, 3*: 493–494.
Epstein, A.N., J.T. Fitzsimons, & B.J. Rolls (1970). Drinking induced by injection by injection of angiotensin into the brain of the rat. *Journal of Physiology, 210,* 457–74.
Epstein, A.N., & S. Hsiao (1975). Angiotensin as dipsogen. In G. Peters, J.T. Fitzsimons & L. Peters-Haefeli (eds)., *Control mechanisms of drinking*. Berlin, Heidelberg: Springer-Verlag.
Epstein, A.N., & R.R. Sakai (1987). Angiotensin-aldosterone synergy and salt intake. In J.P. Buckley & C.M. Ferrario (eds.), *Brain peptides and catecholamines in cardiovascular regulation*. New York: Raven Press.
Espiner, E.A. (1987). The effect of stress on salt and water balance. *Baillier's Clinical Endocrinology and Metabolism, 1,* 375–390.
Falck, B., N.A. Hillarp, G. Thieme, & A. Torp (1962). Fluorescence of catecholamines and related compounds condensed with formaldehyde. *Journal of Histochemical Cytochemistry, 10,* 348–354.
Feldman, S., N. Conforti, & E. Melamed (1986). Norepinephrine depletion in the paraventricular nucleus inhibits the adrenocortical responses to neural stimuli. *Neuroscience Letters, 64,* 191–195.
Felix, D., & M.I. Phillips (1979). Inhibitory effects of luteinizing hormone releasing hormone (LHRH) on neurons in the organum vasculosum lamina terminalis (OVLT). *Brain Research, 169,* 204.
Ferguson, A.V., T.A. Day, & L.P. Renaud (1984). Subfornical organ stimulation excites paraventricular neurons projecting to dorsal medulla. *American Journal of Physiology, 247,* R1088–R1092.
Ferrario, C.M., P.L. Gildenberg, & J.W. McCubbin (1972). Cardiovascular effects of angiotensin mediated by the central nervous system. *Circulation Research, 30,* 257–262.
Feuerstein, G., A.K. Johnson, R.I. Zerbe, R. Davis-Kramer, & A.I. Faden (1984). Anteroventral hypothalamus and hemorrhagic shock: Cardiovascular and neuroendocrine responses. *American Journal of Physiology, 246,* R551–R557.
Fink, G.D., C.A. Bruner, & M.L. Mangiapane (1987). Area postrema is critical for angiotensin-induced hypertension in rats. *Hypertension, 9,* 355–361.

Fink, G.D., D.J. Buggy, J.R. Haywood, A.K. Johnson, & M.J. Brody (1978). Hemodynamic effects of electrical stimulation of forebrain angiotensin II and osmosensitive sites. *American Journal of Physiology, 235*, H445–H451.

Fink, G.D., J. Buggy, A.K. Johnson, & M.J. Brody (1977). Prevention of steroid-salt hypertension in the rat by anterior forebrain lesions. *Circulation, 56*, III–242.

Fink, G.D., C.M. Pawloski, M.L. Blair, & M.L. Mangiapane (1987). Area postrema in deoxycorticosterone-salt hypertension in rats. *Hypertension, 9*, (Suppl.III), III–206–III–209.

Fisher, A.E., & J.N. Coury (1964). Chemical tracing of neural pathways mediating the thirst drive. In M.J. Wayner (Ed.) *Thirst* (pp. 515–529). New York: Pergamon Press.

Fischer-Ferraro, C., V.E. Nahmod, D.J. Goldstein, & D. Finkielman (1971). Angiotensin and renin in rat and dog brain. *Journal of Experimental Medicine, 133*, 353–361.

Fitzsimons, J.T. (1961). Drinking by rats depleted of body fluid without increase in osmotic pressure. *Journal of Physiology, 159*, 297–309.

Fitzsimons, J.T. (1969). The role of a renal thirst factor in drinking induced by extracellular stimuli. *Journal of Physiology, 201*, 349–368.

Fitzsimons, J.T. (1970). The renin-angiotensin system in the control of drinking. In L. Martini, M. Motta, & Fraschini (eds.) *The hypothalamus*, pp. 195–212. New York & London: Academic Press.

Fitzsimons, J.T. (1972). Thirst. *Physiological Reviews, 52*, 468–561.

Fitzsimons, J.T. (1979) *The physiology of thirst and sodium appetite*. Cambridge: Cambridge University Press.

Fitzsimons, J.T., & J. Le Magnen (1969). Eating as a regulatory control of drinking in the rat. *Journal of Comparative and Physiological Psychology, 67*, 273–83.

Fitzsimons, J.T., & B.J. Simons (1969). The effect on drinking in the rat of intravenous angiotensin, given alone or in combination with other stimuli of thirst. *Journal of Physiology, 203*, 45–57.

Foote, S.K., F.E. Bloom, & G. Aston-Jones (1983). Nuelcus locus ceruleus: New evidence of anatomical and physiological specificity. *Physiological Reviews, 63*, 844–914.

Fregly, M.J., & N.E. Rowland (1985). Role of renin-angiotensin-aldosterone system in NaCl appetite of rats. *American Journal of Physiology, 248*, R1–R11.

Fuxe, K, D. Ganten, T. Hokfelt, & P. Bolme (1976). Immunohistochemical evidence for the existence of angiotensin II-containing nerve terminals in the brain and spinal cord of the rat. *Neuroscience Letters, 2*, 229–234.

Gann, D.S., D.G. Ward, & D.E. Carlson (1978). Neural control of ACTH: A homeostatic reflex. In R.O. Greep (Ed.). *Recent Progress in Hormone Research, 34*, 357–400, New York: Academic Press.

Ganten, D., P. Granger, U. Ganten, R. Boucher, & J. Genest (1972). An intrinsic renin-angiotensin system in the brain. *Hypertension*, J. Genest & E. Koiw (Eds.). (pp. 423–432), Heidelberg: Springer-Verlag.

Ganten, D., J.S. Hutchinson, P. Schelling, U. Ganten, & H. Fischer (1976). The iso-renin angiotensin systems in extrarenal tissue. *Clinical and Experimental Pharmacology and Physiology, 3*, 103–126.

Ganten, D., J.L. Minnich, P. Granger, K. Hayduk, H.M. Brecht, A. Barbeau, R. Boucher & J. Genest (1971). Angiotensin-forming enzyme in brain tissue. *Science, 173*, 64–65.

Ganten, D., M. Printz, M.I. Phillips, & B.A. Scholkens (Eds). (1982). *The renin angiotensin system in the brain*, Heidelberg: Springer-Verlag.

Gauer, O.H., & J.P. Henry (1963). Circulatory basis of fluid volume control. *Physiological Reviews, 43*, 423–81.

Gilman, A. (1937). The relation between blood osmotic pressure, fluid distribution and voluntary water intake. *American Journal of Physiology, 120*, 323–328.

Gilman, A., & L. Goodman (1937). The secretory response of the posterior pituitary to the need for water conservation. *Journal of Physiology, 90*, 113–124.

Glasby, M.A., & D.J. Ramsay. (1974). Hepatic osmoreceptors? *Journal of Physiology, 243*, 765–776.

Gordon, F.J., M.J. Brody, G.D. Fink, J. Buggy, & A.K. Johnson (1979). Role of central catecholamines in the control of blood pressure and drinking behavior. *Brain Research, 178*, 161–173.

Gordon, F.J., M.J. Brody, & A.K. Johnson (1985). Regional depletion of central nervous system catecholamines: Effects on blood pressure and drinking behavior. *Brain Research, 345*, 285–297.

Gordon, F.J., J.R. Haywood, M.J. Brody, & A.K. Johnson (1982). Effect of lesions of the anteroventral third ventricle (AV3V) on the development of hypertension in spontaneously hypertensive rats. *Hypertension, 4*, 387–393.

Graham, C.A., D.O. Nelson, & A.K. Johnson (1985). Noradrenergic modulation of subfornical organ input to the nucleus medianus. *Society for Neuroscience Abstracts, 11*, 826.

Grill, J.H., & K.C. Berridge (1985). Taste reactivity as a measure of the neural control of palatability. In J.M. Sprague & A.N. Epstein (eds), *Progress in psychobiology and physiological psychology. Vol 11*, Orlando: Academic Press.

Grill, H.J. & R. Norgren (1978). The taste reactivity test. I. Mimetic responses to gustatory stimuli in neurologically normal rats. *Brain Research, 143*, 263–279.

Gronan, R.J., & D.H. York (1978). Effects of angiotensin II and acetylcholine on neurons in the preoptic area. *Brain Research, 154*, 172–177.

Gross, F. (1974). Effects of aldosterone on blood pressure, water, and electrolytes. In I.H. Page & F.M. Bumpus (eds.), *Angiotensin*. Berlin, Heidelberg: Springer-Verlag.

Grossman, S.P. (1984). A reassessment of the brain mechanisms that control thirst. *Neuroscience and Biobehavioral Reviews, 8*, 95–104.

Gruber, K.A., L.D. Wilkin, & A.K. Johnson (1986). Neurohypophyseal hormone release and biosynthesis in rats with lesions of the anteroventral third ventricle (AV3V) region. *Brain Research, 378*. 115–119.

Guyton, A.C., T.G. Coleman, A.W. Cowley Jr., R.D. Manning, R.A. Norman Jr., & J.D. Ferguson (1974). A systems analysis approach to understanding long-range arterial blood pressure control and hypertension. *Circulation Research, 35*, 159–176.

Haberich, F.J (1968). Osmoreception in the portal circulation. *Federation Proceedings, 27*, 1137–1141.

Hall, J.E., J.P. Montani, L.L. Woods, & H.L. Mizelle (1986). Renal escape from vasopressin: Role of pressure diuresis. *American Journal of Physiology, 250*, F907–F916.

Harris, P.J., & G. Navar (1985). Tubular transport responses to angiotensin. *The American Journal of Physiology, 248*, F621-F630.

Hartle, D.K., & M.J. Brody (1982). Hypothalamic vasomotor pathways mediating the development of hypertension in the rat. *Hypertension, 4*, (Suppl. III), 68–71.

Hartle, D.K., & M.J. Brody (1984). The angiotensin II pressor system of the rat forebrain. *Circulation Research, 54*, 355–366.

Hartle, D.K., R.A. Shaffer, A.K. Johnson, & M.J. Brody (1979). The effect of anteroventral third ventricle (AV3V) lesions on aortic coarctation hypertension in the rat. *Pharmacologist, 21*, 254.

Haywood, J.R., G.D. Fink, J. Buggy, S. Boutelle, & M.J. Brody (1978). Prevention and reversal of two-kidney (2K) renal hypertension in the rat by ablation of anteroventral third ventricle (AV3V) tissue. *Federation Proceedings, 37*, 804.

Healy, D.P., & M.P. Printz (1984). Distribution of immunoreactive angiotensin II, angiotensin I, angiotensinogen and renin in the central nervous system of intact and nephrectomized rats. *Hypertension, 6*, Part II, I-130 — I-136.

Hermann, K., D. Ganten, C. Bayer, T. Unger, R.E. Lang, & W. Rascher. (1982). Definite evidence for the presence of (Ile[5])-angiotensin I and (Ile[5])-angiotensin II in the brain of rats. In. D. Ganten, M. Printz, M.I. Phillips & B.A. Scholkens, (eds.), *The renin angiotension system in the brain*, 192–207, Berlin: Springer-Verglag.

Hermann, K., M.I. Phillips, U. Hilgenfeldt, & M.K. Raizada. (1988). Biosynthesis of angiotensinogen and angiotensins by brain cells in primary culture. *J. Neurochem., 51*, 398–405.

Hermann, K., M.I. Phillips, & M.K. Raizada. (1989). Metabolism of angiotensin peptides by neuronal and gial cultures from rat brain, *J. Neurochem., 52*, 863–868.

Hernesniemi, J., E. Kawana, H. Bruppacher, & C. Sandri. (1972). Afferent connections of the subfornical organ and of the supraoptic crest. *Acta Anatomica, 81*, 321–336.

Hoffman, W.E., & M.I. Phillips. (1976). Regional study of cerebral ventricle sensitive sites to angiotensin II. *Brain Research, 110*, 313–330.

Hoffman, W.E., M.I. Phillips, & P. Schmid. (1977). The role of catecholamines in central antidiuretic and pressor mechanisms. *Neuropharmacology, 16*, 563–369.

Hosutt, J.A., N. Rowland, & E.M. Stricker. (1978). Hypotension and thirst in rats after isoproterenol treatment. *Physiology & Behavior, 21.*, 593–598.

Hosutt, J.A., N. Rowland, & E.M. Stricker. (1981). Impaired drinking responses of rats with lesions of the subfornical organ. *Journal of Comparative Physiological Psychology, 95*, 104–113.

Houpt, K.A., & A.N. Epstein. (1971). The complete dependent of beta-adrenergic drinking on the renal dipsogen. *Physiology and Behavior, 7*, 897–902.

Hsiao, S., A.N. Epstein, & J.S. Camardo. (1977). The dipsogenic potency of peripheral angiotensin II. *Hormones and Behavior, 8*, 129–140.

Hyde, T.M., & R.R. Miselis. (1983). Effects of area postrema/caudal medial nucleus of the solitary tract lesions on food intake and body weight. *American Journal of Physiology, 244*, R577–R587.

Hyde, T.M., & R.R. Miselis. (1984). Area postrema and adjacent nucleus of the solitary tract in water and sodium balance. *American Journal of Pysiology, 247*, R173–R182.

Imaizumi, T., A.R. Granata, E.E. Benarroch, A.F. Sved, & D.J. Reis. (1985). Contributions of arginine vasopressin and the sympathetic nervous system to fulminating hypertension after destruction of neurons of caudal ventrolateral medulla in the rat. *Journal of Hypertension, 3*, 491–501.

Jackson, J.H. (1884). Evolution and dissolution of the nervous system. In J. Taylor (ed.) (1958) *Selected writings of John Hughlings Jackson*, Vol. 2 (pp. 45–75). New York: Basic Books (Croonian Lectures).

Jahr, E., & R.A. Nicoll. (1982). Noradrenergic modulation of dendrodenritic inhibition in the olfactory bulb. *Nature, 297*, 227–229, London.

Jerome, C., & G.P. Smith (1982a). Gastric vagotomy inhibits drinking after hypertonic saline. *Physiological Behavior, 28*, 371–374.

Jerome, C., & G.P. Smith. (1982b). Gastric or coeliac vagotomy decreases drinking after peripheral angiotensin II. *Physiological Behavior, 29*, 533–536.

Jewell, P.A., & E.B. Verney. (1957). An experimental attempt to determine the site of the neurohypophysical osmoreceptors in the dog. *Philosophical Transactions of the Royal Society, 240B*, 197–324.

Johnson, A.K. (1975). The role of the cerebral ventricular system in angiotensin-induced thirst. In G. Peters, J.T. Fitzsimons, & L. Peters-Haefeli (Eds.). *Control mechanisms of drinking*. Berlin-Heidelberg-New York: Springer-Verlag.

Johnson, A.K. (1979). Role of the periventricular tissue of the anteroventral third ventricle in body fluid homeostasis. In P. Mayer & H. Schmitt (Eds.), *Nervous system and hypertension*. New York: John Wiley & Sons.

Johnson, A.K. (1982). Neurobiology of the periventricular tissue surrounding the anteroventral third ventricle (AV3V) and its role in behavior, fluid balance, and cardiovascular control. In O.A. Smith, R.A. Galosy & S.M. Weiss (Eds.), *Circulation, Neurobiology and Behavior* (pp. 277–295). New York: Elsevier.

Johnson, A.K. (1985a). Role of the periventricular tissue surrounding the anteroventral third ventricle (AV3V) in the regulation of body fluid homeostasis. In R.W. Schrier (ed.), *Vasopressin*. New York: Raven Press.

Johnson, A.K. (1985b). The periventricular anteroventral third ventricle (AV3V): Its relationship with the subfornical organ and neural systems involved in maintaining body fluid homeostasis. *Brain Research Bulletin, 15*, 595–601.

Johnson, A.K., & J. Buggy. (1977). A critical analysis of the site of action for the dipsogenic effect of angiotensin II. In J.P. Buckley, C. Ferrario, & M.F. Lokhandwale (Eds.), *Central action of angiotensin and related hormones*. Elmsford, NY: Pergamon Press.

Johnson, A.K., & J. Buggy. (1978). Periventricular preoptic-hypothalamus is vital for third and normal water economy. *American Journal of Physiology, 234*, R122–R129.

Johnson, A.K., & J.T. Cunningham. (1987). Brain mechanisms and drinking: The role of lamina terminalis-associated systems and extracellular thirst. *Kidney International, 32*, S35–S42.

Johnson, A.K., & A.N. Epstein. (1975). The cerebral ventricles as the avenue for the dipsogenic action of intracranial angiotensin. *Brain Research, 86*, 399–418.

Johnson, A.K., & E.A. Fisher. (1973). Taste preferences for sucrose solutions and water under cholinergic and deprivation thirst. *Physiology and Behavior, 10*, 607–612.

Johnson, A.K., W.E. Hoffman, & J. Buggy. (1978). Attenuated pressor responses to intracranially injected stimuli and altered antidiuretic activity following preoptic-hypothalamic periventricular ablation. *Brain Research, 157*, 161–166.

Johnson, A.K., J.F.E. Mann, W. Rascher, J.K. Johnson, & D. Ganten. (1981). Plasma angiotensin II concentrations and experimentally induced thirst. *American Journal of Physiology, 240*, R229–R234.

Johnson, A.K., M.M. Robinson, & J.F.E. Mann. (1986). The role of the renal renin-angiotensin system in thirst. In G. deCaro, A.N. Epstein, & M. Massi (eds.), *The physiology of thirst and sodium appetite*. New York: Plenum Press.

Johnson, A.K., & J.E. Schwob. (1975) Cephalic angiotensin receptors mediating drinking to systemic angiotensin II. *Pharmacology, Biochemistry & Behavior, 3*, 1077–1084.

Johnson, A.K., L.D. Wilkin. (1987). The integrative role of neural systems of the lamina terminalis in the regulation of body fluid homeostasis. In. P. Gross (Ed.), *Circumventricular organs and body fluid homeostasis*. Vol. III (pp. 125–141). Boca Raton, Fla.: CRC Press, Inc.

Jones, M.T., B. Gillham, E.A. Campbell, A.R.H. Al-Taher, T.T. Chuang, & A. DiSciullo. (1987). Pharmacology of neural pathways affecting CRH secretion. In W.F. Ganong, M.F. Dallman & J.L. Roberts (Eds.), *The hypothalamic-pituitary-adrenal Axis revisited: A symposium in honor of Dorothy Krieger & Edward Herberg*. Annals of the New York Acadmey of Sciences, Vol. 512, New York: The New York Academy of Sciences.

Joy, M.D., & R.D. Lowe. (1970). Evidence that the area postrema mediates the central cardiovascular response to angiotensin II. *Nature, 228*, 1303–1304.

Kalia, M. & J.M. Sullivan. (1982). Brainstem projections of sensory and motor components of the vagus nerve in the rat. *The Journal of Comparative Neurology, 211*, 248–264.

Kannan, H., M. Kasai, T. Osaka, & H. Yamashita. (1987). Neurons in the paraventricular nucleus projecting to the median eminence: A study of their afferent connection from peripheral baroreceptors, and from the A_1-catecholaminergic area in the ventrolateral medulla. *Brain Research, 409*, 358–363.

Kannan, H., & H. Yamashita. (1983). Electrophysiological study of paraventricular nucleus neurons projecting to the dorsomedial medulla and their response to baroreceptor stimulation in rats. *Brain Research, 279*, 31–40.

Kapteina, F.W., W. Moltz, D. Schwartz-Porsche, & O.H. Gauer. (1978). Comparison of renal responses to 5% saline infusions into vena porta and vena cava in conscious dogs. *Pflugers Archives, 374* 23–29.

Kasai, M., H. Kannan, Y. Veta, T. Osaka, J. Inenaga, & H. Yamashita. (1988). Effects of iontophoretically applied cortisol on tuberoinfundibular neurons in hypothalamic paraventricular nucleus of anesthetized rats. *Neuroscience Letters, 87*, 35–40.

Kasai, M., & H. Yamashita. (1988). Cortisol suppresses noradrenaline-induced excitatory responses of neurons in the paraventricular nucleus; an in vitro study. *Neurosci. Lett., 9*, 65–70.

Kaufman, S., (1984). Role of right atrial receptors in the control of drinking in the rat. *Journal of Physiology, 349*, 389–396.

Keil, L.D., J. Summy-Long, & W.B. Severs. (1975). Release of vasopressin by angiotensin II, *Endocrinology, 96, 1063*.

Kimura, T., L. Share, B.C. Wang, & J.T. Crofton. (1981). Central effects of dopamine and bromocriptine on vasopressin release and blood pressure. *Neuroendocrinology, 33*, 347–351.

Kiss, J.Z., E. Mezey, & L. Skirboll. (1984). Corticotropin-releasing factor-immunoreactive neurons of the paraventricular nucleus become vasopressin positive after adrenalectomy. *Proceedings of the National Academy of Science USA, 81*, 1854–1858.

Knowles, W.D., & M.I. Phillips. (1980). Angiotensin II responsive cells in the organum vasculosum lamina terminalis (OVLT) recorded in hypothalamic brain slices. *Brain Research, 197*, 256–259.

Knuepfer, M.M., G.F. Gebhart, & M.J. Brody. (1985). Effects of baroreceptor activation on single unit activity of the anteroventral third ventricle region of the rat. *Neuroscience Letters, 56*, 79–85.

Kneupfer, M.M., A.K. Johnson, & M.J. Brody. (1984). Identification of brain stem projections mediating hemodynamic responses to stimulation of the anteroventral third ventricle (AV3V) region. *Brain Research, 294*, 305–314.

Koella, W.P., & J. Sutin. (1967). Extra-blood-brain barrier brain structures. In C.C. Pfeiffer and J.R. Smythier (Eds.), *International Review of Neurobiology*. New York: Academic Press.

Koepke, J.P., S. Jones, & G.F. DiBona. (1986). Hypothalamic beta-2-adrenoceptor control of renal sympathetic nerve activity and urinary sodium excretion in conscious, spontaneously hypertensive rats. *Circulation Research, 58*, No. 2, 241–248.

Kraly, F.S. (1984). Physiology of drinking elicited by eating. *Psychological Reviews, 91*, 478–490.

Kraly, F.S., J. Gibbs, & G.P. Smith. (1975). Disordered drinking after abdominal vagotomy in rats. *Nature, 258*, 226–228.

Kraly, F.S., & K.R. June. (1982). A vagally-mediated histaminergic component of food-related drinking in the rat. *Journal of Comparative and Physiological Psychology, 96*, 89–104.

Kraly, F.S., G.P. Smith, & W.J. Carty. (1978). Abdominal vagotomy disrupts food-related drinking in the rat. *Journal of Comparative Physiological Psychology, 92*, 196–203.

Kuhn, E.R. (1974). Cholinergic and adrenergic release mechanism for vasopressin in the male rat: A study with injections of neurotransmitters and blocking agents into the third ventricle. *Neuroendocrinology, 17*, 255–264.

Leng, G. (1980). Rat supraoptic neurones: The effects of locally applied hypertonic saline. *Journal of Physiology, 304*, 405–414.

Leng, G., W.T. Mason, & R.G. Dyer. (1982). The supraoptic nucleus as an osmoreceptor. *Neuroendocrinology, 34*, 75–82.

Leng, G., R.E.J. Dyball, & W.T. Mason. (1985). Electrophysiology of osmoreceptors. In R.W. Schrier (Ed.), *Vasopressin* (pp. 333–342). New York: Raven Press.

Lenge, G., R.E.J. Dyball, & J.A. Russell. (1988). Neurophysiology of body fluid homeostasis. *Comparative Biochemistry and Physiology, 90A*, 781–788.

Liard, J.F., W. Dolci, & M.B. Vallotton. (1984). Plasma vasopressin levels after infusions of hypertonic saline solutions into the renal, portal, carotid, or systemic circulation in conscious dogs. *Endocrinology, 114*, 986–991.

Lightman, S.L., K. Todd, & B.J. Everitt. (1984). Ascending noradrenergic projections from the brainstem: evidence for a major role in the regulation of blood pressure and vasopressin secretion. *Experimental Brain Research, 55*, 145–151.

Lind, R.W. (1987). Neural connections of the subfornical organ. *Circumventricular Organs and Body Fluids, 1*, 27–42.

Lind, R.W. (1958). Sites of action of angiotensin in the brain. In Harding, J.W., J.W. Wright, R.C. Speth, & C.D. Barnes (Eds.). *Angiotensin and blood pressure regulation* (pp. 135–163), Academic Press.

Lind, R.W., & D. Ganten. (1990). Angiotensin. In: A. Bjorklund, T. Hokfelt, M.J. Kuhar (Eds.) *The Handbook of Chemical Neuroanatomy, Neuropeptides in the CNS, Vol. 9*, New York: Elsevier (in press).

Lind, R.W., & A.K. Johnson. (1982a). Subfornical organ-median preoptic connections and drinking and pressor responses to angiotensin II. *Journals of Neuroscience, 2*, 1043–1051.

Lind, R.W., A.K. Johnson. (1982b). Central and peripheral mechanisms mediating angiotensin-induced thirst. In D. Ganten, M. Printz, M.I. Phillips, B.A. Scholkens (Eds.), *The renin angiotensin system in the brain* (pp. 353–364). Berlin-Heidelberg-New York: Springer-Verlag.

Lind, R.W., & A.K. Johnson. (1983). A further characterization of the effects of AV3V lesions on ingestive behavior. *American Journal of Physiology, 245*, R83–R90.

Lind, H., R.W. Lind, E.E. Shrager, S.L. Bealer, & A.K. Johnson. (1979). Critical tissues within the periventricular region of the anteroventral third ventricle (AV3V) associated with specific thirst deficits. *Society for Neuroscience Abstracts, 5*, 220.

Lind, R.W., L.W. Swanson, D.A. Chin, T.O. Bruhn, & D. Ganten. (1984a). Angiotensin II: An immunohistochemical study of its distribution in the paraventriculohypophysial system and its colocalization with vasopressin and CRF in parvocellular neurons. *Society for Neuroscience Abstracts, 10*, 88.

Lind, R.W., L.W. Swanson, T.O. Bruhn, & D. Ganten. (1985a). The distribution of angiotensin II-immunoreactive cells and fibers in the paraventriculohypophysial system of the rat. *Brain Research, 338*, 81–89.

Lind, R.W., L.W. Swanson, & D. Ganten. (1984b). Angiotensin II immumoreactivity in the neural afferents and efferents of the subfornical organ of the rat. *Brain Research, 321*, 209–215.

Lind, R.W., L.W. Swanson, & D. Ganten. (1985b). Organization of angiotensin II immunoreactive cells and fibers in the rat central nervous system. *Neuroendocrinology, 40*, 2–24.

Lind, R.W., R.L. Thunhorst, & A.K. Johnson. (1984). The subfornical organ and the integration of multiple factors in thirst. *Physiology and Behavior, 32*, 69–74.

Lind, R.W., G.W. Van Hoesen, & A.K. Johnson. (1982). An HRP study of the connections of the subfornical organ of the rat. *Journal of Comparative Neurology, 210*, 265–277.

Loewy, A.D. (1982). Central cardiovascular pathways. In: O.A. Smith, R.A. Galosy & S.M. Weiss (Eds.). *Circulation, Neurobiology and Behavior*, 3–11, New York: Elsevier Biomedical.

Loewy, A.D., & H. Burton. (1978). Nuclei of the solitary tract: Efferent projections to the lower brain stem and spiral cord of the cat. *The Journal of Comparative Neurology, 181*(2), 421–450.

Lynch, KR., C.L. Hawelu-Johnson, & P.G. Guyenet. (1987). Localization of brain angiotensinogen mRNA by hybridization histochemistry. *Molecular Brain Research, 2*, 149–158.

Lynch, K.R., V.I. Simnad, E.T. Ben-Ari, & J.C. Garrison. (1986). Localization of proangiotensinogen messenger RNA sequences in the rat brain. *Hypertension, 8*, 540–543.

Mangiapane, M.L., & M.J. Brody. (1987). Vasoconstrictor and vasodilator sites within anteroventral third ventricle region. *The American Physiological Society, 253*, R827–R831.

Mangiapane, M.L., T.N. Thrasher, L.C. Keil, J.B. Simpson, & W.F. Ganong. (1983). Deficits in drinking and vasopressin secretion after lesion of the nucleus medianus. *Neuroendocrinology, 37*, 73–77.

Mann, J.F.E., A.K. Johnson, & D. Ganten. (1980). Plasma angiotensin II: Dipsogenic levels and angiotensin-generating capacity of renin. *American Journal of Physiology, 238*, R372–R377.

Mann, J.F.E., A.K. Johnson, D. Ganten, & E. Ritz. (1987). Thirst and the renin-angiotensin system. *Kidney International, 32*, (Suppl. 21) S27–S34.

Maran, J.W., & F.E. Yates. (1977). Cortisol secretion during intrapituitary infusion of angiotensin II in conscious dogs. *American Journal of Physiology, 232*, E273–E285.

Mason, W.T. (1980). Supraoptic neurones of rat hypothalamus are osmosensitive. *Nature* (London), *242*, 154–157.

Matsuguchi, H., F.M. Sharabi, F.J. Gordon, A.K. Johnson, & P.G. Schmid. (1982). Blood pressure and heart rate responses to microinjection of vasopressin into the nucleus tractus solitarius region of the heart. *Neuropharmacology, 21*, 687–693.

McAllen, R.M., & W.W. Blessing. (1987). Neurons (presumably A_1-cells) projecting from the caudal ventralateral medulla to the region of the supraoptic nucleus respond to barorectpor inputs in the rabbit. *Neuroscience Letters, 73*, 247–252.

McCloskey, D.I., & J.H. Mitchell. (1972). Reflex cardiovascular and respiratory responses originating in exercising muscle. *J. Physiol., 224*, 173–186.

McGeer, P.L., J.C. Eccles, & E.G. McGeer. (1987). *Molecular neurobiology of the mammalian brain*. New York and London: Plenum Press.

McKinley, M.J., M. Congiu, R.R. Miselis, B.J. Oldfield, & G. Pennington. (1988). The lamina terminalis and osmotically stimulated vasopressin secretion. In S. Yoshida & L. Share (eds.) *Recent progress in posterior pituitary hormones 1988*. Elsevier Science Publishers B.V. (Biomedical Division).

McKinley, M.J., D.A. Denton, R.G. Park, & R.S. Weisinger. (1986). Ablation of subfornical organ does not prevent angiotensin-induced water drinking in sheep. *American Journal of Physiology, 250*, (Regulatory Integrative Comp. Physiol. 19), R1052–R1059.

McKinley, M.J., D.A. Denton, & R.S. Weisinger. Sensors for autidiuresis and thirst—osmoreceptors or CSF sodium detectors? *Brain Research, 141*, 89–103.

McRae-Degueurce, A., S.I. Bellin, S.K. Landas, & A.K. Johnson. (1986). Fetal noradrenergic transplants into amine-depleted basal forebrain nuclei restore drinking to angiotensin. *Brain Research, 374*, 162–166.

McRae-Degueurce, A., J.T. Cunningham, S. Bellin, S. Landas, L. Wilkin, & A.K. Johnson. (1987). Fetal noradrenergic cell suspensions transplanted into amine-depleted nuclei of adult rats. *Annals of the New York Academy of Sciences, 495*, 757–759.

Mendelsohn, F.A.O., R. Quirion, J.M. Saavedra, G. Aguilera, & K.J. Catt. (1984). Autoradiographic localization of angiotensin II receptors in rat brian. *Proceedings of the National Academy of Sciences USA, 81*, 1575–1579.

Meyer, D.K., M.I. Phillips, & L. Eiden. (1982). Studies on the presence of angiotensin II in rat brain. *Journal of Neurochemistry, 38*, 816–820.

Miselis, R.R. (1981). The efferent projections of the subfornical organ of the rat: A circumventricular organ within a neural network subserving water balance. *Brain Research, 230*, 1–23.

Miselis, R.R. (1986). The visceral neuraxis in thirst and renal function. In G. deCaro, A.N. Epstein & M. Massi (Eds.). *The physiology of thirst and sodium and sodium appetite*, New York and London: Plenum Press.

Miselis, R.R., T.M. Hyde, & E.E. Shapiro. (1986). Disturbances in water balance controls following lesions to the area postrema and adjacent solitary nucleus. In G. de Caro, A.N. Epstein & M. Massi (Eds.). *The physiology of thirst and sodium appetite*. New York and London: Plenum Press.

Miselis, R.R., R.E. Shapiro, & P.J. Hand. (1979). Subfornical organ efferents to neural systems for control of body water. *Science, 205*, 1022–1025.

Miselis, R.R., M.L. Weiss, & R.E. Shapiro. (1987). Modulation of the visceral neuraxis. In P.M. Gross (Ed.), *Circumventricular organs and body fluids, Vol. III*, pp. 144–160, Boca Raton, Florida: CRC Press, Inc.

Mitchell, L.D., K. Barron, M.J. Brody, & A.K. Johnson. (1982). Two possible actions for circulating angiotensin II in the control of vasopressin release. *Peptides, 3*, 503–507.

Mitchell, L.D., M.F. Callahan, L.D. Wilkin, S.I. Bellin, & A.K. Johnson. (1985). Systemic angiotensin II,

blood pressure, and supraoptic neuronal activity. *Peptides, 6,* 153–158.
Mitchell, J.H., M.P. Kaufman, & G.A. Iwamoto. (1983). The exercise pressor reflex: Its cardiovascular effects, afferent mechanisms, and Central Pathways. *Ann. Rev. Physiol., 45,* 229–242.
Moffett, B.R., F.M. Bumpus, & A. Husain. (1987). Minireview: Cellular organization of the brain renin-angiotensin system. *Life Sciences, 41,* 1867–1879.
Montani, J.P., J.F. Liard, J. Schoun, & J. Mohring. (1980). Hemodynamic effects of exogenous and endogenous vasopressin at low plasma concentrations in conscious dogs. *Circulation Research, 47,* 346–355.
Mook, D.G. (1963). Oral and postingestinal determinants of the intake of various solutions in rats with esophageal fistulas. *Journal of Comparative and Physiological Psychology, 56,* 645–659.
Moore-Gillon, M.J. (1980). Effects of vagotomy on drinking in the rat. *Journal of Physiology, 308,* 417–426.
Morrison, J.F.B. (1973). Splanchnic slowly adapting mechanoreceptors with punctate receptive fields in the mesentery and gastrointestinal tract of the cat. *Journal of Physiology, 233,* 349–261.
Moss, N.G. (1982). Renal function and renal afferent and efferent nerve activity. *American Journal of Physiology, 243,* F425–F433.
Moss, R.L., I. Urban, & B.A. Cross. (1972). Microelectroporesis of cholinergic and aminergic drugs on paraventricular neurons. *American Journal of Physiology, 232,* 310–318.
Mow, M.T., J.R. Haywood, A.K. Johnson, & M.J. Brody. (1978). The role of the anteroventral third ventricle (AV3V) in development of neurogenic hypertension. *Society for Neuroscience Abstracts, 4,* 23.
Muller, J. (1988). *Regulation of aldosterone biosynthesis.* Berlin, Heidelberg: Springer-Verlag.
Nathan, M.A., & D.J. Reis. (1977). Chronic labile hypertension produced by lesions of the nucleus tractus solitarii in the cat. *Circulation Research, 40*(1), 72–81.
Needleman, P., S.P. Adams, B.R. Cole, M.G. Currie, D.M. Geller, M.L. Michener, C.B. Saper, D. Schwartz, & D.G. Standaert. (1985). Atriopeptins as Cardiac Hormones. *Hypertension, 7,* 469–482.
Nelson, D.O., & A.K. Johnson. (1985). Subfornical organ projections to nucleus medianus: Electrophysiological evidence for angiotensin II synapes. *Federation Proceedings, 44,* 1010.
Nicolaidis, S. (1969). Early systemic responses to orgastric stimulation in the regulation of food and water balance: Functional and electrophysiological Data, *Annals of the New York Academy of Sciences, 157,* 1176–1203.
Niijima, A. (1969). Afferent discharges from osmoreceptors in the liver of the guinea pig. *Science,* 166, 1519–1520.
Norgren, R. (1978). Projections from the nucleus of the solitary tract in the rat. *Neuroscience, 3,* 207–218.
Norgren, R. (1981). The central organization of the gustatory and visceral afferent systems in the nucleus of the solitary tract. In Y. Katsuki, R. Norgren & M. Sato (eds.). *Brain mechanisms of sensation,* (pp. 143–160) New York: Wiley & Sons.
Ohkubo, H., R. Kageyama, M. Ujihara, T. Hirose, S. Inayama, & S. Nakanishi. (1983). *Proceedings of the National Academy of Sciences, USA, 80,* 2196–2200.
Ohkubo, H., J. Nakayama, T. Tanaka, & S. Nakanishi. (1986). Tissue distribution of rat angiotensinogen in RNA and structural analysis of heterogeneity. *Journal of Biological Chemistry, 261,* 319–323.
Ohman, L.E., & A.K. Johnson. (1986). Lesions in lateral parabrachial nucleus enhance drinking to angiotensin II and isoproterenol, *American Journal of Physiology, 251,* R504–R509.
Ohman, L.E., & A.K. Johnson. (1987). Brainstem mechanisms and the inhibition of drinking. *Federation Proceedings,* 46, *1434.*
Ohman, L.E., & A.K. Johnson. (1989). Brain stem mechanisms and the inhibition of angiotensin-induced drinking. *American Journal of Physiology, 256,* R264–R269.
Ohman, L.E., R.E. Shade, & J.R. Haywood. (1988). Parabrachial nucleus involvement in hypotension-induced vasopressin release. *The FASEB Journal,* 2, A1482.
Olsson, K. (1969). Studies on central regulation of secretion and antidiuretic hormone (ADH) in the goat. *Acta Physiologica Scandinavica, 77,* 465–74.
Ono, T., H. Nishino, K. Sasaka, K. Muramoto, I. Yano, & A. Simpson. (1978). Paraventricular nucleus connections to spinal cord pituitary, *Neuroscience Letters, 10,* 141–146.
Palkovits, M. (1966). The role of the subfornical organ in the salt and water balance. *Naturwissenschaften,* 53, 336.
Pamnani, M., S. Hout, J. Buggy, D. Clough, & F. Haddy. (1981). Demonstration of a humoral inhibitor of the Na^+-K^+ pump in some models of experimental hypertension. *Hypertension,* 3, (Suppl 2), II-96–II-101.
Peck, J.W., & E.M. Blass. (1975). Localization of thirst and antidiuretic osmoreceptors by intracranial injections in rats. *American Journal of Physiology, 228,* 1501–1509.
Peck, J.W., & D. Novin. (1971). Evidence that osmoreceptors mediating drinking in rabbits are in the lateral preoptic area. *Journal of Comparative Physiological Psychology, 74,* 134–147.
Pfaffman, C., & J.K. Bare. (1950). Gustatory nerve discharges in normal and adrenalectomized rats. *Journal of Comparative and Physiological Psychology, 43,* 320–324.
Phillips, M.I. (1984). Brain renin-angiotensin and hypertension. In G.P. Guthrie, Jr., & T.A. Kotchen (Eds.). *Hypertension and the brain,* (pp. 63–81). Mount Kisco, New York: Futura.
Phillips, M.I. (1987). Functions of angiotensin in the central nervous system. *Annual Review of Physiology,* 49, 413–435.

Phillips, M.I., & A. Camacho. (1987). Neural connections of the organum vasculosum of that lamina terminalis. In P.M. Gross (Ed.), *Circumventricular organs and body fluids, Vol. 1,* (pp. 158–168), Boca Raton, Florida: CRC Press, Inc.

Phillips, M.I., & B. Stenstrom. (1985). Angiotensin II in rat brain comigrates with authentic angiotensin II in high liquid chromatography. *Cir. Res., 56,* 212–219.

Pittman, Q.J., D. Lawrence, & L. McLean. (1982). Central effects of arginine vasopressin on blood pressure in rats. *Endocrinology, 110,* 1058–1960.

Plotsky, P.M. (1987). Facilitation of immunoreactive corticotropin-releasing factor secretion into the hypophysial-portal circulation after activation of catecholaminergic pathways or central norepinephrine injection. *Endocrinology, 121,* 924–930.

Plotsky, P.M., & W. Vale. (1984). Hemorrhage-induced secretion of corticotropin-releasing factor-like immunoreactivity into the rat hypophysial portal circulation and its inhibition by glucocorticoids. *Endocrinology, 114,* 164–169.

Plunkett, L.M., K. Shigematsu, M. Kurihara, & J.M. Saavedra. (1987). Localization of angiotensin II receptors along the anteroventral third ventricle area of the rat brain. *Brain Research, 405,* 205-212.

Pohl, M., A. Carayon, F. Cesselin, & M. Hamon. (1988). Angiotensin II-like material extracted from the rat brain is distinct from authentic angiotensin II. *Journal of Neurochemistry, 51,* 1407–1413.

Porter, J.P., & M.J. Brody. (1985). Neural projections from paraventricular nucleus that subserve vasomotor functions. *American Journal of Physiology, 248,* R271–R281.

Porter, J.P., & M.J. Brody. (1986). A comparison of the hemodynamic effects produced by electrical stimulation of subnuclei of the paraventricular nucleus, *Brain Research, 375,* 20–29.

Printz, M.P., D. Ganten, T. Unger, & M.I. Phillips. (1982). Minireview: The brain angiotensin system. In D. Ganten, M. Printz, M.I. Phillips, & B.A. Scholkens, (Eds.). The renin angiotensin system in the brain (pp. 3–52) Berlin-Heidelberg: Springer-Verlag.

Quintin, L., J.-Y. Gillon, M. Ghignone, B. Renaud, & J.-F. Pujol. (1987). Baroreceptor-linked variations of catecholamine metabolism in the caudal ventrolateral medulla: An *in vivo* electrochemical study. *Brain Research, 425,* 319–326.

Ramsay, D.J., L.C. Keil, M.C. Sharpe, & J. Shinsako. (1978). Angiotensin infusion increases vasopressin, ACTH and 11-hydroxycorticosteroid secretion. *The American Journal of Physiology, 34,* R66–R71.

Ramsay, D.J. (1982). Effects of circulating angiotensin II on the brain. In W.F. Ganong, & L. Martini (Eds.). *Frontiers in Neuroendocrinology, (Vol. 7),* New York: Raven Press.

Randle, J.C.R., C.W. Bourque, & L.P. Renaud. (1984). Adrenergic activation of rat hypothalamic supraoptic neurons maintained in vitro. *Brain Research, 307,* 374–378.

Reid, I.A. (1979). The brain renin-angiotensin system: A critical analysis. *Federation Proceedings, 38,* 2255–2259.

Renaud, L.P., T.A. Day, J.C.R. Randle, & C.W. Bourque. (1985). In Vivo and In Vitro Electrophysiological evidence that central noradrenergic pathways enhance the activity of hypothalamic vasopressinergic neurosecretory cells. In R.W. Schrier (Ed.). *Vasopressin,* New York: Raven Press.

Rettig, R., D. Ganten, & A.K. Johnson. (1981). Isoproterenol-induced thirst: Renal and extrarenal mechanisms. *American Journal of Physiology, 241,* R152–R157.

Rettig, R., D.P. Healy, & M.P. Printz. (1986). Cardiovascular effects of microinjections of angiotensin II into the nucleus tractus solitarii. *Brain Research, 364,* 233–240.

Rettig, R., & A.K. Johnson. (1986). Aortic baroreceptor deafferentation diminishes saline-induced drinking in rats. *Brain Research, 370,* 29–37.

Ricardo, J.A., & E.T. Koh. (1978). Anatomical evidence of direct projections from the nucleus of the solitary tract to the hypothalamus, amygdala, and other forebrain structures in the rat. *Brain Research, 153,* 1–26.

Richoux, J.-P., J. Bouhnik, E. Clauser, & P. Corvol. (1988). The reninangiotensin system in the rat brain: Immunocytochemical localization of angiotensinogen in glial cells and neurons. *Histochemistry, 89,* 323–331.

Robertson, G.L. (1977). The regulation of vasopressin function in health and disease. *Recent Progress in Hormone Research, 33,* 333–385. New York: Academic Press.

Robinson, M.M. (1987). An increase in mean arterial pressure (MAP) by IV infusion of phenylephrine (PE) inhibits the drinking response to SC injections of hypertonic saline in the rat. *Society for Neuroscience Abstracts, 13,* 1171.

Robinson, M.M., & M.D. Evered. (1987). Pressor action of intravenous angiotensin II reduces drinking response in rats. *American Journal of Physiology, 252,* R754–R759.

Rodriguez, E.M. (1976). The cerebrospinal fluid as a pathway in neuroendocrine integration. *Endocrinology, 71,* 407–443.

Rogers, R.C., D. Novin, & L.L. Butcher. (1979). Electrophysiological and neuroanatomical studies of hepatic portal osmo- and sodium-receptive afferent projections with in the brain. *Journal of the Autonomic Nervous System, 1,* 183–202.

Rolls, B.J., & E.T. Rolls. (1982). Thirst. Cambridge: Cambridge University Press.

Rolls, B.J., R.J. Wood, & R.M. Stevens. (1978). Effects of palatability on body fluid homeostasis. *Physiology and Behavior, 20,* 15–19.

Ross, C.A., D.A. Ruggiero, D.H. Park, T.H. Joh, A.F. Sved, J. Fernandes-Pardal, J.M. Saavedra, & D.J. Reis. (1984). Tonic vasomotor control by the rostral ventrolateral medulla: Effect of electrical or chemical stimulation of the area containing C1 adrenaline neurons on arterial pressure, heart rate, and plasma catecholamines and vasopressin. *The Journal of Neuroscience, 4,* 474–494.

Ross, E.J., & S.B.M. Christie. (1969). Hypernatremia. *Medicine, 48,* 441–473.

Rougeon, F., B. Chambraud, S. Roote, J.J. Panthier, R. Nageotte, & P. Corvol. (1981). *Proceedings of the National Academy of Sciences, USA, 78,* 6367–6371.

Rowland, N. (1980). Impaired drinking to angiotension II after subdiaphragmatic vagotomy in rats. *Physiology and Behavior, 24,* 1177–1180.

Rydin, H., & E.B. Verney. (1983). The inhibition of water-diuresis by emotional stress and by muscular exercise. *Quarterly Journal of Experimental Physiology, 27,* 343–375.

Sanders, B.J., S. Knardahl, & A.K. Johnson. (1989). The effects of lesions of the anteroventral thirst ventricle (AV3V) on the development of stress-induced hypertension in the borderline hypertensive rat (BHR), *Hypertension, 13,* 817–821.

Saper, C.B., K.M. Hurley, M.M. Moga, H.R. Holmes, S.A. Adams, K.M. Leahy, & P. Needleman. (1989). Brain natriuretic peptides: differential localization of a new family of neuropeptides. *Neuroscience Letters, 96,* 29–34.

Saper, C.B., & Levisohn, D. (1983). Afferent connections of the median preoptic nucleus in the rat, anatomical evidence for a cardiovascular integrative mechanism in the anteroventral third ventricular, AV3V region, *Brain Research, 288,* 21–31.

Saper, CB., & Loewy, A.D. (1980). Efferent connections of the parabrachial nucleus in the rat. *Brain Res., 197,* 291–317.

Saper, C.B., D.J. Reis, & T. Joh. (1983). Medullary catecholamine inputs to the anteroventral third ventricular cardiovascular regulatory region in the rat. *Neuroscience Letters, 42,* 285–291.

Saper, C.B., D.G. Standaert, M.G. Currie, D. Schwartz, D.M. Geller, & P. Needleman. (1985). Atriopeptin-immunoreactive neurons in the brain: presence in cardiovascular regulatory areas. *Science, 277,* 1047–1049.

Sarnoff, S.J., & S.I. Yamada. (1959). Evidence for reflex control of arterial pressure from abdominal receptors with special reference to the pancreas. *Circulation Research, 7,* 325–335.

Satinoff, E. (1978). Neural organization and evolution of thermal regulation in mammals. *Science, 201,* 16–21.

Sawchenko, P.E., & L.W. Swanson. (1983). The organization of forebrain afferents to the paraventricular and supraoptic nuclei of the rat. *Journal of Comparative Neurology, 218,* 121–144.

Sawchenko, P.E., L.W. Swanson, W.W. Vale. (1984). Co-expression of corticotropin-releasing factor and vasopressin immunoreactivity in parvocellular neurosecretory neurons of the adrenalectomized rat. *Proceedings of the National Academy of Sciences USA, 81,* 1883–1887.

Schneider, E.G., J.O, Davis, C.A. Robb, J.A. Baumber, J.A. Johnson, & F.S. Wright. (1970). Lack of evidence for a hepatic osmoreceptor mechanism in conscious dogs. *American Journal of Physiology, 218,* 42–45.

Severs, W.B., & A.E. Daniels-Severs. (1973). Effects of angiotensin on the central nervous system. *Pharmacological Reviews, 25,* No. 3, 415–445.

Severs, W.B., J. Summy-Long, J.S. Taylor, & J.D. Connor. (1970). A central effect of angiotensin: release of pituitary pressor material, *Journal of Pharmacology and Experimental Therapeutics, 174,* 27–34.

Shapiro, R.E., & R.R. Miselis. (1985). The central neural connections of the area postrema of the rat. *Journal of Comparative Neurology, 234,* 344–364.

Share, L. (1974). Blood pressure, blood volume, and the release of vasopressin. In R.O. Greep, E.B. Astwood, E. Knobil, W.H. Sawyer, & S.R. Geiger. (Eds.). *Handbook of Physiology, Sec. 6. Endocrinology: Vol. IV. The pituitary gland and its neuroendocrine control. Part I.* Washington, D.C.: American Physiological Society.

Share, L., (1983). Centrally acting humoral factors in the control of vasopressin release. In B.A. Cross & G. Leng (Eds), *The neurohypophysis: Structure, function and control, progress in brain research, Vol. 60* (pp. 425–435. Amsterdam: Elsevier.

Share, L. & M.N. Levy. (1962). Cardiovascular receptors and blood titer of antidiuretic hormome. *American Journal of Physiology, 203,* 425–428.

Sharpe, D.M., G.J. Mogenson, & F.R. Calareso. (1978). The role of renal nerves in the response to dipsogenic stimuli in the rat. *Canadian Journal of Physiological Pharmacology,* 56, 731–734.

Shrager, E.E. (1981). *The contribution of periventricular structures of the laminia terminalis to the control of thirst.* Unpublished doctoral dissertation. The University of Iowa, Iowa City.

Shrager, E.E., M.J. Osborne, A.K. Johnson, & A.N. Epstein. (1975). Entry of angiotensin into cerebral ventricles and circumventricular structures. In D.S. Davies & J.L. Reid (Eds.). *Central action of drugs in blood pressure regulation.* Baltimore, MD: University Park Press.

Sibbald, J.R., J.I. Hubbard, & N.E. Sirett. (1988) Responses from osmosensitive neurons of the rat Subfornical organ in vitro. *Brain Research,* 461, 205–214.

Simpson, J.B. (1981). The circumventricular organs and the central actions of angiotensin. *Neuroendocrinology, 32* 248–256.

Simpson, J.B., A.N. Epstein, & J.S. Camardo, Jr. (1978). Localization of receptors for the dipsogenic action of angiotensin II in the subfornical organ of rat. *Journal of Comparative Physiological Psychology, 92*, 581–601.

Simpson, J.B., & A. Routtenberg. (1973). Subfornical organ: Site of drinking elicited by angiotensin II. *Science, 181*, 1172–1175.

Sklar, A.H. & R.W. Schrier. (1983). Central nervous system mediators of vasopressin release. *Physiological Review, 63*, 1243–1279.

Skultety, F.M., & R.J. Joynt. (1963). Clinical implications of adipsia. *Journal of Neurosurgery, 20*, 793–800.

Sladek, C.D., & W.E. Armstrong. (1987). Effect of neurotransmitters and neuropeptides on vasopressin release. In D.M. Gash & G.J. Boer (Eds.). *Vasopressin: Principles and properties* (pp. 275–334). New York: Plenum Press.

Sladek, C.D., & A.K. Johnson. (1983). The effect of anteroventral third ventricle lesions on vasopressin release by organ-cultured hypothalamo-neurohypophyseal explants. *Neuroendocrinology, 37*, 78–84.

Smith, H.W. (1957). Salt and water volume receptors: An exercise in physiologic apologetics. *American Journal of Medicine, 23*, 623–651.

Songu-Mize, E., S.L. Bealer, & R.W. Caldwell. (1982). Effect of AV3V lesions on development of DOCA-salt hypertension and vascular Na^{+}-pump activity. *Hypertension, 4*, 575–580.

Spoerri, V. (1963). Uber die gefassversorgung des subfornikalorgans der ratte. *Acta Anatomica* (Basel), *54*, 333.

Standaert, D.G., P. Needleman, & C.B. Saper. (1986). Organization of atriopeptin-like immunoreactive neurons in the central nervous system of the rat. *The Journal of Comparative Neurology, 253*, 315–341.

Stricker, E.M. (1966). Extracellular fluid volume and thirst. *American Journal of Physiology, 211*, 232–238.

Stricker, E.M. (1969). Osmoregulation and volume regulation in rats: inhibition of hypovolemic thirst by water. *American Journal of Physiology, 217*, 98–105.

Swanson, L.W. (1977). Immunohistochemical evidence for a neurophysin-containing autonomic pathway arising in the paraventricular nucleus of the hypothalamus, *Brain Research, 128*, 346–353.

Swanson, L.W., J. Kucharczyk, & G.J. Mogenson. (1978). Autoradiographic evidence for pathways from the medial preoptic area to the midbrain involved in the drinking response to angiotensin II. *The Journal of Comparative Neurology, 178*, 645–660.

Swanson, L.W., & R.W. Lind. (1986). Neural projections subserving the initiation of a specific motivated behavior in the rat: New projections from the subfornical organ. *Brain Research, 379*, 399–403.

Swanson, L.W., & G.J. Mogenson. (1981). Neural mechanisms for the functional coupling of autonomic, endocrine and somatomotor responses in adaptive behavior. *Brain Research, 3*, 1–34.

Swanson, L.W., & P.E. Sawchenko. (1983). Hypothalamic integration: Organization of the paraventricular and supraoptic nuclei. *Annual Review of Neuroscience, 8*, 269–324.

Swingle, W.W., J.P. Da Vanzo, D. Glenister, H.C. Crossfield, & G. Wagle. (1959). Role of gluco- and mineralocorticoids in salt and water metabolism of adrenalectomized dogs. *Journal of Physiology, 196*, 283–286.

Tanaka, J., H. Kaba, H. Saito, & K. Seto. (1985). Inputs from the A1 noradrenergic region to hypothalamic paraventricular neurons in the rat. *Brain Research, 335*, 368–371.

Tanaka, J., H. Saito, & H. Kaba. (1987). Subfornical organ and hypothalamic paraventricular nucleus connections with median preoptic nucleus neurons: an electrophysiological study in the rat. *Experimental Brain Research, 68*, 579–585.

Tanaka, J., H. Saito, H. Kaba, & K. Seto. (1987). Subfornical organ neurons act to enhance the activity of paraventricular vasopressin neurons in reponse to intravenous angiotensin II. *Neuroscience Research, 4*, 424–427.

Teitelbaum, P. & A.N. Epstein. (1962). The lateral hypothalamic syndrome: Recovery of feeding and drinking after lateral hypothalamic lesions. *Psychology Reviews, 69*, 74–90.

Thornton, S.N., A. Jevlin, R. de Beurepaire, & S. Nicolaidis. (1985). Iontophoretic application of angiotensin II, vasopressin and oxytocin in the region of the anterior hypothalamus in the rat. *Brain Research Bulletin, 14*, 211–215.

Thrasher, T.N., C.J. Brown, L.C. Keil, & D.J. Ramsay. (1980). Thirst and vasopressin release in the dog: An osmoreceptor or sodium receptor mechanism? *American Journal of Physiology, 238*, R333–R339.

Thrasher, T.N., & L.C. Keil. (1987). Regulation of drinking and vasopressin secretion: role of organum vasculosum laminae terminalis. *American Journal of Physiology*, 253, R108–R120.

Thrasher, T.N., L.C. Keil, & D.J. Ramsay. (1982). Lesions of the organum vasculosum of the lamina terminalis (OVLT) attenuate osmotically-induced drinking and vasopressin secretion in the dog. *Endocrinology, 110*, 1837–1839.

Thrasher, T.N., J.F. Nistal-Herrea, L.C. Keil, & D.J. Ramsay. (1981). Satiety and inhibition of vasopressin secretion after drinking in dehydrated dogs. *Am. J. Physiol., 240*, E394–E401.

Thrasher, T.N., J.B. Simpson, & D.J. Ramsay. (1982). Lesions of the subfornical organ block angiotensin-induced drinking in the dog. *Neuroendocrinology, 35*, 68–72.

Tordoff, M.G., J. Schulkin, & M.I. Friedman. (1986). Hepatic contribution to satiation of salt appetite in rats. *American Journal of Physiology, 251*, R1095–R1102.

Tuttle, R.S., & M. McCleary. (1975). Mesenteric baroreceptors. *American Journal of Physiology, 229*, 1514–1519.

Ueda, H., S. Katayama, & R. Kato. (1972). Area postrema — Angiotensin-sensitive site in brain. In T.A. Assaykeen (Ed.), *Control of renin secretion: Advances in experimental medicine and biology, 17,* 109–116, New York: Plenum Press.
Undesser, K.P., E.M. Hasser, J.R. Haywood, A.K. Johnson, & V.S. Bishop. (1985). Interactions of vasopressin with the area postrema in arterial baroreflex function in consicous rabbits, *Circulation Research, 56,* 410–417.
Vallet, P., & A.J. Baertschi. (1980). Sodium-chloride sensitive receptors located in hepatic portal vein of the rat. *Neuroscience Letters, 17,* 283–288.
Vallet, P.G., & A.J. Baertschi. (1982). Spinal afferents for peripheral osmoreceptors in the rat. *Brain Research, 239,* 271–174.
Van der Kooy, D., & L.Y. Koda. (1983). Organization of the projections of a circumventricular organ: The area postrema in the rat. *Journal of Comparative Neurology, 219,* 328–338.
Verney, E.B. (1946). Absorption and excretion of water. *Lancet, 251,* 739–744.
Verney, E.B. (1947). The antidiuretic hormone and the factors which determine its release. *Proceedings of the Royal Society, 135B,* 25–106.
Wakerly, J.B., R. Noble, & G. Clarke. (1983). *In vitro* studies of the control of phasic discharge in neurosecretory cells of the supraoptic nucleus. In B.A. Cross & G. Leng (Eds.) *The Neurohypophysis: Structure, function and control. Progress in Brain Research, 60,* 53–59.
Weindl, A. (1973). Neuroendocrine aspects of circumventricular organs. In W.F. Ganong & L. Martini (Eds.), *Frontiers in Neuroendocrinology,* New York, Oxford University Press.
Weiner, R.I., & W.F. Ganong. (1978). Role of brain monoamines and histamine in regulation of anterior pituitary secretion. *Physiological Reviews, 58,* 905–959.
Weyhenmeyer, J.A., & M.I. Phillips. (1982). Angiotensin-like immunoreactivity in the brain of the spontaneously hypertensive rat. *Hypertension, 4,* 514–523.
Wilkin, L.D., K.A. Gruber, & A.K. Johnson. (1986). Changes in magnocellular-neurophypophyseal vasopressin following anteroventral third ventricle (AV3V) Lesions, *Cardiovascular Pharmacology, 8,* (Suppl. 7), 570–575.
Wilkin, L.D., L.D. Mitchell, D. Ganten, & A.K. Johnson. (1989). The supraoptic nucleus: Afferents from areas involved in control of body fluid homeostatis, *Neuroscience, 28,* 573–584.
Wilkin, L.D, K.P. Patel, P.G. Schmid, & A.K. Johnson. (1987). Increased norepinephrine turnover in median preoptic nucleus following reduced extracellular fluid volume, *Brain Research, 423,* 369–372.
Willoughby, J.O, P.M. Jervois, M.F. Menadue, & W.W. Blessing. (1987). Noradrenaline, by activation of alpha-1-adrenoreceptors in the region of the supraoptic nucleus, causes secretion of vasopressin in the unanesthetised rat. *Neuroendocrinology, 45,* 219–226.
Wise, B.L. & W.F. Ganong. (1960.) Effect of brain stem stimulation on renal function. *American Journal of Physiclogy, 198,* 1291–1295.
Witt, D.M., A.D. Keller, H.L. Batsel, & J.R. Lynch. (1952). Absence of thirst and resultant syndrome associated with anterior hypothalamectomy in the dog. *American Journal of Physiology, 171,* 780.
Wolf, A.V. (1958). *Thirst: Physiology of the Urge to Drink and Problems of Water Lack.* A.V. Wolf, (Ed.). Springfield, IL: Charles C. Thomas.
Wolfson, B., R.W. Manning, L.G. Davis, R. Arentzen, & F. Baldino, Jr. (1985). Co-localization of corticotropin releasing factor and vasopressin mRNA in neurones after adrenalectomy. *Nature, 315,* 59–61.
Woodward, D.J., H.C. Moises, B.D. Waterhouse, B.J. Hoffer, & R. Freedman. (1979). Modulating actions of norepinephrine in the central nervous system. *Federation Proceedings, 38,* 2109–2116.
Wright, J.W., S.L. Morseth, R.H. Abhold, & J.W. Harding. (1985). Pressor action and dipsogenicity induced by angiotensin II and III in rats. *American Journal of Physiology, 249,* R514–R521.
Yamashita, H., H. Kannan, K. Inenaga, & K. Koizumi. (1984). The role of cardiovascular and muscle afferent systems in control of body water balance. *J. Autonomic Nervous System, 10,* 305–316.
Young, P.T. (1967). Palatability; the hedonic response to foodstuffs. In C.F. Code & W. Heidel (Eds.), *Handbook of physiology: Sec. 6. Alimentary canal: Vol. 1. Control of food and water intake.* Washington, D.C.: American Physiological Society.
Zardetto-Smith, A.M., & T.S. Gray, (1987). A direct neural projections from the nucleus of the solitary track to the subfornical organ in the rat. *Neuroscience Letters, 80,* 163–166.

ACKNOWLEDGEMENTS

Studies from the author's laboratory discussed in this chapter were supported in part by USPHS grants HLP 14388, HL 33447, HL 35600, and MH 00064 and by the Iowa Affiliate of the American Heart Association.

The author is grateful for the constructive comments that were provided by Michael Brody, Gaylen Edwards, Carl Gisolfi, Paul Gross, Ian Phillips, and Kathy Travis on earlier drafts of the manuscript and for the excellent editorial and secretarial assistance of Ms. Norma Mottet. The author, also, wishes to thank R. W. Lind for providing a preprint of Lind and Ganten (1990), for his colleagueship over the years, and for his contributions to furthering the understanding of the brain-renin angiotensin system.

DISCUSSION

PHILLIPS: I think the central question that Kim has very nicely analyzed is, "how does the brain know when to induce thirst or to induce drinking?" It comes down to two major stimuli; the osmotic stimulus and the hypovolemic stimulus. The osmotic stimulus has two primary mechanisms; one is through sodium acting on sodium receptors, and the other is through neurotransmitter action. If you inject carbachol or NaCl into the brain of rats, they drink because the osmotic pathway in the brain is activated.

The message for hypovolemia comes from afferent inputs that enter the brain stem from baroreceptors telling the brain essentially that we have a state of hypovolemia. The neurotransmitter appears to be norepinephrine. It's very interesting that Kim has the experiments with norepinephrine because we found that norepinephrine releases brain angiotensin. This is an element Kim didn't have much time to review, but in the brain, angiotensin is made independently of peripheral levels of angiotensin. We have found that brain angiotensin is cyclic — it rises at night and falls during the day. It responds to situations such as hemorrhage with an increase. At least in rats, where the angiotensin cyclicity is up at night and down during the day, rats drink at night and drink less during the day. It fits with the angiotensin cycle. Thus, brain angiotensin and norepinephrine may play important roles in thirst. I would say that on a moment-to-moment basis, the osmotic stimulus is probably the most important and that the situation of hypovolemia is not frequently met unless you're an athlete out running or someone having a hemorrhage or an astronaut with fluid compartment shifts.

Now when you have a state of hypovolemia, you will, of course, get release of peripheral angiotensin and as the angiotensin levels rise, they will induce thirst, but there is a caution here. Angiotensin in the blood itself is not, as far as I can tell, just a cause for drinking. There is a threshold for the level of plasma angiotensin II before it will cause drinking. Many of us tried to get rats to drink with infusions of IV angiotensin II and that proved quite difficult unless you used a high dose. If you measure the actual amounts of angiotensin II in plasma after you have infused angiotensin IV to produce drinking, we find that levels are about 450 pg mL or more. So there is a fairly precise threshold for blood angiotensin to cause drinking.

Kim has a graph showing angiotensin levels correlated to different states of dehydration. One of them is 48 h of dehydration and that's at about the level of 450 pg/mL. So for angiotensin in the blood to act as a dipsogen and induce thirst, it has to be at levels that normally would be experienced under 48 h dehydration, which would be an emergency level. So, I would say that angiotensin in the blood is more for an emergency state which would certainly come in athletes and astronauts and during severe dehydration or hemorrhage, but would not drive normal day-to-day drinking. On the other hand, brain angiotensin, because it is cyclic, could elicit day-to-day drinking. Lastly, moment-to-moment drinking is probably controlled by osmotic and sodium stimuli through the cholinergic system.

The next question is "why does blood angiotensin have a dipsogenic threshold?" What is holding it back? I think the onset of thirst is registered in the circumventricular organs. These organs are very small regions of the brain that do not have a blood brain barrier; but they are full of glial cells which have angiotensin II receptor cells. Presumably the glial cells do not relay the message of thirst; neurons relay the thirst message. The hypothesis we are currently working on is that in circumventricular organs, angiotensin from the blood, which can get into circumventricular organs, has to bind up all the glial receptors before it can move into the brain. At a high level, angiotensin would overpower those receptors or the number of binding site, and then move into the brain and have effects on thirst. That would account for the threshold and that would be why angiotensin in the blood would not be important until it reached that high level.

JOHNSON: I will begin by making a few comments with regard to the role of circulating angiotensin II (ANG II) in thirst. This has been a hotly contested question since Fitzsimon's implication of the renin-angiotensin system in drinking behavior. I think it is fair to begin by emphasizing the fact that thirst results from the input of various classes of stimuli into the central nervous system. Under experimental conditions, either cellular dehydration alone or a 'pure" extracellular dehydration can produce drinking. However, under normal conditions, such as water deprivation or during exercise, water loss accrues in both body fluid compartments. Therefore, receptors and afferent input from both compartments signal the brain of dehydration. I think it is fair to say that the threshold for drinking to cellular dehydration is probably lower than that for drinking to extracellular depletion so that when comparing cellular versus extracellular mechanisms in the control of drinking, it is probably the cellular receptors and pathways that are biologically more "relevant."

When considering mechanisms involved in mobilizing homeostatic responses to extracellular depletion, it is important to emphasize the existence of both a humoral (i.e., ANG II) and afferent neural input into the central nervous system. Under conditions of extracellular hypovolemia, both afferent neural and humoral input into the nervous system is activated. Therefore, it is unlikely that ANG II is ever required to act as a sole dipsogenic hormone under physiological conditions. It is best considered as a participant in the processes that generate thirst.

When one considers the experimental approaches that have been employed to evaluate the role of ANG II in the circulation as a dipsogen, it is important to recognize that intravenous infusions of ANG II raise systemic blood pressure. Recent work by Marilyn Robinson and Mark Everd at the University of Western Ontario has shown that hypertension inhibits water intake. Therefore, one has to be very careful in making judgments about the efficacy of systemically administered angiotensin in infusion studies in which the elevation in pressure is not controlled or taken into account.

WADE: What is the role of low pressure receptors in drinking to hypovolemia?

JOHNSON: In most species it is impossible to test the role of input from low pressure receptors simply because cervical vagotomy is incompatible with a behaviorally viable preparation. We have studied the effects of removal of high pressure baroreceptor input (i.e., sinoaortic denervation [SAD]) on drinking to hypovolemia in rats and find no effect of SAD.

Susan Kaufman of the University of Alberta has used a balloon placed in the right atrium to investigate the effect of atrial stretch on the inhibition of experimentally induced thirst. Her results indicate that drinking to extracellular fluid depletion is inhibited by atrial expansion.

SUMMERS: I just wanted to ask Ian about these glial cells. What is their role? Why do they have receptors?

PHILLIPS: Glial cell receptors from cultured cells have binding sites and low affinity for angiotensin II. They bind it and rapidly metabolize it. Neurons do not metabolize angiotensin. The glial cells have something like angiotensin receptors that take up angiotensin.

CONVERTINO: I'd like to go back to your previous comment on the role of the low pressure baroreflex. As acute exercise is repeated daily during exercise training, the plasma volume is not merely replaced through thirst and renal mechanisms, but it is expanded. The obvious questions are "Where does the added plasma volume go? How can it be expanded and remain in the same vascular space?" With the evidence that you have presented, it occurs to me that blood volume expansion resulting from chronic exercise may occur because of a resetting of the pressure/volume response relation controlled by the cardiopulmonary baroreflex and the CNS.

JOHNSON: When considering the role of both high and low pressure baroreceptor derived input into the CNS in the control of fluid balance, I think that there are two things that must be emphasized. First, is the fact that one of the most notable aspects of pressure/volume receptor systems is that they have a tremendous capacity to reset. There have been several experimental demonstrations that baroreceptors reset in the order of minutes. Therefore, baroreceptors in all likelihood are reset in the course of exercise or conditioning.

The second aspect of pressure/volume receptors that must be appreciated is the capacity of these two systems to interact and the fact that there is a great deal of redundancy in these two systems. Experimentally, it has been demonstrated that, if you measure vasopressin release or sympathetic activation after removal of just high pressure input (e.g., sinoaortic denervation) or just after removal of low pressure input (e.g., cold block of the vagus), there is little effect in comparison to when both afferent mechanisms are blocked simultaneously. The neural mechanisms responsible for pressure/volume baroreceptor mechanisms resetting and the nature of the interaction of high and low pressure afferent systems will prove to be a thoroughly provocative and challenging area for future research.

HUBBARD: I would like to thank you for a marvelous presentation and to make a comment regarding our concept that thirst is related to the consequences of sodium pumping such as cellular energy depletion during hyperthermia. A metabolic component exists in ADH release (and presumably thirst) because hypoglycemia stimulates it. Although ADH is also released as a function of body osmolality and plasma sodium, potassium deficiency and hypokalemia stimulate ADH and thirst, as well. I'm wondering if there is any way, within your scheme of looking at thirst, that hypernatremia and hypokalemia stimulate thirst — that's one question. Another relates to the work of Stricker in which rats made hypovolemic by osmotic dehydration (injecting colloid subcutaneously) will drink water immediately as well as increasing amounts of concentrated saline after a 4- to 5-h delay. However, if the rats are first made sodium-deficient, they drink the hypertonic saline immediately. I'm wondering if that effect relates to a hormone that stimulates sodium appetite or are we talking about a situation that represents a profound level of hyponatremic hypovolemia?

JOHNSON: In states of high osmolality and/or high extracellular sodium, it is generally agreed that an osmoreceptor or sodium receptor mechanism is likely to mediate the drinking response. What puzzled physiologists during the late 30s, 40s and into the 50s was the observation that sodium depletion also induced drinking. Reduced sodium is an effective stimulus for the activation of the renin-angiotensin system, and Fitzsimons' implication of the renin-angiotensin system as a mediator of thirst in the 1960s gave a logical explanation of why sodium depletion would induce thirst and provided a logical candidate (ANG II) as a mediator of the drinking response. I only mention this because it serves to illustrate that there are multiple factors involved in the generation of a drinking response and, although the behavior is identical in both cases, the physiological mechanisms mediating the response are quite different.

Regarding the point about Stricker's work in which he demonstrated that animals placed on a low sodium diet show a shorter latency for the onset of a sodium appetite in the face of hypovolemia, Stricker has made the point that laboratory rats (on standard laboratory chow) should be considered to be on a high sodium diet. It is necessary to remove what might be considered a reservoir of sodium by placing the animal on a low sodium diet in order to activate afferent pathways when hypovolemia is experimentally induced.

TIPTON: With regard to thirst mechanism, e.g. water or sodium, where does palatability fit and is it common to higher animals?

JOHNSON: What I'm talking about was the way that we give therapy for animals that are completely adipisic after AV3V lesions. All we have to do is offer them a sweet solution and they love it. This demonstrates that there is no motor impairment per se produced by the AV3V lesion. The adipisic AV3V-lesioned rats ingest the fluid just as if it were water in terms of the motor patterns action required to drink. However, these dehydrated rats will not drink water. The intake of sucrose solution is purely driven by the sweet nature of the fluid. The way that we handle these animals post lesion is to start out with a 10% sucrose solution and wean them over subsequent days to water.

11

Clinical Implications of Fluid Imbalance

JOHN R. SUTTON, M.D.

INTRODUCTION

Fluid imbalance will have clinical implications if it produces symptoms or results in a sequence of events that cause pathophysiological derangements. The clinical manifestations of fluid imbalance may be the result of a general depletion of body fluids; an excess of fluid; a change of fluid composition within body compartments with respect to electrolytes, acid-base or osmolality; and/or a derangement of an organ-specific fluid. The clinical manifestations will vary depending on the following:

1. the magnitude of the fluid imbalance,

2. the rate of change of fluid imbalance,
3. the effects on central and local hemodynamics,
4. the consequences for thermoregulation, and
5. the accompanying changes in metabolites, electrolytes, acid-base balance, and the products of organ malfunction.

Many of the thermal illnesses are associated with dehydration; however, as has been recently noted, even heat stroke can occur in the absence of severe dehydration (Hales et al., 1986) if fluid distribution is inappropriate.

DEHYDRATION

Although heat stroke has been shown to occur in the absence of significant dehydration, it is well known that heat-dissipating mechanisms are further compromised by dehydration (Adolph, 1947; Gisolfi & Copping, 1971; Greenleaf & Castle, 1971; Strydom & Holdsworth, 1968). However, it was the work of Sawka and associates (1985) which systematically quantified the physiological responses to four separate degrees of dehydration in the same subjects. In a study of eight subjects who underwent dehydration equivalent to 3%, 5%, and 7% of their body weights, a predictable and progressive increase in heart rate and rectal temperature responses to a heat stress test was demonstrated. With progressive dehydration, the sweat rates decreased and the rectal temperatures at the onset of sweating increased. All eight subjects were able to complete 120 min of exercise when they were normally hydrated and when dehydrated by 3%. At 5% dehydration, one subject withdrew because of multiple premature ventricular contractions, and at 7% dehydration, six subjects stopped—one because of premature ventricular contractions and the other five because they were "exhausted."

In the past, considerable emphasis has been placed on distinguishing the signs and symptoms of heat exhaustion on the basis of salt depletion versus water depletion. However, Hubbard and Armstrong (1988) have emphasized that the pure forms of salt and water depletion are rare and in support of Dinman and Horvath (1984), that such a distinction in signs and symptoms of heat exhaustion was not clinically feasible.

The predominant heat exhaustion symptoms that may differ according to the degree of salt versus water depletion are: 1) thirst—more common in water depletion, 2) muscle cramps—more common in salt depletion, and 3) vomiting—more common in salt depletion.

HEAT-RELATED DISORDERS, WITH OR WITHOUT DEHYDRATION

Heat Syncope

Heat syncope is the abrupt loss of consciousness usually observed in unacclimatized people in the upright position (Weiner & Horne, 1958).

Dehydration is not a prerequisite, and the mechanisms whereby heat syncope occurs are well understood. Most commonly, it results from venous pooling of blood in the vasodilated periphery. This results in a diminished venous return, reduced cardiac output, and impaired cerebral perfusion with resultant syncope. The clinical settings in which heat syncope is most commonly found are:

1. suddenly standing from a lying or sitting position,
2. standing for a prolonged time in the heat (e.g., a soldier on guard duty),
3. stopping at the end of a foot race when the muscle pump is no longer working to enhance venous return, and
4. being adversely affected by: a) cardiovascular disease, b) autonomic neuropathy such as diabetes or the Shy-Dreger syndrome, c) hypokalemia, d) dehydration or salt depletion, and e) drugs such as diuretics, peripheral vasodilators, beta blockers, and calcium channel antagonists.

Heat Cramps

Heat cramps are spasms of skeletal muscle, commonly in the legs, arms, or the abdominal wall, which usually occur several hours after exercise when the subjects are cooling down or have already cooled down. Classically, the subjects have sweated profusely and consumed copious amounts of fluid without replacing the lost sodium. They also tend to pass little urine. These conditions were well described earlier this century during the construction of the Boulder Dam (Talbot, 1933). Although the diagnosis is usually obvious, the muscle cramps associated with heat are similar to those induced by hyperventilatory alkalosis (Boyd & Beller, 1972). When the muscles of the abdominal wall are involved, the differential diagnosis may include an acute surgical abdomen, acute gastroenteritis, or exercise-induced peritonitis (Sutton and Sauder, 1989). Although Knochel and Reed (1987) have suggested that heat-acclimatized individuals are more susceptible to heat, this has not been the experience with Israeli soldiers (Shibolet, 1976) or the Indian army (Malhotra & Venkataswamy, 1974), nor was it the experience of Talbot (1933) with the workers on the Boulder Dam or with the Youngstown, Ohio, steelworkers (1935).

Although the precise mechanism responsible for the heat-induced cramps is not understood, there seems to be general agreement that sodium depletion with a relative hyponatremia is almost universally associated with heat-induced cramps (Ladell, 1949; Leithead & Gunn, 1964; Talbot, 1935).

Heat Exhaustion and Heat Stroke

These two conditions are probably part of a continuum with relatively minor non-serious changes in the former but with loss of consciousness, possibly leading to death, in the latter. Normally, plasma volume decreases during moderate to intense exercise as increased hydrostatic pressure forces water out of capillaries and into the muscle interstitium. This decrease in plasma volume exacerbates problems of blood flow distribution between skin and muscle in the heat. The competition between the skin and the muscle for blood flow is accentuated by exercise, and for a comparable external heat stress, skin blood flow is lower in the resting state (Rowell, 1971). If significant dehydration occurs, heat-dissipating mechanisms will be compromised even further, but heat stroke may occur without significant dehydration.

As has been demonstrated, exertional heat stroke is reported more and more frequently during fun runs and marathons when the environmental conditions are not particularly hot (Sutton et al., 1972). Hales (1986) has shown that during severe heat stress, skin blood flow begins to fall; this phenomenon is rather similar to that found when central venous pressure is reduced by lower body negative pressure (Nadel, 1988). From his detailed circulatory studies under a variety of environmental conditions, Rowell (1974) concluded that a hierarchy of homeostatic mechanisms favored the maintenance of arterial pressure in the circulation to vital organs at the expense of skin vasodilatation and thermoregulation. This hypothesis was supported by a recent finding of Hales and coworkers (1986) in collapsed fun runners. These runners had a marked reduction in skin blood flow compared to their controls.

Heat stroke. Serious central nervous system dysfunction such as delirium and coma are the main distinguishing features of heat stroke. Anhydrosis, a rectal temperature greater than 40.6°C or 41°C (105°F), and a hot, dry skin were once considered essential components for the diagnosis of heat stroke but are no longer regarded as prerequisites (O'Donnell, 1977; Shibolet et al., 1976). In fact, to regard the presence of these features as essential may confound the diagnosis and delay treatment (Hart & Sutton, 1987). Knochel (1974) brought attention to the major distinctions between classical heat stroke observed after several days where the ambient temperature was particularly high (37.9°C, 100°F) and that associated with exertion. Classical heat stroke occurred in the very young and the old, often when they were unwell and sedentary. Many of the elderly patients, in particular, who suffered classical heat stroke were using drugs that might impair thermoregulation, and they also appeared not to be sweating. Exertion-associated heat stroke occurs when any combination of the heat produced by an exercising individual and the ability to lose heat to the environment is such that body temperature continues to rise (Table 11-1). Such a problem is well known in endurance events such as the marathon (McKechnie et al., 1967; Pugh et al., 1967) and in cyclists (Bernhein & Cox, 1960). It was first recognized in fun runners in 1972 by Sutton et al. This finding has since been confirmed

TABLE 11-1. *Characteristics of "classical" and "exertion-induced" heat stroke. (Reproduced from* Heat Stroke and Temperature Regulation, *edited by M. Khogali and J.R.S. Hales. Sydney: Academic Press Australia, 1983, p. 3, with permission of the authors and editors.)*

Characteristics	Classical	Exertional
Age	Older	Young
Occurrence	Epidemic form	Isolated cases
Pyrexia	Very high	High
Predisposing illness	Frequent	Rare
Sweating	Often absent	Usually present
Acid-base disturbance	Resp. alkalosis	Lactic acidosis
Rhabdomyolysis	Rare	Common
Disseminated intravascular coagulation	Rare	Common
Acute renal failure	Rare	Common
Hyperuricemia	Mild	Marked
Enzymes elevation	Mild	Marked

many times in short races in "fun runners" (Hanson & Zimmerman, 1979; Hart et al., 1980; Hughson et al., 1980; Richards et al., 1979a); military recruits (Beller & Boyd, 1975; Brahams, 1988; Costrini et al., 1979; O'Donnell & Clowes, 1972; Shibolet et al., 1976); and football players (Knochel, 1975). Potentially disastrous situations can arise in which there is a need to "make weight" for events such as rowing or wrestling and the athlete runs in track suits or impervious plastic such as garbage bags or as in one instance, a wet suit (Brahams, 1988). As Knochel and Reed pointed out (1987), there is sometimes the misconception that water denial accelerates physical conditioning; worse still is the situation in which fluid restriction is used as a disciplinary measure, as reported in 13 young military recruits with heat stroke by Knochel and Reed (1987). Factors which predispose to heat stroke are summarized in Table 11-2.

Pathophysiology of heat stroke. Knochel and Reed (1987) suggest that for a comparable rectal temperature, the tissue damage to various organs is greater in exertional rather than in classical heat stroke. There is considerable inter-individual variation in the temperature required to provoke abnormalities. Presumably, part of these individual differences are associated with the duration of hyperthermia and the rate of increase of body core temperature. Some people have survived with temperatures of 46.5°C (115.7°F) (Slovis et al., 1982), whereas others have died of exertional heat stroke with a temperature not above 40.6°C (Knochel & Reed, 1987). Nevertheless, Richards and colleagues (1979b) have reported many cases in which the recorded rectal temperature ranged from 42–43°C and, following prompt treatment, the patients recovered without any serious sequelae. In addition to the core temperature, its duration, and rate of change, the most important determinant of organ damage is the state of circulation. As long as perfusion continues to all organs, heat and waste products will be removed and ischemic injury is unlikely.

TABLE 11-2. *Factors that predispose to heat stroke.*

Personal	Environmental
Young	Hot
Old	Humid
Dehydrated	Windless
Ill - Febrile illness	Polluted
Obese	Unseasonably hot
Unfit	
Unacclimatized to heat	
Predisposed to malignant hyperthermia	

On the other hand, hypotension and ischemia may well be the common thread which results in major organ damage in the presence of hyperthermia. A variety of drugs which may be prescribed by the athlete's physician may also increase the risk of heat stroke (Table 11-3).

1. *Cardiovascular impairment:* The most common clinical finding in heat stroke is that of sinus tachycardia; there may be transient hypertension and less commonly, hypotension with clinical shock. Rarely, there is acute left heart failure. Electrocardiographic changes include sinus tachycardia, nonspecific flattening and inversion of the T-waves, and various transient conduction disturbances (Costrini et al., 1979; Hart et al., 1980). Costrini and coworkers (1979) demonstrated prolonged or borderline Q-T intervals in 6 of 12 patients with heat stroke. There was right bundle branch block in one patient, left bundle branch block in another, and left axis deviation in two patients. Two patients had S-T segment

TABLE 11-3. *Drugs that increase the risk of environmental heat injury. (Reproduced from Knochel, J.P., and G. Reed. Disorders of heat Regulation. In:* Clinical Disorders, Fluid and Electrolyte Metabolism, *edited by C. K. Kleeman, M. H. Maxwell and R. G. Narin. New York: McGraw-Hill, 1987, p. 1210, with permission of the authors and editors.)*

Drug Class	Examples	Mechanism
Diuretics	Benzodiathiazines, furosemide, ethacrynic acid, acetazolamide	Salt depletion and dehydration
Anticholinergics	Atropine, belladonna	Suppression of sweating
Anti-Parkinsonians	Procyclydine-HCl benztropine mesylate	Suppression of sweating
Phenothiazines	Chlorpromazine, promethazine	Suppression of sweating and possibly distrubed hypothalamic temperature regulation
Tricyclics	Tranylcypromine	Increased motor activity and increased heat production
Antihistamines	Diphenhydramine	Suppression of sweating
Butyrophenones	Haloperidol	Possibly disturbed hypothalamic temperature regulation and failure to recognize thirst
Sympathomimetic amines	Dextroamphetamine, phenmetrazine	Increased psychomotor activity.

depression compatible with anterolateral ischemia. This S-T segment change resolved within hours in one patient but took three weeks to resolve in the second patient. Kew and associates (1969) noted a high incidence of S-T segment and T-wave changes in a group of patients in whom coronary disease was extremely unlikely. These authors concluded that this was a heat-related injury and not the result of ischemia. Detailed studies of cardiac pathology in heat stroke have been described (Malamud et al., 1946; Wilson, 1940) and include dilatation of the right heart, particularly the atrium, and the appearance of subendocardial, subpericardial, and myocardial hemorrhages that are most common in the intraventricular septum and on the posterior wall of the left ventricle. Fragmentation and ruptured muscle fibers are also common when interstitial edema is present. In a recent report of a young football player dying of heat stroke, a hemorrhagic infarction in the anterior papillary muscle was noted (Barschenas et al., quoted in Knochel and Reed, 1987). The specific pathophysiological mechanisms causing the myocardial changes are unknown.

Renal impairment: Mild proteinuria occurs in virtually all patients with heat stroke, and up to 25% may later exhibit oliguria, anuria, and acute renal insufficiency with acute tubular necrosis (Clowes & O'Donnell, 1974; Hart et al., 1980; Knochel & Reed, 1987; Schiff et al., 1978; Schrier et al., 1967; Vertel & Knochel, 1967). Knochel and Reed (1987) made the point that acute renal failure is much more common in exercise-related heat stroke than in classical heat stroke, probably because of the much higher incidence of rhabdomyolysis. They pointed out that rhabdomyolysis in the dehydrated subject, particularly with increased uric acid from purine breakdown, is important in the pathophysiology of renal impairment. Many of these patients will recover well (Hart et al., 1980; Vertel & Knochel, 1967) although they may require a prolonged period of peritoneal and/or hemodialysis. Nevertheless, some patients may have progressive renal impairment following recovery from heat stroke. Kew and colleagues (1970a) have demonstrated interstitial nephritis in renal biopsies of such patients.

Liver dysfunction: Herman and Sullivan (1959) showed a frequent occurrence of jaundice in patients who survived heatstroke for more than two days. An increased bilirubin (direct and indirect), marked increases in leakage of liver enzymes (AST, ALT, GGT) into the blood (indicating hepatocellular damage), as well as increased serum alkaline phosphatase (indicating impairment of the liver's excretory function), are usually found. Later impairment of the liver's synthetic function may occur, with decreases in serum albumin together with decreases in coagulation factors, although a consumption coagulopathy is more common. Pathological findings in the liver include perisinusoidal edema and a predominantly centrilobular necrosis. Kew and coworkers (1970b; 1978) have demonstrated degeneration or desquamation of sinusoidal and lining cells and ballooning and flattening of the microvilli as well as changes in the mitochondria.

Central nervous system disorders: A number of CNS changes are common with heat stroke; these include delirium, hallucinations, status epilepticus, oculogyric crisis, opisthotonos, coma, cerebellar syndromes, and hemiplegia. There may also be decerebrate posturing (Clowes & O'Donnell, 1974; Hart et al., 1980; Knochel & Reed, 1987).

Pathological changes documented by Malamud and colleagues (1946) consist of edema, patchy congestion, and diffuse petechial hemorrhages. In cases of severe coagulopathy, cerebral hemorrhage may occur.

Hematological disorders: Meikle and Graybill (1967) demonstrated fibrinolysis and hemorrhage in a fatal case of heat stroke. This is best diagnosed in the laboratory with the use of euglobulin lysis time. Disseminated intravascular coagulation (DIC), a coagulopathy characterized by consumption of fibrinogen factor VIII and factor V, is more commonly seen and is usually due to circulating thrombin; thrombocytopenia is usually seen within 24 h of the onset of heat stroke. Laboratory determinations of fibrinogen, fibrin split products, and factors V and VIII will discriminate DIC from fibrinolysis. Clinical manifestations of DIC include petechial hemorrhages and ecchymoses. In fact, the hemorrhage associated with DIC is a major cause of death in patients with severe heat stroke who succumb several days after the injury (Knochel & Reed, 1987).

Pulmonary dysfunction: Tachypnea and alveolar hyperventilation are common in heat stroke. If patients develop a DIC, pulmonary edema, usually of an adult respiratory distress syndrome (ARDS) type, occurs. In this state, pulmonary artery wedge pressure is low, distinguishing it from cardiogenic pulmonary edema. Such patients have a reduced lung compliance with severe arterial hypoxemia and a low arterial PCO_2. As ventilation becomes more difficult, PCO_2 may rise; if these patients are also in circulatory failure, they may develop lactic acidosis. With both respiratory and metabolic acidosis, the prognosis is poor. At postmortem examination, pulmonary edema and hemorrhages are usually noted (Chao, 1987).

Biochemical and acid-base changes: Changes in serum calcium and phosphorus are often seen in victims of heat stroke. These are usually associated with renal impairment. The serum enzymes associated with muscle breakdown have also been observed with heat stroke; in severe cases, creatine kinase readings over 100,000 U/L have been reported (Hart et al., 1980). The acid-base changes noted in patients with heat stroke are extremely variable and depend on the time of sampling and the nature of the patient's condition. Taken shortly after the collapse of the patient, a metabolic-acidosis due to lactic acid is common, and there is often an independent or accompanying respiratory alkalosis, with a low PCO_2 which usually resolves. In patients who develop circulatory failure or renal impairment, there are often several causes of metabolic acidosis. One is associated with renal failure and results in increased phosphate and sulphate. Another cause is tissue ischemia because of circulatory failure; this leads to increased lactate production and lactic acidosis. This lactic acidosis may be further complicated if there is hepatic damage resulting in an inability to metabolize lactate.

OVERHYDRATION

Overhydration is relatively uncommon but increasingly recognized in ultramarathons (Noakes et al., 1985) and triathlons (Hiller et al., 1985). This situation arises in athletes who consume excess fluids without replacing their electrolyte losses. They are often the slower athletes who gain weight during the event and exhibit cerebral manifestations of delirium, changes in personality, deteriorating states of consciousness, and seizures. These persons characteristically have hyponatremia, which is dilutional in origin (Table 11-4).

Maintenance of weight and consumption of electrolyte-containing solutions during a prolonged event will reduce the likelihood of hyponatremia. Treatment of such patients will depend on the severity of the clinical condition and may require infusion of hypertonic saline.

Localized Edema In Limbs, Lung, and Brain

Ankle edema is common during exercise at sea level, especially during the first few days in a hot environment (Knochel & Reed, 1987). However, reports of pulmonary (McKechnie et al., 1979; Noakes et al., 1985) and cerebral (Young et al., 1987) edema in athletes exercising at sea level represent serious and potentially fatal episodes of fluid imbalance (Figure 11-1).

In the latter case report, a 21-year-old white student developed pulmonary and cerebral edema some hours after completing a 42-km marathon. He had clinical, radiological, and hemodynamic evidence of low

TABLE 11-4. *Estimated water and sodium chloride balance in 4 athletes who developed water intoxication during prolonged exercise. (Reproduced from Noakes et al,* Med. Sci. Sports Exer. *17: 373, 1985, with permission of the authors and editors.)*

Age	Sex	Body Wt. (kg)	Exercise Duration (h:min)	Post-race serum Sodium Concentration (mM)
46	F	49	± 7:00	115
37	M	75	10:10	118
20	M	73	± 9:00	124
29	F	57	9:56	125

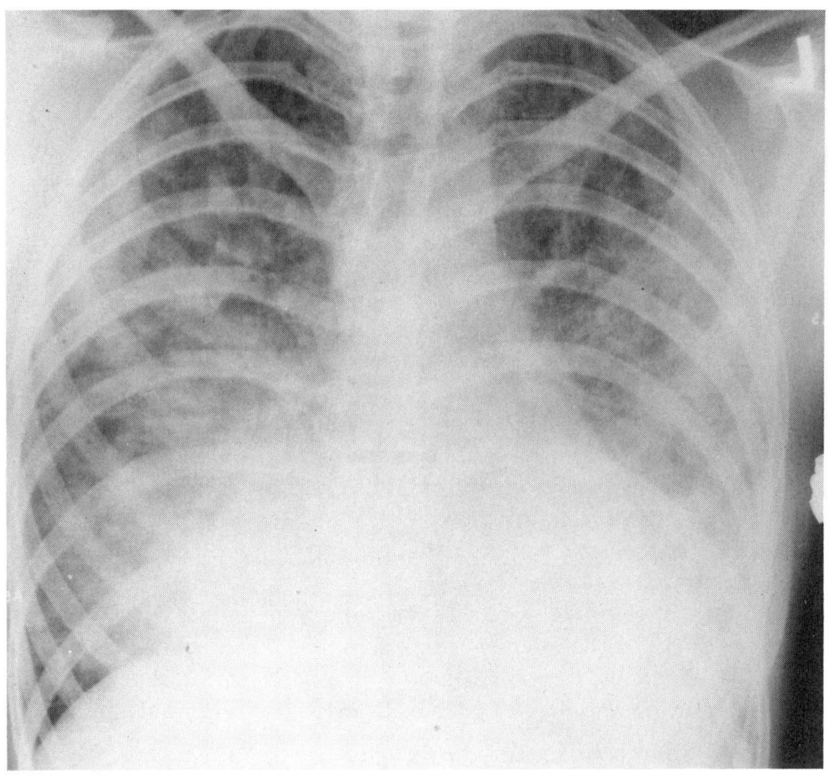

FIGURE 11-1. *Non-cardiogenic pulmonary edema (chest x-ray).*

pressure, non-cardiogenic pulmonary edema, and a CT scan of the brain showed small ventricles, consistent with generalized cerebral edema (Figure 11-2). A lumbar puncture confirmed increased pressure. The pulmonary function, blood gases, and hemodynamics are shown in Table 11-5).

Although the mechanisms of the exercise-related pulmonary and cerebral edema are speculative, they are consistent with those proposed for the hemodynamic altitude syndromes (Sutton and Lessen, 1979). Mechanisms underlying this edema may be of neural origin (Malik, 1985) or may be associated with water intoxication (Anastossiades, 1983; Arieff, 1984; Swanson & Iser, 1958). The rapid clinical and radiological clearing of the edema suggests that it is not a variant of ARDS, which will occur in fulminant heat stroke. These exercise-associated edemas may also be caused by increased-capillary permeability with an increased protein in the edema fluid, as is the case with high altitude pulmonary edema (Schoene et al., 1988). A recent finding by Bosenberg and colleagues (1988) could explain an increased capillary permeability that results in

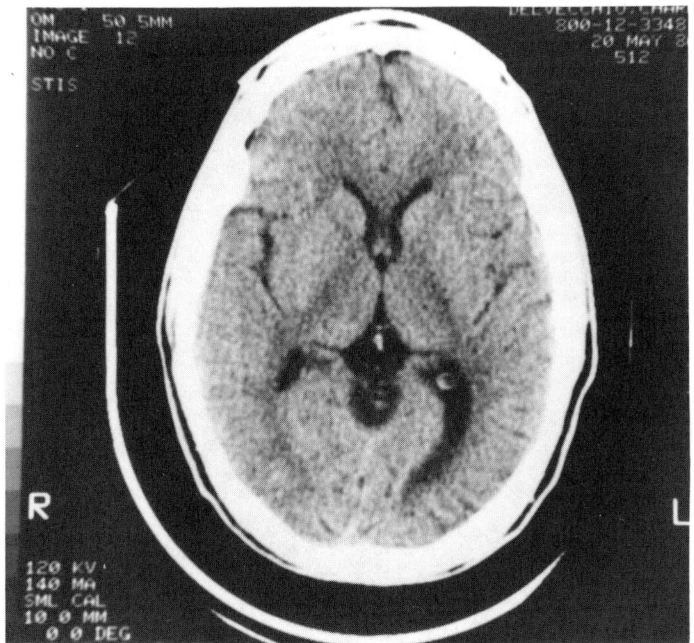

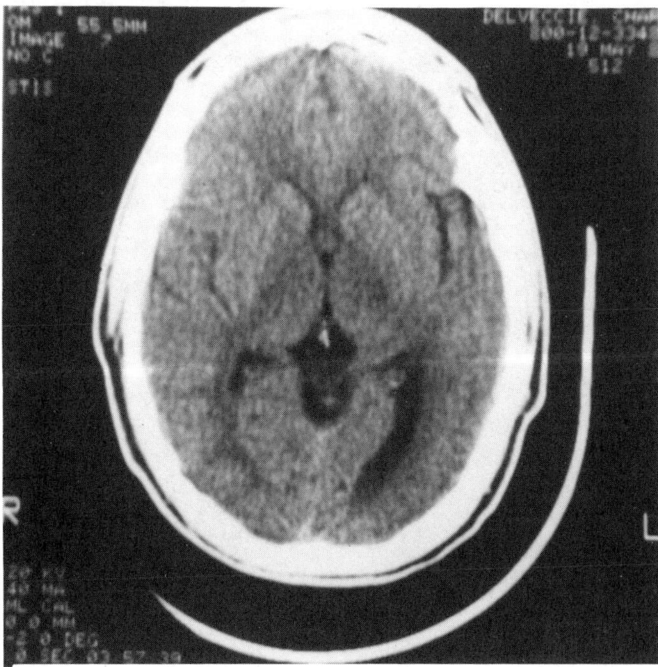

FIGURE 11-2. *a. Computerized tomography (CT) scan of the brain showing compressed lateral ventricles, consistent with cerebral edema. b. Repeat CT scan of the brain with clearing and expansion of ventricles concomitant with the clinical improvement. (Photos courtesy of M. Young.)*

TABLE 11-5. *Time Course of Clinical Events*

	Hours after Conclusion of Marathon										
	4	5	6	6	7	9	15	19	24	48	72
Event	Found	Arrives E.R.	Pulmonary Edema	ETT	↓BP Dopamine	Catheter Placed	Dopamine Off	Spontaneous Diuresis	ETT out		
Vent mode		Spon	Spon	PPV	PPV	PPV	PPV	PPV	Spon	Spon	Spon
$F_{I}O_2$		Room Air	4 1 NC	1.0	1.0	0.6	0.7	0.4	0.4 FM	2 1 NC	Room Air
PEEP				0.0	20.0	20.0	7.5	0.0			
pH		7.4	7.2	7.3	7.3	7.4	7.4	7.4	7.4	7.5	7.5
Pco_2		33.0	49.0	52.0	45.0	34.0	31.0	37.0	35.0	35.0	38.0
Po_2		56.0	30.0	57.0	64.0	73.0	181.0	67.0	93.0	75.0	73.0
Hemodynamic data											
CVP						4.0	9.0				
Ppa						26/14*	28/12				
Ppcw						12†	12				
CI						2.8	3.6				
$C(a\text{-}v)O_2$						6.7	4.0				
PVRI						114	118				
PVRI						1600	1600				
$\dot{Q}s/\dot{Q}_T$						0.20	0.17				
$P\dot{V}O_2$						30	41				
Mental status	Confused Agitated						intermit oriented			fully oriented	
Neuro tests						Head Ct LP	EEG			Head Ct EEG	

Definition of abbreviations: ETT = endotracheal tube; BP = blood pressure; PPV = positive pressure ventilation; CVP = central venous pressure; Ppa = pulmonary artery pressure in mm Hg; Ppcw = pulmonary capillary wedge pressure; CI = cardiac Index; $C(a\text{-}v)O_2$ = arteriovenous oxygen content difference; PVRI = pulmonary vascular resistance index ($dyne \cdot s \cdot cm^{-5} \cdot M^2$); SVRI = systemic vascular resistance index; $\dot{Q}s/\dot{Q}_T$ = calculated shunt fraction; $P\dot{V}O_2$ = mixed venous oxygen tension.

*Without PEEP = 20/10.

†Without PEEP = 7.

Reproduced from Young et al, Am. Rev. Resp. Dis. 136: 738, 1987, with permission of the authors and editors.

edema at sea level. In 18 triathletes, endotoxin and plasma lipopolysaccharide (LPS) concentrations in the blood serum increased and anti-LPS immunoglobulin decreased after a triathalon. Normally, endotoxins and large numbers of gram negative bacteria are present in the intestines. It is conceivable that in the dehydrated athlete, a reduction in splanchnic blood flow (Rowell et al., 1971) would result in a relative bowel ischemia and enhance the release of these endotoxins into the circulation, predisposing the subject to high premeability edema.

MANAGEMENT OF EXERTIONAL HEAT STROKE

> "I am of the opinion that in healthy subjects the only serious potential risk to life from violent exercise is heat stroke — a danger well exhibited by examples I have seen of alarming collapse and, on one occasion, death. The correct precaution would be to prohibit the race in circumstances in which an occurrence might be expected — a moisture-laden atmosphere, a following wind and the early afternoon of a day with a shade temperature of 85°F (29.5°C) or higher."

This opinion of Sir Adolphe Abrahams was published in the "Athletics" section of the 1950 edition of the *British Encyclopaedia of Medical Practice.* It is as relevant today as it was 40 years ago. With the advent of mass participation events such as marathons, which may attract 20,000 participants, and fun runs with 30,000–50,000 participants, the potential for large-scale disaster is very real. Yet many organizers of such events fail to take even elementary precautions to prevent and treat possible victims of heat stroke. Richards and Richards (1986a; 1986b) and Dobbin (1986) believe such planning should be done on the scale of a civil disaster exercise. Most importantly, all authors emphasize that heat stroke is a medical emergency; the sooner the diagnosis is made and treatment commenced, the better. Treatment must begin immediately *on site* (American College of Sports Medicine, 1984; Richards et al., 1979b; Richards et al., 1979c; Sutton, 1984; Sutton et al., 1972).

Following the first "City-to-Surf" race in 1971, an analysis of the predisposing factors enabled us to suggest improvement in three general areas: 1) race organization, 2) medical support, and 3) competitor education.

These recommendations have been refined over the years as experience has grown (Sutton & Harrison, 1977). It is also clear that to stage a fun run requires an enormous amount of logistical and medical support. The days are over in which one could simply advertise a "fun run for charity" and see who turned up to run.

It is ideal to have a medical director who is responsible for the coordination of all the preventive and therapeutic aspects related to the fun run. This person works closely with the race director and is involved in many aspects of the race planning.

Organization Of The Race

Ideally, races should be organized to avoid the hottest summer months and the hottest part of the day. Organizers should be very cautious of unseasonably hot days in the early spring, particularly in North America, as entrants will almost certainly not be heat acclimatized.

Competitor Education

The education of fun runners has increased greatly in recent years, owing largely to the popularity of runners' magazines for lay audiences. Distributing sample runners' guidelines at the time of registration, if preregistration occurs, and also holding clinics before runs are valuable. In particular, all competitors should be advised of the following facts.

1. Adequate training and fitness are important for full enjoyment of the run and also to prevent heat stroke.
2. Prior training in the heat will produce heat acclimatization and also reduce the risk of heat injury. It is wise to do as much training as possible at the time of day at which the race will be held.
3. Fluid consumption before and during the race will also reduce the risk of heat injury, particularly in the longer runs such as the marathon.
4. Splashing with water or running under hoses during a race will make competitors feel cooler, although these tactics will not lower core temperature.
5. Illness prior to or at the time of the event should preclude competition. This applies to any febrile condition (e.g., gastroenteritis or upper respiratory tract infection).
6. Competitors should understand the early symptoms of heat injury. These include excessive sweating, headache, nausea, dizziness, and any gradual impairment of consciousness.
7. Competitors should choose a comfortable pace and not run faster than they have run during training.
8. Competitors should run with a partner, each being responsible for the other's well-being.

Medical Organization

Race organizers should alert local hospitals and ambulance services about the event and should make prior arrangements with medical personnel for the care of casualties, especially those suffering from heat injury. The mere fact that an entrant signs a waiver in no way absolves the organizers of moral and/or legal responsibility.

Medical Facilities

Medical care facilities should be available at the race site, staffed with personnel capable of instituting immediate and full-scale resuscitation. Apart from the routine resuscitation equipment, ice packs and fans for cooling are required. People trained in first aid should be stationed along the course with the right to stop runners who exhibit signs of impending heat stroke or other abnormalities. One or more ambulances or vans with accompanying medical personnel should follow the competitors at intervals.

Although the emphasis has been on the management of hyperthermia, athletes will be cold and require "space blankets" and warm drinks to prevent hypothermia on cold, wet, and windy days (Sutton, 1972). Especially vulunerable are the slower athletes who, when lightly clad, will lose heat faster than their rate of metabolic heat production.

The importance of a measurement of rectal temperature to an accurate diagnosis cannot be overemphasized. Too frequently, problems have occurred when oral or axillary temperatures have been taken or when the clinical condition of the patient, who may have cold and clammy skin, suggests that that individual may not be suffering heat stroke. The initial assessment must include measurements of rectal temperature, central nervous system function, and cardiovascular function. The insertion of an intravenous catheter and care of the airway, if appropriate, must also be instituted.

Experience from the "City to Surf" race suggests that treatment is far better begun on site than in a remote hospital. Since instituting this approach in fun runs, there has been little need for subsequent hospitalization (Figure 11-3). In the experience with several hundreds of thousands of runners, no serious sequelae have resulted when resuscitation and cooling were begun at the race site. This has not been the case in other circumstances. Furthermore, we are aware of more than one dozen fatalities that have occurred when resuscitation facilities were not available immediately.

Detailed advice for on-site management has been previously documented, with rehydration and cooling the cornerstones of treatment. Kielblock (1987) has recently compared various cooling strategies (Table 11-6) and noted that whole body immersion in water at 12°C produced the most rapid cooling (0.262°C/min) compared with evaporative cooling, the "Mecca" cooling method (0.081°C/min). The use of endorphin antagonists is of no proven value as I-V naloxone in a double-blind, placebo control, crossover study had no effect on the thermoregulatory or cardiovascular response to 45 min of exercise in a warm, humid environment (Sutton et al., 1990; Figure 11-4.

Thus, it would seem that complications from heat stroke can be pre-

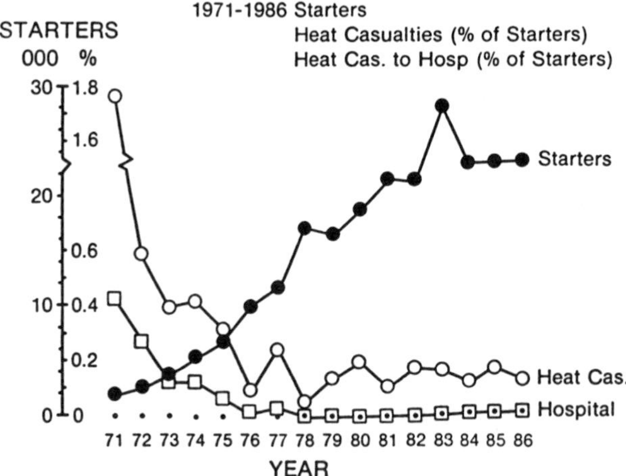

FIGURE 11-3. *Closed circles indicate the numbers of starters for the years 1971–1986 (left side of ordinate, in thousands) in the Sydney* Sun *"City-to-Surf" fun run. Open circles indicate the incidence of heat casualties as a percentage of starters (right side of discontinuous ordinate). Open squares indicate the incidence of heat casualties taken to hospital as a percentage of starters (right side of ordinate). (Reproduced from Richards and Richards in* Heat Stress, *J.R.S. Hales and D.A.B. Richards, eds., Amsterdam: Elsevier, 1987, p. 519, with permission of the authors and editors.)*

vented if cooling is commenced immediately; however, should complications arise, the patients will require transfer to a critical care unit of a hospital. Here, the management of the unconscious, seizing, ventilated patient in pulmonary edema with DIC, liver failure, dehydration, and acute renal failure is routine, but beyond the scope of this paper.

SUMMARY

Fluid imbalance may be generalized, as with dehydration and overhydration, or organ-specific. The clinical implications arise when the physiological homeostasis is disturbed to such an extent that symptoms occur and pathophysiological changes ensue.

TABLE 11-6. *Efficacies of different body cooling procedures relative to passive cooling*

Method of Cooling	Cooling Rate	
	Relative[1]	$^{0}C\ min^{-1}$
Passive	1	0.054
Ice packs on 6 major arteries	−9	0.049
Body covered with ice packs	+35	0.074
Evaporative cooling	+50	0.081
Evaporative plus 6 ice packs	+59	0.086
Whole body immersion (25°C)	+39	0.075
Whole body immersion (12°C)	+385	0.262

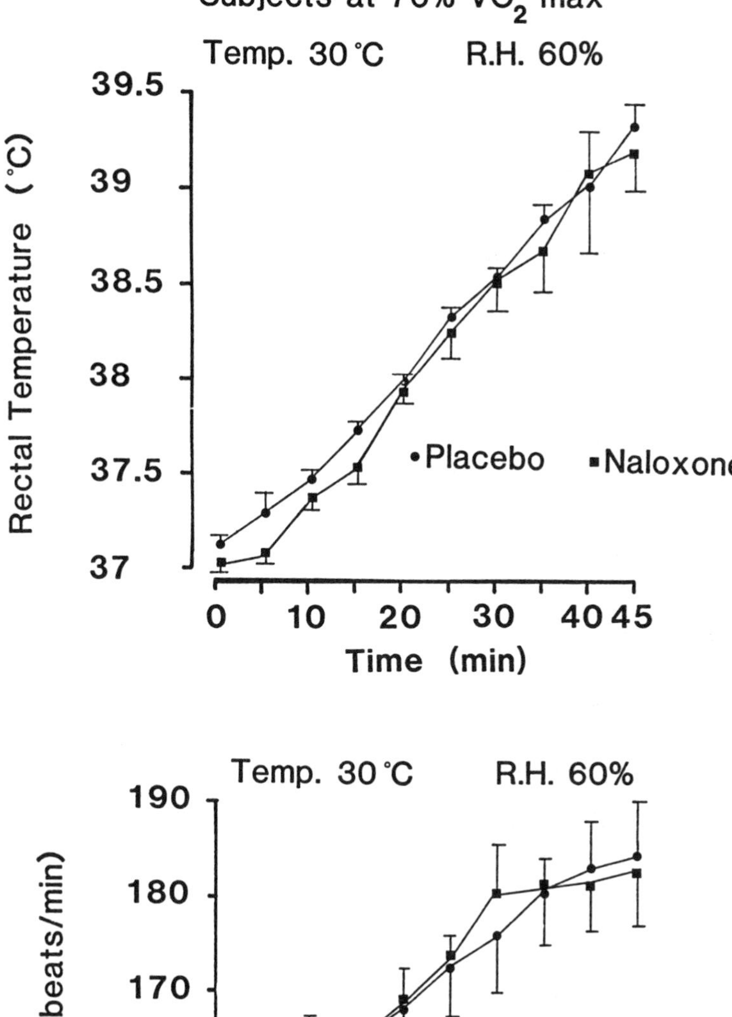

FIGURE 11-4. *Effect of naloxone, 2 mg i.v. on (a) rectal temperature and (b) heart rate response to 45 min exercise at 70% VO_2max while in an environment of 30°C and 60% relative humidity.*

Overhydration results in a dilutional hyponatremia which, if severe, will impair brain function. Organ-specific overhydration is most serious when it affects the lungs with pulmonary edema and the brain with cerebral edema.

Strict attention to fluid and electrolyte balance can minimize the risk of developing these syndromes. In their severe form, each is potentially fatal and requires immediate recognition and treatment. It is imperative that the treatment of these disorders begin on-site and not be delayed until the patient is transferred to the hospital.

BIBLIOGRAPHY

Adolph, E.F. *Physiology of Man in the Desert*. New York: Interscience, 1947.

American College of Sports Medicine. Position stand on prevention of thermal injuries during distance running. *Med. Sci. Sports Exer.* 16:ix–xiv, 1984.

Anastossiades, E. Fatal brain oedema due to accidental water intoxication. *Br. Med. J.* 287:1181–1182, 1983.

Arieff, A.I. Central nervous system manifestations of disordered sodium metabolism. *Clin. Endocrinol. Metab.* 13:269–294, 1984.

Beller, G.A., and A.E. Boyd. Heatstroke: a report of 13 consecutive cases without mortality despite severe hyperpyrexia and neurologic dysfunction. *Mil. Med.* 140:464–467, 1975.

Bernheim, I.T., and J.N. Cox. Cours de chaleur et intoxication amphetamine chez un sportif. *Schweiz Med. Wochenscher.* 90:322–331, 1960.

Bosenberg, A.T., J.G. Brock-Utne, S.L. Gaffin, M.T.B. Wells, and G.T.W. Blake. Strenuous exercise causes systemic endotoxemia. *J. Appl. Physiol.* 65:106–108, 1988.

Boyd, A.E., and G.A. Beller. Acid-base changes in heat exhaustion during basic training. *Proc. Army Sci. Conf.* 1:114–125, 1972.

Brahams, D. Death of a soldier: accident or neglect? *Lancet* 1:485, 1988.

Chao, T.C. Post-mortem findings of heat stroke. In: J.R.S. Hales and D.A.B. Richards eds. *Heat Stress.* Amsterdam: Elsevier. 297–301, 1987.

Clowes, G.H.A., and T.F. O'Donnell. Heat stroke. *N. Engl. J. Med.* 291:564–567, 1974.

Costrini, A.M., H.A. Pitt, A.B. Gustafson, and D.E. Uddin. Cardiovascular and metabolic manifestations of heat stroke and severe heat exhaustion. *Am. J. Med.* 66:296–302, 1979.

Dinman, B.D., and S.M. Horvath. Heat disorders in industry: a reevaluation of diagnostic criteria. *J. Occupat. Med.* 26:489–495, 1984.

Dobbin, S.W. Providing medical services for fun runs and marathons in North America. In: J.R. Sutton and R.M. Brock (eds.) *Sports Medicine for the Mature Athlete.* Indianapolis: Benchmark Press. 193–204, 1986.

Gisolfi, C.V., and J.R. Copping. Thermal effects of prolonged treadmill exercise in the heat. *Med. Sci. Sports* 6:108–113, 1971.

Greenleaf, J.E., and B.L. Castle. Exercise temperature regulation in man during hypohydration and hyperhydration. *J. Appl. Physiol.* 30:847–853, 1971.

Hales, J.R.S. A case supporting the proposal that cardiac filling pressure is the limiting factor in adjusting to heat stress. *Yale J. Biol. Med.* 59:237–245, 1986.

Hales, J.R.S., F.R.N. Stephens, A.A. Fawcett, R.A. Westerman, J.D. Vaughan, D.A.B. Richards, and C.R.B. Richards. Lowered skin blood flow and erythrocyte sphering in collapsed fun-runners. *Lancet* 1:1494–1495, 1986.

Hanson, P.G., and S.W. Zimmerman. Exertional heatstroke in novice runners. *J. Am. Med. Assoc.* 242:154–157, 1979.

Hart, L.E., and J.R. Sutton. Environmental considerations for exercise. *Cardiol. Clin.* 5:245–258, 1987.

Hart, L.E., B.P. Egier, A.G. Shimizu, P.J. Tandan, and J.R. Sutton. Exertional heat stroke: the runner's nemesis. *Can. Med. Assoc. J.* 122:1144–1150, 1980.

Herman, R.H., and B.H. Sullivan, Jr. Heatstroke and jaundice. *Am. J. Med.* 27:154–166, 1959.

Hiller, W.D.B., M.L. O'Toole, F. Massimino, R.E. Hiller, and R.H. Laird. Plasma electrolyte and glucose changes during the Hawaiian Ironman Triathlon. *Med. Sci. Sports Exerc.* 17:219, 1985.

Hubbard, R.W., and L.E. Armstrong. The heat illnesses: biochemical, ultrastructural, and fluid-electrolyte considerations. In: K.B. Pandolf, M.N. Sawka and R.R. Gonzalez, eds. *Human Performance Physiology and Environmental Medicine at Terrestrial Extremes.* Indianapolis: Benchmark Press. 305–359, 1988.

Hughson, R.L., H.J. Green, M.E. Houston, J.A. Thomson, D.R. MacLean, and J.R. Sutton. Heat injuries in Canadian mass participation runs. *Can. Med. Assoc. J.* 122:1141–1144, 1980.

Kew, M.C., C. Abrahams, and H.C. Seftel. Chronic interstitial nephritis as a consequence of heatstroke. *Quart. J. Med.* 39:189–199, 1970a.
Kew, M.C., I. Bersohn, H.C. Seftel, and E. Kent. Liver damage in heat stroke. *Am. J. Med.* 49:192–202, 1970b.
Kew, M.C., O.T. Minick, R.M. Bahu, J. Stein, and G. Kent. Ultrastructural changes in the liver in heatstroke. *Am. J. Pathol.* 90:609–614, 1978.
Kew, M.C., R.B.K. Tucker, I. Bersohn, and H.C. Seftel. The heart in heatstroke. *Am. Heart J.* 77:324–335, 1969.
Kielblock, A.J. Strategies for the prevention of heat disorders with particular reference to the efficacy of body cooling procedures. In: J.R.S. Hales and D.A.B. Richards eds. *Heat Stress.* Amsterdam: Elsevier. 489–497, 1987.
Knochel, J.P. Environmental heat illness. An eclectic review. *Arch. Intern. Med.* 133:841–864, 1974.
Knochel, J.P. Dog days and siriasis: how to kill a football player. *J. Am. Med. Assoc.* 233:513–515, 1975.
Knochel, J.P. and G. Reed. Disorders of heat regulation. In: C.R. Kleeman, M.H. Maxwell, and R.G. Narin eds. *Clinical Disorders, Fluid and Electrolyte Metabolism.* New York: McGraw-Hill. 1197–1232, 1987.
Ladell, W.S.S. Heat cramps. *Lancet* 2:836–839, 1949.
Leithead, C.S., and E.R. Gunn. The aetiology of cane cutter's cramps in British Guiana. In: *Environmental Physiology and Psychology in Arid Conditions.* Liege, Belgium: UNESCO. 13–17, 1964.
Malamud, N., W. Haymaker, and R.P. Custer. Heatstroke: a clinico-pathologic study of 125 fatal cases. *Mil. Surg.* 99:397–449, 1946.
Malhotra, M.S., and Y. Venkataswamy. Heat casualties in the Indian Armed Forces. *Ind. J. Med. Res.* 62:1293–1302, 1974.
Malik, A.B. Mechanisms of neurogenic pulmonary edema. *Circ. Res.* 57:1–19, 1985.
McKechnie, J.K., W.P. Leary, and O.M. Joubert. Some electrocardiographic and biochemical changes in marathon runners. *S. Afr. Med. J.* 41:722–725, 1967.
McKechnie, J.K., W.P. Leary, T.D. Noakes, J.C. Kallmeyer, E.T.M. MacSearraigh, and L.R. Olivier. Acute pulmonary oedema in two athletes during a 90-km running race. *S. Afr. Med. J.* 56:261–265, 1979.
Meikle, A.W., and J.R. Graybill. Fibrinolysis and hemorrhage in a fatal case of heat stroke. *N. Engl. J. Med.* 276:911–913, 1967.
Nadel, E.R., G.W. Mack, H. Nose, and A. Tripathi. Tolerance to severe heat and exercise. Peripheral vascular responses to body fluid changes. In: J.R.S. Hales and D. Richards eds. *Heat Stress.* Amsterdam: Elsevier. 117–131, 1988.
Noakes, T.D., N. Goodwin, B.L. Rayner, T. Branken, and R.K.N. Taylor. Water intoxication: a possible complication during endurance exercise. *Med. Sci. Sports Exer.* 17:370–375, 1985.
O'Donnell, T.F. The hemodynamic and metabolic alterations associated with acute heat stress injury in marathon runners. *Ann. N.Y. Acad. Sci.* 301:262–269, 1977.
O'Donnell, T.F., and G.H. Clowes. The circulatory abnormalities of heat stroke. *N. Engl. J. Med.* 287:734–737, 1972.
Pugh, L.G.C.E., J.L. Corbett, and R.H. Johnson. Rectal temperatures, weight losses, and sweat rates in marathon running. *J. Appl. Physiol.* 23:347–352, 1967.
Richards, C.R., and D. Richards. Prevention of exercise-induced heat stroke. In: J.R. Sutton and R.M. Brock eds. *Sports Medicine for the Mature Athlete.* Indianapolis: Benchmark Press. 151–166, 1986a.
Richards, C.R., and D. Richards. Providing medical care in fun runs and marathons in Australasia. In: J.R. Sutton and R.M. Brock eds. *Sports Medicine for the Mature Athlete.* Indianapolis: Benchmark Press, 167–180, 1986b.
Richards, R., D. Richards, P. Schofield, V. Ross, and J.R. Sutton. Reducing the hazards in Sydney's *The Sun* "City-to-Surf" runs, 1971–1979. *Med. J. Aust.* 2:453–457, 1979a.
Richards, R., D. Richards, P. Schofield, V. Ross, and J.R. Sutton. Management of heat exhaustion in Sydney's *The Sun* "City-to-Surf" fun runners, 1971–1979. *Med. J. Aust.* 2:457–461, 1979b.
Richards, R., D. Richards, P. Schofield, V. Ross, and J.R. Sutton. Organization of *The Sun* "City-to-Surf" fun run, Sydney. *Med. J. Aust.* 2:470–474, 1979c.
Rowell, L.B. Human cardiovascular adjustments to exercise and thermal stress. *Physiol. Rev.* 54:75–159, 1974.
Rowell, L.B., J.M.R. Detry, G.R. Profant, and C. Wyss. Splanchnic vasoconstriction in hyperthermic man: role of falling blood pressure. *J. Appl. Physiol.* 31:864–869, 1971.
Sawka, M.N., A.J. Young, R.P. Francesconi, S.R. Muza, and K.B. Pandolf. Thermoregulatory and blood responses during exercise at graded hypohydration levels. *J. Appl. Physiol.* 59:1394–1401, 1985.
Schiff, H.B., E.T. MacSearraigh, and J.C. Kallmeyer. Myoglobinuria, rhabdomyolysis, and marathon runners. *Quart. J. Med.* 47:463–472, 1978.
Schoene, R.B., E.R. Swenson, C.J. Pizzo, P.H. Hackett, R.C. Roach, W.J. Mills, Jr., W.R. Henderson, Jr., and T.R. Martin. The lung at high altitude: bronchoalveolar lavage in acute mountain sickness and pulmonary edema. *J. Appl. Physiol.* 64:2604–2613, 1988.
Schrier, R.W., H.S. Henderson, C.C. Ticher, and R.T. Tannen. Nephropathy associated with heat stress and exercise. *Ann. Intern. Med.* 67:356–376, 1967.
Shibolet, S., M.C. Lancaster, and Y. Danon. Heatstroke: a review. *Aviat. Space Environ. Med.* 47:280–301, 1976.

Slovis, C.M., G.F. Anderson, and D.P. Solightly. Survival in a heatstroke victim with a core temperature in excess of 46.5°C. *Ann. Emerg. Med.* 11:269–271, 1982.
Strydom, N.B., and L.D. Holdsworth. The effects of different levels of water deficit on physiological responses during heat stress. *Int. Z. Angew Physiol. Einschl. Arbeitsphysiol.* 26:95–102, 1968.
Sutton, J.R. Community jogging versus arduous running. *N. Engl. J. Med.* 286:951, 1972.
Sutton, J.R. Heat illness. In: R.H. Strauss, ed. *Sports Medicine*. Philadelphia: W.B. Saunders. 307–322, 1984.
Sutton, J.R., A. Brown, and J.D. MacDougall. The influence of intravenous naloxone on the thermoregulatory responses to exercise. (In press, 1990).
Sutton, J., M.J. Coleman, A.P. Millar, L. Lazarus, and P. Russo. The medical problems of mass participation in athletic competition. The "City-to-Surf" Race. *Med. J. Aust.* 2:127–133, 1972.
Sutton, J.R., and H.C. Harrison. Health hazards in community jogs and fun runs. *Med. J. Aust.* I:193, 1977.
Sutton, J.R, and N. Lassen. Pathophysiology of acute mountain sickness and high altitude pulmonary oedema. *Bull. europ. Physiopath. Resp.* 15:1045–1052, 1979.
Sutton, J.R., and D.N. Sauder. Fever and abdominal pain following exercise. *Med. Sci. Sports Exerc.* 21:S103, 1989.
Swanson, A.G., and O.A. Iser. Acute encephalopathy due to water intoxication. *N. Engl. J. Med.* 208:831–834, 1958.
Talbot, J.H. Heat cramps. In: *Medicine*. Baltimore: Williams and Wilkins. 323–376, 1935.
Talbot, J.H., and J. Michelsen. Heat cramps. *J. Clin. Invest.* 12:533–535, 1933.
Vertel, R.M., and J.P. Knochel. Acute renal failure due to heat injury. An analysis of ten cases associated with a high incidence of myoglobinuria. *Am. J. Med.* 43:435–451, 1967.
Weiner, J.S., and G.O. Horne. A classification of heat illness. *Br. Med. J.* 1:1533–1535, 1958.
Wilson, G. The cardiopathology of heatstroke. *J. Am. Med. Assoc.* 114:557–567, 1940.
Young, M., F. Sciurba, and J. Rinaldo. Delirium and pulmonary edema after completing a marathon. *Am. Rev. Respir. Dis.* 136:737–739, 1987.

DISCUSSION

HARVEY: I think a very important point, John, is the differentiation between head injury and heat illness. Many times a cyclist can become hyperthermic, become dizzy, and fall off his bike. The assumption is made that he has had an accident, and the focus is on the head injury. Similarly, when a football player wanders to the distant sideline in a somewhat disoriented manner, the assumption is often made that he has a head injury, and everyone misses the diagnosis of heat stroke. I think that it is really important to have an index of suspicion.

I am also dismayed about the lack of emphasis on the use of i.v. fluids in resuscitation of these poeple. We make a big to-do about whether we should fan them or not, give them iced fluids or not, or put ice packs on their groin or all over their head; but secondarily we talk about i.v. fluids. There is a recently published paper from which I quote: "If ice and chilled water are unavailable, i.v. fluids are indicated." The use of i.v. fluids in the Canadian Iron Man race and the Iron Man race of the Boston Marathon have certainly increased throughout the years. I think that you do no harm if you infuse 1–2 L of saline while you are taking rectal temperature. I know of cases in which people have gotten a liter of fluids, and in 15–20 min were alert. I am going to make a plea that i.v. fluids need to be the cornerstone of treatment in hyperthermia, and not relegated to a secondary role.

SUTTON: I think those are excellent points. The first one is expecting the problem; that's a key in medicine. Unless the thought crosses your mind, you'll never make the diagnosis of heat stroke. Sadly, that has been the history of this type of problem, i.e., people do not think that the person is going to be hyperthermic. The heat stroke patients that we see in fun runs are sweating, and they usually feel cold and clammy; it is a totally different clinical picture from that described in classical heat stroke seen in the desert. That is why a lot of physicians and physiologists remain ignorant about it. But it has been in the literature for almost two decades. I think we do have a very important education program ahead of us. It really is an unbelievable tragedy that these athletes die unnecessarily.

Your next point about intravenous fluids is also very important; they can be important even in short runs (less than one hour). At the finish line of the City to Surf race, casualties are triaged into an intensive care unit area or to an area for less serious problems. The intensive care unit area is staffed by professional, intensive-care-unit physicians and nurses. There are clerks, nurses, and physicians allotted to a total of 30 different beds. The casualty comes in, and the documentation and baseline measurements are made. Simultaneously, a blood sample is taken and a liter of fluid is given intravenously. There is a theoretical concern that some people might have heart failure, and you'd put them into pulmonary edema, but this has never happened in all our years of experience. Everyone has recovered, and everyone's temperature was reduced to 38°C within a short time (most within 30 min), even though some of them have started as high as 42–43°C. There have been more than 30 of these cases with temperatures of 43°C; that's pretty hot. It doesn't matter what i.v. fluid is given as long as it contains sodium, because sodium will stay in the vascular space. We give dextrose saline because some of these people will be hypoglycemic. The range of blood glucose varies from about 1–18 mM, in other words, from about 18 mg/100 mL to 324mg/100mL. There is no way to predict it when you look at these people clinically, because the causes of unconsciousness are as long as your arm. If in doubt, give the glucose. Suspect the problem, treat it immediately, and treat it on site. Thus, no time is lost in cooling the patient or in correcting hypoglycemia.

SCHEDL: I was interested to see the word "euphoric" applied to the people who were getting into complications. I recently read an article about the euphoria of well-trained people. I've never experienced it myself. I wonder, do you get the euphoria if you are well-trained and also if you are going to collapse?

SUTTON: There is often a mismatch between one's perception of these things and the real world. A lot of these people do feel quite euphoric; they tell you how great they feel as they're about to hit the pavement.

PHILLIPS: In treatment, one needs to address the underlying pathophysiology. Generally, a conservative approach is to treat the hyperthermia first. Where that situation becomes compromised is in the field, especially with the military, where ice packs are not readily available. In those situations, you have to be conservative with the i.v. fluid. I suggest 1.5 L of any i.v. solution except on those who have obvious head wounds. The assumption is made that almost everyone is at least 1 L hypohydrated, and this treatment has proven to be a valid and lifesaving maneuver. In most circumstances, we are dealing with a young, healthy population. Where the situation becomes muddy is when heat stroke is not the underlying problem. For example, an older person may have fluid electrolyte imbalances; if you fill them with fluids and then cool them, they may become worse. That's a risk. I think you have to characterize your treatable population at risk and then do what is best.

SUTTON: The question about giving intravenous fluids is a fairly crucial one. In a fun run lasting 1–1.5 h, dehydration is not nearly as important as in the longer races. Nevertheless, the clinical experience in what is now over half a million people is that no one has run into trouble in this relatively young, athletic, trained population by giving a liter of fluid intravenously, even though it contains a lot of sodium. Having said that, I should point out that those who administer this type of treatment are all experienced intensive care physicians with the ability to put in a central venous catheter and monitor central venous pressure. I maintain that if there is any question about fluid administration, you can monitor central pressure and put in as much fluid as you like until that pressure comes up. You can titrate the pressure, and that is totally safe. I think the key thing about cooling these people is that if they are hyperthermic and hypovolemic, you can only help them by restoring an adequate circulation. This is not to say that you don't need to institute other measures. Most of the fun runs now use things like ice packs or atomized sprays, but the most dramatic findings were those of Costrini, who threw military personnel into a bath of 12°C and had by far the greatest cooling rate. Many people organizing fun runs have said that this is too drastic; what happens if they have a cardiac arrest? Again, experience in 50,000 fun runners is that it is so uncommon that it should be of minor concern. The only ones to have heart trouble were those who were known to have heart disease and who actually had premonitory signs that they chose to ignore.

I accept the point that one needs to be cautious. In the intensive care unit, we can sometimes check variables such as blood pressure and heart rate on a minute-to-minute basis; if we find that the stimulus has been more than is needed, we then ease off.

SAWKA: In Florida, heat exhaustion is common. I wonder if people who are exposed to nearly constant air conditioning have ruined their natural ability for heat acclimation. The amount of heat acclimation that you obtain is relative to how much you increase your core temperature, either by exercising or by being exposed to heat. If you are living in air conditioning and not exercising, you probably infrequently raise your core temperature and thus fail to get thermoregulatory acclimation. Since a large portion of the population in Florida is older, age could be an additional factor in heat exhaustion.

Another question is, what happens with wheelchair athletes who have a decreased ability to thermoregulate? Particularly when exercising in a hot environment, don't they have a very large disadvantage?

NADEL: In wheelchair athletes, we found a dissociation between rectal temperature, which was quite stable during heavy exercise for 40–60 min, and the esophageal temperature, which climbed quite high. You can imagine why there is a disparity between the two. In wheelchair athletes, the heavy energy is produced in the upper body, and the primary circulation is in the upper body. A rectal probe (in an area with a very poor circulation) doesn't reveal the extent to which the heat has occurred. Another problem with wheelchair athletes is that they tend to have their lower bodies clothed during the exercise. They don't like to expose their withered legs, so they don't have the advantages for heat exchange that occurs when the skin surface is exposed.

SAWKA: Are there any reports of increased incidence of heat injury in these individuals?

SUTTON: I've heard of instances occurring, but I have no idea of the incidence rate.

NADEL: Characteristically, in the large heat waves that have occurred in the U.S., it is always the heat waves that are early in the summer that have the greatest number of excess deaths. I might add that most of these deaths occur in people in the inner city, i.e., the ones without air conditioning who are not heat-acclimated. The second heat wave of the summer causes relatively fewer excess deaths because, presumably these people have become more heat acclimated.

TIPTON: How common is the pulmonary edema seen in runners?

SUTTON: Pulmonary edema in fun runs is rare. I wouldn't want people to get the message that pulmonary and cerebral edema are frequent in athletes; that is not the case.

HUBBARD: I'd like to discuss a feature that might characterize a subject that is prone to reinjury. One Scandinavian study included liver biopsies of heat stroke athletes, and it was found that liver abnormalities were present a year after they were determined to be "clinically normal." We've recently completed a study of 10 heat stroke subjects, and all of them were certified as clinically normal before coming to the lab for the acclimatization procedure. At least 3 or 4 of these subjects exhibited acclimatization abnormalities up to 3–5 months after injury after a very mild 3-mph treadmill walk. One of them failed to acclimatize for up to 9 months after heat injury. Although they appear clinically normal, we doubt that they are physiologically normal when subjected to heat exposure.

I get a little nervous about the lack of follow-up observations of athletes or others who suffer heat stroke and apparently recover quickly. This is a problem because it has been shown that heat stroke patients may appear to recover in the first 24–48 h and 24 h later may experience secondary hyperthermia.

SUTTON: I'm glad you brought up that point of the likelihood of prolonged problems. One of my patients had markedly increased serum creatine kinase values after very gentle jogs for more than one year after heat stroke. Other patients for years after a heat injury have a much higher core temperature during standardized exercise.

One point I think that we probably have not emphasized is to distinguish between the clinical scenarios that occur with a fun run that lasts an hour where athletes are hyperthermic for a short time, versus those running for a longer time who have a heat injury where the temperature remains elevated for a prolonged time. I don't know the answer to this, but I suspect that the extent of organ damage, the ability to recover from it, and the subsequent long-term effects may be very different in a person who spikes 43°C for a few minutes compared to someone who remains hyperthermic for several hours or more.

HUBBARD: In a recent symposium at ACSM, there was an Australian who stood up and said that they always treat heat stroke with 1 or 2 L of i.v. fluids, and the subjects are always up and about. However, our responsibilities are to have adequate cooling available for someone that might come in at a core temepration of 110–112°F. I suggest at that point, i.v. fluids may not save the person. Although they may help, they are still no substitute for other emergency therapy.

SUTTON: When you have people who are hot, you have to cool them. If you don't treat them properly, they'll either die or be severely impaired. Renal dialysis is no fun. We're talking about severe, significant, clinical problems that have a major mortality. It's not either i.v. fluid or cooling, but rather cooling *and* fluids that should be administered.

Final Discussion

GISOLFI: The objective of this final discussion is to determine if we can come to some agreement with regard to the formulation of an oral rehydration solution for use during prolonged exercise in a warm environment. Let's begin with carbohydrate content. In Dave Costill's last slide, he suggested that the concentration of carbohydrate in such a beverage should be in the range of 8 to 12%. In terms of intestinal absorption, studies have indicated that you can increase glucose concentration in the lumen up to 500 mM, which is almost a 10% solution, and still have a linear increase in water and glucose absorption. I think 12% is too high. Some of the work by Mark Davis suggests that 12% is high. We found no significant difference in gastric emptying between water and a 10% carbohydrate beverage. I don't know if we want to recommend a solution with a carbohydrate content as high as 10%, but I do think that 12% is a little high. Dave, do you want to comment?

COSTILL: The reason I put that broad range in my recommendation was to show that we had some individuals who could empty a 12% solution just as well as one of lower concentration. To say that there is a finite line where that determination ought to be made is misleading. We are dealing with wide individual variations, making it very difficult to draw that line. I don't think that an 11 or 12% solution will be acceptable by most people. There are, of course, some individuals who can't tolerate even an 8% solution.

NADEL: If one takes in fluid at a rate of 1 L/h which is a near-maximal rate for gastric emptying, then a 6 to 9% glucose solution will match the rate of glucose oxidation in the muscles at exercise intensities that can be sustained for prolonged periods. In other words, maximal glucose oxidation for prolonged periods is between 1 and 2 g/min. It doesn't seem necessary to provide glucose at a rate greater than is being oxidized. At a National Research Council meeting on fluid replacement last February, my recollection is that the consensus of an optimal level for glucose in fluid was 6–8%.

JOHNSON: I'm a little surprised that we are supposed to consider "a" fluid replacement beverage. We know about the behavior of animals — they are marvelously well equipped to determine the appropriate beverage if they are given the opportunity to select from different choices. It might be most appropriate to consider the range or alternatives of formulations that should be offered and available to the individual.

GISOLFI: I don't think that we can zero in on a particular figure. A range would be fine.

JOHNSON: No. I mean an athlete should have access to water and also one or more electrolyte solutions as alternatives. In other words, given different states of dehydration and different amounts of electrolyte loss, it is likely the individual may select the appropriate solution to replenish those losses if the choice is available.

GISOLFI: I would agree. We may be talking about a series of solutions, depending upon how dehydrated an individual is.

COYLE: If I understand the question correctly, we are talking about the optimal fluid replacement solution and not the optimal solution for replacement of carbohydrates. Those might be two different solutions.

GISOLFI: My question was primarily concerned with fluids. What formulation will maximize water absorption?

TIPTON: I like Johnson's concept. It seems to me that in the early stages only water should be replaced, whereas in the middle stages we should replenish both water and electrolytes, and in the final stages (after 2 h) water, electrolytes, and glucose should be consumed by the exercising subject.

WADE: One of the problems is the translation of observations in animals to humans. Animals have a very good salt appetite. If you offer them a hypertonic salt solution and water, they will drink from each solution in quantities that result in isotonic fluid replacement. Humans do not seem to do that very well. In our work with prolonged exercise, hyponatremia can occur even with adequate salt available for intake. If a loss of total body electrolytes occurs, you have to tell humans to replace it. They don't have that same capability that the animal does. I think this is important.

COSTILL: In a cool environment where carboydrate is the limiting factor, the more carbohydrate you feed them, the better they will perform. Up to almost 100 g/h, subjects tend to perform better. Feedings of less than 40 g/h do not appear to produce significant improvements in performances. I think that large carbohydrate feedings help maintain a greater source of blood-borne glucose.

MEYER: Carl, your interest is in intestinal absorption of a salt and water mix. The problem with triple lumen tube analysis is that another dimension is overlooked, i.e., how far fluid volume spreads along the G.I. tract determines the absorption area. When one considers that, a lower carbohydrate concentration in a beverage to facilitate gastric emptying would probably be advantageous. It is so complicated that it is difficult to find the answer. The only way to find out is to do studies like those using deuterium uptake. I don't think you can figure it out from taking an intestinal absorption study and a gastric emptying study and putting them together.

SHERMAN: Relative to the question of what the appropriate fluid is to deliver water during exercise, we should keep in mind that in the real world people do not consume just fluids. It goes back to providing energy sources during exercise to enhance performance, or at least maintain performance. In the context of the question that you proposed, athletes are consuming solid foods with carbohydrate beverages before exercise. They are also consuming them during exercise.

HUBBARD: I'd like to follow up on a point initially discussed in Marriot's classic text on water and salt balance. He made the point that there is a very strong anorexia component to progressive salt depletion. Whether we are dealing with wrestlers or soldiers who become salt depleted, once that anorexic state is established, it is a very difficult cycle to break. In these circumstances, prevention is worth a ton of cure. In my experience in this field, people who skip a meal are more at risk or susceptible to heat illness symptoms during a 4-h event, whatever that event may be, than someone who had 200–300 mEq of sodium in his gut already. It's very important to establish whether the solution you are designing is to replace a prior meal that has been skipped or to supplement salt losses due to sweating only and assume a prior meal was eaten.

GISOLFI: Perhaps we should start with a euhydrated individual and talk about what we would do when faced with the problem of someone exercising for 3–4 h in a warm environment. Does that help?

ZAMBRASKI: I'd like to support a practice rather than a reactive response with regard to hydration during exercise. By maintaining a hydrated state this may decrease the complications associated with rehydration. I think it would be advantageous to consume fluids with the appropriate solutes early during exercise in anticipation of a deficit.

GISOLFI: Is there any consensus on that point? We have had a lot of discussion so far and a lot of different opinions, but that seems to be a good starting point. Is there any consensus on that?

COYLE: That is a good idea. I have one point from way back regarding adding glucose to a solution for intestinal absorption. Why do you need it?

GISOLFI: Why do you need glucose?

COYLE: Yes. In your solution as far as fluid absorption is concerned.

GISOLFI: Glucose does stimulate sodium absorption and therefore stimulates water absorption. You don't need much to do that. The Km for active glucose transport is only 5 to 10 mM.

COYLE: But whatever is leaving the stomach is eventually, and rather rapidly, going to be absorbed in the intestines. So what you are ingesting is not going to be accumulated in your intestines and cause diarrhea. So why put glucose in a drink designed solely for fluid replacement?

DAVIS: The question perhaps is not why you would add glucose to enhance fluid absorption as much as perhaps why not add it. It complicates the issue if you try to design a drink "just to replace fluids" or "just to supply carbohydrate." Why not formulate an optimal fluid replacement beverage that has glucose and will be readily utilized by the muscle?

GISOLFI: In general, the rationale for including glucose and salt in replacement beverages is that these solutes are utilized and lost, respectively, during exercise. Moreover, the inclusion of sodium provides far more rapid rehydration than if you ingest plain water. Is there anyone that would like to speak against the proposal that we try to offset the deficit by starting with a solution that contains some salt and some glucose? If that is acceptable, would anyone disagree with a beverage that contained between 6% and 10% carbohydrate?

NADEL: Carl, I want to make certain that everyone understands the possibility of reactive hypoglycemia if glucose is consumed within a certain time prior to the initiation of exercise. In some people, reactive hypoglycemia will occur. This is because the glucose load stimulates insulin release from the pancreas. The combined effects of high plasma insulin and exercise will cause plasma glucose to drop substantially in sensitive people.

SHERMAN: I don't think that is as much of a problem as we generally seem to think that it is. A series of studies done over the last three years suggests that reactive hyperglycemia is not common and when it does occur, it is quite transient.

NADEL: I tried to qualify this point. Reactive hypoglycemia occurs during exercise in *some* people following a glucose load taken prior to exercise.

GISOLFI: What about electrolytes? Should we include them in this beverage? Some of the things that we have said around this table over the last three days would certainly indicate that we should include sodium. What about potassium? Should we include potassium in a beverage? Is there any compelling reason to do that?

NADEL: We all recognize that potassium is the intracellular cation. To provide for optimal rehydration of the intracellular fluid compartment, it would seem likely that potassium should be provided in any rehydration drink. I can provide some preliminary results from experiments that are in progress in my laboratory right now. For the five subjects whose data we have, they appear to lose less plasma volume during a 2-h exercise bout when taking sodium and potassium capsules than when taking placebo capsules. When taking sodium alone, they fall in between. It seems that there is some benefit to have sodium and potassium in the rehydration drink. I stress that these are preliminary data.

SUTTON: How much potassium are you talking about?

NADEL: We are giving 5 mEq/L.

SUTTON: So how much are they getting totally?

NADEL: Drinking 800 mL/h, they are receiving around 8 mEq in 2 h.

GISOLFI: How much sodium was ingested? In that study, was it the total cation that was important, or was it potassium?

NADEL: We don't know the answer because obviously the total cation was greater in the latter case.

GISOLFI: Bob, do we know anything about the effects of potassium on palatability?
MURRAY: Whenever minerals are present in a fluid replacement beverage, there is a risk of generating some negative taste perceptions. Potassium is one of the candidates for that, because of its characteristically bitter off-taste. That perception is related to the absolute amount of potassium used, the ions to which potassium is attached, and other factors such as flavor type and level, which can be manipulated to mask the taste of potassium. The potassium content of sports drinks is relatively low and is easily masked by the flavorings.
COSTILL: Listening to the discussions about the value of sodium, it is clear that this cation does play a major role, not only in replacing the ions that are lost, but in transport and a number of other things. The problem I am always faced with is finding documentation of potassium deficiency in relatively short-term work, that is, in exercise bouts of 6–8 h or less. If anything, you get hyperkalemia. I think we often forget that, unlike animal studies, humans produce a hypotonic sweat that produces an increase in body ion concentration. Body tissues can't sense total ion loss. They can only sense concentration changes. So as far as the body is concerned, you have too much ion because the concentrations are elevated. Even using biopsy studies, we have never observed conditions where hypokalemia really exists. I am not opposed to putting it in, but it's like adding vitamins. It probably won't do you any harm, but I'm not sure from a scientific point of view that it will do any good.
NADEL: Theoretically, to provide for adequate rehydration one would have to restore the potassium to restore the intracellular fluid space.
COSTILL: They are already hyperosmotic.
NADEL: I'm talking about rehydration.
COSTILL: Do you mean after the exercise?
NADEL: Yes.
COSTILL: But one meal will replace everything you are going to lose.
NADEL: Of course. We are discussing whether the rehydration drink should provide for complete rehydration. If this is the goal, the drink should contain some potassium.
SUTTON: I think that we have to do the mathematics on this. If you look at the total body potassium, the tiny bit that you lose in sweat is really negligible. If you only replace 8 to 10 mEq over 2 h, that is not important. Theoretically, it looks tidy because you lose about that amount in the sweat, but in terms of complimenting the total body intracellular stores of potassium, you'll have a hard time convincing me that it is going to make any difference.
NADEL: A portion of the intracellular water loss will accompany the loss of muscle glycogen.
WADE: I just wanted to note that the kidneys have adequate ability to

conserve potassium, and you can increase potassium reabsorption to limit losses incurred in sweat.

HARVEY: I'd like to make mention of Hubbard's talk where if the fluid was cold, subjects drank twice as much. I think that when we provide the fluid, we need to figure out some recommendations on how *best* to provide it. You can have the best fluid in the world, but if nobody drinks it because it is hot and tastes terrible, it doesn't help anyone.

GISOLFI: I'd like to try to summarize here very quickly. There seems to be relative agreement that we should include some salt, that being sodium chloride. We're not so sure about potassium. Although if you try to have some combination of sodium and potassium, the total amount of salt we have may be critical. The question then becomes — going back to some of Ethan's experiments — What about this business of salt tablets? Is that a way of replacing salt? Should we seriously consider that? They are apparently back on the market, people are using them; they are in football locker rooms; people are being advised to take them. What does this group think about that?

NADEL: Jack Harvey gave me the amounts of sodium chloride that are recommended by various companies manufacturing salt tablets. I did a calculation based upon these recommendations, considering what may be lost during the day. Bob Murray did the same calculation independently, and remarkably, we came up with similar values. For people who sweat on the order of 1–2 L/h with sweat concentrations of sodium around 50 mEq/L or 1150 mg/L, roughly 3–6 g of sodium chloride would be lost each hour. These salt tablets contain between 400 mg and 450 mg per pill. Thus, one has to calculate how much sodium to replace based upon the given conditions. Weighing oneself and assuming a sweat sodium of 50 mEq/L will provide the answer.

GISOLFI: The concerns in the past with salt tablets have been that people have taken too many or too few, depending on the amount of water they ingested. This is one problem. The other problem is that a lot of them, at least those that were made earlier on, were coated and never dissolved, they passed out of the system so that the individual never really got the salt. Perhaps some of these problems are still with us. That's always going to be the case with athletes; they are either going to take too much, which could lead to gastric distress, or too little and not replace what they lost. I'd like to hear some compelling reasons for us to endorse taking salt tablets and going back to the way things were years ago.

PHILLIPS: I'd like to add to your list of why you should not take salt tablets. The fact is that if they take the tablets to reduce hypo-osmolality, the tablets are taken at a time when they are not thirsty. However, they will need to take more water to titrate their osmotic balance, but the increased hyperosmolality may occur when they do not have access to water while running. Consequently, the runner swings from hypo-osmotic to hyperosmotic conditions, which could be dangerous to brain cells.

GISOLFI: Would it be fair to say that this group would not favor going back to recommending salt tablets?

NADEL: Carl, I think you said it very clearly. The problem with salt tablets is that you must read the label correctly and dilute the tablets properly. I think that you are relying a lot on the individual, and most of the time this just isn't adequate.

GISOLFI: Let's return to the original question again. I think we agree that glucose should be included. We suggested the value of 6–10%. There also seems to be some agreement that we should include some salt. We didn't talk about the amount of salt. In a preliminary study that we performed, there wasn't any advantage to doubling the salt concentration from 25 to 50 mEq/L in terms of enhancing salt absorption, water absorption, or glucose absorption from a glucose-electrolyte solution. Considering the amount of sodium lost in the sweat, there is no need to add as much as 50–60 mEq of sodium in a L of replacement beverage. I think that in most fluid replacement beverages on the market, the range is from 10 to 30 mEq/L. Is there any discussion on this point?

HARVEY: Dave, you said you were giving how much?

COSTILL: We were giving 25 mEq.

GISOLFI: As we mentioned earlier, salt also effects palatability. Some salt enhances palatability, but too much is unpalatable. To prevent hyponatremia, only 20–30 mEq/L is necessary if fluid intake is less than or matches fluid loss in sweat. If 20–30 mEq/L is palatable, it seems that this quantity would be a reasonable amount to include in a replacement beverage.

Index

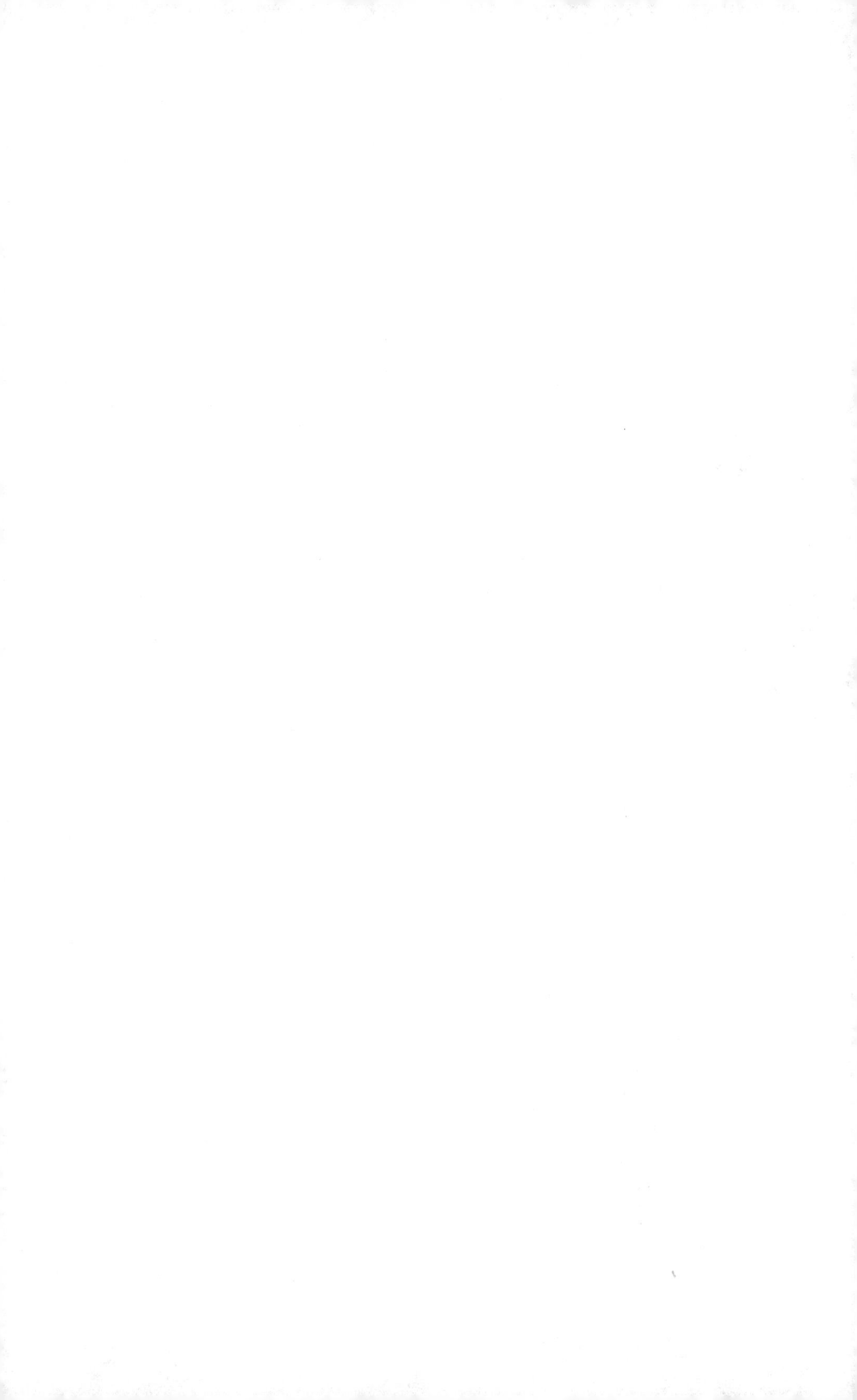

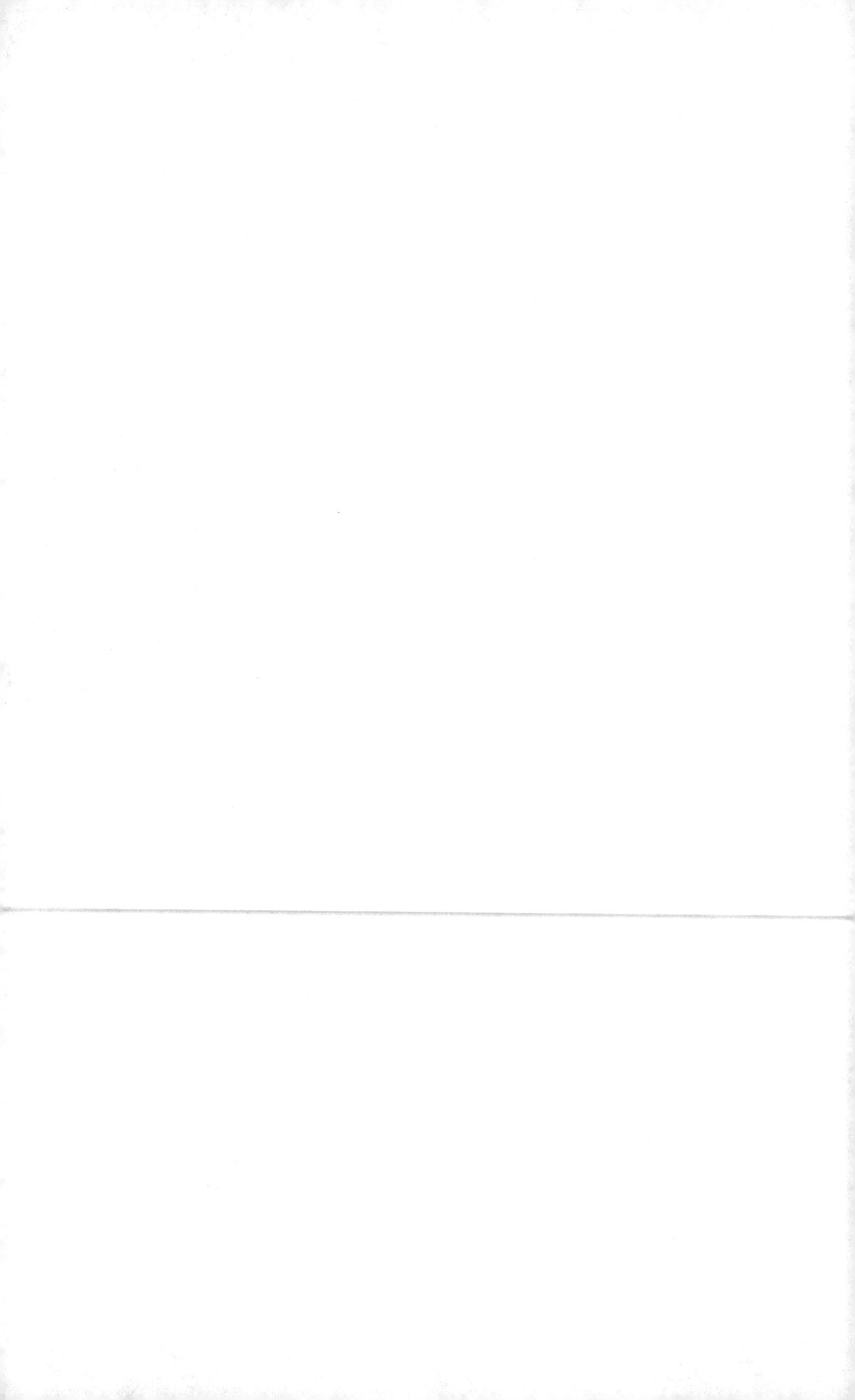